TESTING

BCPS test deadline: 11:59 p.m. (Central) on May 15, 2015.
ACPE test deadline: 11:59 p.m. (Central) on January 14, 2018.

Online errata: Go to www.accp.com/docs/products/psap1315/errata.pdf. **Be sure to check the online errata before submitting a posttest.**

For information on passing levels, assignment of credits, and credit reporting, see Continuing Pharmacy Education and Recertification Instructions on page v.

IMPORTANT NOTICE ON BCPS RECERTIFICATION
Submitting the required posttest for BCPS recertification attests that you have completed the test as an individual effort and not in collaboration with any other individual or group. Failure to complete this test as an individual effort may jeopardize your ability to use PSAP for BCPS recertification.

BOOK FORMATS

Online book: All purchasers have access to the online book (interactive PDFs). To access, go to your My Account page on www.accp.com and sign in using your e-mail address and password (technical assistance is available). You will find your book and the required posttests under My Online Products.

Print books: If you have purchased a print version of this book, it will be delivered on or near the release date to the address of record on your ACCP account. If you have not received the print book within 1 week of the release date, contact customer service by e-mailing accp@accp.com.

E-Media Package: If you have purchased this package, follow these instructions to load the text and self-assessment questions in this book onto your e-reader, tablet, or Android phone. This package includes the PSAP Audio Companion: follow these instructions to download these files onto a listening device or burn them onto an audio CD.

BOOK CONTENT

Electronic annotation: The online book can be saved to the desktop or printed. The latest version of Adobe Reader (available free) offers functionality such as highlighting or adding "sticky notes" to the text.

Hyperlinks: This book contains both internal and external hypertext links (visible as underlined text in the print book). Clicking on the intra-document/internal links in the Table of Contents will take you to the page containing the selected content. Clicking on external hyperlinks will take you away from the ACCP Web site to the outside resource, guidelines, tools, or other information you have selected.

NOTE: To facilitate further learning and research, this publication incorporates print and live hyperlinks to Web sites administered by other organizations. The URLs provided are those of third parties not affiliated in any way with ACCP. ACCP assumes no liability for material downloaded from or accessed on these Web sites. It is the responsibility of the reader to examine the copyright and licensing restrictions of linked pages and to secure all necessary permissions.

Laboratory Reference Values: The last page of this book contains a table with reference ranges and abbreviations for many common laboratory tests. Use this table as a resource in completing the required posttest.

NOTE: The editors and publisher of PSAP recognize that the development of this volume of material offers many opportunities for error. Despite our best efforts, some errors may persist into print. Drug dosage schedules are, we believe, accurate and in accordance with current standards. Readers are advised, however, to check package inserts for the recommended dosages and contraindications. This is especially important for new, infrequently used, and highly toxic drugs.

Director of Professional Development: Nancy M. Perrin, M.A., CAE
Associate Director of Professional Development: Wafa Y. Dahdal, Pharm.D., BCPS
Recertification Project Manager: Edward Alderman, B.S., B.A.
Desktop Publisher/Graphic Designer: Mary Ann Kuchta, B.S.
Medical Editor: Kimma Sheldon, Ph.D., M.A.
Information Technology Project Manager: Brent Paloutzian, A.A.S.

For ordering information or questions, write or call:
Pharmacotherapy Self-Assessment Program
American College of Clinical Pharmacy
13000 W. 87th St. Parkway
Lenexa, KS 66215-4530
Telephone: (913) 492-3311
Fax: (913) 492-4922
E-mail: accp@accp.com

Library of Congress Control Number: 2014958542
ISBN-13: 978-1-939862-10-5 (PSAP 2015 BOOK 1, *Infectious Diseases*)

Print versions are produced in the United States of America.

To cite PSAP properly:

Authors. Chapter name. In: Murphy JE, Lee MW, eds. Pharmacotherapy Self-Assessment Program, 2015 Book 1. Infectious Diseases. Lenexa, KS: American College of Clinical Pharmacy, 2015:page range.

PSAP™ is a registered trademark of the American College of Clinical Pharmacy.

Table of Contents

Skin and Soft Tissue Infections

By Elias B. Chahine, Pharm.D., BCPS (AQ-ID); and Allana J. Sucher, Pharm.D., BCPS

Intra-Abdominal Infections

By David T. Bearden, Pharm.D.

Bone and Joint Infections

By Sandy J. Estrada, Pharm.D., BCPS (AQ-ID)

Antimicrobial Resistance

By Kristi M. Kuper, Pharm.D., BCPS; and Amy N. Schilling, Pharm.D., BCPS

Invasive Fungal Infections

By Russell E. Lewis, Pharm.D., FCCP, BCPS (AQ-ID)

Tuberculosis

By Alexandria Garavaglia Wilson, Pharm.D., BCPS (AQ-ID)

PREFACE

The start of a new edition of the Pharmacotherapy Self-Assessment Program (PSAP) is truly an exciting time. Our mission remains the same today as for the first edition – to provide evidence-based updates that will improve clinical pharmacy practice and patient outcomes. However, to accomplish this, PSAP must reflect the changes in practice models, patient populations, and the overall health care environment. This new edition introduces features and formats designed to enhance information access while accommodating individual learning styles.

PSAP remains a labor of love for the faculty panel chairs, authors, and expert and professional reviewers, as well as for us, the series editors. We contribute to this endeavor because we are committed to the board certification process and the national recognition of the expertise of clinical pharmacists. We are also dedicated to sharing the most up-to-date knowledge with our colleagues, and we are driven to create opportunities for board-certified clinicians to participate in scholarly activity. The PSAP 2013–2015 releases are each carefully developed to identify clinically relevant content, solid case-based examples, and fair but challenging self-assessment questions that allow the tester to demonstrate mastery of this important material.

For individual chapters, the focus continues to be on significant new information rather than a review of common knowledge about a topic. Authors incorporate the latest national or international guidelines for management, landmark clinical trials, and content, which integrate concepts of biostatistics, epidemiology, and health systems to cover all identified domains for the pharmacotherapy specialist. In response to feedback from PSAP users, many authors have included case-based examples demonstrating the application of concepts, a treatment algorithm or decision tree, and a summative box with practice points or pearls. On the first page of each chapter is listed the baseline knowledge presumed on the part of the reader as well as open-access literature resources that can provide this knowledge, if needed. The process for developing self-assessment questions has been revised by carefully tying the questions to objectives and material presented in the books and incorporating a field-test process using panels of specialists. It is our hope that these efforts will build on and improve PSAP's reputation as a quality professional development tool for Board Certified Pharmacotherapy Specialists.

We extend our heartfelt appreciation to all the faculty panel chairs, authors, and reviewers for lending their time and expertise to this new series and to ACCP Publications staff members for their ever-present willingness to help and guide the development of this new series.

John E. Murphy and Mary W. Lee, *series editors*

DISCLOSURE OF POTENTIAL CONFLICTS OF INTEREST

Consultancies: Craig R. Ballard (Janssen, ViiV Healthcare); Sandy Bartlett (Sunflower Developmental Solutions); David T. Bearden (Society of Infectious Diseases Pharmacists); Chi Duong (Warm Springs Health & Wellness Center); Sandy J. Estrada (Astellas); Monica V. Mahoney (Cubist Pharmaceuticals), (Forest Laboratories); Russell E. Lewis (Merck & Co., Inc.), (Gilead); Wilson O. Ly (Pacific AIDS Education Training Center); Christopher McCoy (Durata, Astra Zeneca);

Stock Ownership: Jennifer Cocohoba (Arena Pharmaceuticals [spouse or significant other]);

Royalties:

Grants: David T. Bearden (Cubist Pharmaceuticals); Elias B. Chahine (Cubist Pharmaceuticals, Inc.); Jennifer Cocohoba (National Institutes of Mental Health); Christopher R. Frei (Bristol-Myers Squibb [2 grants], Forest, Pfizer); Katie J. Suda (Intel Corporation); Christopher McCoy (Forest/Cerexa)

Honoraria: Craig R. Ballard (Janssen, Gilead Sciences, Merck, ViiV Healthcare, Simply Speaking HIV); Scott J. Bergman (Sanofi-Pasteur); P. Brandon Bookstaver (Merck and Co, Inc.); Elias B. Chahine (Cubist Pharmaceuticals, Inc., Forest Pharmaceuticals, Inc., Optimer Pharmaceuticals, Inc.); Sandy J. Estrada

(Cubist); Lucas Hill (International Antiviral Society-USA); Vanthida Huang (Forest Pharmaceutical, Inc.); Wilson O. Ly (Gilead Sciences); Allana J. Sucher (AbbVie)

Other:

Nothing to Disclose: Matthew F. Ambury, Melissa Badowski, Kimberli M. Burgner, Jessica Cottreau, Paulina Deming, Eric A. Dietrich, Nancy E. Flentge, Alexandria Garavaglia-Wilson, Taylor K. Gill, Shellee A. Grim, Carol Heunisch, Shaun P. Keegan, Thomas J. Kleyn, Kristi M. Kuper, Becky S. Linn, Kim G. Luk, Kathleen A. Lusk, Michelle T. Martin, Kari A. McCracken, Ian R. McNicholl, April Miller Quidley, Carolyn Orendorff, Michael Ott, Jennifer Phillips, Abby Rivas Marrero, Amy N. Schilling, Douglas Slain, Inna S. Tsuker

ROLE OF BPS: The Board of Pharmacy Specialties (BPS) is an autonomous division of the American Pharmacists Association (APhA). BPS is totally separate and distinct from ACCP. The Board, through its specialty councils, is responsible for specialty examination content, administration, scoring, and all other aspects of its certification programs. PSAP has been approved by BPS for use in BCPS recertification. Information about the BPS recertification process is available at www.bpsweb.org/recertification/general.cfm.

Other questions regarding recertification should be directed to:

Board of Pharmacy Specialties
2215 Constitution Avenue NW
Washington, DC 20037
(202) 429-7591
www.bpsweb.org

Continuing Pharmacy Education and Recertification Instructions

 Continuing Pharmacy Education Credit: The American College of Clinical Pharmacy is accredited by the Accreditation Council for Pharmacy Education (ACPE) as a provider of continuing pharmacy education (CPE).

Available CPE credits: Purchasers who successfully complete all posttests for PSAP 2014 Book 2 (Infectious Diseases) can earn 25.5 contact hours of CPE credit. The universal activity numbers are as follows: Infectious Diseases I – 0217-0000-15-001-H01-P, 5.5 contact hours; Infectious Diseases II – 0217-0000-15-002-H01-P, 7.0 contact hours; Infectious Diseases III – 0217-0000-15-003-H01-P, 7.0 contact hours; and Infectious Diseases IV – 0217-0000-15-004-H01-P, 6.0 contact hours. You may complete one or all three modules for credit. Tests may not be submitted more than one time.

BCPS test deadline: 11:59 p.m. (Central) on May 15, 2015.
ACPE test deadline: 11:59 p.m. (Central) on January 14, 2018.

Posttest access: Go to www.accp.com and sign in with your e-mail address and password. Technical support is available from 8 a.m. to 5 p.m. (Central) weekdays by calling (913) 492-3311. PSAP products are listed under My Online Products on your My Account page.

BCPS Recertification Credit: To receive BCPS recertification CPE credit, a PSAP posttest must be submitted within the 4-month period after the book's release. The first page of each print and online book lists the deadline to submit a required posttest for BCPS recertification credit. Only completed tests are eligible for credit; no partial or incomplete tests will be processed. Tests may not be submitted more than once. The passing point for BCPS recertification is based on a statistical analysis of the answers submitted for each posttest module.

ACPE CPE Credit: To receive ACPE CPE credit for a PSAP module, a posttest must be submitted within 3 years after the book's release. The appropriate CPE credit will be awarded for test scores of 50% and greater.

Credit Assignment and Reporting: All required posttests that meet the 50% score standard will be awarded the appropriate ACPE CPE credit within 3 days of test submission. For statements of CPE credit, visit www.mycpemonitor.net.

Required posttests that are submitted before the BCPS test deadline and that meet the passing point set by statistical analysis will earn BCPS recertification credits. These credits will be posted **within 30 days after the BCPS test deadline.** For statements of CPE credit, visit www.mycpemonitor.net.

All BCPS recertification credits are forwarded by ACCP to the Board of Pharmacy Specialties (BPS). Questions regarding the number of hours required for BCPS recertification should be directed to BPS at (202) 429-7591 or www.bpsweb.org. The ACCP Recertification Dashboard is a free online tool that can track recertification credits as they are earned through ACCP and schedule new opportunities for credits from upcoming ACCP professional development programs.

Posttest answers: The explained answers – with rationale and supporting references – will be posted **1 week after the BCPS test deadline** and will be available to anyone who has submitted a posttest or waived his or her right to receive credit (see below) from a posttest. Go to www.accp.com and sign in with your e-mail address and password. Click the PSAP book on your My Account page and you will see a link to the explained answers.

Test Waivers: To access the explained answers without submitting a posttest, sign in to your My Account page, select the PSAP book, and click on the waiver link for that module. By completing the waiver form for a module, you waive the opportunity to receive CPE credit for that module. After you submit a waiver, you will see a link to the PDF file that contains the answers for the module you waived. Answers will be available **starting 1 week** after the BCPS test deadline. ROLE OF BPS: The Board of Pharmacy Specialties (BPS) is an autonomous division of the American Pharmacists Association (APhA). BPS is totally separate and distinct from ACCP. The Board, through its specialty councils, is responsible for specialty examination content, administration, scoring, and all other aspects of its certification programs. PSAP has been approved by BPS for use in BCPS recertification. Information about the BPS recertification process is available at www.bpsweb.org/recertification/general.cfm.

INFECTIOUS DISEASES I PANEL

SERIES EDITORS:

John E. Murphy, Pharm.D., FCCP, FASHP
Professor of Pharmacy Practice and Science
Associate Dean for Academic Affairs and Assessment
University of Arizona College of Pharmacy
Tucson, Arizona

Mary Wun-Len Lee, Pharm.D., FCCP, BCPS
Vice President and Chief Academic Officer
Pharmacy and Health Sciences Education
Midwestern University
Professor of Pharmacy Practice
Midwestern University
Chicago College of Pharmacy
Downers Grove, Illinois

Faculty Panel Chair

Ian R. McNicholl, Pharm.D., FCCP,
BCPS (AQ-ID), AAHIVP
Associate Director, Medical Affairs
Gilead Sciences
Foster City, California

SKIN AND SOFT TISSUE INFECTIONS

Authors

Elias B. Chahine, Pharm.D., BCPS (AQ-ID)
Associate Professor of Pharmacy Practice
Department of Pharmacy Practice
Palm Beach Atlantic University
Lloyd L. Gregory School of Pharmacy
West Palm Beach, Florida
Clinical Pharmacist
Department of Pharmacy
JFK Medical Center
Atlantis, Florida

Allana J. Sucher, Pharm.D., BCPS
Associate Professor of Pharmacy Practice
Department of Pharmacy Practice
Regis University
Rueckert-Hartman College for Health Professions
Denver, Colorado

Reviewers

Christopher R. Frei, Pharm.D., M.Sc., FCCP, BCPS
Associate Professor
Head, Division of Pharmacotherapy
The University of Texas at Austin College of Pharmacy
Austin, Texas
Adjoint Associate Professor
Director, Pharmacotherapy Education
and Research Center
University of Texas Health Science
Center School of Medicine
San Antonio, Texas

Eric Dietrich, Pharm.D., BCPS
Clinical Assistant Professor
Department of Pharmacotherapy and Translational
Research; Community Health and Family Medicine
University of Florida Colleges of
Pharmacy and Medicine
Gainesville, Florida

INTRA-ABDOMINAL INFECTIONS

Author

David T. Bearden, Pharm.D.
Clinical Associate Professor and Chair
Department of Pharmacy Practice
Oregon State University College of Pharmacy
Portland, Oregon
Clinical Assistant Director
Department of Pharmacy Services
Oregon Health & Science University
Portland, Oregon

Reviewers

Wilson Ly, Pharm.D., BCPS, AAHIVP
HIV and Hepatitis C Clinical Pharmacist
Department of Santa Clara Valley Medical Center,
Partners In AIDS Care and Education (PACE) Clinic
Santa Clara Valley Medical Center
San Jose, California
Medical Student
Department of University of California San
Francisco School of Medicine and University of
California Berkeley School of Public Health
University of California San Francisco and
University of California Berkeley
San Francisco, California

Kathleen A. Lusk, Pharm.D., BCPS
Assistant Professor
Department of Pharmacy Practice
University of the Incarnate Word
Feik School of Pharmacy
Clinical Pharmacy Specialist
South Texas Veterans Health Care System
San Antonio, Texas

Bone and Joint Infections

Authors

Sandy J. Estrada, Pharm.D., BCPS (AQ-ID)
Clinical Specialist – Infectious Diseases
Lee Memorial Health System
Fort Myers, Florida

Reviewers

Scott Bergman, Pharm.D., BCPS (AQ-ID)
Associate Professor
Department of Pharmacy Practice
Southern Illinois University
Edwardsville School of Pharmacy
Edwardsville, Illinois
*PGY2 Infectious Diseases Pharmacy
Residency Program Director*
HSHS St. John's Hospital
Springfield, Illinois

Shaun P. Keegan, Pharm.D, BCPS
Clinical Pharmacy Specialist, Critical Care
UC Health - University Hospital
Department of Pharmacy Services
Cincinnati, Ohio

The American College of Clinical Pharmacy and the authors thank the following individuals for their careful review of the Infectious Diseases I chapters:

Judy Cheng, Pharm.D., MPH, BCPS (AQ Cardiology)
Professor of Pharmacy Practice
Department of Pharmacy Practice
MCPHS University
Clinical Pharmacy Specialist
Department of Pharmacy
Brigham and Women's Hospital
Boston, Massachusetts

Marisel Segarra-Newnham, Pharm.D., MPH, FCCP, BCPS
Clinical Pharmacy Specialist, Infectious Diseases Pharmacy Service
Veterans Affairs Medical Center
West Palm Beach, Florida
Clinical Assistant Professor of Pharmacy Practice
University of Florida College of Pharmacy
Gainesville, Florida

Ralph H. Raasch, Pharm.D., BCPS
Associate Professor of Pharmacy (retired)
Division of Practice Advancement
and Clinical Education
Eshelman School of Pharmacy
The University of North Carolina at Chapel Hill
Chapel Hill, North Carolina

Skin and Soft Tissue Infections

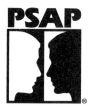

By Elias B. Chahine, Pharm.D., BCPS (AQ-ID);
and Allana J. Sucher, Pharm.D., BCPS

Reviewed by Christopher R. Frei, Pharm.D., M.Sc., FCCP, BCPS; and Eric Dietrich, Pharm.D., BCPS

Learning Objectives

1. Given a patient's clinical presentation and risk factors, distinguish between the various types of skin and soft tissue infections.
2. Given a patient's profile, develop a pharmacotherapeutic plan to treat a skin or soft tissue infection.
3. Assess the safety profiles of antimicrobials commonly used for the treatment of skin and soft tissue infections.
4. Justify prevention measures to reduce the recurrence and transmission of a patient's skin and soft tissue infections.

Introduction

Skin and soft tissue infections (SSTIs), also referred to as *skin and skin structure infections*, represent a group of infections that are diverse in their clinical presentations and degrees of severity. They are generally classified into two categories: purulent infections (e.g., furuncles, carbuncles, abscesses) nonpurulent infections (e.g., erysipelas, cellulitis, necrotizing fasciitis). They are then further classified into three subcategories: mild, moderate, and severe. Mild infections present with local symptoms only, whereas moderate to severe infections are associated with systemic signs of infection such as temperature higher than 38°C, heart rate higher than 90 beats/minute, respiratory rate higher than 24 breaths/minute, or WBC higher than 12 x 10³ cells/mm³. Patients with immunocompromising conditions, clinical signs of deeper infection, or infection that fails to improve with incision and drainage (I&D) plus oral antibiotics are also classified as severe cases. Purulent infections are treated with I&D and antibiotic administration in moderate and severe cases. Nonpurulent infections are treated with antibiotic administration, with the addition of surgical debridement in severe cases (Stevens 2014).

The majority of SSTIs are caused by bacteria and are referred to as acute bacterial skin and skin structure infections (ABSSSIs). Some cases are caused by viruses—most notably, varicella zoster virus (VZV), which is the causative

---

Baseline Knowledge Statements

Readers of this chapter are presumed to be familiar with the following:
- Basic knowledge of skin and soft tissue infections
- Pharmacology—including mechanisms of action, adverse effects, and drug interactions—of antimicrobials used in the treatment of skin and soft tissue infections

Additional Readings

The following free resources are available for readers wishing additional background information on this topic.
- Infectious Diseases Society of America (IDSA). Guidelines for skin and soft tissue infections, 2014.
- IDSA. Guidelines for diabetic foot infections, 2012.
- IDSA. Guidelines for methicillin-resistant *Staphylococcus aureus* infections, 2011.
- Centers for Disease Control and Prevention (CDC). Methicillin-resistant *Staphylococcus aureus* (MRSA) infections, 2014 [homepage on the Internet].
- CDC. Shingles (herpes zoster), 2014 [homepage on the Internet].
- CDC. Prevention of herpes zoster, 2008 [homepage on the Internet].

organism of chickenpox and shingles. Similarities in clinical presentation and limitations in the ability to identify the causative organisms in a timely manner make the diagnosis and treatment of SSTIs initially challenging. Therefore, careful assessment of risk factors and degree of severity, as well as obtaining a detailed medical history and performing a physical examination are required to appropriately diagnose and manage a patient presenting with an SSTI. Antimicrobial regimens are often selected empirically based on host characteristics, most likely pathogens, and local susceptibility patterns, with streamlining according to microbiology culture and sensitivity if the causative organisms are isolated.

This chapter provides an update on the epidemiology, pathophysiology, risk factors, causative organisms, and clinical features of the most common ABSSSIs, as well as of herpes zoster, and focuses on the pharmacologic management of those infections in both the outpatient and inpatient settings. Antimicrobial stewardship, infection control, and prevention options are also discussed.

EPIDEMIOLOGY

The true prevalence of SSTIs is unknown because mild infections are typically self-limiting and patients do not seek medical attention. Nonetheless, SSTIs are encountered often in both the outpatient and inpatient settings. According to the 2011 National Statistics of the Healthcare Cost and Utilization Project, SSTIs accounted for 3.4 million emergency department visits, or 2.6% of all emergency department visits, with 13.9% of visits resulting in hospitalization (DHHS 2011a). Skin and soft tissue infections also accounted for 500,000 hospital discharges, or 1.4% of total discharges, with a mean length of stay of 3.7 days and

a mean charge of $18,299 per case (DHHS 2011b). Those numbers are on the rise because the prevalence of community-associated methicillin-resistant *Staphylococcus aureus* (CAMRSA) increased in the past decade (Merritt 2013; Talan 2011; Edelsberg 2009; Gerber 2009). A recent prospective study demonstrated that 1 in 5 patients presenting to a primary care clinic for an SSTI caused by methicillin-resistant *S. aureus* (MRSA) require additional interventions at an associated cost of almost $2000 per patient (Labreche 2013). The incidence of herpes zoster is also increasing, and there are more than 1 million cases each year in the United States, with an annual rate of 3 to 4 cases per 1000 persons (Rimland 2010).

Pathophysiology

Intact skin provides protection from the external environment by serving as a physical barrier and maintaining a normal flora that is not conducive to the growth of pathogenic organisms. *Primary SSTIs* occur when microorganisms invade otherwise healthy skin, whereas *secondary SSTIs* occur when, because of underlying disease or trauma, microorganisms infect already damaged skin. In both cases, pathogenic microorganisms cause damage to the surrounding tissues, which leads to an inflammatory response characterized by warmth, erythema, and pain. Such damage is more complicated in patients with diabetes because long-term hyperglycemia leads to motor and autonomic neuropathy, cellular and humoral immunopathy, and angiopathy. Reactivation of latent VZV at the spinal root or cranial nerve neurons causes the inflammatory response associated with herpes zoster. Figure 1-1 illustrates human skin structures and the corresponding locations of various SSTIs.

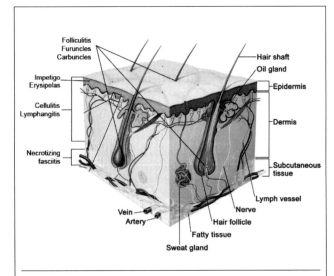

Figure 1-1. Skin structures.

Image from National Cancer Institute. Skin anatomy [homepage on the Internet].

Risk Factors

Acute bacterial skin and skin structure infections occur when skin integrity is compromised as a result of high bacterial load on the skin, the availability of bacterial nutrients, excessive skin moisture, inadequate blood supply, immunosuppression, or damage to the corneal layer. Poor hygiene, the sharing of personal items, physical contact, and crowded living conditions facilitate the spread of contagious infections such as furuncles, carbuncles, and impetigo. Peripheral vascular disease and pre-existing skin diseases increase the risk of erysipelas and cellulitis. Poorly controlled diabetes often leads to diabetic foot infection (DFI). Traumatic events such as cuts and bites and injection drug use result in wounds that increase the risk of skin infections and abscesses. The risk of surgical site infection (SSI) depends on the category of operation, with clean and low-risk operations having the smallest risk of infections and contaminated and high-risk operations having the highest risk.

Colonization with *S. aureus* in the anterior nares and *Streptococcus pyogenes* on the skin increases the risk of those skin infections. Skin-to-skin contact from playing sports, attendance at day care or school, and living in close quarters (e.g., military barracks) are risk factors for CAMRSA skin infections. Risk factors for health care–associated methicillin-resistant *S. aureus* (HAMRSA) skin infections include recent exposure to antibiotics or the health care system (Herman 2008).

Herpes zoster is associated with advanced age and immunosuppressive conditions. The risk is higher for women, whites, and those with family histories of herpes zoster (Cohen 2013).

Causative Organisms

Acute bacterial skin and skin structure infections are caused primarily by gram-positive cocci—particularly, *S. aureus* and *S. pyogenes*. *S. aureus* is the most common cause of furuncles, carbuncles, cutaneous abscesses, and impetigo. *S. pyogenes* is the most common cause of erysipelas, lymphangitis, and cellulitis in patients without penetrating trauma, evidence of MRSA infection elsewhere, nasal colonization with MRSA, injection drug use, or systemic inflammatory-response syndrome. Gram-negative rods and anaerobic bacteria can also cause ABSSSIs, particularly in patients with deep long-standing ulcers, immunocompromising conditions, or recent antibiotic exposure (Stevens 2014).

In the past decade, MRSA has become the most common identifiable cause of purulent SSTIs among patients presenting to emergency departments in the United States (Merritt 2013; Talan 2011). The CAMRSA isolates are predominantly pulsed-field type USA300 or USA400, with staphylococcal chromosome cassette type IV or V, and are most likely to be producers of Panton-Valentine leucocidin toxin (Herman 2008). These CAMRSA

isolates typically remain susceptible to trimethoprim/sulfamethoxazole, clindamycin, and tetracycline (Talan 2013; Herman 2008). The HAMRSA isolates are predominantly pulsed-field type USA100, USA500, or USA800, with staphylococcal chromosome cassette type I, II, or III, and are less likely to be producers of Panton-Valentine leucocidin toxin (Herman 2008). They are often resistant to older, non-β-lactam antibiotics (Herman 2008). Figure 1-2 depicts a cutaneous abscess caused by MRSA.

Infected dog and cat bite wounds are polymicrobial, with *Pasteurella* spp., *Streptococcus* spp., *Staphylococcus* spp., and *Moraxella* spp. as the most common aerobic organisms, and with *Fusobacterium* spp., *Porphyromonas* spp., *Prevotella* spp., and *Bacteroides* spp. as the most common anaerobic organisms. Pasteurella spp. is the most common etiology of dog and cat bite infections, and many infections are caused by both aerobic and anaerobic microorganisms. Such organisms often reflect the oral flora of the biting animal and, to a lesser extent, the victim's own skin flora (Abrahamian 2011). Infected human bite wounds are also polymicrobial, with *Streptococcus* spp., *Staphylococcus* spp., *Corynebacterium* spp., *Eikenella* spp., and oral anaerobic flora as the most common organisms (Pettitt 2012).

Necrotizing SSTIs are either monomicrobial or polymicrobial. Monomicrobial infections are often caused by hypervirulent strains of *S. pyogenes* and to a lesser extent by *S. aureus*, *Clostridium perfringens*, *Vibrio vulnificus*, or *Aeromonas hydrophila*. Infection with streptococci and staphylococci can occur simultaneously, and infection with *C. perfringens* is referred to as *clostridial gas gangrene* or *myonecrosis* (Stevens 2014). Polymicrobial infections are caused by a variety of organisms, with *Streptococcus*

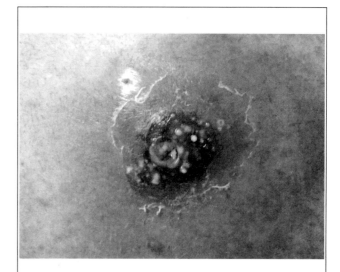

Figure 1-2. Cutaneous abscess caused by methicillin-resistant *Staphylococcus aureus*.

Image from the Centers for Disease Control and Prevention. Methicillin-resistant Staphylococcus aureus (MRSA) infections [homepage on the Internet].

spp. and *Staphylococcus* spp. as the most common Gram-positive cocci; Enterobacteriaceae as the most common gram-negative rods; and *Bacteroides* spp., *Clostridium* spp., and *Peptostreptococcus* spp. as the most common anaerobic organisms (Anaya 2007).

TREATMENT

The goals of therapy for ABSSSIs are to eradicate the causative organism(s), alleviate signs and symptoms, avoid complications, and prevent recurrences (Figure 1-3). Incision and drainage represents the mainstay of therapy for all purulent SSTIs. Table 1-1 lists dosing regimens in adults and children, adverse effects, and significant drug interactions for common antibiotics used in the treatment of SSTIs.

Mild purulent infections are treated with I&D and do not require systemic antibiotic therapy. Moderate purulent infections are treated with I&D and oral antibiotics. Severe purulent infections are treated with I&D and an initial course of intravenous antibiotics followed by oral antibiotics when appropriate.

Mild nonpurulent infections are treated with oral antibiotics. Moderate nonpurulent infections are treated with an initial course of intravenous antibiotics followed by oral antibiotics when appropriate. Severe nonpurulent infections are treated with surgical debridement and intravenous antibiotics (Stevens 2014).

The goals of therapy for herpes zoster are to alleviate signs and symptoms and avoid complications. Moderate to severe infections are often treated with antivirals that target VZV. Table 1-2 lists dosing regimens in adults, adverse effects, and significant drug interactions for antivirals commonly used in the treatment of herpes zoster.

INFECTIONS IN THE OUTPATIENT SETTING

Folliculitis, Furuncles, Carbuncles, and Cutaneous Abscesses

Folliculitis is an infection of one or more hair follicles that may affect any area of the body (excepting the palms and soles, where there is no hair). It presents as a red dot that ultimately becomes a white tip, and it may be associated with rash or pruritus. Furuncles are deeper than folliculitis and result in painful swollen boils on the skin. Carbuncles and cutaneous abscesses are larger than furuncles and have openings that drain pus; they are often associated with fever, swollen lymph nodes, and fatigue. Diagnosis of these SSTIs is based on clinical presentation. Gram stain and culture of the pus from carbuncles and abscesses are recommended, but treatment without those studies is reasonable in typical cases (Stevens 2014).

In mild cases, I&D is recommended without systemic antibiotic therapy. Conditions for which antibiotic therapy is recommended after I&D are summarized in Box 1-1. In moderate cases, oral antibiotics directed

against CAMRSA (e.g., trimethoprim/sulfamethoxazole, doxycycline, clindamycin) are recommended in addition to I&D. A recent multicenter randomized double-blind controlled trial of clindamycin versus trimethoprim/sulfamethoxazole in the treatment of uncomplicated SSTIs found no differences in efficacy and tolerability between the two agents (Miller 2013).

When methicillin-sensitive *S. aureus* (MSSA) is isolated, oral dicloxacillin or cephalexin is recommended. In severe cases, intravenous antibiotics directed against MRSA (e.g., vancomycin, daptomycin, linezolid) are recommended in addition to I&D. When MSSA is isolated, intravenous nafcillin, cefazolin, or clindamycin is recommended in severe cases (Singer 2014; Stevens 2014; Forcade 2012). The duration of therapy is 5–10 days for outpatients and 7–14 days for inpatients but should be individualized based on a patient's clinical response (Liu 2011).

In all cases, application of warm moist compresses facilitates pus elimination. Recurrent abscesses should be drained, cultured, and treated for 5–10 days with an antibiotic directed against the isolated organism. A decolonization regimen with mupirocin intranasally twice daily for 5 days, chlorhexidine washes daily, and decontamination of personal items should be considered (Stevens 2014). Patients in need of education about SSTIs caused by MRSA may be provided with a link to an online video.

Impetigo

Impetigo occurs mostly in children and is characterized by multiple erythematous, vesicular, and pruritic lesions on the face and the extremities. Nonbullous impetigo presents with small fluid-filled vesicles that soon develop into pustules that rupture, leaving golden-yellow crusts. Bullous impetigo presents with vesicles that develop into yellow fluid-filled bullae that rupture, leaving brown crusts. Rarely, streptococcal impetigo leads to

Continued on page 10

Box 1-1. Conditions in Which Antibiotic Therapy is Recommended After Incision and Drainage

---

- Abscess in area difficult to drain completely
- Associated comorbidities or immunosuppression
- Associated septic phlebitis
- Extremes of age
- Lack of response to incision and drainage alone
- Severe or extensive disease
- Signs and symptoms of systemic illness

Information from: Liu C, Bayer A, Cosgrove SE, et al; Infectious Diseases Society of America. Clinical practice guidelines by the Infectious Diseases Society of America for the treatment of methicillin-resistant *Staphylococcus aureus* infections in adults and children. Clin Infect Dis 2011;52:e18-55.

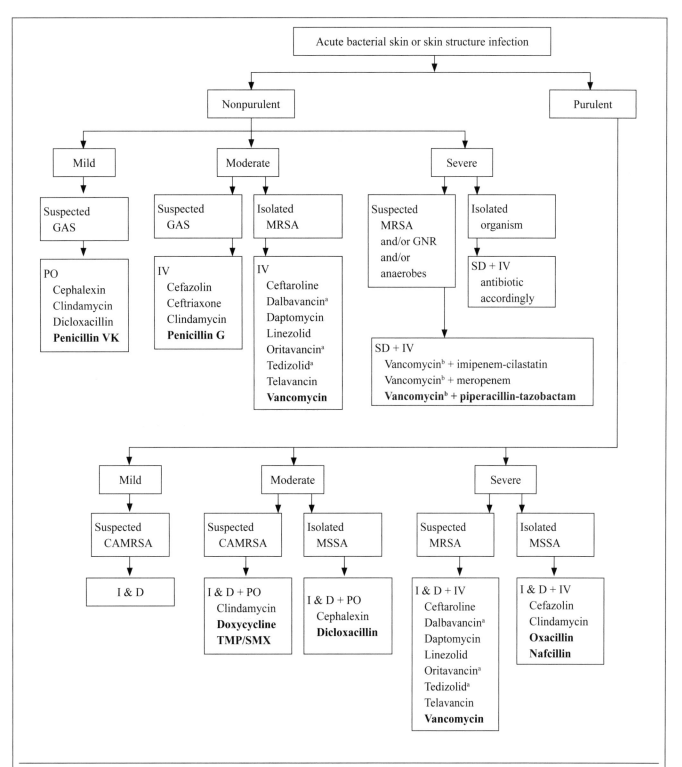

Figure 1-3. General approach to the management of acute bacterial skin and skin structure infections. Bolding indicates antibiotic of choice.

[a]Not included in the 2014 IDSA guidelines for the management of skin and soft tissue infections.
[b]An alternative new anti-MRSA antibiotic can also be used.
CAMRSA = community-associated methicillin-resistant *Staphylococcus aureus*; GAS = Group A β-hemolytic *Streptococcus*; GNR = gram-negative rods; I & D = incision and drainage; IV = intravenous; MRSA = methicillin-resistant *Staphylococcus aureus*; MSSA = methicillin-sensitive *Staphylococcus aureus*; PO = oral; SD = surgical debridement.
Information from: Stevens DL, Bisno AL, Chambers HF, et al. Practice guidelines for the diagnosis and management of skin and soft tissue infections: 2014 update by the Infectious Diseases Society of America. Clin Infect Dis 2014;59:e10-52.

Table 1-1. Common and New Antibiotics Used for Skin and Soft Tissue Infections

Agent	Clinically Useful Activity Against MRSA	Dosing Regimen[a,b]	Adverse Effects	Drug Interactions
Topical Antibiotics				
Mupirocin (ointment, cream)	Yes	Skin infections for adults and children ≥ 2 months: Apply to affected area twice daily for 5 days MRSA decolonization for adults and children ≥ 12 years: Apply to anterior nares twice daily for 5 days	Hypersensitivity reactions, skin irritation, pruritus, burning	None significant
Retapamulin (ointment)	Yes	Impetigo for adults and children ≥ 9 months: Apply to affected area twice daily for 5 days	Hypersensitivity reactions, skin irritation, eczema, pruritus	None significant
Systemic Antibiotics				
Amoxicillin/ clavulanic acid	No	Adults and children ≥ 40 kg: 875 mg of amoxicillin PO twice daily Children < 40 kg: 25 mg/ kg/day of amoxicillin PO divided into 2 doses	Hypersensitivity reactions, gastrointestinal upset	None significant
Cefazolin	No	Adults: 1 g IV three times daily Children: 50 mg/kg/day IV divided into 3 doses	Hypersensitivity reactions	None significant
Ceftaroline	Yes	Adults: 600 mg IV twice daily	Hypersensitivity reactions	None significant
Ceftriaxone	No	Adults: 1 g IV daily Children: 50–75 mg/kg/day IV divided into 1 to 2 doses	Hypersensitivity reactions	None significant
Cephalexin	No	Adults and children > 15 years: 250 to 500 mg PO 4 times daily Children ≤ 15 years: 25 to 50 mg/ kg/day PO divided into 3 to 4 times	Hypersensitivity reactions	None significant
Clindamycin	Yes[c]	Adults: 300–450 mg PO four times daily Adults: 600 mg IV three times daily Children: 20–40 mg/kg/day IV/ PO divided into 3 doses	*Clostridium difficile* infection, gastrointestinal upset	None significant
Dalbavancin	Yes	Adults: 1000 mg on day 1 followed by 500 mg on day 8	Hypersensitivity reactions, infusion reactions, gastrointestinal upset	None significant
Daptomycin	Yes	Adults: 4 mg/kg IV daily	Elevated creatine phosphokinase, eosinophilic pneumonia	Statins
Dicloxacillin	No	Adults and children ≥ 40 kg: 250– 500 mg PO four times daily Children < 40 kg: 25–50 mg/kg/ day PO divided into 4 doses	Hypersensitivity reactions	None significant

Table 1-1. Common and New Antibiotics Used for Skin and Soft Tissue Infections (*continued*)

Agent	Clinically Useful Activity Against MRSA	Dosing Regimen[a,b]	Adverse Effects	Drug Interactions
Doxycyline[d]	Yes[c]	Adults and children > 45 kg: 100 mg PO twice daily Children ≥ 8 years and ≤ 45 kg: 2 mg/kg PO twice daily	Gastrointestinal upset, photosensitivity, permanent tooth discoloration in children < 8 years, not recommended for pregnant women and children < 8 years	Oral cations
Linezolid	Yes	Adults and children ≥ 12 years: 600 mg IV/PO twice daily Children < 12 years: 10 mg/kg/day IV/PO twice daily	Myelosuppression, neuropathy, serotonin syndrome	Serotonergic agents
Minocycline[d]	Yes[c]	Adults: 200 mg PO on day 1 followed by 100 mg twice daily Children ≥ 8 years: 4 mg/kg PO on day 1 followed by 2 mg/kg twice daily	Gastrointestinal upset, photosensitivity, permanent tooth discoloration in children < 8 years, not recommended for pregnant women and children < 8 years	Oral cations
Nafcillin	No	Adults: 1–2 g IV six times daily Children: 100–150 mg/kg/day divided into 4 doses	Hypersensitivity reactions	None significant
Oritavancin	Yes	Adults: 1200 mg IV single dose	Hypersensitivity reactions, infusion reactions, gastrointestinal upset	Warfarin, heparin, coagulation tests
Oxacillin	No	Adults: 1–2 g IV 6 times daily Children: 100–150 mg/kg/day divided into 4 doses	Hypersensitivity reactions	None significant
Penicillin G	No	Adults: 2–4 million units IV four to six times daily Children: 60,000 to 100,000 units/kg/dose IV four times daily	Hypersensitivity reactions	Probenecid
Penicillin VK	No	Adults: 250–500 mg PO four times daily Children: 25–50 mg/kg/day PO divided into 2 to 4 doses	Hypersensitivity reactions	Probenecid
Piperacillin-tazobactam	No	Adults and children > 40 kg: 3.375 g IV three or four times daily Children ≤ 40 kg: 100 mg/kg of piperacillin IV three times daily	Hypersensitivity reactions	None significant
Tedizolid	Yes	Adults: 200 mg IV/PO daily	Myelosuppression, neuropathy, serotonin syndrome	Serotonergic agents
Telavancin	Yes	Adults: 10 mg/kg IV daily	Infusion reactions, QT prolongation, nephrotoxicity, foamy urine, dysgeusia, gastrointestinal upset, headache, dizziness, not recommended for pregnant women	QT prolonging agents, nephrotoxic agents

Table 1-1. Common and New Antibiotics Used for Skin and Soft Tissue Infections *(continued)*

Agent	Clinically Useful Activity Against MRSA	Dosing Regimen[a,b]	Adverse Effects	Drug Interactions
Trimethoprim/ sulfamethoxazole[d]	Yes[c]	Adults: 1 to 2 DS tablet(s) PO twice daily Children: 8–12 mg/kg/day of trimethoprim divided into 4 doses IV or 2 doses PO	Hypersensitivity reactions, nausea, vomiting, myelosuppression, hyperkalemia, hepatotoxicity, not recommended for women in the third trimester of pregnancy	Warfarin, renin-angiotensin-aldosterone system inhibitors
Vancomycin	Yes	Adults: 30 mg/kg/day divided into 2 doses Children: 40 mg/kg/day divided into 4 doses	Infusion reactions, red man syndrome, nephrotoxicity	Nephrotoxic agents

[a]Doses recommended for patients with skin and soft tissue infections and are based on normal kidney and liver functions.
[b]Pediatric regimens exclude dosing for neonates and infants.
[c]Commonly used to treat community-associated methicillin-resistant *Staphylococcus aureus* infections.
[d]Not active against *Streptococcus pyogenes*.
DS = double strength (160 mg of trimethoprim and 800 mg of sulfamethoxazole); IV = intravenously; MRSA = methicillin-resistant *Staphylococcus aureus*; PO = by mouth.

Information from: Stevens DL, Bisno AL, Chambers HF, et al. Practice guidelines for the diagnosis and management of skin and soft tissue infections: 2014 update by the Infectious Diseases Society of America. Clin Infect Dis 2014;59:e10-52; and Liu C, Bayer A, Cosgrove SE, et al. Clinical practice guidelines by the Infectious Diseases Society of America for the treatment of methicillin-resistant *Staphylococcus aureus* infections in adults and children. Clin Infect Dis 2011;52:285-92.

Continued from page 6

complications such as acute rheumatic fever and glomerulonephritis. Diagnosis of impetigo is based on clinical presentation. Gram stain and culture of the pus or exudates are recommended to identify whether *S. pyogenes* or *S. aureus* is the cause, but treatment without those studies is reasonable in typical cases (Stevens 2014).

The mainstay of therapy for both nonbullous and bullous impetigo is topical mupirocin or retapamulin twice daily for 5 days. Oral antibiotics directed against MSSA (e.g. dicloxacillin or cephalexin for 7 days) are recommended for patients with many lesions and in the setting of an outbreak. If the cultures reveal only streptococci, oral penicillin VK is recommended. When MRSA is suspected or confirmed, oral trimethoprim/ sulfamethoxazole, doxycycline, or clindamycin is recommended (Stevens 2014). In all cases, soaking in soapy warm water facilitates crust removal.

Bite Wound Infections

A comprehensive history, including how and when a bite occurred; the patient's medical history, allergies, and tetanus immunization status; immunization history of the animal; and medical history of the biter (for viral hepatitis, HIV, and other transmissible diseases) should be obtained. Patients should be evaluated for type of wound, presence of damage to surrounding or underlying structures, and signs of infection (e.g., erythema, swelling, discharge), which may not develop until 24–72 hours after injury. Patients may also present with enlargement of the lymph nodes adjacent to the wound, fever, or leukocytosis. Gram stain and culture are usually not performed on wounds. Radiography is used to assess for septic arthritis or osteomyelitis when damage to a bone or joint is suspected (Brook 2009).

Preemptive early antibiotic therapy for 3–5 days is recommended for patients with immunocompromising conditions (e.g., asplenia, advanced liver disease). Preemptive therapy is also recommended in patients with edema in the affected area; injuries to the face, hands, or feet; or joint or bone injuries. Antibiotic therapy directed against both aerobic and anaerobic bacteria (e.g., amoxicillin/clavulanate) should be initiated. Alternative agents include second- or third-generation cephalosporin or fluoroquinolone or trimethoprim/sulfamethoxazole plus clindamycin or metronidazole. Doxycycline, moxifloxacin, or a carbapenem is also appropriate. Because of the high prevalence of *Pasteurella multocida*, antistaphylococcal penicillins, first-generation cephalosporins, and macrolides are not recommended (Stevens 2014).

For infected animal or human bites in patients who can receive oral outpatient therapy, a 5- to 10-day course of antibiotic therapy is commonly used. Intravenous therapy for 7–14 days (extended to 4 weeks for septic arthritis and 6 weeks for osteomyelitis) is recommended for serious injuries, clenched-fist bite injuries, or injuries initially treated in the outpatient setting that have infection that progresses after 24 hours of oral therapy. Intravenous options include ampicillin/sulbactam, a cephamycin, or ertapenem. In patients allergic to penicillins, either doxycycline or a fluoroquinolone may be used in combination with metronidazole or clindamycin.

All bite wounds should be thoroughly irrigated and cleansed with sterile normal saline. Primary closure of wounds is not recommended except for wounds to the face. Patients should be evaluated for rabies prophylaxis—particularly in geographic areas with high prevalence—and for bites from feral and wild animals. Patients should also be evaluated for tetanus prophylaxis, and tetanus toxoid should be administered to patients without toxoid vaccination in the previous 10 years. The tetanus, diphtheria, and acellular pertussis vaccine is preferred for patients who have not received a pertussis-containing vaccine as adults (Stevens 2014).

Herpes Zoster

Herpes zoster is characterized by a unilateral rash localized to one or two adjacent dermatomes without crossing the body's midline. It initially presents as an erythematous, maculopapular rash that transforms into vesicles and is followed by pustules that crust over and heal after 2–4 weeks. The rash may be preceded by a prodrome of episodic or continuous symptoms of pain, itching, and/or tingling. Patients with immunocompromising conditions may present with disseminated rash and the appearance of new lesions for up to 2 weeks. Postherpetic neuralgia—characterized by the persistence of pain for weeks, months, or several years after resolution of rash—is the most common complication of herpes zoster. Patients who scratch lesions are at risk of bacterial superinfection caused by skin flora, including *S. aureus* and *S. pyogenes*. Herpes zoster is usually diagnosed on the basis of its characteristic clinical presentation. Diagnostic testing (e.g., polymerase chain reaction to detect VZV DNA from skin lesions, direct fluorescent antibody staining of VZV-infected cells, serologic methods) may be used for patients with atypical presentations or to rule out infection with herpes simplex virus.

In addition to therapy for acute-pain control, the systemic antivirals listed in Table 1-2 are strongly recommended for the treatment of herpes zoster in patients with immunocompromising conditions or patients with one or more of the following: age 50 years or older, moderate or severe pain or rash, nontruncal involvement, or complications. An antiviral agent should be started as early as possible—ideally, within 72 hours of the onset of rash.

Table 1-2. Common Antivirals Used in the Treatment of Herpes Zoster

Drug	Clinically Useful Activity Against Acyclovir-Resistant VZV	Dosing Regimen[a]	Adverse Effects	Drug Interactions
Acyclovir	No	Immunocompetent: 800 mg PO 5 times daily. Immunocompromised: 10 mg/kg IV three times daily	Malaise, nephrotoxicity	Nephrotoxic agents, zoster vaccine
Famciclovir	No	Immunocompetent: 500 mg PO three times daily	Headache, nausea	Zoster vaccine
Foscarnet[b]	Yes	Immunocompromised: 40 mg/kg IV three times daily	Fever, electrolyte disturbances, nausea, vomiting, diarrhea, headache, anemia, granulocytopenia	Nephrotoxic agents, QT prolonging agents
Valacyclovir	No	Immunocompetent: 1 g PO three times daily	Headache, nausea, abdominal pain, hepatotoxicity, nasopharyngitis	Zoster vaccine

[a]Doses recommended for patients with herpes zoster and are based on normal kidney and liver functions.
[b]Not approved for the treatment of herpes zoster by the FDA.
IV = intravenously; PO = by mouth; VZV = varicella zoster virus.
Information from: Cohen JI. Herpes zoster. N Engl J Med 2013;369:255-63.

There is still benefit to initiation of treatment after that time frame for those with continued formation of new lesions or complications. Famciclovir and valacyclovir are typically given for a 7-day course of treatment, whereas acyclovir is given for 7–10 days, with consideration given to extending treatment in those who experience continued formation of new lesions or complications after the recommended duration of therapy. Valacyclovir or famciclovir is preferred to acyclovir because of less frequent dosing, higher bioavailability, and higher and more consistent antiviral drug concentrations in the blood (Cohen 2013; McDonald 2012; Dworkin 2007). In a large randomized double-blind study, valacyclovir significantly accelerated the resolution of acute neuritis compared with acyclovir, and the proportion of patients with postherpetic neuralgia was lower in the valacyclovir arm compared with the acyclovir arm (Beutner 1995).

INFECTIONS IN BOTH THE OUTPATIENT AND INPATIENT SETTINGS

Erysipelas and Cellulitis

Erysipelas is characterized by a bright red erythematous lesion of the superficial layers of the skin; the lesion has a raised border and a well-demarcated margin. Erysipelas is often preceded by flu-like symptoms and is associated with burning pain. Cellulitis is an acute inflammation of the epidermis, dermis, and sometimes the superficial fascia, and it can be purulent or nonpurulent. The lesion is characterized by erythema and edema of the skin and has nonelevated and poorly defined margins. Cellulitis is considered a serious infection because of the propensity of the microorganism(s) to invade lymphatic tissue and blood. If left untreated, cellulitis can progress to adjacent tissue and cause an abscess, septic arthritis, or osteomyelitis. Diagnosis is based on clinical presentation, and cultures of blood or cutaneous aspirates, biopsies, or swabs are not routinely recommended, except in patients with immersion injuries or in those who with immunocompromising conditions (Stevens 2014).

Mild and typical cases with no focus of purulence are treated in the outpatient setting with oral antibiotics directed primarily against streptococci (e.g., penicillin VK) but could also include coverage against MSSA (e.g., dicloxacillin, cephalexin, or clindamycin). The recommended duration of therapy is 5 days, but treatment should be extended if the infection has not improved. Moderate cases with systemic signs of infection (e.g., fever, leukocytosis, extensive lesions) require a short hospitalization for administration of intravenous penicillin G, cefazolin, ceftriaxone, or clindamycin, with a switch to oral agents upon clinical response. For patients whose cellulitis is associated with penetrating trauma, evidence of MRSA infection elsewhere, nasal colonization with MRSA, injection drug use, or systemic inflammatory-response

syndrome, intravenous vancomycin or another antibiotic effective against both MRSA and streptococci is recommended.

Broad-spectrum antibiotic therapy with vancomycin plus either piperacillin-tazobactam or a carbapenem is a reasonable empiric regimen in severe cases, such as those occurring in patients whose cellulitis has failed oral antibiotic therapy, those occurring in immunocompromised patients, those with clinical signs of deeper infection, or those associated with systemic inflammatory-response syndrome. Other antibiotics commonly used in this setting are third- and fourth-generation cephalosporins, fluoroquinolones, and metronidazole. Because of increased risk of resistance among Enterobacteriaceae, ampicillin-sulbactam is rarely used, and aminoglycosides are considered less desirable alternative options because of their unfavorable adverse effect profiles. To hasten clinical improvement, the use of systemic corticosteroids such as prednisone 40 mg daily for 7 days could be considered in patients who do not have diabetes (Stevens 2014).

In all cases, immobilization and elevation of the affected extremity facilitate drainage. Treating fissuring, scaling, and maceration in the interdigital toe spaces reduces the incidence of recurrent lower-leg infections. Treating predisposing conditions such as obesity, edema, venous insufficiency, and eczema reduces the risk of recurrent infections. Lastly, prophylactic administration of penicillin VK or erythromycin orally twice daily or benzathine penicillin intramuscularly every 2 to 4 weeks should be considered in patients who have three or four episodes of cellulitis per year despite attempts to treat predisposing factors (Stevens 2014).

Diabetic Foot Infections

Diabetic foot infection presents as a deep abscess, cellulitis of the dorsum, or a mal perforans ulcer after a history of penetrating trauma or extension of local infection. Although reports of swelling, edema, warmth, tenderness, and purulence are common, pain is often absent because of peripheral neuropathy. Diabetic foot infections are often much more extensive than they appear, and systemic signs of infection are rare, except in severe limb-threatening cases. Table 1-3 describes the classification of DFIs. Diagnosis is based on clinical presentation, medical history of diabetes, imaging, and cultures obtained from deep tissue samples post-debridement. Diabetic foot infection can be complicated by the presence of concomitant osteomyelitis, which must be assessed by bone imaging. Osteomyelitis is best diagnosed by bone culture and histology (Lipsky 2012).

Treatment

The general approach to the management of DFI is highlighted in Figure 1-4. Wounds without evidence of soft tissue infection or bone infection do not require antibiotic therapy. Infected wounds require antibiotic therapy that targets aerobic gram-positive cocci. Coverage for MRSA should be considered in patients with histories of MRSA infections, when the local prevalence of MRSA infection or colonization is high, or for severe infections. Broad-spectrum antibiotic therapy is prescribed for patients at risk of infection with antibiotic-resistant organisms, including patients with chronic, previously treated, or severe infections. Coverage for *Pseudomonas aeruginosa* is usually unnecessary except when the local prevalence of *Pseudomonas* infection is high, in the setting of a warm climate, or in patients whose feet are frequently exposed to water. Anaerobic coverage is needed in patients with ischemic, necrotic, or foul-smelling wounds.

In addition to antibiotic therapy, most DFIs require surgical interventions ranging from debridement to

---

Patient Care Scenario

Three days ago, a 50-year-old man was admitted to the hospital for the management of purulent left lower leg cellulitis. He has been receiving vancomycin 1000 mg intravenously every 12 hours. The lesion associated with cellulitis has shrunk, the erythema has improved, and the pain is much more manageable. His medical history is significant for hypertension, atrial fibrillation, and congestive heart failure. In addition to vancomycin, his home drugs include lisinopril 40 mg orally daily, warfarin 5 mg orally daily, spironolactone 25 mg orally daily, furosemide 20 mg orally daily, carvedilol 25 mg orally twice daily, and oxycodone/acetaminophen 5 mg/325 mg 1 tab orally every 6 hours as needed for pain. Blood cultures are negative so far, but the culture obtained from aspiration of the edge of the lesion revealed *Staphylococcus aureus*, abundant growth, with the following microbiology and sensitivity report:

Antibiotic	MIC (mcg/mL)	Interpretation
Clindamycin	≥ 8	R
Oxacillin	≥ 4	R
Rifampin	≤ 0.5	S
Tetracycline	≤ 1	S
Trimethoprim/ sulfamethoxazole	≤ 10	S
Vancomycin	0.5	S

Upon admission, his temperature was 38°C, WBC count was 12,520 cells/mm³, and his INR was 2.6. Today, his temperature is 37.2°C, his WBC is 7.1 x 10³ cells/mm³, and his INR is 2.9. What is the most appropriate antibiotic regimen for the patient to take upon discharge?

Answer

The patient is hospitalized for the management of purulent cellulitis caused by methicillin-resistant *Staphylococcus aureus* sensitive to rifampin, tetracycline, trimethoprim/sulfamethoxazole, and vancomycin, but resistant to clindamycin. The patient responded favorably to a 3-day course of parenteral vancomycin as evidenced by improvement in signs and symptoms and normalization of temperature and WBC count. Therefore, the clinician should discharge the patient on an oral antibiotic regimen to complete the course of therapy. Clindamycin should not be used because the sensitivity report shows resistance to clindamycin. Although the sensitivity report is showing susceptibility to rifampin, rifampin should not be used as monotherapy for the management of staphylococcal infections because resistance can quickly develop during treatment. In addition, vancomycin should not be used orally for the treatment of staphylococcal infections because it is not systemically absorbed. The only remaining options are trimethoprim/sulfamethoxazole, doxycycline, minocycline, tedizolid, and linezolid. Trimethoprim/sulfamethoxazole is known to interact with warfarin resulting in an increase in INR. In the absence of monitoring and dosage adjustment for warfarin, trimethoprim/sulfamethoxazole may not be the best option because it can increase the risk of bleeding particularly in this patient whose INR is already at the upper limit of the desired range of 2 to 3. Linezolid and tedizolid are considered expensive agents compared with generic antibiotics and may not be covered by this patient's insurance. This will leave minocycline or doxycycline orally twice daily for at least 4 days as the best options for the patient. This case illustrates the importance of taking into account the microbiology culture and sensitivity report as well as concomitant medications and patient-specific factors before switching to a different antibiotic regimen for a given patient.

1. Stevens DL, Bisno AL, Chambers HF, et al. Practice guidelines for the diagnosis and management of skin and soft tissue infections: 2014 update by the Infectious Diseases Society of America. Clin Infect Dis 2014;59:e10-52.
2. Liu C, Bayer A, Cosgrove SE, et al. Clinical practice guidelines by the Infectious Diseases Society of America for the treatment of methicillin-resistant *Staphylococcus aureus* infections in adults and children. Clin Infect Dis 2011;52:285-92.
3. Howard PA, Ellerbeck EF, Engelman KK, et al. The nature and frequency of potential warfarin drug interactions that increase the risk of bleeding in patients with atrial fibrillation. Pharmacoepidemiol Drug Saf 2002;11:569-76.

resection and amputation. Most DFIs also require wound care, including debridement to remove necrotic tissue, off-loading to redistribute pressure off the wound, and appropriate dressings to allow for moist wound healing. Bed rest and leg elevation are recommended initially to decrease swelling and edema, and glycemic control is crucial to the healing process and for the prevention of future infections. Although bioengineered skin equivalents, growth factors, granulocyte-colony-stimulating factors, hyperbaric oxygen therapy, and negative-pressure wound therapy have not been shown to consistently facilitate resolution of infection, they may be used on a case-by-case basis at the clinician's discretion (Lipsky 2012).

Infections in the Inpatient Setting
Surgical Site Infections

Surgical site infections are divided into three categories: superficial incisional SSI, deep incisional SSI, and organ or space SSI. Diagnosis is based on purulent incisional discharge; positive culture of aseptically obtained material; local signs of pain, swelling, erythema, and tenderness; or assessment by the attending surgeon or an experienced physician. The majority of SSIs occur more than 4 days after operation (Stevens 2014).

Suture removal plus incision and drainage is the mainstay of therapy for SSIs. In addition, antibiotics are beneficial for patients presenting with erythema and induration extending more than 5 cm from the wound edge, temperature higher than 38.5°C, heart rate higher than 110 beats per minute, or WBC higher than 12 x 10³ cells/mm³. An antistaphylococcal penicillin or a first-generation cephalosporin is recommended if MSSA is suspected or isolated. Vancomycin or another intravenous anti-MRSA antibiotic is recommended if MRSA is suspected (e.g., nasal colonization with MRSA, prior MRSA infection, recent hospitalization, recent antibiotic exposure). A cephalosporin or a fluoroquinolone in combination with metronidazole is recommended if gram-negative or anaerobic bacteria are suspected (e.g., surgery on the axilla, gastrointestinal or genital tracts, or perineum) (Stevens 2014).

Necrotizing fasciitis

Patients with necrotizing fasciitis present initially with erythema, tenderness, warmth, swelling, and pain out of proportion to physical findings. As the infection progresses, blistering, skin crepitus, skin discoloration, and necrosis occur. Polymicrobial necrotizing fasciitis presents with relatively intact skin and spreads in 3–5 days. Streptococcal necrotizing fasciitis (what the lay press terms *flesh-eating bacteria*) can progress quickly within 1–2 days. Clostridial gas gangrene is characterized by gas production and muscle necrosis. Diagnosis is based on clinical presentation, recent history of penetrating or blunt trauma, laboratory abnormalities, and surgical exploration. Cultures should be obtained from tissue samples and blood. Once the diagnosis is established, necrotizing fasciitis is considered a medical emergency (Lancerotto 2012).

Immediate and aggressive surgical debridement is essential in the management of necrotizing fasciitis. Polymicrobial infections must be empirically treated with broad-spectrum antibiotics such as vancomycin, linezolid, or daptomycin plus piperacillin-tazobactam or a

Table 1-3. Classification of Diabetic Foot Infections

Clinical Manifestation of Infection	IDSA	PEDIS
No signs or symptoms of infection	Uninfected	1
Local infection[a] involving only the skin and the subcutaneous tissue If erythema is present, must be 0.5–2 cm around the ulcer Exclude other causes of an inflammatory response of the skin	Mild	2
Local infection[a] as described above with erythema >2 cm or involving structures deeper than skin and subcutaneous tissues No SIRS	Moderate	3
Local infection[a] as described above with signs of SIRS as manifested by ≥2 of the following: • T 38°C to 36°C • HR >90 beats/minute • RR >20 breaths/minute or PaCO$_2$ <32 mm Hg • WBC count >12,000 or <4000 cells/mcL or ≥10% bands	Severe	4

[a]Infection defined by the presence of at least two of the following: erythema, local swelling or induration, local tenderness or pain, local warmth, and purulent discharge.

HR = heart rate; IDSA = Infectious Diseases Society of America; PEDIS = perfusion, extent/size, depth/tissue loss, infection, and sensation; RR = respiratory rate; SIRS = systemic inflammatory response syndrome; T = temperature; WBC = white blood cells.

Information from: Lipsky BA, Berendt AR, Cornia PB, et al. 2012 Infectious Diseases Society of America clinical practice guideline for the diagnosis and treatment of diabetic foot infections. Clin Infect Dis 2012;54:e132-73; and Chahine EB, Harris S, William II R. Diabetic foot infections: an update on treatment. US Pharm 2013;38:23-6.

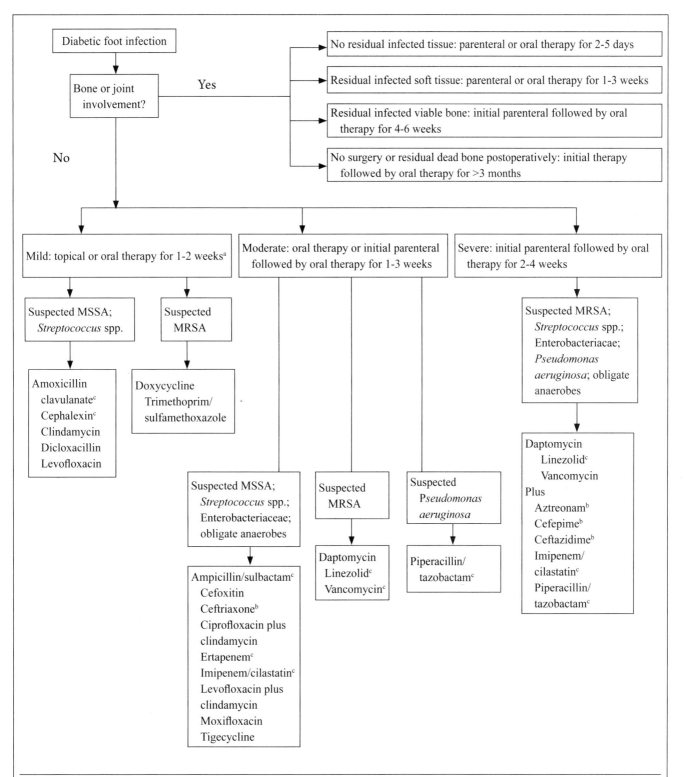

Figure 1-4. General approach to the management of diabetic foot infection. Note: agents similar to those listed in this algorithm can be substituted based on clinical, epidemiologic, and financial considerations.

[a]May extend up to 4 weeks if slow to resolve.
[b]Consider adding an antibiotic with activity against obligate anaerobes
[c]Agents commonly used as comparators in clinical trials for the treatment of diabetic foot infections.
MRSA = methicillin-resistant *Staphylococcus aureus*; MSSA = methicillin-sensitive *Staphylococcus aureus*.
Information from: Lipsky BA, Berendt AR, Cornia PB, et al. 2012 Infectious Diseases Society of America clinical practice guideline for the diagnosis and treatment of diabetic foot infections. Clin Infect Dis 2012;54:e132-73.

carbapenem or ceftriaxone plus metronidazole that are directed against gram-positive cocci, Enterobacteriaceae, and anaerobes. Group A streptococcal and clostridial infections are treated with parenteral aqueous penicillin G plus clindamycin. Adding clindamycin to β-lactam therapy provides several advantages, including additional coverage against streptococci and staphylococci, an immunomodulatory effect, and inhibition of toxin production. Pyomyositis caused by MSSA is treated with nafcillin or oxacillin or cefazolin. The recommended total duration of therapy is 2–3 weeks. Hyperbaric oxygen therapy is not recommended because it has not been proved effective and because it may delay resuscitation and surgical debridement (Stevens 2014).

Monitoring
Efficacy

For the majority of SSTIs, patients should note improvement in clinical symptoms of infection within 3 days of appropriate treatment; improvement may take up to 1 week for patients with impetigo. For any patient not responding to therapy within that period, additional culture and sensitivity testing should be performed, with therapy modified toward the specific infecting pathogen(s) and/or further surgical debridement for infections such as necrotizing fasciitis. Mild cases of folliculitis or furuncles without improvement after 2 to 3 days of moist heat or use of a topical agent likely require incision and drainage. Methicillin-resistant *Staphylococcus aureus* should be considered for any patient who has not had improvement after 3 days of antimicrobial therapy with an anti-staphylococcal penicillin or first-generation cephalosporin. When vancomycin is used, it should be dosed according to a patient's actual body weight to achieve a target trough of 10–15 mcg/mL for most SSTIs. A target trough of 15–20 mcg/mL is recommended for patients with necrotizing fasciitis or whose infection has progressed to osteomyelitis (Rybak 2009). Although this dosing strategy has not consistently correlated with improved outcomes, the traditional vancomycin dosing of 1 g every 12 hours is unlikely to achieve a sufficient concentration to eradicate MRSA in many patients and should no longer be recommended.

Safety

See Table 1-1 for adverse effects and significant drug interactions of antibiotics commonly used in the treatment of SSTIs, and Table 1-2 for antiviral agents used for the treatment of herpes zoster. Clinicians are seeing more nephrotoxicity with the aggressive dosing of vancomycin. A recent large retrospective study showed that vancomycin trough concentrations higher than 12.1 mg/L were associated with increased risk of nephrotoxicity (Han 2014). Another retrospective study showed that the concomitant use of piperacillin-tazobactam was associated with increased risk of nephrotoxicity (adjusted odds ratio [OR] of 5.36; 95% confidence interval (CI) 1.41–20.5) (Meaney

2014). The main safety concerns with daptomycin are creatine phosphokinase elevation and myalgia. A recent meta-analysis of six randomized controlled trials of daptomycin versus other antibiotics for the treatment of SSTIs showed that patients receiving daptomycin had elevated creatine phosphokinase compared with control groups (OR 1.95; 95% CI, 1.04–6.65). However, this adverse event was reversible upon therapy discontinuation (Wang 2014).

Finally, the main safety concerns with linezolid are myelosuppression, neuropathy, and serotonin syndrome. A recent retrospective-analysis study showed that receiving linezolid therapy for 14 or more days was a significant risk factor for thrombocytopenia (OR 13.3; 95% CI, 3.2–55.6). Also, the incidence of thrombocytopenia was significantly higher in patients with CrCl less than 30 mL/minute than in patients with normal renal function (p=0.014) (Hirano 2014). Because linezolid is a weak monoamine oxidase inhibitor, the U.S. Food and Drug Administration (FDA) recommends avoiding its use with other serotonergic drugs. In fact, the incidence of linezolid-associated serotonin toxicity is 0.5% to 18.2%, and most cases occurred in patients receiving selective serotonin reuptake inhibitors or multiple serotonergic drugs (Woytowish 2013).

NEW ANTIBIOTICS

The FDA recently released guidance to assist sponsors in developing antibiotics for the treatment of ABSSSIs. For the purpose of this guidance, ABSSSIs include cellulitis/erysipelas, wound infection, and major cutaneous abscess and have a minimum lesion surface area of about 75 cm^2. The FDA has designated more stringent efficacy end points and stricter timing of assessments. The primary end point is cessation of spread of skin lesion erythema and absence of fever at 48–72 hours after treatment initiation (FDA 2013). The FDA recently approved five antibiotics for the treatment of ABSSSIs: ceftaroline, dalbavancin, oritavancin, tedizolid, and telavancin.

Ceftaroline

Ceftaroline is a fifth-generation cephalosporin active against MRSA, drug-resistant *Streptococcus pneumoniae*, and Enterobacteriaceae and was recently approved by the FDA for the treatment of ABSSSIs and community-acquired bacterial pneumonia. Results from two phase-3 multicenter randomized double-blind clinical trials, with clinical cure rates as primary outcome, have shown that ceftaroline 600 mg administered intravenously for 60 minutes is noninferior to vancomycin plus aztreonam administered intravenously for 5–14 days for the treatment of ABSSSIs (CANVAS 1: 91.1% with ceftaroline and 93.3% with vancomycin/aztreonam, 95% CI, –6.6–2.1; CANVAS 2: 92.2% with ceftaroline and 92.1% with vancomycin/aztreonam, 95% CI, –4.4–4.5). The most common adverse events associated with ceftaroline in those trials were positive Coombs test without hemolysis and gastrointestinal upset (Corey 2010a, 2010b, Wilcox 2010). Ceftaroline is currently the only β-lactam antibiotic approved for the treatment of ABSSSIs caused by MRSA. Because of its broad spectrum of activity and because it can replace combination therapy in this setting, ceftaroline is particularly useful when used empirically for the treatment of SSTIs when both MRSA and Enterobacteriaceae are suspected.

Dalbavancin

Dalbavancin is a new lipoglycopeptide antibiotic with activity against MRSA; it was recently approved by the FDA for the treatment of ABSSSIs. Results from two phase-3 multicenter randomized double-blind clinical trials with early clinical response as primary outcome showed that dalbavancin 1000 mg administered intravenously for 30 minutes on day 1 followed by 500 mg on day 8 is noninferior to vancomycin administered intravenously for at least 3 days, with an option to switch to oral linezolid for the treatment of ABSSSIs (DISCOVER 1: 83.3% with dalbavancin and 81.8% with vancomycin/linezolid, 95% CI, –4.6–7.9; DISCOVER 2: 76.8% with dalbavancin and 78.3% with vancomycin/linezolid, 95% CI, –7.4–4.6). The most common treatment-related adverse events associated with dalbavancin in these trials were nausea, diarrhea, and pruritus (Boucher 2014).

Dalbavancin is currently the only antibiotic with once-weekly dosing (2 total doses) for the treatment of SSTIs; this enables clinicians to avoid or shorten the hospitalization of selected patients and potentially reduce health care costs.

Oritavancin

Oritavancin is a new lipoglycopeptide antibiotic active against MRSA; it was recently approved by the FDA for the treatment of ABSSSIs. Results from a phase-3 multicenter randomized double-blind clinical trial with early clinical response as primary outcome demonstrated that oritavancin 1200 mg administered intravenously as a single dose over a 3-hour infusion is noninferior to vancomycin administered intravenously twice daily for 7–10 days for the treatment of ABSSSIs (SOLO 1: 82.3% with oritavancin 78.9% with vancomycin, 95% CI, –1.6–8.4). Although the overall frequency of adverse events was similar between the two treatment arms, nausea was more common among those treated with oritavancin (Corey 2014).

Oritavancin is the first antibiotic with a single-dose formulation for the treatment of SSTIs, potentially enabling clinicians to avoid or shorten the hospitalization of selected patients and potentially reduce health care costs.

Tedizolid

Tedizolid is a new oxazolidinone antibiotic active against MRSA. It was recently approved by the FDA for the treatment of ABSSSIs. Results from two phase-3

multicenter randomized double-blind clinical trials with early clinical response as primary outcome showed that tedizolid 200 mg administered intravenously or orally daily for 6 days is noninferior to linezolid administered intravenously or orally twice daily for 10 days for the treatment of ABSSSIs (ESTABLISH 1: 79.5% with tedizolid and 79.4% with linezolid, 95% CI, –6.1–6.2; ESTABLISH 2: 85% with tedizolid and 83% with linezolid, 95% CI, –3.0–8.2). Treatment-emergent adverse events were similar between the two treatment groups, with fewer gastrointestinal disorders reported in the tedizolid group than in the linezolid group (Moran 2014; Prokocimer 2013). Tedizolid is the second antibiotic with both oral and parenteral formulations to be indicated for the treatment of MRSA infections.

Telavancin

Telavancin is a lipoglycopeptide antibiotic active against MRSA; it was recently approved by the FDA for the treatment of ABSSSIs and hospital-acquired and ventilator-associated bacterial pneumonia. Results from two phase-3 multicenter randomized double-blind clinical trials with clinical cure rates as primary outcome showed that telavancin 10 mg/kg administered intravenously for 60 minutes is noninferior to vancomycin administered intravenously for at least 7 days for the treatment of ABSSSIs (ATLAS 1: 84.3% with telavancin and 82.8% with vancomycin, 95% CI, –4.3–7.3; ATLAS 2: 83.9% with telavancin and 87.7% with vancomycin, 95% CI, –9.2–1.5). The most common adverse events associated with telavancin in these trials were taste disturbance, gastrointestinal upset, headache, and foamy urine (Stryjewski 2008). Telavancin was the first lipoglycopeptide antibiotic to be approved by the FDA for the treatment of ABSSSIs. It carries two boxed warnings: (1) new onset or worsening renal impairment and potential adverse developmental outcomes in pregnant women based on animal data; and (2) precautions related to QTc prolongation and potential for decreased efficacy in those with a CrCL of 50 mL/minute or greater. Because of its unfavorable safety profile, telavancin should be used as an alternative to vancomycin and other anti-MRSA agents for the treatment of SSTIs suspected to be caused by MRSA.

PREVENTION

General Measures

All patients with SSTIs should be counseled on hygiene and wound care measures to prevent the spread of infection. Patients should (1) cover any draining wounds with clean and dry bandages, (2) bathe regularly, (3) clean their hands regularly, (4) clean their hands after touching the area of infection or any item that has been in contact with a draining wound, and (5) avoid reusing or sharing any personal items that may have contacted the site of infection.

Because early recognition and management of risk factors for ulcers or amputations can prevent or delay adverse outcomes, all patients with diabetes mellitus should have an annual comprehensive foot examination, including inspection, assessment of foot pulses, and testing for loss of protective sensation. All patients with diabetes should also be educated on the importance of daily foot monitoring, proper nail and skin care of the foot, and the selection of appropriate footwear. Patients with loss of protective sensation should be counseled on alternative ways to assess for early foot problems, such as hand palpation, visual inspection, or assistance from another person (ADA 2014). A recently published update describes the detection and prevention of SSIs in acute-care hospitals (Anderson 2014).

Pharmacologic Measures

Because of an association between colonization and subsequent MRSA infection, different strategies for decolonization may be used in the outpatient setting for patients with recurrent infections (typically defined as two or more SSTIs at different body sites within 6 months) despite appropriate preventive measures (Liu 2011). A common decolonization strategy is intranasal mupirocin twice daily for 5–10 days, either alone or in combination with a skin antiseptic solution such as chlorhexidine or hexachlorophene for 5–14 days (Liu 2011). A recent study found that a 5-day regimen of hygiene, intranasal mupirocin, and 4% chlorhexidine body washes for all household members significantly reduced the incidence of self-reported recurrent SSTI in children during a 12-month period compared with decolonization of the index patient alone (72% vs. 52%, p=0.02) (Fritz 2012).

Oral antibiotics are not routinely recommended for decolonization, but a 5- to 10-day course of rifampin in combination with trimethoprim/sulfamethoxazole or doxycycline may be considered for recurrent infections despite other preventive (appropriate personal and environmental hygiene) and decolonization measures (use of nasal and/or topical decolonization). A recent study showed a reduction in mean number of CAMRSA infections (0.03 vs. 0.84 infections/month, p< 0.0001) when patients with recurrent infection were given 10-day regimens of intranasal mupirocin, daily hexachlorophene body wash, and an oral anti-MRSA agent (either trimethoprim/sulfamethoxazole, doxycycline, or minocycline) compared with placebo before the intervention (Miller 2012).

Several decolonization strategies have been used in the inpatient setting. Typically, patients undergoing surgical procedures, especially open-heart surgery or procedures involving implants, are preoperatively screened for MRSA; patients found to be carriers are given intranasal mupirocin and chlorhexidine baths. A recent study found that universal decolonization (intranasal mupirocin for 5 days plus daily bathing with 2% chlorhexidine-impregnated cloths for duration of ICU stay for all patients) was more effective than either targeted decolonization (5 days of intranasal mupirocin and daily bathing with 2% chlorhexidine-impregnated cloths for those who screened positive for MRSA) or screening and isolation in preventing infections in the ICU setting (Huang 2013).

Varicella Zoster Vaccine

To prevent shingles, the Advisory Committee on Immunization Practices (ACIP) recommends routine vaccination with a single dose of zoster vaccine for all eligible persons 60 years and older, regardless of history with herpes zoster (CDC 2014). The ACIP's recommendation comes primarily from the Shingles Prevention Study, a double-blind, placebo-controlled trial designed to assess the efficacy of the zoster vaccine in 38,546 persons aged 60 years and older (Oxman 2005). The vaccine significantly reduced the incidence of herpes zoster by 51% overall, with reduction rates of 54% and 41% in those aged 60–69 years and 70–79 years, respectively. The zoster vaccine was also 66.5% effective overall at preventing postherpetic neuralgia.

Although the zoster vaccine is licensed by the FDA for use in persons aged 50 years and older, the ACIP does not recommend its routine use in patients younger than 60 years. Because it is a live, attenuated vaccine, its use is contraindicated in those who are pregnant, severely immunosuppressed, or severely immunodeficient, including those with malignancies, those who are HIV positive with a CD4$^+$ cell count less than 200 cells/mm^3, or those who have been receiving the equivalent of 20 mg of prednisone daily for at least 2 weeks. In addition, the zoster vaccine is contraindicated in those with histories of anaphylaxis to gelatin, neomycin, or any other vaccine components. Because antivirals against VZV may interfere with replication of the live vaccine, clinicians should stop chronic antiviral treatment at least 24 hours before immunization if possible; and therapy should be restarted at least 14 days after vaccine administration. Vaccination should be deferred for at least 1 month after the discontinuation of immunosuppressive therapy and administered at least 14 days (with some recommending a delay of 1 month if possible) before the start of immunosuppressive therapy (Harpaz 2008).

ANTIMICROBIAL STEWARDSHIP

Pharmacists play an integral role in antimicrobial stewardship programs, with the overall goal of selecting the most appropriate antimicrobial agent(s), dose, route, frequency, and duration of therapy to achieve clinical cure or prevention of infection while limiting the development of resistance, adverse drug events (e.g., *Clostridium difficile* infection), and cost (Dellit 2007). Because of the high incidence of SSTIs in both outpatient and inpatient settings, there are many opportunities for stewardship in the management of those infections.

In terms of selecting the most appropriate agent, although vancomycin is considered the gold standard for many types of SSTIs caused by MRSA, there is controversy over use of vancomycin for the treatment of certain systemic infections—particularly if they are caused by isolates that have a minimum inhibitory concentration (MIC) close to 2 mcg/mL, which is the upper limit of what is defined as sensitive (Van Hal 2013; Rybak 2009). For SSTIs caused by *S. aureus* with a vancomycin MIC of 2 or more mcg/mL, clinical response should be considered for determining whether its use should be continued. For patients who have had adequate debridement and any other foci of infection removed but who still have not had a clinical or microbiological response, it is recommended to change therapy to an alternate anti-MRSA agent. For the treatment of SSTIs caused by *S. aureus* isolates with a vancomycin MIC more than 2 mcg/mL, clinicians should use an alternative antimicrobial agent for treatment.

CONCLUSION

Skin and soft tissue infections are commonly encountered in both outpatient and inpatient settings. Nonpharmacologic therapy such as cleansing and irrigation and I&D is just as important as pharmacologic therapy and can be used in mild purulent infections without any additional pharmacologic therapy. Pharmacists often assist prescribers in selecting the most-appropriate antimicrobial regimens for patients presenting with SSTIs. Pharmacists play an important role in educating both patients and health care professionals about the judicious and appropriate use of antimicrobials to optimize the outcomes of patients presenting with SSTIs. Pharmacists also assist in preventing DFIs by educating patients on the importance of optimal glycemic control and regular foot examination.

REFERENCES

Abrahamian FM, Goldstein EJ. Microbiology of animal bite wound infections. Clin Microbiol Rev 2011;24:231-46.

American Diabetes Association. Standards of medical care in diabetes. Diabetes Care 2014;37 (Suppl 1):S14-S80.

Anaya DA, Dellinger EP. Necrotizing soft-tissue infection: diagnosis and management. Clin Infect Dis 2007;44:705-10.

Anderson DJ, Podgorny K, Berríos-Torres SI, et al. Strategies to prevent surgical site infections in acute care hospitals: 2014 update. Infect Control Hosp Epidemiol 2014;35:605-27.

Beutner KR, Friedman DJ, Forszpaniak C, et al. Valacyclovir compared with acyclovir for improved therapy for herpes zoster in immunocompetent adults. Antimicrob Agents Chemother 1995;39:1546-53.

Practice Points

In determining the optimal management of a patient with a skin or soft tissue infection, the clinician must consider the following important points:

- Determine first whether the infection is purulent or nonpurulent, and second whether the infection is mild, moderate, or severe.
- Most purulent infections are treated with incision and drainage first, followed by administration of oral antibiotics directed against MRSA in moderate cases and intravenous antibiotics directed against MRSA in severe cases.
- Most nonpurulent infections are treated with oral antibiotics directed against GAS in mild cases and intravenous antibiotics directed against GAS in moderate cases. Severe nonpurulent infections are treated with surgical debridement and intravenous broad spectrum antibiotics that cover MRSA.
- Employ nonpharmacologic therapy particularly cleansing and irrigation and incision and drainage whenever possible. Nonpharmacologic therapy is sufficient alone without antibiotics to treat mild purulent infections.
- The type of SSTIs, extent and severity of the infection, risk factors for MRSA, and comorbid conditions contribute to the most likely cause(s) of the infection. These elements, along with host factors such as allergies, hepatic and renal functions, and concomitant medications, should serve as the basis for selecting an antibiotic regimen to treat SSTIs.
- Keep in mind safety and drug interaction concerns before selecting an antimicrobial regimen for the treatment of SSTIs.
- Monitor for the cessation of the spread of the infection and for the reduction of inflammation within 48 to 72 hours after antibiotic administration. Otherwise, re-evaluate the diagnosis and/or the antibiotic regimen.
- Educate patients presenting with diabetic foot infections about the importance of achieving optimal glycemic control and keeping the feet clean and dry to prevent foot ulcers and subsequent infections.
- In the absence of any contraindications, encourage patients aged 60 years and older to receive the zoster vaccine to decrease the risk of herpes zoster.

Boucher HW, Wilcox M, Talbot GH, et al. Once-weekly dalbavancin versus daily conventional therapy for skin infection. N Engl J Med 2014;370:2169-79.

Brook I. Management of human and animal bite wound infection: an overview. Curr Infect Dis Rep 2009;11:389-95.

Centers for Disease Control and Prevention. Recommended adult immunization schedule, United States, 2014.

Cohen JI. Clinical practice: Herpes zoster. N Engl J Med 2013;369:255-63.

Corey GR, Kabler H, Mehra P, et al; SOLO I Investigators. Single-dose oritavancin in the treatment of acute bacterial skin infections. N Engl J Med 2014;370:2180-90.

Corey GR, Wilcox MH, Talbot GH, et al; CANVAS 1 investigators. CANVAS 1: the first Phase III, randomized, double-blind study evaluating ceftaroline fosamil for the treatment of patients with complicated skin and skin structure infections. J Antimicrob Chemother 2010;65(Suppl4):iv41-51.

Corey GR, Wilcox M, Talbot GH, et al. Integrated analysis of CANVAS 1 and 2: phase 3, multicenter, randomized, double-blind studies to evaluate the safety and efficacy of ceftaroline versus vancomycin plus aztreonam in complicated skin and skin-structure infection. Clin Infect Dis 2010;51:641-50.

Dellit TH, Owens RC, McGowan JE Jr, et al; Infectious Diseases Society of America; Society for Healthcare Epidemiology of America. Infectious Diseases Society of America and the Society for Healthcare Epidemiology of America guidelines for developing an institutional program to enhance antimicrobial stewardship. Clin Infect Dis 2007;44:159-77.

Dworkin RH, Johnson RW, Breuer J, et al. Recommendations for the management of herpes zoster. Clin Infect Dis 2007;44(Suppl 1):S1-26.

Edelsberg J, Taneja C, Zervos M, et al. Trends in US hospital admissions for skin and soft tissue infections. Emerg Infect Dis 2009;15:1516-8.

Forcade NA, Wiederhold NP, Ryan L, et al. Antibacterials as adjuncts to incision and drainage for adults with purulent methicillin-resistant Staphylococcus aureus (MRSA) skin infections. Drugs 2012;72:339-51.

Fritz SA, Hogan PG, Hayek G, et al. Household versus individual approaches to eradication of community-associated Staphylococcus aureus in children: a randomized trial. Clin Infect Dis 2012;54:743-51.

Gerber JS, Coffin SE, Smathers SA, et al. Trends in the incidence of methicillin-resistant Staphylococcus aureus infection in children's hospitals in the United States. Clin Infect Dis 2009;49:65-71.

Han H, An H, Shin KH, et al. Trough concentration over 12.1 mg/L is a major risk factor of vancomycin-related nephrotoxicity in patients with therapeutic drug monitoring. Ther Drug Monit 2014 Feb 26. [Epub ahead of print]

Harpaz R, Ortega-Sanchez IR, Seward JF; Advisory Committee on Immunization Practices Centers for Disease Control and Prevention. Prevention of herpes zoster: recommendations of the Advisory Committee on Immunization Practices. MMWR Recomm Rep 2008;57(RR-5):1-30;quiz CE2-4.

Herman RA, Kee VR, Moores KG, et al. Etiology and treatment of community-associated methicillin-resistant Staphylococcus aureus. Am J Health Syst Pharm 2008;65:219-25.

Hirano R, Sakamoto Y, Tachibana N, et al. Retrospective analysis of the risk factors for linezolid-induced thrombocytopenia in adult Japanese patients. Int J Clin Pharm 2014;36:795-9.

Huang SS, Septimus E, Kleinman K, et al. Targeted versus universal decolonization to prevent ICU infection. New Engl J Med 2013;368:2255-65.

Labreche MJ, Lee GC, Attridge RT, et al. Treatment failure and costs in patients with methicillin-resistant Staphylococcus aureus skin and soft tissue infections: a South Texas Ambulatory Research Network (STARNet) study. J Am Board Fam Med 2013;26:508-17.

Lancerotto L, Tocco I, Salmaso R, et al. Necrotizing fasciitis: classification, diagnosis, and management. J Trauma Acute Care Surg 2012;72:560-6.

Lipsky BA, Berendt AR, Cornia PB, et al; Infectious Diseases Society of America. 2012 Infectious Diseases Society of America clinical practice guideline for the diagnosis and treatment of diabetic foot infections. Clin Infect Dis 2012;54:e132-73.

Liu C, Bayer A, Cosgrove SE, et al; Infectious Diseases Society of America. Clinical practice guidelines by the Infectious Diseases Society of America for the treatment of methicillin-resistant Staphylococcus aureus infections in adults and children. Clin Infect Dis 2011;52:e18-55.

McDonald EM, de Kock J, Ram FS. Antivirals for management of herpes zoster including ophthalmicus: a systematic review of high-quality randomized controlled trials. Antivir Ther 2012;17:255-64.

Meaney CJ, Hynicka LM, Tsoukleris MG. Vancomycin-associated nephrotoxicity in adult medicine patients: incidence, outcomes, and risk factors. Pharmacotherapy 2014;34:653-61.

Merritt C, Haran JP, Mintzer J, et al. All purulence is local – epidemiology and management of skin and soft tissue infections in three urban emergency departments. BMC Emerg Med 2013;13:26.

Miller L, Daum R, Creech C, et al. A multi-center randomized double blind controlled trial of clindamycin versus trimethoprim/sulfamethoxazole for uncomplicated skin and soft tissue infection (L-337). Presented at the 53rd Interscience Conference on Antimicrobial Agents and Chemotherapy. Denver, CO. September 10, 2013.

Miller LG, Tan J, Eells SJ, et al. Prospective investigation of nasal mupirocin, hexachlorophene body wash, and systemic antibiotics for prevention of recurrent community-associated methicillin-resistant Staphylococcus aureus infections. Antimicrob Agents Chemother 2012;56:1084-86.

Moran GJ, Fang E, Corey GR, et al. Tedizolid for 6 days versus linezolid for 10 days for acute bacterial skin and skin-structure infections (ESTABLISH-2): a randomized, double-blind, phase 3, non-inferiority trial. Lancet Infect Dis 2014;14:696-705 .

Oxman MN, Levin MJ, Johnson GR, et al. A vaccine to prevent herpes zoster and postherpetic neuralgia in older adults. N Eng J Med 2005;352:2271-84.

Pettitt DA, Molajo A, McArthur P. A human bite. BMJ 2012;345:e4798.

Prokocimer P, De Anda C, Fang E, et al. Tedizolid phosphate vs linezolid for treatment of acute bacterial skin and skin structure infections: the ESTABLISH-1 randomized trial. JAMA 2013;309:559-69.

Rimland D, Moanna A. Increasing incidence of herpes zoster among veterans. Clin Infect Dis 2010;50:1000-5.

Rybak M, Lomaestro B, Rotschafer JC, et al. Therapeutic monitoring of vancomycin in adult patients: a consensus review of the American Society of Health-System Pharmacists, the Infectious Diseases Society of America, and the Society of Infectious Diseases Pharmacists. Am J Health Syst Pharm 2009;66:82-98.

Singer AJ, Talan DA. Management of skin abscesses in the era of methicillin-resistant Staphylococcus aureus. N Engl J Med 2014;370:1039-47.

Stevens DL, Bisno AL, Chambers HF, et al; Practice guidelines for the diagnosis and management of skin and soft tissue infections: 2014 update by the Infectious Diseases Society of America. Clin Infect Dis 2014;59:e10-52.

Stryjewski ME, Graham DR, Wilson SE, et al; Assessment of Telavancin in Complicated Skin and Skin-Structure Infections Study. Telavancin versus vancomycin for the treatment of complicated skin and skin-structure infections caused by gram-positive organisms. Clin Infect Dis 2008;46:1683-93.

Talan DA, Krishnadasan A, Gorwitz RJ, et al; EMERGEncy ID Net Study Group. Comparison of Staphylococcus aureus from skin and soft-tissue infections in US emergency department patients, 2004 and 2008. Clin Infect Dis 2011;53:144-9.

U.S. Department of Health & Human Services. Agency for Healthcare Research and Quality. 2011 National Statistics.

U.S. Department of Health & Human Services. Agency for Healthcare Research and Quality. 2011 National Statistics.

U.S. Food and Drug Administration. Guidance for Industry. Acute Bacterial Skin and Skin Structure Infections: Developing Drugs for Treatment.

Van Hal SJ, Fowler VG. Is it time to replace vancomycin in the treatment of methicillin-resistant Staphylococcus aureus infections? Clin Infect Dis 2013;56:1779-88.

Wang SZ, Hu JT, Zhang C, et al. The safety and efficacy of daptomycin versus other antibiotics for skin and soft-tissue infections: a meta-analysis of randomised controlled trials. BMJ Open 2014;4:e004744.

Wilcox MH, Corey GR, Talbot GH, et al. CANVAS 2 investigators. CANVAS 2: the second Phase III, randomized, double-blind study evaluating ceftaroline fosamil for the treatment of patients with complicated skin and skin structure infections. J Antimicrob Chemother 2010;65 (Suppl4):iv53-65.

Woytowish MR, Maynor LM. Clinical relevance of line-zolid-associated serotonin toxicity. Ann Pharmacother 2013;47:388-97.

Self-Assessment Questions

Questions 1–3 pertain to the following case.

R.F., a 54-year-old man, presents to the emergency room with a 2-day history of left lower extremity edema, redness, and pain that limits his normal daily activities. The lesion is not elevated and has poorly defined margins. His weight has not changed. His physical examination is notable for temperature 38°C, blood pressure 148/92 mm Hg, heart rate 88 beats/minute, respiratory rate 18 breaths/minute, and 1+ lower extremity edema. His laboratory values include sodium 138 mEq/L, potassium 4.4 mEq/L, BUN 18 mg/dL, SCr 0.9 mg/dL, WBC 16 x 10^3 cells/mm³, hemoglobin 13 g/dL, hematocrit 39%, and platelet count 240,000 cells/mm³. R.F.'s medical history includes hypertension (HTN), dyslipidemia, and depression. His home drugs include hydrochlorothiazide 25 mg/day, atorvastatin 20 mg/day, fluoxetine 40 mg/day, and duloxetine 60 mg/day. R.F. is admitted to the hospital for intravenous antibiotic administration and nasal swab is positive for methicillin-resistant *Staphylococcus aureus* (MRSA).

1. Which one of the following is the most likely cause of R.F.'s lesions?
   A. Cellulitis.
   B. Erysipelas.
   C. Furuncle.
   D. Impetigo.

2. Which one of the following regimens is the best empiric therapy for R.F.?
   A. Ciprofloxacin 400 mg intravenously every 12 hours.
   B. Linezolid 600 mg intravenously every 12 hours.
   C. Penicillin G 2 million units intravenously every 6 hours.
   D. Vancomycin 15 mg/kg intravenously every 12 hours. (MRSA + streptococci)

3. Which one of the following topical antibiotics is the best option to decolonize R.F. from nasal MRSA carriage?
   A. Clindamycin.
   B. Retapamulin.
   C. Metronidazole.
   D. Mupirocin.

4. A 65-year-old man was bitten in his leg by a dog while walking in the park. His wounds are infected. He has had uncontrolled type 2 diabetes mellitus for the past 5 years, for which he takes metformin 1000 mg PO twice daily. He developed hives when he received sulfa drugs. He received the full primary vaccine series of tetanus immunization and had a tetanus toxoid-containing booster 12 years ago. In addition to cleansing and irrigation, which one of the following is the most appropriate treatment for this patient?
   A. Amoxicillin-clavulanate.
   B. Amoxicillin-clavulanate plus a tetanus toxoid-containing vaccine.
   C. Ciprofloxacin plus clindamycin.
   D. Moxifloxacin plus a tetanus toxoid-containing vaccine.

Questions 5 and 6 pertain to the following case.

F.R., a 64-year-old woman, presents to the emergency room with a 2-week history of left lower extremity edema, redness, and pain that limits her normal daily activities. She has a lesion close to her small toes that is is macerated and foul-smelling. The erythema is close to 3 cm around the ulcer. She thinks she might have stepped on a nail while walking on the beach in South Florida. Her physical examination is notable for temperature 38.2°C, blood pressure 145/90 mm Hg, heart rate 92 beats/minute, respiratory rate 19 breaths/minute, and 1+ lower extremity edema. Her laboratory values include sodium 139 mEq/L, potassium 4.3 mEq/L, BUN 19 mg/dL, SCr 0.9 mg/dL, glucose 180 mg/dL, A1C 8%, WBC 14 x 10^3 cells/mm³, hemoglobin 12 g/dL, hematocrit 36%, and platelet count 290,000 cells/mm³. F.R.'s medical history is significant for HTN, type 2 diabetes, painful diabetic neuropathy, and a recent history of diabetic foot infection (DFI). Her home drugs include hydrochlorothiazide 25 mg/day, lisinopril 20 mg/day, glyburide 10 mg/day, metformin 1000 mg twice daily, pregabalin 75 mg twice daily, and aspirin 81 mg/day. F.R is admitted to the hospital for intravenous antibiotic administration and nasal swab is positive for MRSA.

5. In addition to cleansing, irrigation, and surgical debridement, which one of the following is the most appropriate empiric antibiotic treatment for F.R.'s DFI?
   A. Levofloxacin plus vancomycin.
   B. Piperacillin-tazobactam.
   C. Piperacillin-tazobactam plus metronidazole.
   D. Piperacillin-tazobactam plus vancomycin.

6. Which one of the following treatment durations would be best for F.R's DFI?
   A. 5 days
   B. 7 days
   C. 21 days
   D. 42 days

7. A 61-year-old woman presents to your clinic with a 3-day history of rash. She has vesicles and pustules on the left side of the forehead, a few lesions on the left side of the nose, and blurry vision in the left eye. The rash is associated with moderate to severe burning pain and was preceded by a tingling sensation on the left side of the face. She has diabetes and hypothyroidism for which she takes glyburide 5 mg/day and levothyroxine 25 mcg/day. Which one of the following is the most likely cause of this patient's lesions?

    A. Cellulitis.
    B. Erysipelas.
    C. Impetigo.
    D. Shingles.

8. A 66-year old man presents to your clinic with a moderate to severe case of herpes zoster. The primary care physician decides to treat the patient with antivirals and is asking you to recommend the most appropriate regimen. The patient is currently taking aspirin 81 mg/day, naproxen 500 mg twice daily, and oxycodone/acetaminophen 10 mg/325 mg 2 tablets three times daily. His CrCl is 60 mL/minute. Which one of the following is best to recommend for this patient?

    A. Acyclovir 400 mg orally five times daily for 7 days.
    B. Acyclovir 800 mg orally five times daily for 5 days.
    C. Famciclovir 500 mg orally three times daily for 5 days.
    D. Valacyclovir 1 g orally three times daily for 7 days.

9. A 48-year-old woman is in your pharmacy asking if she is a candidate for the herpes zoster vaccine. She had an episode of severe herpes zoster 3 years ago. She also has asthma for which she takes fluticasone propionate and salmeterol 100 mcg/50 mcg per inhalation 1 inhalation twice daily and levalbuterol 2 puffs q4–6h PRN shortness of breath. She is currently on day 5 (last day) of a tapered dose of oral methylprednisolone for an acute asthma exacerbation. Which one of the following best explains why this patient is not a candidate for herpes zoster vaccination?

    A. She has asthma and is currently on fluticasone and salmeterol.
    B. She has had an episode of severe herpes zoster in the past.
    C. She is currently on methylprednisolone for asthma exacerbation.
    D. She is too young for herpes zoster vaccination.

Questions 10 and 11 pertain to the following case.

M.I. is an 18-year-old man who presents to your clinic with a small purulent tender mass on his thigh that looks like a spider bite. The middle of the lesion is filled with pus and debris. The area is painful and warm to touch. M.I. has no chills and no other complaints. He is very active and exercises on a daily basis with a group of athletes. Physical examination reveals the following: temperature 37°C, blood pressure 120/70 mm Hg, heart rate 60 beats/minute, and respiratory rate 16 breaths/minute.

10. Which of the following is the most likely cause of M.I's clinical presentation?

    A. *Clostridium perfringens.*
    B. Methicillin resistant *Staphylococcus aureus.*
    C. Methicillin sensitive *Staphylococcus aureus.*
    D. *Streptococcus pyogenes.*

11. Which one of the following is best to recommend for M.I.?

    A. Clindamycin.
    B. Incision and drainage.
    C. Penicillin G plus clindamycin.
    D. Penicillin VK.

Questions 12 and 13 pertain to the following case.

M.N., a 40-year-old man, is admitted to the hospital for the management of an infection on the right side of his face. The area is red, elevated, and clearly demarcated. He thinks he may have scratched his face a couple of days ago. His physical examination is notable for temperature 38.6°C, blood pressure 135/80 mm Hg, heart rate 80 beats/minute, and respiratory rate 17 breaths/minute. M.N.'s laboratory values include sodium 140 mEq/L, potassium 4.2 mEq/L, BUN 20 mg/dL, SCr 1.1 mg/dL, WBC 17 x 10³ cells/mm³, hemoglobin 14 g/dL, hematocrit 42%, and platelet count 310,000 cells/mm³. M.N. has a history of anaphylactic shock caused by penicillin VK when he was 11 years old.

12. Which one of the following is the most likely cause of M.N.'s lesions?

    A. Cellulitis.
    B. Cutaneous abscess.
    C. Erysipelas.
    D. Impetigo.

13. Which of the following is best to recommend for M.N.?

    A. Aztreonam 1 g intravenously three times daily
    B. Cefazolin 1 g intravenously three times daily.
    C. Trimethoprim/sulfamethoxazole 1 double-strength tablet orally twice daily.
    D. Vancomycin 15 mg/kg intravenously twice daily.

14. A 30-year-old man presents to the emergency department with fever and severe pain in his right hand with erythema, tenderness, warm skin, and swelling. Two days ago, he had a minor scratch to his hand while gardening. He is admitted to the hospital for further evaluation and management. Twenty-hours later, blisters, crepitus, and necrosis become apparent on his right hand, and the patient is rushed to the operating room for surgical debridement and removal of necrotic tissues. Pertinent laboratory values are WBC 19 x 10³ cells/mm³, creatine kinase 301 IU/L, and albumin 3 g/dL. Blood cultures reveal group A β-hemolytic streptococci susceptible to all antibiotics tested. Nasal swab is negative for MRSA. Which one of the following is the most appropriate antibiotic treatment for this patient?

    A. Imipenem-cilastatin.
    B. Imipenem-cilastatin plus vancomycin.
    C. Penicillin G.
    D. Penicillin G plus clindamycin.

15. A 65-year-old woman is in the hospital for management of an infected wound, a complication of a surgery on the trunk. She is currently receiving telavancin 10 mg/day pending microbiology culture and sensitivity report. Her other hospital medications include methadone 20 mg three times daily, oxycodone/acetaminophen 10 mg/325 mg 1 tablet three times daily PRN pain, bisacodyl 5 mg/day, docusate 100 mg twice daily, enoxaparin 40 mg subcutaneously daily, and omeprazole 20 mg/day. Which one of the following is this patient most at risk of because of her medications?

    A. Hepatotoxicity.
    B. Hypothyroidism.
    C. QTc prolongation.
    D. Seizures.

16. You wish to measure the degree of patient satisfaction in the prevention of herpes zoster in patients who were referred to the pharmacist-run immunization clinic and those who received standard care. Patients are asked to indicate their satisfaction level using a Likert scale (1 = strongly dissatisfied, 5 = strongly satisfied). Which one of the following statistical tests would be best to compare these data?

    A. McNemar's test.
    B. Paired t test.
    C. Wilcoxon rank sum.
    D. Wilcoxon signed rank.

17. You are asked to implement an antimicrobial stewardship initiative to decrease the incidence of *Clostridium difficile* infection (CDI) after several patients who were treated with clindamycin for skin and soft tissue infections (SSTIs) came back to the emergency

department with CDI. Physicians in your department have recently switched from cephalexin to clindamycin because of the sharp increase in the incidence of community-associated MRSA (CAMRSA) infections. In addition to incision and drainage, which one of the following would be best to recommend for the treatment of moderate purulent SSTIs?

    A. Continue the use of clindamycin if the double disk diffusion test is positive.
    B. Use cephalexin instead of clindamycin.
    C. Use linezolid instead of clindamycin.
    D. Use trimethoprim/sulfamethoxazole instead of clindamycin.

18. You are asked to implement a strategy to reduce the incidence of recurrent SSTIs caused by MRSA in a long-term care facility. Despite emphasizing personal and environmental hygiene, a large percentage of residents still present with MRSA infections. After treating the infections, which one of the following would be best to administer to residents to prevent recurrences?

    A. Mupirocin intranasally twice daily for 5 days.
    B. Retapamulin intranasally twice daily for 7 days.
    C. Rifampin 600 mg orally daily for 5 days.
    D. Trimethoprim/sulfamethoxazole 1 DS tablet orally twice daily for 7 days.

19. A 7-year-old girl was ready to be discharged after a 2-day course of vancomycin therapy for the treatment of a carbuncle in her right buttock. The culture from the abscess grew MRSA sensitive to all antibiotics tested except erythromycin and oxacillin, and the double disk diffusion test was positive. Which one of the following would best complete the course of antibiotic therapy for this patient?

    A. Clindamycin.
    B. Doxycycline.
    C. Levofloxacin.
    D. Trimethoprim/sulfamethoxazole.

20. A 51-year-old man is expected to receive a 3-week-course of outpatient daptomycin therapy for the treatment of DFI. He has a history of myocardial infarction for which he has been taking aspirin 81 mg/day, lisinopril 40 mg/day, metoprolol 25 mg twice daily, and simvastatin 20 mg/day at bedtime for 5 years with no complaints. His SCr is 0.8 mg/dL. Which one of the following monitoring parameters would best ensure the safety of this patient's antibiotic regimen?

    A. Creatine kinase.
    B. Liver function tests.
    C. QTc interval.
    D. Serum creatinine.

Learner Chapter Evaluation: Skin and Soft Tissue Infections.

As you take the posttest for this chapter, also evaluate the material's quality and usefulness, as well as the achievement of learning objectives. Rate each item using this 5-point scale:

- Strongly agree
- Agree
- Neutral
- Disagree
- Strongly disagree

1. The content of the chapter met my educational needs.
2. The content of the chapter satisfied my expectations.
3. The author presented the chapter content effectively.
4. The content of the chapter was relevant to my practice and presented at the appropriate depth and scope.
5. The content of the chapter was objective and balanced.
6. The content of the chapter is free of bias, promotion, or advertisement of commercial products.
7. The content of the chapter was useful to me.
8. The teaching and learning methods used in the chapter were effective.
9. The active learning methods used in the chapter were effective.
10. The learning assessment activities used in the chapter were effective.
11. The chapter was effective overall.

Use the 5-point scale to indicate whether this chapter prepared you to accomplish the following learning objectives:

12. Given a patient's clinical presentation and risk factors, distinguish between the various types of skin and soft tissue infections.
13. Given a patient's profile, develop a pharmacotherapeutic plan to treat a skin or soft tissue infection.
14. Assess the safety profiles of antimicrobials commonly used for the treatment of skin and soft tissue infections.
15. Justify prevention measures to reduce the recurrence and transmission of a patient's skin and soft tissue infections.
16. Please provide any specific comments relating to any perceptions of bias, promotion, or advertisement of commercial products.
17. Please expand on any of your above responses, and/or provide any additional comments regarding this chapter:

Intra-Abdominal Infections

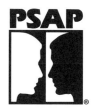

By David T. Bearden, Pharm.D.

Reviewed by Wilson Ly, Pharm.D., BCPS, AAHIVP; and Kathleen A. Lusk, Pharm.D., BCPS

Learning Objectives

1. Distinguish the microbiologic differences typical among major intra-abdominal infections arising from different sites of the gastrointestinal tract.
2. Classify disease severity, likelihood of resistant pathogens, and infection site for a patient with intra-abdominal infection.
3. Design an appropriate empiric antimicrobial regimen (including duration) for the patient with intra-abdominal infection.
4. Assess microbiology reports, patient response to therapy (including adverse events related to pharmacotherapy) and appropriately alter empiric therapy regimens for the patient with intra-abdominal infection.
5. Compose appropriate antimicrobial stewardship practices pertinent to patients with intra-abdominal infections.

Introduction

Intra-abdominal infections represent a diverse set of infectious processes within the abdominal cavity. An understanding of the likely etiology of the infection is a key to treatment pathways and the ultimate selection of empiric anti-infective therapy. Intra-abdominal infections are common, with appendicitis alone resulting in more than 300,000 infections and 1 million patient-days of hospitalization per year in the United States (Solomkin 2010).

Pathophysiology

Intra-abdominal infections are commonly classified in four major ways: by the primary organ infected, presence and source of peritonitis, infection acquisition location (hospital or community acquired), and severity of illness. Infections extending beyond a single organ and spreading into the abdominal cavity with peritonitis or abscess are termed *complicated* by the Infectious Diseases Society of America (IDSA). Complicated infections are the most common intra-abdominal infections and can be separated into three classes: primary, secondary, and tertiary peritonitis.

Primary Peritonitis

Primary peritonitis is associated with two typical patient types: (1) patients with hepatic failure and ascites; and (2) patients undergoing peritoneal dialysis. The two disparate groups share the common feature of the infectious organisms' arising without another underlying organ infection. Pathogens are introduced into the peritoneal space directly by translocation of the organisms from an intact gut in a patient with hepatic disease or from exogenous

---

Baseline Knowledge Statements

Readers of this chapter are presumed to be familiar with the following:

- National rates of antimicrobial resistance for pathogens typical in intra-abdominal infections
- Pediatric and adult antimicrobial dosing and antimicrobial pharmacodynamic profiles
- Guidelines for the treatment of complicated intra-abdominal infections as specified by the Infectious Diseases Society of America
- Antimicrobial stewardship recommendations as outlined by the Infectious Diseases Society of America and the Society for Healthcare Epidemiology of America
- Guidelines for the treatment of intraperitoneal-dialysis-related peritonitis as set forth by the International Society of Peritoneal Dialysis

introduction (peritoneal catheters). The disease burden in primary peritonitis is very high, representing 18% of infection-related mortality in patients on peritoneal dialysis and a 43% mortality rate in spontaneous bacterial peritonitis related to cirrhosis (Pleguezuelo 2013; Li 2010).

Secondary Peritonitis

Secondary peritonitis is so termed because of the initial presence of another organ infection that spread to include a more diffuse intra-abdominal process. The spread can occur by direct extension from a current infection; or perforation of the gastrointestinal (GI) or biliary tracts, resulting in spillage of pathogens into the abdomen. A primary example of the second route would be the rupture of an infected appendix that spills fecal matter into the abdomen, causing widespread infection of the peritoneal lining. Finally, an abscess in the peritoneal space or an abscess formation and rupture can lead to secondary peritonitis.

Tertiary Peritonitis

Tertiary peritonitis is a controversial classification for a complicated and difficult-to-control case of secondary peritonitis. In tertiary peritonitis, severe infections continue when source control of the initial organ infection cannot be achieved. In such cases, the peritonitis fails antimicrobial therapy multiple times because the infectious source cannot be eradicated by medical treatment alone or by surgical procedures. Some practitioners advocate that a tertiary infection be labeled as a *complicated secondary peritonitis*, but both designations are used clinically and in the literature.

Diagnosis and Prognosis

Abdominal pain is the primary distinguishing clinical feature of most intra-abdominal infections, but general presentation varies widely with the infectious source. Serum laboratory monitoring reveals usual infection-related elevation of white blood cells and sepsis-associated chemistries (e.g., decreased serum pH, elevated lactate, low partial pressure of arterial oxygen). Imaging, including ultrasound and computed tomography scans, is vital in early diagnosis. For more severe infections, surgical repair or peritoneal inspection is often required for definitive diagnoses; in treatment trials, the need for a surgical procedure is pathognomonic for complicated infection. The wide range of severity observed with intra-abdominal infections produces major differences in morbidity and mortality. Simple organ infections like diverticulitis are rarely fatal, whereas more severe infections may lead to sepsis, which has a mortality rate that ranges from 17% to 63% (de Ruiter 2009).

The microbiology of intra-abdominal infections depends on the initial infection site. In general, upper GI infections are dominated by gram-positive and gram-negative aerobes and increasing amounts of anaerobic flora that cause infection from the small to large intestine. Most infections—especially those with organ infection extending into the peritoneum—are caused by a mixture of aerobes and anaerobes, typically with three or four organisms isolated. Figure 2-1 outlines the major bacterial groups isolated in secondary infections.

Increasing antimicrobial resistance—particularly within the enteric gram-negative pathogens—is complicating the choice of treatment regimens. A study of 1442 gram-negative aerobes from intra-abdominal infections in U.S. hospitals revealed extended-spectrum β-lactamase production in 12.7% of *Klebsiella pneumonia* and 9.7% of *Escherichia coli* (Hawser 2014). Those enteric species are commonly isolated in culture and are targets of most empiric therapy. A study of 2049 patients with intra-abdominal infections was conducted to best identify those at high risk of having a pathogen resistant to broad-spectrum antimicrobials (e.g., piperacillin/tazobactam or imipenem) (Swenson 2009). The most-important risk factors identified included health care acquisition, corticosteroid use, organ transplantation, underlying pulmonary or hepatic disease, and duodenal source of infection. Mortality rates among nontransplant patients associated with susceptible pathogens were 49/584 (8.4%) versus 54/386 (14.0%) with resistant infections (p=0.008). High local rates of resistance in a health care system may require broadened antibiotic coverage or unique therapy recommendations.

TREATMENT

The general goals of treatment for patients with intra-abdominal infections include restoring and maintaining patient vital signs and organ function, controlling the source of infection, eliminating the infecting organisms, and restoring health for a return to normal functioning.

Surgery and Drainage

Surgical repair of perforations and resection or removal of infected organs is imperative for the successful treatment of many intra-abdominal infections. Drainage of abscesses, when possible, is also a mainstay of treatment. Failure to control the source of infection can lead to increased morbidity and mortality and limit the effectiveness of any pharmacotherapy. A recent review of eight clinical trials comprising nearly 5000 patients found that adequate source control was not evaluated uniformly. The data from smaller trials showed that 5% to 29% of patients were not adequately surgically controlled (Solomkin 2013); this is important because poor surgical control can lead to under-estimation of antimicrobial efficacy. More careful scrutiny is recommended by regulators reviewing clinical trial data. In additional, readers should look in all studies for evidence that source control was reviewed or addressed when this may affect patient outcomes. However, those data may be lacking in many retrospective studies.

Pharmacotherapy
General Patient Support

General supportive care is critical for patients with intra-abdominal infections. The need for aggressive fluid and hemodynamic support is common, with intra-abdominal infections often resulting in sepsis. Intravenous fluid and vasopressor choices should be driven by common practice for patients with sepsis, as defined by the Surviving Sepsis Campaign (Dellinger 2012). Specialized nutrition support is often required for patients with long-term GI dysfunction, although early enteral feeding has been advocated, even for patients with repaired perforations. Most patients should receive nothing by mouth during a portion of their treatment course so as to limit GI activity postsurgery. Therefore, both acute and maintenance drugs may need to be adjusted to intravenous options and then back to oral regimens once the patient's status has improved.

Empiric Antimicrobial Therapy
Timing

Appropriate empiric antimicrobial therapy is crucial for patients with intra-abdominal infections. Although microbiologic data are helpful in guiding targeted antimicrobial therapy, nearly all patients require empiric therapy based on probable pathogens. An IDSA expert panel recommended 8 hours as a maximal time frame from presentation to a health care setting to receipt of antimicrobials in patients who are nonseptic—a recommendation that is very achievable in most instances (Solomkim 2010). In septic patients, increased urgency for early therapy is necessary, with a goal of treatment within 1 hour. Newer data from a trial of 17,990 septic patients, 3505 of whom had abdominal infection sources, suggest that each hour of delay in implementation of antimicrobial therapy during the first 6 hours of care increases absolute mortality by more than 1% (Ferrer 2014).

Whether or not the patient has sepsis, it is ideal to obtain cultures before antimicrobials are initiated. Once administered, antimicrobials can alter the flora present and may reduce the yield of clinically important pathogens. Pharmacists in both emergency departments and hospital units can positively influence antimicrobial therapy and culture timing by recognizing the needs for both while making patient-specific recommendations for optimal therapy and ensuring its timely delivery and administration.

Specific Organ Infections

Specific organ infections without secondary peritonitis should be treated according to the prevailing pathogens in that anatomic region (see Figure 2-1). Antimicrobial considerations for a number of localized infections that spread to a more generalized intra-abdominal peritonitis

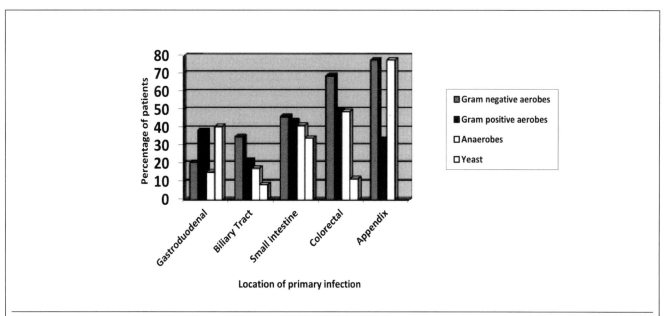

Figure 2-1. Percentage of patients with various organisms identified from abdominal cultures by primary infection site in critically ill patients with peritonitis.

Information from: de Ruiter J, Weel J, Manusama E, et al. The epidemiology of intra-abdominal flora in critically ill patients with secondary and tertiary abdominal sepsis. Infection 2009;37:522-7.

Patient Care Scenario

A 44-year-old woman presents to the emergency department with complaints of diffuse abdominal pain and nausea that have increased over the last 24 hours. Her vital signs are mildly abnormal with a current temperature of 100.2°F, HR 90 beats/minute, RR 14 breaths/minute, and BP 100/60. Her medical history is non-contributory and she has no medication allergies. Physical abdominal examination is not conclusive. Radiography reveals no obvious abnormalities or perforations and a CT scan is ordered. The patient is admitted to a general medicine floor to await further evaluation. Early differential diagnoses include cholecystitis and pancreatitis as most likely causes, pending further testing. Upon transfer to the medicine service after a 2 hour stay in the ED, the discussion turns to the need for empiric antimicrobial therapy for this patient. What antimicrobial therapy should be recommended in this patient presently?

Answer

Abdominal pain is a common complaint in medicine. The hallmarks of diagnosis are largely based on diagnostic imaging. While that imaging is being processed, empiric antimicrobial need should be based on the likelihood of infection and severity of illness. This patient does not appear septic, which makes delay of therapy reasonable at present. A septic patient should not have therapy delayed, as it increases morbidity and mortality. In a non-septic patient like this, the case patient, an 8-hour window for antimicrobial(s) initiation is generally acceptable. Primary peritonitis is not likely because this patient does not have hepatic disease or a dialysis catheter. The fact that this patient does not appear to have any gastrointestinal perforation furthers the likelihood that this is not a secondary peritonitis. The stated working diagnoses of pancreatitis or cholecystitis are also helpful. If pancreatitis, there is no need for any antimicrobial therapy in most cases. If cholecystitis, perioperative antimicrobials would be suggested, but could wait for diagnosis. In this patient, no empiric antimicrobials should be recommended at this time. Results of the pending imaging and other laboratory tests should be gathered before making an antimicrobial decision. Further results suggestive of an alternative infectious diagnosis or a rapid decline in patient status would be reasons to re-evaluate this decision. The first question of antimicrobial management – "is this patient infected?" needs to be answered first.

1. McNamara R, Dean AJ. Approach to acute abdominal pain. Emerg Med Clin North Am 2011;29:159-73.
2. Blot S, De Waele JJ, Vogelaers D. Essentials for selecting antimicrobial therapy for intra-abdominal infections. Drugs 2012;72:e17-32.
3. Strasberg SM. Clinical practice. Acute calculous cholecystitis. N Engl J Med 2008;358:2804-11.

are listed in Table 2-1. Drug selections are based on the suspected microbiology, the severity of the patient's infection, and the acquisition location (hospital or community acquired). Individual regimen choice is also driven by the adverse effect profiles of the drugs and any patient-specific factors such as drug interactions or hepatic or renal function. In general, the likelihood of resistance expands the need for additional agents like vancomycin or aminoglycosides.

Appendicitis

Appendicitis is the most common intra-abdominal infection requiring emergency surgery. A simple infection without perforation or necrosis requires only 24 hours of broad-spectrum perioperative antimicrobials. Data from a systematic review suggest that a single preoperative antibiotic dose may be sufficient in simple cases (Daskalakis 2014). The IDSA guidelines recommend a 24-hour period of prophylaxis; recent pediatric guidelines from the American Pediatric Surgical Association are less conservative, suggesting only a single preoperative dose. Using the minimum required coverage is most practical, but further data are needed to make a definitive case. Perforation is always treated more aggressively with 5 days of antimicrobial therapy that targets gram-positive and gram-negative aerobes and anaerobes (see Table 2-1).

Considerable debate is in process on the possible use of antibiotics as a primary treatment for acute, uncomplicated appendicitis—without the usual surgical appendectomy. A meta-analysis of five trials in adults comparing antibiotics alone versus appendectomy and antibiotics showed increased risk for the need of further interventions (40.3% vs. 8.5%, respectively) but some studies showed favorable outcomes for reduced complications and faster return to work (Mason 2012). A more recent study, with strict inclusion criteria for observation instead of surgery, reported that amoxicillin/clavulanate 1 g orally three times daily for 5–7 days was effective in preventing surgery in 88.1% patients (Di Saverio 2014). Antimicrobials remain a mainstay of therapy and are being increasingly seen as possible alternatives to surgery in selected patients. That trend may continue as methods improve to better identify the most appropriate patients to observe without surgery. The trend will also require better pharmacist understanding of the variable pre- or postoperative states of patients with appendicitis.

Cholecystitis/Cholangitis

In the absence of any direct perforation or connection with the upper GI tract, infections of the biliary tract are caused predominantly by aerobic pathogens. Surgical removal of the gallbladder is often the primary therapy, with antimicrobials used for surgical prophylaxis. Prophylaxis is continued for more than 24 hours unless more extensive infection outside the gallbladder is observed. Recent data have begun to challenge universal antimicrobial treatment after cholecystectomy for mild infections, with a small randomized study (n=82) finding no difference in length of stay (5.6 days vs. 5.1 days) or readmissions (19% vs. 13%) with and without antimicrobial therapy (Mazeh 2012). In mild cases of biliary infections, intravenous cephalosporins such as cefazolin, cefuroxime, and ceftriaxone are indicated. With increasing severity or perforation, extended coverage for anaerobic pathogens is required (see Table 2-1).

Diverticulitis

Diverticulitis is generally divided into uncomplicated and complicated infections, with complicated infections resulting in perforation or abscess. A study of 623 patients with CT-confirmed uncomplicated diverticulitis randomized patients to a minimum of 7 days of either prescriber-chosen antibiotic therapy or no antibiotic therapy. No differences in subsequent perforation, length of hospital stay, or long-term recurrence were observed (Chabok 2012). A Cochrane review of the treatment of diverticulitis, which included the Chabok study, cautiously suggests that few data exist for recommending any antimicrobial use in uncomplicated diverticulitis (Shabanzadeh 2012). That finding is being increasingly accepted and has been echoed in recent national reviews on the subject. Complicated diverticulitis treatment would still mirror that of secondary peritonitis when perforation of the colon would require broad-spectrum coverage for both aerobic and anaerobic pathogens (see Table 2-1).

Severe/Necrotizing Pancreatitis

Simple or so-called typical pancreatitis is not typically an infectious process and does not require antimicrobial therapy. Antimicrobial therapy is reserved for severe, secondary infections of the pancreas and possible subsequent peritonitis. Data suggest limited benefit to the antimicrobial prophylaxis of even severe pancreatitis. Instead, broad-spectrum therapy against aerobes and anaerobes should be initiated only when infection is confirmed—typically by surgical exploration and debridement (see Table 2-1). Pancreatic infections are notoriously difficult to treat because of the challenges of source control within the pancreas and its inherent enzymatic properties that can cause severe parenchymal damage to surrounding tissues. A longitudinal study from 1998 to 2010 included more than 1700 patients nationwide undergoing pancreatic debridement and revealed a slowly declining mortality rate that was still 17.8% from 2006 to 2010. (Wormer 2014).

Primary Peritonitis

Because of disparate etiologies, the major types of primary peritonitis are best treated as two separate entities. Primary peritonitis in patients with hepatic failure and ascites, usually termed spontaneous bacterial peritonitis (SBP), is typically caused by a single pathogen that translocates through the gut. Common organisms include enteric gram-negative rods, *Streptococcus pneumoniae*, other streptococci, and enterococci. The incidence of enterococcal infections has increased. A 12-year, single-site study reported significant increases from 11% to 35% of all SBP cases. The investigators completed a multivariate analysis and found that major risk factors for enterococcal infections include nosocomial infection and recent antimicrobial therapy (Reuken 2012).

Table 2-1. Recommended Empiric Antibiotic Regimens for Intra-abdominal Infections

Regimen		Single Agents	Combination Therapy
Community-associated	Mild-moderate infection	Cefoxitin Ertapenem Moxifloxacin Ticarcillin/clavulanic acid	Cefazolin Cefuroxime Ceftriaxone Ciprofloxacin Levofloxacin Plus Metronidazole
	Severe infection	Imipenem/cilastatin Meropenem Doripenem Piperacillin/tazobactam	Cefepime Ceftazidime Ciprofloxacin Levofloxacin Plus Metronidazole
Health care–associated		Same as for severe community-associated with consideration of aminoglycosides and vancomycin	Same as for severe community-associated with consideration of aminoglycosides and vancomycin

Information from: Solomkin JS, Mazuski JE, Bradley JS, et al. Diagnosis and management of complicated intra-abdominal infection in adults and children: guidelines by the Surgical Infection Society and the Infectious Diseases Society of America. Clin Infect Dis 2010;50:133-64.

Cefotaxime and ceftriaxone are commonly recommended for initial therapy, with alternatives based on final specific cultures and susceptibilities. Risk factors for enterococci or other resistant pathogens should be considered in initial antimicrobial selection. Access to ascitic fluid makes culture and diagnosis rapid enough to postpone expanding coverage in patients who are not severely ill. Treatment durations as short as 5 days have demonstrated efficacy, but the usual duration of treatment is 10–14 days. Lifelong secondary antimicrobial prophylaxis with oral fluoroquinolones is still recommended for patients with previous SBP, as is short-term primary prophylaxis with oral fluoroquinolones or intravenous ceftriaxone (while hospitalized) for those at high risk (e.g., with presence of ascites, malnutrition, encephalopathy, high bilirubin). The most effective duration of primary prophylaxis is unknown, with 7–10 days suggested for individuals with GI bleeds and long-term suppression in patients awaiting liver transplant. Risk-benefit analyses must be individualized.

A recent meta-analysis of eight studies that included more than 3800 patients suggests that acid-suppressive therapy increases the risk of SBP. The meta-analysis found a 3-fold increase in SBP risk in patients with hepatitis taking proton-pump inhibitors (Deshpande 2013). Although these findings are still debatable, it is worth evaluating the need for proton-pump inhibitor therapy in both outpatient and inpatient settings in patients with hepatic failure. Less-intensive acid suppression with H2-antagonists was associated with lower rates of SBP (Deshpande 2013) and might be a more appropriate alternative.

Peritonitis associated with peritoneal dialysis represents the second major group of patients with primary disease. Both gram-positive and gram-negative aerobes (e.g., *Staphylococcus aureus*, coagulase-negative staphylococci, enteric gram-negative pathogens) are introduced through the percutaneous dialysis catheter, and infections are typically monomicrobial. Empiric coverage of both pathogen groups can generally be achieved with a combination of third-generation cephalosporins and vancomycin. The intraperitoneal route of delivery is preferred in such patients (Table 2-2). Special attention needs to be paid to the compatibility and stability of any agents instilled into the peritoneum and to the unique dosing regimens dependent on dialysis schedules, with either single daily doses or continuous doses being equally efficacious. Treatment duration depends on speed of resolution and the organism isolated but is usually 1–3 weeks.

Secondary/Tertiary Peritonitis

Secondary peritonitis is caused by an initial intraabdominal source, often the perforation of an abdominal organ. The bacteriology is diverse and should be expected to include a mix of gram-positive and gram-negative aerobes and anaerobes, including Enterobacteriaceae, streptococci, enterococci, *S. aureus*, and *Bacteroides* species. In selecting a regimen, this broad coverage should be considered, as well as infection severity and whether the

---

Table 2-2. Intraperitoneal Antimicrobial Dosing for Continuous Ambulatory Peritoneal Dialysis Patients[a]

Antimicrobial	Intermittent Dosing (per exchange, once daily)	Continuous (all exchanges)
Cefazolin	15 mg/kg	Loading dose 500 mg/L; maintenance 125 mg/L
Ceftazidime	1000–1500 mg	Loading dose 500 mg/L; maintenance 125 mg/L
Ciprofloxacin	No data	Loading dose 50 mg/L; maintenance 25 mg/L
Fluconazole	200 mg every 24–48 hours	No data
Gentamicin, tobramycin	0.6 mg/kg	Loading dose 8 mg/L; maintenance 4 mg/L
Nafcillin	No data	Maintenance 125 mg/L
Vancomycin	15–30 mg/kg every 5–7 days	Loading dose 1000 mg/L; maintenance 25 mg/L

[a]For dosing renally cleared drugs in patients with residual renal function (>100 mL urine/day), dose should be increased by 25%.

Adapted from: Li PK, Szeto CC, Piraino B, et al; International Society for Peritoneal Dialysis. Peritoneal dialysis-related infections recommendations: 2010 update. Perit Dial Int 2010;30:393-423.

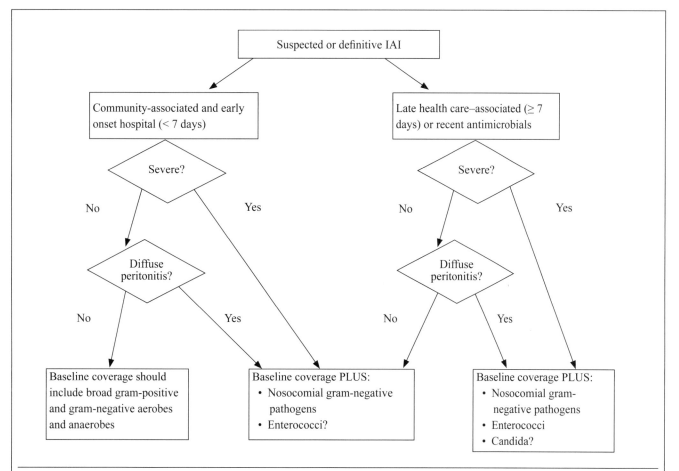

Figure 2-2. Algorithm for empiric drug selection in intraabdominal infections (IAI). Consideration of MRSA risk factors should be considered in all patients and would necessitate specific coverage. Severe infection is defined as infection in a patient with major vital sign abnormalities and hypotension and hypoperfusion resistant to fluid resuscitation (septic shock). Diffuse peritonitis is generally defined as peritonitis involving more than one abdominal quadrant.

Information from Blot S, De Waele JJ, Vogelaers D. Essentials for selecting antimicrobial therapy for intra-abdominal infections. Drugs 2012 16;72:e17-32.

infection was community or hospital acquired. Figure 2-2 presents a treatment algorithm for appropriately selecting the type and depth of antibacterial coverage.

Severe infections have been classified by both poor source control and general predictors of mortality (e.g., APACHE scores of 15 or higher, delays in therapy, advanced age [70 years or older], organ dysfunction, low albumin, poor nutritional status, malignancy, diffuse peritonitis). The presence of septic shock is considered severe by most definitions available in the guideline literature. Additional factors suggestive of a higher risk of resistant pathogens, including prior antimicrobial administration, should be considered in antimicrobial selection (see Table 2-1).

Although listed in the IDSA guidelines, moxifloxacin has been considered by some clinicians as a more questionable single agent for peritonitis, in part because of concerns about the depth of anaerobic coverage. A large analysis (642 anaerobic isolates from four clinical trials comparing moxifloxacin with other antimicrobial agents)

found high levels of moxifloxacin susceptibility (87.4% ≤ 2 mcg/mL) with limited full resistance (7.3% ≥ 8 mcg/mL). The clinical outcomes of infected patients did not differ until very high levels of resistance (≥ 32 mcg/mL) were observed (Goldstein 2011). It is difficult to determine the role of anaerobic minimum inhibitory concentration alone in these mixed infections, but the data support moxifloxacin use in those populations.

Another recent study of 699 patients with mild to moderate infection confirmed clinical noninferiority, finding similar clinical success for moxifloxacin (89.5%) and ertapenem (93.4%) (De Waele 2013). An additional published meta-analysis and other pooled data suggest similar safety and efficacy when moxifloxacin was compared with other agents, including ceftriaxone plus metronidazole and piperacillin/tazobactam. These data suggest that early concern for moxifloxacin use in mild to moderate disease may not have been warranted, although many clinicians still prefer more aggressive anaerobic coverage.

Tigecycline has been included in both the IDSA guidelines and European guidelines for intra-abdominal infections. However, recent pooled results from 13 studies that included 7424 patients in comparative trials revealed an absolute 0.7% increased rate of mortality (30% relative increase vs. comparators) in tigecycline-treated patients, which also included an additional increase in the rates of patients with unresolved infections (Prasad 2012). That finding has since led to a U.S. Food and Drug Administration (FDA) boxed warning suggesting tigecycline be used only in life-threatening cases when other alternative antimicrobials are unavailable.

Empiric antifungal therapy in secondary peritonitis is under considerable scrutiny, with difficulty in defining the most appropriate population for this aggressive early therapy. In general, severely ill patients with risk factors for fungal infections (e.g., recurrent abdominal surgery, recurrent or slowly treated GI tract perforations, GI anastomosis leaks) are considered at highest risk. Additional typical risk factors for *Candida* infections (e.g., central lines, receipt of total parenteral nutrition or broad-spectrum antibacterials) are also important to consider. For patients in whom empiric antifungal therapy is selected, the echinocandins are recommended for their fungicidal activity and superior coverage of more resistant *Candida* species compared with the azoles. The IDSA guidelines suggest that fluconazole may be appropriate for *Candida albicans* infections. The azole antifungals have been widely studied in candidiasis and candidemia, and a justifiable case can be made to continue fluconazole rather than choosing an echinocandin.

Definitive Antimicrobial Therapy

The use of microbiology reports to guide subsequent therapy is commonplace in all infections and is a usual step in antimicrobial therapy for intra-abdominal sources. It should be noted that few clinical data are available to suggest that alterations in therapy for intra-abdominal infections based on culture data improve outcomes; however, consensus suggests this method is useful. Direct cultures from surgical sites, with an emphasis on tissues and fluid rather than on microbiologic swabs, are recommended for all hospital-associated and severe infections. Percutaneous drains may be useful in early cultures, but because colonization is likely at this point, within 24 hours they lose their effectiveness in identifying organisms from the abdominal site. Pharmacists should inquire about exact specimen location and the timings of specimen collection and antibiotic administration when interpreting any cultures and determining the need to alter coverage. Anaerobic pathogens are usually difficult to culture and therefore may be under-identified. More than 30% of patients with secondary and tertiary peritonitis may not have any positive cultures identified (de Ruiter 2009). Coverage of typical aerobes and anaerobes should generally be continued in any patient with intra-abdominal infection regardless of the presence of those aerobes and anaerobes in cultures. Initial blood cultures are rarely helpful in community-acquired infections and should be reserved for more severe nosocomial infections or in cases where sepsis is identified.

Debate exists on the need to adjust therapy to cover all isolates from intra-abdominal cultures. The relative importance of individual pathogens in mixed flora is variable. Recommendations in 2013 from the IDSA and the American Society for Microbiology guidelines detail the appropriate use of cultures and results in intra-abdominal infections (Baron 2013). In mixed infections, laboratories may report only susceptibilities on isolates with known resistance concerns. Patients with mild to moderate disease who are clinically improving may not need alterations in therapy for pathogens lacking coverage by empiric regimens. It is well established that the finding of enterococci in cultures from patients treated without enterococcal therapy (e.g., cephalosporins) did not change outcomes in many patients. However, poor clinical response would generally dictate targeted therapy for those pathogens. In patients with severe infections, prompt change to agents with microbiologic activity against the isolated pathogens is recommended. Any intra-abdominal pathogen isolated from the blood should also be covered immediately.

Monitoring

Patients should be monitored for resolution of signs and symptoms of infection; improvement is typically observed within 48 to 72 hours in appropriately treated patients. As stated above, microbiology reports may be useful in guiding therapy. Patients who are not improving should be evaluated for both appropriate source control and appropriate antimicrobial therapy. Expansion of coverage to include more-resistant pathogens may be prudent in poorly responding patients—even in the absence of positive cultures.

In severely ill patients (particularly surgical patients), antimicrobial dosing should be reevaluated often. Pharmacokinetic changes may be rapid and marked with (1) fluid overload, (2) third-spacing altering volume of distribution, and (3) organ dysfunctions because of hypoperfusion in sepsis-altering clearance. Further severe organ dysfunction and procedures such as renal replacement therapy can further alter antimicrobial dosing needs.

QUALITY IMPROVEMENT

Antimicrobial Stewardship

Antimicrobial stewardship is vitally important in limiting resistance and improving antimicrobial usage and patient outcomes. All of the traditional mechanisms for stewardship apply in both the individual patient and systemwide treatment of intra-abdominal infections. Only a single study was found directly addressing intra-abdominal infections. That stewardship study sought to align therapy in 626 patients with IDSA guideline recommendations but found only limited benefit (Dubrovskaya

2012). Although significant changes were observed in antimicrobials selected, no differences were observed in length of hospital stay, *Clostridium difficile* rates, or readmissions. Nonsignificant increases were observed in the streamlining of therapy and appropriate therapy choice against isolated pathogens. Even though that study did not lead to major advances, it should be noted that it focused only on empiric guideline adherence. The use of guideline-directed therapies remains a mainstay of larger stewardship efforts but is only one of many tools for improving the use of antimicrobials.

Other traditional stewardship efforts should be applied to intra-abdominal infections when possible. Switching to oral antimicrobial therapy, when appropriate, has been used to contain costs, limit catheter use, and at times narrow spectrums. Those efforts are often difficult to conduct in patients with variable gut functionality caused by infection and surgery. In general, all patients able to tolerate oral diets can receive oral antibiotics. There is some concern for perforation, but once a rupture has been repaired and intestinal function has returned, there is little need for concern. Because treatment durations are usually short, many patients with more severe infections may complete therapy before GI tract function improves, limiting the ability to switch to oral options.

Optimal Duration of Therapy

Treatment duration varies with the specific site and extent of infection, as well as with patient-specific factors. Table 2-3 lists general recommendations for a variety of intra-abdominal infections. Slow response and the need for alterations in therapy should be considered in selecting final duration. Patients with lengthy, complicated cases may require many weeks of therapy. In those instances, the optimal timing of cessation of therapy is unknown, and treatment is sometimes stopped before complete resolution of symptoms.

Interprofessional Patient Care

To obtain optimal patient outcomes, pharmacists treating patients with intra-abdominal infections must interact professionally with physicians, nurses, respiratory therapists, microbiologists, and many other health care personnel. An understanding of surgical findings, procedures, and cultures obtained is generally the purview of a surgeon—and is vital for both selection of therapy and its monitoring. Nurses provide a vital link to subtle patient disposition, including patient clinical deterioration and improvements, and they are the key links in medication administration. Microbiologists and technicians can provide the pharmacist with important information and interpretation of microbiology reports. Finally, the patient and the patient's family should be included as

---

Table 2-3. Duration of Antimicrobial Therapy According to Primary Infection Site

Infection Site	Additional Data	Duration of Therapy
Abscess	Drained	3–7 days after surgery or drainage
	Un-drained	Weeks, based on clinical context
Appendicitis	No perforation	Perioperative prophylaxis, single dose to 24 hours
	Perforation	4–7 days
Cholecystitis	Nonoperative approach	5–10 days
	Operative approach:	
	No perforation	Up to 24 hours
	Perforation	4–7 days
Diverticulitis	Uncomplicated	No antimicrobials recommended
	Moderate/severe	4–7 days
Gastro-duodenal perforation	Early intervention (< 24 hours)	Perioperative prophylaxis only
	Late intervention (> 24 hours)	4–7 days
Pancreatitis	Non-necrotic and necrotic without infection	No antimicrobials recommended
	Necrotic with infection	4–7 days
Peritonitis	Generalized or localized	4–7 days

Information from: Blot S, De Waele JJ, Vogelaers D. Essentials for selecting antimicrobial therapy for intra-abdominal infections. Drugs 2012;72:e17-32; Solomkin JS, Mazuski JE, Bradley JS, et al. Diagnosis and management of complicated intra-abdominal infection in adults and children: guidelines by the Surgical Infection Society and the Infectious Diseases Society of America. Clin Infect Dis 2010;50:133-64; and Shabanzadeh DM1, Wille-Jørgensen P. Antibiotics for uncomplicated diverticulitis. Cochrane Database Syst Rev. 2012 Nov 14;11:CD009092.

---

central members of the health care team because they can provide insight into medical history and current medical function better than most other team members can. Pharmacists have extensive training in patient history taking and patient counseling and can apply these skills to investigations of patient and family histories regarding past antimicrobial use or allergic events. A clear understanding of (1) roles, (2) professional responsibilities, and (3) the need for strong interprofessional communication is imperative.

Conclusion

Intra-abdominal infections present a wide range of processes with variable degrees of severity. Antimicrobial therapy is important in most intra-abdominal infections, but surgical source control is also required. Microbiology is often mixed, with polymicrobial infections predominating. Appropriate antimicrobial selection is based on patient characteristics, site of infection, and severity of illness, with heavy reliance on empiric therapy. Antimicrobial stewardship is important in providing appropriate coverage and dosing while limiting resistance and adverse events.

References

Baron EJ, Miller JM, Weinstein MP, et al. A guide to utilization of the microbiology laboratory for diagnosis of infectious diseases: 2013 recommendations by the Infectious Diseases Society of America (IDSA) and the American Society for Microbiology (ASM). Clin Infect Dis 2013;57:e22-e121.

Chabok A, Påhlman L, Hjern F, et al; AVOD Study Group. Randomized clinical trial of antibiotics in acute uncomplicated diverticulitis. Br J Surg 2012;99:532-9. Cochrane Database Syst Rev 2012;11:CD009092.

Daskalakis K, Juhlin C, Pahlman L. The use of pre- or postoperative antibiotics in surgery for appendicitis: a systematic review. Scand J Surg 2014;103:14-20.

de Ruiter J, Weel J, Manusama E, et al. The epidemiology of intra-abdominal flora in critically ill patients with secondary and tertiary abdominal sepsis. Infection 2009;37:522-7.

De Waele JJ, Tellado JM, Alder J, et al. Randomised clinical trial of moxifloxacin versus ertapenem in complicated intra-abdominal infections: results of the PROMISE study. Int J Antimicrob Agents 2013;41:57-64.

Dellinger RP, Levy MM, Rhodes A, et al; Surviving Sepsis Campaign Guidelines Committee including the Pediatric Subgroup. Surviving sepsis campaign: international guidelines for management of severe sepsis and septic shock: 2012.Crit Care Med 2013;41:580-637.

Deshpande A, Pasupuleti V, Thota P, et al. Acid-suppressive therapy is associated with spontaneous bacterial peritonitis in cirrhotic patients: a meta-analysis. J Gastroenterol Hepatol. 2013;28:235-42.

Di Saverio S, Sibilio A, Giorgini E, et al. The NOTA Study (Non Operative Treatment for Acute Appendicitis): prospective study on the efficacy and safety of antibiotics (amoxicillin and clavulanic acid) for treating patients with right lower quadrant abdominal pain and long-term follow-up of conservatively treated suspected appendicitis. Ann Surg 2014 Mar 18. [Epub ahead of print]

Dubrovskaya Y, Papadopoulos J, Scipione MR, et al. Antibiotic stewardship for intra-abdominal infections: early impact on antimicrobial use and patient outcomes. Infect Control Hosp Epidemiol 2012;33:427-9.

Ferrer R, Martin-Loeches I, Phillips G, et al. Empiric antibiotic treatment reduces mortality in severe sepsis and septic shock from the first hour: Results from a guideline-based performance improvement program. Crit Care Med 2014 Apr 8 [Epub ahead of print]

Goldstein EJ, Solomkin JS, Citron DM, et al. Clinical efficacy and correlation of clinical outcomes with in vitro susceptibility for anaerobic bacteria in patients with complicated intra-abdominal infections treated with moxifloxacin. Clin Infect Dis 2011;53:1074-80..

Hawser SP, Badal RE, Bouchillon SK, et al. Susceptibility of gram-negative aerobic bacilli from intra-abdominal pathogens to antimicrobial agents collected in the United States during 2011. J Infect 2014;68:71-6.

Practice Points

In patients with complicated intra-abdominal infections, including secondary peritonitis, the following factors should be considered in empiric antimicrobial selection:

- Primary source of infection – the site of initial infection guides the need for aerobic or anaerobic pathogen coverage.
- Healthcare association – patients with recent healthcare exposure need coverage of nosocomial pathogens, as do those with infections acquired during hospitalization.
- Local resistance – unique pathogen susceptibilities should be considered for commonly encountered organisms.
- Need for specific pathogen coverage
  - Enterococcus – coverage should be initiated in only severely ill patients, for definitive therapy when isolated in the blood, and in patients not responding to other therapies.
  - MRSA – consider with patient risk factors, but deescalate if not isolated
  - Candida – important if found in the blood, or multiple risk factors are identified, but limited empiric needs.
- Severity of illness –severely ill patients should be covered more broadly with considerations of double gram-negative coverage.
- Patient comorbidities, including allergy –should be considered, as with all therapy selections, in both improving outcomes and minimizing toxicities

Li PK, Szeto CC, Piraino B, et al; International Society for Peritoneal Dialysis. Peritoneal dialysis-related infections recommendations: 2010 update. Perit Dial Int 2010;30:393-423.

Mason RJ, Moazzez A, Sohn H, et al. Meta-analysis of randomized trials comparing antibiotic therapy with appendectomy for acute uncomplicated (no abscess or phlegmon) appendicitis. Surg Infect (Larchmt) 2012;13:74-84

Mazeh H, Mizrahi I, Dior U, et al. Role of antibiotic therapy in mild acute calculus cholecystitis: a prospective randomized controlled trial. World J Surg 2012;36:1750-9.

Pleguezuelo M, Benitez JM, Jurado J, et al. Diagnosis and management of bacterial infections in decompensated cirrhosis. World J Hepatol 2013;5:16-25.

Prasad P, Sun J, Danner RL, et al. Excess deaths associated with tigecycline after approval based on noninferiority trials. Clin Infect Dis 2012;54:1699-709.

Reuken PA, Pletz MW, Baier M, et al. Emergence of spontaneous bacterial peritonitis due to enterococci - risk factors and outcome in a 12-year retrospective study. Aliment Pharmacol Ther 2012;35:1199-208.

Shabanzadeh DM1, Wille-Jørgensen P. Antibiotics for uncomplicated diverticulitis. Cochrane Database Syst Rev 2012 Nov 14;11:CD009092.

Solomkin JS, Mazuski JE, Bradley JS, et al. Diagnosis and management of complicated intra-abdominal infection in adults and children: guidelines by the Surgical Infection Society and the Infectious Diseases Society of America. Clin Infect Dis 2010;50:133-64.

Solomkin JS, Ristagno RL, Das AF, et al. Source control review in clinical trials of anti-infective agents in complicated intra-abdominal infections. Clin Infect Dis 2013;56:1765-73.

Swenson BR, Metzger R, Hedrick TL, et al. Choosing antibiotics for intra-abdominal infections: what do we mean by "high risk"? Surg Infect (Larchmt) 2009;10:29-39.

Wormer BA, Swan RZ, Williams KB, et al. Outcomes of pancreatic debridement in acute pancreatitis: analysis of the nationwide inpatient sample from 1998 to 2010. Am J Surg 2014;208:350-62.

SELF-ASSESSMENT QUESTIONS

Questions 21 and 22 pertain to the following case.

J.Z. is a 73-year-old man who is brought to the emergency department (ED) at 0800 from a long-term care facility. J.Z. has a 2-day history of appetite loss and increasing lethargy and confusion. His vital signs remain stable. J.Z. presents with complaints of abdominal pain and is sent to surgery from the emergency room after diagnostic imaging reveals possible small bowel necrosis. He is given a dose of imipenem before surgery at 1000. Surgical exploration reveals necrotic small intestine, which is successfully resected, and localized peritonitis. Appropriate intraoperative cultures and blood cultures are obtained. Postoperatively at 1300, J.Z.'s condition is deteriorating with a blood pressure of 80/60 mm Hg, a respiratory rate of 21 breaths/minute, a heart rate of 88 beats/minute, and Tmax of 39°C. His WBC is 14×10^3 cells/mm^3, with a stable SCr of 0.7 mg/dL. J.Z. has no known drug allergies.

21. Which one of the following is the most important to address for J.Z.'s care at present?

    A. Redose cefoxitin 2 g intravenous every 6 hours.
    B. Begin piperacillin-tazobactam 3.375 g intravenous every 8 hours.
    C. Begin gentamicin 7 mg/kg intravenous every 24 hours.
    D. Begin aggressive fluid therapy with 1L of NS.

22. Twenty-four hours later, J.Z. continues to deteriorate clinically although he is receiving an appropriate antibacterial regimen. Intraoperative cultures return with mixed bacteria susceptible to the regimen selected. Additionally, *C. albicans* is isolated from the intra-abdominal cultures, with susceptibilities pending. Blood cultures remain negative. Which one of the following is best to recommend for J.Z.?

    A. No additional therapy is recommended.
    B. Fluconazole 200 mg intravenous once, then 100 mg intravenous every 24 hours.
    C. Amphotericin B deoxycholate 0.8 mg/kg intravenous every 24 hours.
    D. Micafungin 100 mg intravenous every 24 hours.

23. A 53-year-old man with a history of alcoholism presents to his primary care provider with increased abdominal pain. He has a mild fever of 37.4°C and a WBC of 10×10^3 cells/mm^3. His LFTs and serum chemistries are normal, and he has no ascites. After diagnostic imaging, the patient is diagnosed with diverticulitis. He has no known drug allergies. Which one of the following is best to recommend for this patient?

    A. Begin ceftriaxone 1 g intravenous every 24 hours.
    B. Begin ciprofloxacin 400 mg intravenous every 12 hours and metronidazole 500 mg intravenous every 8 hours.
    C. Begin vancomycin 1 g intravenous every 12 hours and cefuroxime 1.5 g intravenous every 8 hours.
    D. Do not initiate antimicrobial therapy.

Questions 24–26 pertain to the following case.

P.D. is a 44-year-old trauma patient admitted to the SICU after multiple stab wounds. He has been in the ICU for 6 days since his admission and has had two subsequent surgeries for multiple visceral repairs, including lung and peritoneal punctures. On hospital day 7, P.D. begins to spike a fever of 39°C with increasing abdominal tenderness and distension. Other vital signs and chemistries remain within high-normal ranges. P.D. developed a minor diffuse rash postoperatively, possibly caused by pre-operative cefazolin. Exploratory abdominal surgery reveals a small unrepaired leak in the colon and diffuse peritonitis. Intraoperative cultures are obtained and pending.

24. Which one of the following postoperative antimicrobials is best to recommend for P.D.?

    A. Ertapenem 1 g intravenous every 24 hours.
    B. Piperacillin/tazobactam 4.5 g intravenous every 8 hours.
    C. Meropenem 1 g intravenous every 8 hours.
    D. Ceftriaxone 1 g intravenous every 24 hours plus metronidazole 500 mg intravenous every 12 hours.

25. P.D. remains stable postoperatively for 48 hours with no major improvement in symptoms. Additional cultures are taken from an external abdominal drain and are pending. The most recent intraoperative cultures return with multiple organisms and the following susceptibilities.

Enterococcus faecalis	Ampicillin -S
	Vancomycin -S
Staphylococcus aureus –MRSA	Linezolid -S
	Vancomycin -S
	TMP/SMX -S
Klebsiella oxytoca	Ceftriaxone -S
	Gentamicin -S
	Piperacillin/tazobactam -S
	Ciprofloxacin -S
	Meropenem -S

Which one of the following is best to recommend for P.D.?

   A. Vancomycin 1 g intravenous every 12 hours plus ceftriaxone 1 g intravenous every 24 hours.

   B. Vancomycin 1 g intravenous every 12 hours plus meropenem 1 g intravenous every 8 hours.

   C. Ampicillin 2 g intravenous every 6 hours plus gentamicin 7 mg/kg intravenous every 24 hours plus metronidazole 500 mg intravenous every 8 hours.

   D. Moxifloxacin 400 mg intravenous every 24 hours.

26. Over the next 72 hours, P.D. continues to improve clinically with an absence of major abdominal pain and normalized vital signs and chemistries. Cultures from the abdominal drain placed during surgery return with *Bacteroides fragilis* (susceptibilities not provided) and *Candida glabrata* (susceptibilities pending). Which one of the following is best to recommend for P.D.?

   A. Maintain the current antimicrobial course.

   B. Discontinue therapy because he has received an adequate 5 total days of treatment.

   C. Change all agents to a new regimen that covers the five isolated organisms.

   D. Maintain bacterial coverage and add therapy to include coverage of *C. glabrata*.

27. A 42-year-old woman with hypertension and renal failure has been on continuous ambulatory peritoneal dialysis for the past 3 years. She reports no drug allergies. She presents to the renal clinic with abrupt severe abdominal pain and cloudy exchange fluid. The fluid is sent for cell count and culture, with a preliminary diagnosis of peritonitis. Which one of the following is best to recommend as empiric therapy for this patient?

   A. Intraperitoneal vancomycin and intraperitoneal ceftazidime.

   B. Intraperitoneal tobramycin.

   C. Intraperitoneal cefepime and intravenous metronidazole.

   D. Intravenous moxifloxacin.

Questions 28–30 pertain to the following case.

L.P. is a 52-year-old woman (weight 290 pounds) with a medical history of type 2 diabetes, hypertension, and sleep apnea. She underwent successful gastric bypass surgery 1 week ago and has been recovering at home for the past 3 days. She received cefazolin preoperatively. She presents to her surgeon with complaints of increasing abdominal pain and a low fever. Her operative site looks to be healing well. Imaging of her abdomen is completed with concern for perforation of the intestine. She is to be sent for exploratory surgery to repair the probable leak.

28. Which one of the following is best to recommend as empiric therapy for L.P.?

   A. Moxifloxacin.

   B. Ampicillin/sulbactam.

   C. Amoxicillin/clavulanate.

   D. Cefepime and metronidazole.

29. L.P. has her anastomosis repaired intra-operatively and is found to have localized peritonitis. Appropriate tissue cultures were obtained during surgery. L.P. was maintained on appropriate empiric coverage pending the culture results. Culture results are returned on hospital day 2 and reveal MSSA (susceptible to all antibiotics tested but penicillin), *Pseudomonas aeruginosa* (susceptible to meropenem and gentamicin, and resistant to ciprofloxacin, piperacillin/tazobactam, ceftazidime, and cefepime), and mixed anaerobes. Which one of the following is best to recommend for L.P.?

   A. Meropenem.

   B. Vancomycin and meropenem.

   C. Gentamicin and clindamycin.

   D. Meropenem and gentamicin.

30. L.P. has been on the above regimen for 72 hours with continued improvement of her clinical signs and symptoms and discharge planning for her has begun. Which one of the following is best to recommend as duration of treatment for L.P.?

   A. Her current regimen should be stopped now for 3 days of therapy.

   B. Her current regimen should continue for 5 days total.

   C. Her current regimen should continue for 14 days total.

   D. No duration of therapy should be suggested without follow-up cultures.

31. A 46-year-old woman presents to the ED with a 36-hour history of diffuse abdominal pain and vomiting. Her medical history includes hypertension, renal insufficiency (CrCL 40 mL/minute), and gout. Physical examination, laboratories, and abdominal ultrasonography are ongoing, but results are not yet available. Based on her presentation, which one of the following conditions requiring empiric antimicrobial therapy is most likely to be diagnosed in this patient?

   A. Pancreatitis.

   B. Primary peritonitis.

   C. Secondary peritonitis.

   D. Tertiary peritonitis.

Questions 32 and 33 pertain to the following case.

A.M. is a 39-year-old woman who was admitted to the hospital with a diagnosis of appendicitis. She works as a carpenter and has been in her normal state of health before her present illness started 48 hours ago. She has no pertinent medical history. She has just returned from laparoscopic resection, which identified localized peritonitis but no perforation of the appendix. Her current vital signs are Tmax 100.9°F, blood pressure 130/92 mm Hg, respiratory rate 16 breaths/minute, and heart rate 88 beats/minute. She has no known drug allergies.

32. Which one of the following is best to recommend for A.M.?

    A. Moxifloxacin.
    B. Meropenem.
    C. Piperacillin/tazobactam.
    D. Tigecycline.

33. A.M. is started on the regimen above postoperatively and continues to improve clinically over the next 48 hours. No intraoperative or blood cultures have returned positive. She is being considered for discharge if clinically appropriate. Which one of the following is the best option for continuation of therapy for A.M.?

    A. Remain an inpatient to complete 7 days of therapy.
    B. Discharge without additional therapy.
    C. Oral therapy as an outpatient to complete 5 days of therapy. *Diet ?*
    D. Receive outpatient intravenous therapy to complete 5 days of therapy.

34. Your hospital is implementing an antimicrobial stewardship effort to improve appropriate selection of antimicrobial therapy for intra-abdominal infections. The first initiative is a guideline for treatment of appendicitis. Which one of the following describes the most important elements of this pathway for stewardship-related efforts?

    A. Limit antimicrobials to single preoperative doses for uncomplicated resected appendices.
    B. Ensure 5 days of intravenous therapy for complicated infections.
    C. Initiate antimicrobial courses with oral therapy for patients who are able to swallow. X
    D. Limit anaerobic coverage on an order set by listing cefazolin as the preferred agent for treatment of perforations.

35. You are using your hospital antibiogram and current formulary to create an order-set recommending optimal antimicrobial regimens for patients being prescribed intra-abdominal infection treatment. You are considering the selection of antimicrobials targeted against enterococci. Your hospital has a 78%

ampicillin susceptibility rate and a 20% vancomycin resistant enterococci rate. In which one of the following scenarios is the empiric therapy suggested most appropriate with regard to necessary enterococcal coverage?

    A. Required use of at least one enterococcal active agent for mild and moderate community-acquired infections.
    B. Linezolid containing regimens for severe community-acquired infections.
    C. Piperacillin/tazobactam for hospital-acquired infections.
    D. Cefepime and metronidazole containing regimens for severe community-acquired infections.

Questions 36 and 37 pertain to the following case.

K.K. is 12-year-old girl being examined in the emergency room for possible appendicitis. She has no significant medical history. Her father reports she had hives as 4-year-old when treated with amoxicillin/clavulanate for a recurrent ear infection. Upon examination and radiologic reports, K.K. is diagnosed with appendicitis with a suspicion of perforation and is scheduled for surgical resection.

36. With careful observation, which one of the following is best to recommend for K.K. before surgery?

    A. Cefoxitin.
    B. Piperacillin/tazobactam.
    C. Ciprofloxacin plus clindamycin.
    D. Meropenem.

37. K.K.'s surgery is uneventful and no perforation or peritoneal involvement is observed. Post-operatively, she is noticed to have a new rash appearing on her upper chest. She has been scheduled to receive two more doses of antibiotics. Which one of the following is best to recommend for K.K.?

    A. Discontinue all antimicrobials.
    B. Continue the present regimen for two more doses.
    C. Change therapy to aztreonam and metronidazole.
    D. Change therapy to moxifloxacin.

38. A 54-year-old man with a history of worsening hepatic insufficiency and significant ascites is admitted for suspected intra-abdominal infection. He was recently treated for an upper respiratory tract infection with moxifloxacin, but had been in his usual state of poor health in the past 2 weeks until feeling ill 2 days ago. His ascitic fluid is sent for analysis and returns suggestive of spontaneous bacterial peritonitis. Which one of the following is best to recommend for this patient?

A. Ciprofloxacin.
B. Cefotaxime.
C. Ampicillin/sulbactam.
D. Imipenem.

Questions 39 and 40 pertain to the following case.

G.B. is a 61-year-old man who has been in the ICU for the past 9 days. He required three surgical procedures during his first week of hospitalization to fix a recurrent large bowel perforation. His antimicrobial therapy has been changed from piperacillin/tazobactam at day 5 to vancomycin, ceftazidime, and metronidazole as a result of poor response to initial therapy and microbiology reports. His initial intraoperative cultures revealed MRSA and *E. coli*. G.B. was noted to have diffuse peritonitis visualized intra-operatively. Blood and operative cultures have been ordered. His clinical status has remained critical, but stable, with an elevated WBC and intermittent fevers.

39. Which one of the following is the most appropriate classification for G.B.'s condition?

A. Complicated spontaneous bacterial peritonitis.
B. Primary peritonitis.
C. Secondary peritonitis.
D. Tertiary peritonitis.

40. G.B. remains on vancomycin, ceftazidime, and metronidazole. Today his blood cultures return positive for an extended spectrum β-lactamase-producing (ESBL) *E. coli*. Which one of the following is best to recommend for G.B.?

A. Discontinue ceftazidime and begin ertapenem.
B. Discontinue vancomycin and begin doripenem.
C. Discontinue ceftazidime and metronidazole and begin meropenem.
D. Add ertapenem to the regimen above.

LEARNER CHAPTER EVALUATION: INTRA-ABDOMINAL INFECTIONS.

As you take the posttest for this chapter, also evaluate the material's quality and usefulness, as well as the achievement of learning objectives. Rate each item using this 5-point scale:

- Strongly agree
- Agree
- Neutral
- Disagree
- Strongly disagree

18. The content of the chapter met my educational needs.
19. The content of the chapter satisfied my expectations.
20. The author presented the chapter content effectively.
21. The content of the chapter was relevant to my practice and presented at the appropriate depth and scope.
22. The content of the chapter was objective and balanced.
23. The content of the chapter is free of bias, promotion, or advertisement of commercial products.
24. The content of the chapter was useful to me.
25. The teaching and learning methods used in the chapter were effective.
26. The active learning methods used in the chapter were effective.
27. The learning assessment activities used in the chapter were effective.
28. The chapter was effective overall.

Use the 5-point scale to indicate whether this chapter prepared you to accomplish the following learning objectives:

29. Distinguish the microbiologic differences typical among major intra-abdominal infections arising from different sites of the gastrointestinal tract.
30. Classify disease severity, likelihood of resistant pathogens, and infection site for a patient with intra-abdominal infection.
31. Design an appropriate empiric antimicrobial regimen (including duration) for the patient with intra-abdominal infection.
32. Assess microbiology reports, patient response to therapy (including adverse events related to pharmacotherapy) and appropriately alter empiric therapy regimens for the patient with intra-abdominal infection.
33. Compose appropriate antimicrobial stewardship practices pertinent to patients with intra-abdominal infections.
34. Please provide any specific comments relating to any perceptions of bias, promotion, or advertisement of commercial products.
35. Please expand on any of your above responses, and/ or provide any additional comments regarding this chapter:

Bone and Joint Infections

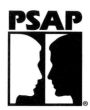

By Sandy J. Estrada, Pharm.D., BCPS (AQ-ID)

Reviewed by Scott Bergman, Pharm.D., BCPS (AQ-ID); and Shaun P. Keegan, Pharm.D., BCPS

Learning Objectives

1. Design a treatment plan for a patient with bone and joint infection.
2. Evaluate the role of newer antimicrobials in the treatment of bone and joint infections.
3. Detect adverse effects related to antimicrobials used for treatment of bone and joint infections.
4. Develop a monitoring plan for antimicrobials used in the treatment of bone and joint infection.
5. Demonstrate an understanding of the role of outpatient antimicrobial therapy for patients with bone and joint infections.

Introduction

Bone and joint infections cause significant morbidity and require complex treatment strategies that often involve both surgical management and long-term intravenous antimicrobials. This chapter reviews the treatment of septic arthritis, osteomyelitis, and prosthetic joint infection, including duration of therapy, oral treatment options, and opportunity to provide intravenous antimicrobials in the outpatient setting as a means to increase patient quality of life and decrease use of health care resources. Although gram-positive organisms remain the most common causes of bone and joint infections, the rise of resistant gram-negative organisms is of concern in the formulation of treatment strategies. Extended-spectrum β-lactamase–producing organisms and carbapenemases are of special concern.

Septic Arthritis

Epidemiology and Diagnosis

Septic arthritis is an infection of the joint space; usually related to bacterial infection, it can also include fungal and mycobacterial infections. Predisposing factors are listed in Box 3-1. Hematogenous spread is the most common source of bacterial septic arthritis. Additional causes include animal bites, other trauma, or direct inoculation during surgery. Bacterial septic arthritis generally presents as a painful, usually swollen joint with fever. The knee is the joint affected most commonly. Symptoms may be minimal in patients who are older, immunosuppressed, or debilitated. Gram-positive organisms (including *Staphylococcus*, *Streptococcus*, and *Enterococcus*) are the most common pathogens causing bacterial septic arthritis.

Baseline Knowledge Statements

Readers of this chapter are presumed to be familiar with the following:
- Basic pathophysiology of osteomyelitis
- Basic microbiology concepts
- Spectrum of activity of antimicrobials used in the treatment of bone and joint infections
- Common adverse effects associated with bone and joint infections

Additional Readings

The following free resources are available for readers wishing additional background information on this topic.
- Conterno LO, Turchi MD. Antibiotics for treating chronic osteomyelitis in adults (review). Cochrane Collaboration, 2013.
- Osmon DR, Berbari EF, Berendt AR, et al. Diagnosis and management of prosthetic joint infection: clinical practice guidelines by the Infectious Diseases Society of America. Clin Infect Dis 2013;56:e1-25.

Box 3-1. Predisposing Factors for Septic Arthritis in Adults

- Age >80 years
- Diabetes mellitus
- Rheumatoid arthritis
- Prosthetic joint
- Recent joint surgery
- Skin infection, cutaneous ulcers
- IV drug abuse
- Alcoholism
- Previous intra-articular corticosteroid injection

Information from Margaretten ME, Kohlwes J, Moore D, et al. Does this adult patient have septic arthritis? JAMA 2007;297:1478.

Gram-negative organisms should be suspected in intravenous-drug users, neonates, older patients, and patients with immunosuppression. Gonococcal infections are also of concern and present with polyarthralgias, fever, and joint pain with effusion. Two-thirds of patients with gonococcal infection have rash and tenosynovitis of small distal joints. Gonococcal septic arthritis should be suspected in patients with recent exposure to sexually transmitted diseases or concurrent mucosal gonococcal infection.

Synovial fluid analysis is required for definitive diagnosis of septic arthritis. Synovial fluid aspiration should be performed at initial suspicion of joint infection. Gram stain, culture, leukocyte count, and differential should be performed. Table 3-1 details synovial fluid analysis interpretation. Negative synovial fluid cultures may be encountered in patients already on antimicrobial therapy or with organisms such as streptococci. Gout should be ruled out by means of synovial fluid analysis because many patients with this diagnosis also present with fever and leukocytosis. The presence of urate crystals on synovial fluid analysis is indicative of gout. Blood cultures are positive in 50% of septic arthritis cases and should be obtained in all patients with suspected bacterial arthritis. Baseline radiography should be performed to rule out osteomyelitis and for future comparison. Elevations in nonspecific diagnostic markers, C-reactive protein (CRP), and erythrocyte sedimentation rate (ESR) may be seen as well (Hariharan 2011, Ernst 2010)}

Treatment and Monitoring

The initial choice of antimicrobial therapy must be made based on the most likely organisms suspected, the Gram stain, and clinical presentation. If gram-positive cocci are present, treatment with vancomycin should be initiated unless contraindicated. If vancomycin cannot be used, alternate therapies include daptomycin and linezolid. If gram-negative bacilli are present, a third-generation cephalosporin such as ceftriaxone should be initiated. If the Gram stain is negative, then vancomycin plus ceftriaxone should be initiated.

Table 3-1. Synovial Fluid Analysis

Measure	Normal	Inflammatory/Gout	Septic
Volume (knee)	< 3.5 mL	Often > 3.5 mL	Often > 3.5 mL
Clarity	Transparent	Translucent-opaque	Opaque
Color	Clear	Yellow to opalescent	Yellow to green
Viscosity	High	Low	Variable
WBC	< 200/mm³	1000–100,000/mm³	25,000 to >100,000/mm³
PMNs	< 25%	≥ 50%	≥ 75%
Culture	Negative	Negative	Often positive
Total protein	1–2 g/dL	3–5 g/dL	3–5 g/dL
Glucose	Nearly equal to blood	> 25 mg/dL, lower than blood	< 25 mg/dL, much lower than blood

PMN = polymorphonuclear neutrophil.

There are limited data defining appropriate treatment duration for septic arthritis. A total of 14–28 days is generally recommended depending on the organism. Parenteral antibiotics are usually recommended for the first 14 days. Gonococcal septic arthritis can be treated for 2 weeks. Staphylococcal infections and other gram-negative infections require 28 days of therapy; switching to an oral agent such as linezolid or clindamycin can be considered after the first 2 weeks of therapy. Fluoroquinolones are appropriate oral options for the treatment of gram-negative infections once the sensitivity of the organism is known (MMWR 2011). In general, a switch to an oral fluoroquinolone can occur for the final 1–2 weeks of therapy. Table 3-2 lists specific dosing recommendations. Patients should be monitored for resolution of signs and symptoms of infection, as well as for antimicrobial toxicities.

Osteomyelitis

Epidemiology and Diagnosis

Osteomyelitis is an infection of the bone that develops in one of several ways. *Hematogenous osteomyelitis* is secondary to bacteremia, and *contiguous osteomyelitis* is related to an adjacent soft tissue infection—most commonly a diabetic foot infection. Osteomyelitis can also be caused by direct inoculation (e.g., trauma, surgical procedure).

An acute case of osteomyelitis is commonly defined as being diagnosed 2 weeks or less from onset of signs and symptoms; chronic osteomyelitis represents infections with onset longer than 2 weeks before presentation. Chronic osteomyelitis can persist for years, with failures to treatment and/or relapses being common. Long-term recurrence rates are around 20%. Historically, treatment has consisted of long-term parenteral, high-dose, antibiotic therapy. The extended duration of antimicrobial therapy stems from concerns of relapse secondary to bacterial evasion of host defenses while contained within biofilm. That approach must be balanced against concerns of antimicrobial resistance related to long-term therapy, risk associated with intravenous catheters, and costs accompanying intravenous therapy. *Staphylococcus aureus* is the most prevalent causative microorganism, followed by coagulase-negative *Staphylococcus, Streptococcus, Enterococcus,* and gram-negative organisms. As with septic arthritis, mycobacterium and fungal organisms are possible causes of osteomyelitis, although rare.

Diagnosis is made with a combination of clinical suspicion, imaging, and isolation of an organism by blood culture or bone biopsy. The imaging of choice is MRI for diagnosis of osteomyelitis. In patients who cannot have MRI, CT may be used. Radiography is not recommended for the detection of acute osteomyelitis but may reveal the findings associated with chronic osteomyelitis. Reliable cultures are necessary for appropriate diagnosis and treatment strategy. Because of the high prevalence of skin flora isolated in patients with osteomyelitis, superficial samples

Patient Care Scenario

A 67-year-old white man (height 71 in, weight 106 kg) is admitted for I&D of left knee. He had been complaining of left knee pain and swelling for the past 3 days. He received an injection in his knee 5 days ago; 70 mL of thick yellow fluid was aspirated and sent for cell count, crystals and culture and sensitivity. Initial report is positive for uric acid crystals and patient was started on colchicine and sent home. He returned for follow-up in the morning and the Gram stain is negative but his WBC is 80 x 10³ cells/mm³. A repeat aspiration was performed. As he was leaving the office the lab called and identified gram-positive cocci in yesterday's sample. The patient is admitted and taken for I&D of knee. His other medical history includes type 2 diabetes mellitus. His home drugs include metformin 1000 mg twice daily, lisinopril 10 mg daily, atorvastatin 40 mg daily. His SCr is 0.65 mg/dL. The patient is afebrile and other vital signs are normal. Preliminary culture results show coagulase-negative staphylococci. What is the best treatment to start for this patient?

Answer

This patient presents with classic symptoms of septic arthritis. His calculated CrCl is normal and he has no known medication allergies. His preliminary culture shows coagulase-negative staphylococci with no specific identification or antimicrobial susceptibilities. He should be started on vancomycin because the majority of coagulase negative staphylococci isolates are methicillin resistant. He does not need to have empiric coverage for gram-negative organisms because he does not have any known risk factors for gonococcal or health-care associated organisms. Most septic arthritis cases are monomicrobial and an organism has already been identified in this case. Once the susceptibilities of the organism are known, the vancomycin can be de-escalated.

1. Margaretten ME, Kohlwes J, Moore D, et al. Does this adult patient have septic arthritis? JAMA 2007;297:1478-88
2. Sharff KA, Richards EP, Townes JM. Clinical management of septic arthritis. Curr Rheumatol Rep 2013;15:332
3. Mathews CJ, Weston VC, Jones A, et al. Bacterial septic arthritis in adults. Lancet 2010;375:846-55.

cannot be relied on for the diagnosis. The WBC may be elevated in acute osteomyelitis but is often normal in chronic cases. The ESR and CRP may be elevated and usually normalize during the therapy course.

The microbiological etiology of osteomyelitis is highly dependent on the type or source of osteomyelitis. Hematogenous osteomyelitis is usually *monomicrobial,* whereas contiguous osteomyelitis or that following trauma is more likely to be *polymicrobial.* Gram-negative bacteria and anaerobic organisms are commonly involved in osteomyelitis evolving secondary to diabetic foot infections. Gram-positive bacteria remain the most commonly isolated organisms in osteomyelitis. Specifically, *S. aureus* is the most common pathogen in patients with diabetic foot infections, who have fractures, or who use intravenous drugs.

Treatment and Monitoring

Goals of therapy include eradication of infection, restoration of function, and pain relief. If the patient is stable, antimicrobials should not be started until cultures are obtained during debridement or bone biopsy. Surgical debridement is usually required for long-bone, open-fracture, or foot osteomyelitis and early postoperative spine infection associated with hardware. Therapy is determined

based on suspected organisms and is modified based on Gram stain, cultures, and sensitivities when available. The duration of therapy is at least 4–6 weeks. A minimal duration of 8 weeks is recommended if methicillin-resistant *Staphylococcus aureus* (MRSA) is the infecting pathogen. If the infection is chronic or debridement is not performed, consideration can be given to an additional 1–3 months of oral combination therapy with rifampin plus an additional susceptible oral agent (Liu 2011).

Vertebral Osteomyelitis

Vertebral osteomyelitis is an infection of the spine and often includes extension to the disk space between

Table 3-2. Antimicrobials Used in the Treatment of Bone and Joint Infections

Antibiotic	Recommended Dosage and Route	Laboratory Monitoring Parameters	Adjustment for Kidney Impairment
Cefazolin	2 g IV q8h	CBC, BMP	Yes
Ceftaroline	600 mg IV 8–12h	CBC, BMP	Yes
Cefepime	2 g IV q8–12h	CBC, BMP	Yes
Ceftazidime	2g IV q8h	CBC, BMP	Yes
Ceftriaxone	2 g IV daily	CBC, BMP	No
Ciprofloxacin	400 mg IV q8–12h 750 mg PO BID 250–500 mg PO BID (chronic suppression)	CBC, BMP	Yes
Clindamycin	900 mg IV q8h	CBC, LFT	Yes
Daptomycin	6 mg/kg IV daily	CBC, BMP, CPK	Yes
Doxycycline	100 mg PO BID	CBC, BMP	No
Ertapenem	1 g IV daily	CBC, BMP, LFT	Yes
Levofloxacin	750 mg IV/PO daily 250-500 mg PO daily (chronic suppression)	CBC, BMP	Yes
Linezolid	600 mg IV/PO BID	CBC	No
Meropenem	1–2 g IV q8h	CBC, BMP	Yes
Minocycline	100 mg PO BID	LFT, BMP	Yes
Moxifloxacin	400 mg IV/PO daily	CBC, BMP, LFT	No
Nafcillin	2 g IV q4h	CBC, BMP, LFT	No
Piperacillin/tazobactam	4.5 g IV q6h	CBC, BMP	Yes
Rifampin	600 mg PO daily	LFT	No
Telavancin	10 mg/kg IV q24h	CBC, BMP, Pregnancy	Yes
Trimethoprim/ sulfamethoxazole	4 mg/kg per dose IV BID; 1 DS tablet PO daily (chronic suppression)	CBC, BMP	Yes
Vancomycin	15–20 mg/kg IV q 8-12 h	CBC, BMP, Trough	Yes

BID = two times/day; BMP = basic metabolic panel; CBC = complete blood count; CPK = creatinine phosphokinase; DS = double strength; h = hours; IV = intravenously; LFT = liver function test; PO = orally; q = every.

Adapted from Winner JS. Bone and Joint Infections. In Richardson M, Chant C, Chessman KH, et al, eds. Pharmacotherapy Self-Assessment Program, 7th ed. Infectious Diseases. Lenexa, KS: American college of Clinical Pharmacy, 2012, 164.

vertebrae (i.e., discitis). Significant morbidity and mortality are associated with vertebral osteomyelitis and discitis. Risk factors include age, diabetes, intravenous drug use, immunocompromise, indwelling intravascular devices, and increased prevalence of orthopedic prosthetic joint devices. Infection can spread to the spine from transient bacteremia or bacteremia from a distant focus of infection. Trauma and surgery are also possible causes.

Clinical presentation is often vague, with back or neck pain being the most common symptom. Fever may or may not be present. The majority of patients will have positive blood cultures and elevated ESR and CRP. Diagnosis is initially based on clinical presentation and is confirmed by aspiration of the disk space or vertebral bone. _S. aureus_ remains the most common organism to cause osteomyelitis in this area of the body. In patients with urinary tract infection, gram-negative bacilli and _Enterococcus_ could be causative. Vertebral osteomyelitis practice guidelines from the Infectious Diseases Society of America (IDSA) are in progress. Current recommendations are to treat based on pathogen similar to osteomyelitis at other sites of infection. The recommended duration of therapy is 6–12 weeks.

Prosthetic Joint Infections

Epidemiology and Diagnosis

Infection of a prosthetic joint is one of the most concerning complications of orthopedic device placement. Placement procedures significantly improve quality of life, but infection has a significant impact and prolongs the recovery period. Additional surgical procedures and extended courses of intravenous antimicrobial therapy are the mainstays of treatment. As the numbers of prosthetic joint implantations rise, the numbers of prosthetic joint infections (PJIs) are expected to rise. In 2009, the incidence of PJI in the United States was estimated to be 1%–2% over the lifetime of the prosthetic joint. The IDSA definition of PJI is listed in Box 3-2. Diagnosis of PJI is possible even if none of the criteria are met based on clinical presentation and other available evidence. Presence of microorganisms commonly considered contaminants must be carefully evaluated in the context of other available evidence.

A PJI should be suspected in patients with persistent wound drainage over a joint prosthesis, acute onset of pain at the prosthesis, or chronic pain unresolved by joint replacement. A complete patient history that includes details on type of prosthesis placed, dates of surgical intervention, history of wound healing or infection-related problems, and microbiology results is necessary to develop an optimal treatment plan. Previous antimicrobial therapy is also an important part of the history and decision-making for future antimicrobial therapy options. An ESR or CRP should be obtained if the diagnosis is not clinically evident; ioth are abnormal, there is high sensitivity and specificity for the diagnosis of PJI.

Diagnostic arthrocentesis should be performed in suspected acute PJI and chronic painful prosthesis with unexplained elevated ESR or CRP or other clinical suspicion of PJI. Diagnostic arthrocentesis does not need to be performed if surgery is planned and the results will not alter current management. The analysis of synovial fluid collected should include aerobic and anaerobic cultures, as well as total cell count and differential leukocyte count. If the patient is medically stable, there is an increased likelihood of recovering organisms if antimicrobial therapy is held for at least 1 week before the synovial fluid collection. Blood cultures are recommended only if the patient is febrile, experiences an acute onset of symptoms, or has a suspected pathogen that would make bloodstream infection more likely. Imaging scans are not routinely recommended for the diagnosis of PJI.

Surgical Strategies

Intraoperative inspection with histopathologic sampling is a highly reliable diagnostic strategy for PJI. Optimally, five or six operative tissue samples or the explanted prosthesis should be submitted for aerobic and anaerobic culture at the time of surgical debridement or prosthesis removal.

Once PJI has been diagnosed, choice of surgical strategy is made based on time since prosthesis implantation, duration of symptoms, presence or absence of sinus tract, susceptibility of oral antimicrobial agents, and how well the prosthesis is fixed in place. Ultimately, the decision regarding surgical management is made by the orthopedic surgeon in consultation with other specialists when necessary.

Debridement and retention of the prosthesis can be considered in a patient with a well-fixed prosthesis without a sinus tract and who is either in the first 30 postoperative days or less than 3 weeks from onset of infection. This strategy can also be considered in patients at an unacceptably high risk for alternative procedures.

Box 3-2. Definition of Prosthetic Joint Infection

- Presence of a sinus tract that communicates with the prosthesis
- Presence of acute inflammation on histopathology examination of periprosthetic tissue at the time of surgical debridement or prosthesis removal (highly suggestive)
- Presence of purulence without another known etiology surrounding the prosthesis (definitive evidence)
- Two or more intraoperative cultures or combination of preoperative aspiration and intraoperative cultures that yield the same organism (definitive evidence)
- Growth of a virulent microorganism in a single specimen of a tissue biopsy or synovial fluid

Information from Osmon DR, Berbari EF, Berendt AR, et al. Diagnosis and management of prosthetic joint infection: clinical practice guidelines by the Infectious Diseases Society of America. Clin Infect Dis 2013;56:1-25..

Relapse of infection is more likely in this situation. If the prosthesis cannot be retained, it can be removed in a one-stage exchange whereby the prosthesis is removed and a new prosthesis is placed during one surgical procedure. One-stage exchange is considered in patients with a total hip arthroplasty if the identity of the pathogens is known and they are susceptible to appropriate oral antimicrobials. Failure is a risk if bone grafting is required or if an effective antibiotic-impregnated bone cement cannot be used. This procedure is not commonly used in the United States.

A two-stage exchange procedure is commonly used in the United States and is indicated in patients medically able to undergo multiple surgeries when the surgeon believes reimplantation arthroplasty is feasible. In this procedure, the prosthesis is removed in one surgery, and the new prosthesis is implanted several weeks or months later after antimicrobials have been administered. Amputation is the last-resort surgical option and should be considered only after the patient has been evaluated at a center with specialist experience in the evaluation and management of PJI.

Treatment
Debridement and Retention of the Prosthesis
For staphylococcal PJI, 2–6 weeks of pathogen-specific intravenous antimicrobial therapy plus rifampin is recommended, followed by an oral antimicrobial and rifampin for 3 months (for hip) or 6 months (for knee). A β-lactam or vancomycin plus rifampin remain the antimicrobials of choice for staphylococcal PJI. Rifampin should always be used in combination therapy because of its biofilm activity and its propensity to develop resistance when used as monotherapy. Rifampin should be coadministered with both the intravenous and oral therapy.

Elbow, shoulder, and ankle infections are managed similarly to hip infection. Options for the oral antimicrobial to be used in combination with rifampin include fluoroquinolones, minocycline, doxycycline, trimethoprim/sulfamethoxazole, cephalexin, or dicloxacillin. A fluoroquinolone plus rifampin is recommended as first-line therapy based on a randomized clinical trial of susceptible staphylococcal infections of prosthetic joints and fracture fixation devices. There was a statistical benefit in using combination therapy with ciprofloxacin and rifampin in patients who completed therapy (Zimmerli 1998). Table 3-3 describes the dosing and frequency of antimicrobials used in the treatment of bone and joint infections.

For PJI caused by organisms other than Staphylococcus, current guidelines recommend 4–6 weeks of pathogen-specific intravenous or oral therapy (highly bioavailable). Chronic oral suppression may follow the same recommendations as for staphylococcal infections based on sensitivities, allergies, and tolerability or toxicity of the regimens.

Treatment After Resection Arthroplasty
Whether or not reimplantation is planned, 4–6 weeks of pathogen-specific intravenous or highly bioavailable

Table 3-3. Bone Penetration of Antibiotics with High Oral Bioavailability

Antibiotic	Dose (mg)	Route	Serum Level Mean (mcg/mL)	Bone Level, Mean (Range) mcg/g	Serum-Bone Ratio (%)
Ciprofloxacin	500	PO	1.4-2	0.4-0.7	30-35
Ciprofloxacin	750	PO	2.6-2.9	0.7-1.4	27-48
Ciprofloxacin	200	IV	NA	2[a]/1.4[b]	66[a]/47[b] ([d])
Clindamycin	600	IV	7.3-8.5	2.6-3.8	40-45
Doxycycline	200	IV	6	0.13	2
Levofloxacin	500	IV	7.5	7.4[a]/3.9[b]	99[a]/50[b]
Linezolid	600	PO	23	8.5	37
Metronidazole	500	IV	NA	14	100([e])
Moxifloxacin	400	IV	4.9	1.9[a]/1.3[b]	39[a]/27[b]
Moxifloxacin	400	PO	3.7	1.8[a]/1.6[b]	43
Trimethoprim/ sulfamethoxazole	1 DS tab twice Daily x 2 days	PO	7.4/143	3.7/19[c]	50/15

[a]Medullary.

[b]Cortical.

[c]Trimethoprim/sulfamethoxazole levels respectively.

[d]Assuming peak serum levels of 3 mcg/mL for ciprofloxacin.

[e]Assuming peak serum levels of 14 mcg/mL for metronidazole.

Information from Spellberg B, Lipsky BA. Systemic antibiotic therapy for chronic osteomyelitis in adults. Clin Infect Dis 2012;54:393-407.

oral therapy is recommended. Longer duration (6 weeks) is recommended when a highly virulent pathogen such as *S. aureus* is the causative organism. Rifampin combination therapy is not necessary because there is no retained prosthetic providing the environment for biofilm formation.

ANTIMICROBIAL SELECTION CONSIDERATIONS

Organism-Specific Therapy
Staphylococci

An antistaphylococcal penicillin (e.g., nafcillin) or first-generation cephalosporin (e.g., cefazolin) is appropriate therapy for methicillin-susceptible strains. The use of ceftriaxone for methicillin-sensitive *Staphylococcus aureus* (MSSA) bone and joint infections remains controversial because of concerns about achieving adequate bone concentrations and because of the agent's broad spectrum of activity including gram-negative bacteria. The U.S. Food and Drug Administration (FDA) considers MSSA isolates susceptible at a breakpoint of less than 4 mcg/mL compared with an 8-mcg/mL breakpoint for susceptibility, as set forth by the Clinical and Laboratory Standards Institute.

Minimal inhibitory concentrations (MICs) are not routinely tested for staphylococci in the microbiology laboratory because susceptibility is predicted from antistaphylococcal penicillins. Target time above the typical MIC can be attained for susceptible MSSA isolates when ceftriaxone is dosed at 2 g/day. Recent retrospective reviews have suggested that ceftriaxone at a dosage of 2 g/day is effective in the treatment of MSSA bone and joint infections (Sharff 2014). However, IDSA guidelines for the treatment of PJI could not reach consensus on this issue. In most cases in which ceftriaxone has been used successfully, an antistaphylococcal penicillin or cefazolin has been the initial therapy and was transitioned to ceftriaxone for outpatient therapy. Therefore there are no available data on the use of ceftriaxone in the initial treatment of potentially high-inoculum infections (Sharff 2014, Wieland 2012)

Vancomycin remains the drug of choice for methicillin-resistant strains of *S. aureus* when the MIC is 1 mcg/mL or less. However, the utility of vancomycin in MRSA strains with an MIC of 2 has been challenged based on the difficulty of achieving the recommended area-under-the-curve/MIC ratio of higher than 400—without exposing the patient to risk for toxicity (Lodise 2009). Alternatives to vancomycin include linezolid, daptomycin, tigecycline, telavancin, and ceftaroline. Those agents are discussed further in the section on therapy selection.

Streptococcus and Enterococcus

Streptococcal osteomyelitis may be treated by using ampicillin or ceftriaxone as first-line antimicrobials. Ceftriaxone is often chosen because its once-daily

---

Pivotal Study That May Change Practice

Wieland BR, Marcantoni JR, Bommarito KM et al. A retrospective comparison of ceftriaxone vs. oxacillin for osteoarticular infections due to methicillin-susceptible *Staphylococcus aureus*. Clin Infect Dis 2012;54:585-90.

Setting: Treatment of bone and joint infections require long durations of antimicrobials and often involve treatment in the outpatient setting. The treatment options for bone and joint infections caused by methicillin-susceptible *S. aureus* (MSSA) include oxacillin, nafcillin, and cefazolin. Ceftriaxone is an effective treatment option for MSSA infections and is attractive because of once-daily administration, no renal dosage adjustment, and excellent tolerability. The use of ceftriaxone for bone and joint infections is controversial because of concerns of failure given MIC (90) concentrations of 4 mcg/mL against MSSA. This study compared patient outcomes of MSSA osteoarticular infections with ceftriaxone versus oxacillin.

Design: 124 patients were enrolled in a retrospective cohort study of patients with MSSA osteoarticular infections at a tertiary care hospital. Successful treatment was compared at 3-6 months and >6 months after completion of antimicrobial therapy.

Outcomes: Data for 97 patients (3–6 months) and 88 patients (> 6 months) were available for analysis. Treatment success was similar in both groups at 3–6 months (83% vs 86% respectively) and > 6 months (77% vs 81% respectively), however the study was not powered to demonstrate noninferiority. Discontinuation because of toxicity was higher in the oxacillin group (18% vs 4%, p=0.01). Approximately one-half of the patients had orthopedic hardware involvement. In this subset, 81% of ceftriaxone treated patients vs 93% (p=0.4) of oxacillin treated patients had treatment success at early follow up and 74% vs 85% (p=0.7) at late-follow up. Forty-three patients (29 ceftriaxone and 14 oxacillin) were discharged with hardware in place. At early followup, treatment success was 76% in these ceftriaxone treated patients vs 100% (p=0.08) in oxacillin treated patients and 69% versus 93% (p=0.2) at late follow-up.

Impact: The IDSA PJI guideline authors could not reach consensus on the use of ceftriaxone to treat MSSA bone and joint infections. This is the first case-control retrospective cohort study to compare ceftriaxone with an antistaphylococcal penicillin for the treatment of osteoarticular infections. Findings were similar to previous retrospective cohort studies, suggesting that ceftriaxone 2 g daily was similar to oxacillin 4 g every 6 hours. These findings give additional evidence to support use of ceftriaxone 2 g daily to treat osteoarticular infections. Failure rates may be higher in patients with retained hardware, and this is an area that requires additional investigation.

administration is convenient, especially in an ambulatory setting. Ampicillin remains the antimicrobial of choice for susceptible enterococcal infections. In the case of β-lactam allergies, clindamycin (for *Streptococcus*) or vancomycin (for *Streptococcus* or *Enterococcus*) may be used.

Gram-negative Bacilli

Antimicrobial choice for treatment of gram-negative pathogens depends on the specific organism and susceptibility pattern. A β-lactam/β-lactamase inhibitor such as piperacillin/tazobactam or ampicillin/sulbactam is often chosen as empiric therapy. Carbapenem therapy may be necessary in the case of highly resistant gram-negative bacteria such as Enterobacteriaceae producing extended-spectrum β-lactamases. Ertapenem is a once-daily carbapenem that can be used in cases when treatment for *Pseudomonas*, *Enterococcus*, or MRSA is not required. Fluoroquinolones are often used because of proven efficacy and the ease of switch to oral therapy. However, they generally are not appropriate as empiric therapy because of high resistance rates among gram-negative pathogens. In the case of carbapenem-resistant Enterobacteriaceae, alternative antimicrobials such as colistin or tigecycline should be considered in conjunction with expert consultation.

Parenteral Therapy
β-Lactams

Beta-lactams remain the antimicrobials of choice for bone and joint infections because of susceptible organisms, and these agents should be used unless prohibited by allergy or other contraindications. Bone penetration of β-lactam antibiotics ranges from 5% to 20%; however, because of high serum concentrations, bone concentrations above the MIC of the pathogen are still possible. Because of the relatively poor bioavailability of β-lactams, their use in the treatment of bone and joint infections is generally limited to intravenous therapy. For monitoring parameters, see Table 3-2.

Vancomycin

Vancomycin remains the antimicrobial of choice for MRSA and is also used to treat MSSA infections in patients with β-lactam allergies. When compared with β-lactam antimicrobials, vancomycin has slower bactericidal activity and therefore should be used only in patients who cannot be treated with a β-lactam. Vancomycin penetration into bone is relatively poor but is thought to be sufficient in MRSA infections with an MIC of less than 2 mcg/mL, with goal trough concentration of 15–20 mcg/mL. In a study of outpatient antimicrobial therapy for osteomyelitis caused by *S. aureus*, treatment with vancomycin (compared with a β-lactam for MSSA) resulted in an odds ratio for infection recurrence of 2.5 by multivariate analysis (Tice 2003). That finding reinforces the importance of using β-lactams when possible. Patients receiving vancomycin must be monitored for leukopenia, ototoxicity, and nephrotoxicity.

Linezolid

Linezolid has bacteriostatic activity against MRSA and MSSA and has FDA label approval for the treatment of skin and soft tissue infections, including diabetic foot infections. It is not typically used as initial treatment for osteomyelitis because a therapy duration if 4 weeks or less is usually recommended because of adverse effects. However, success with longer durations of therapy has been reported (Pea 2012). Linezolid is highly bioavailable and can be considered in patients who are not at risk of drug interactions or adverse effects.

A compassionate-use study evaluating linezolid included 89 treatment courses for bone infection (Birmingham 2003). In a study evaluating the tolerability of prolonged linezolid therapy in bone and joint infections, 48% of patients receiving linezolid alone developed thrombocytopenia (defined as a reduction in platelet count to less than 75% of baseline) (Legout 2010). Clinicians should monitor for cytopenias, peripheral neuropathy, lactic acidosis, and optic neuritis along with serotonin syndrome in patients treated concurrently with interacting agents. Complete blood counts should be monitored weekly in patients receiving linezolid for longer than 2 weeks.

Daptomycin

Daptomycin is an intravenous antimicrobial option for treatment of bone and joint infections caused by MSSA or MRSA. Daptomycin has bactericidal activity and exhibits bone penetration similar to that of β-lactams and vancomycin (Traumuller 2010). There is concern about the development of resistance, specifically with pretreatment with vancomycin and high inoculum infections (when surgical intervention was not done or foreign body is present).

Animal models and in vitro biofilm models have suggested that both high-dose daptomycin (10 mg/kg) and combination therapy with rifampin might be necessary to maximize the killing effect of daptomycin within biofilm (Parra Ruiz 2012, Garrigos 2010). Several reviews analyzed the use of daptomycin for both osteomyelitis and prosthetic joint infections, with cure rates ranging from 65% to 75% (Gallagher 2012, Holtom 2007, Lamp 2007). An open-label, randomized, controlled trial compared daptomycin 6 mg/kg and 8 mg/kg with standard of care in 75 patients undergoing two-stage revision arthroplasty. Clinical cure and microbiologic success rates were similar in both daptomycin groups (Byren 2012).

Weekly monitoring of creatine phosphokinase is necessary because of the risk of rhabdomyolysis. The manufacturer recommends consideration be given to holding statins during daptomycin therapy; however, that practice may cause detrimental cardiovascular effects and has not been confirmed to decrease the incidence of creatine phosphokinase elevation (Berg 2014). Neuropathy and eosinophilic pneumonia are other, rarely reported adverse effects.

Lipoglycopeptides

Telavancin is a once-daily intravenous lipoglycopeptide with bactericidal activity against MSSA and MRSA, including organisms with high vancomycin MICs. Telavancin had excellent activity in bone infections in an animal model (Yin 2009). Clinical trials showed higher rates of nephrotoxicity compared with vancomycin, which may limit its role in therapy. However, telavancin may have a role in the treatment of patients after vancomycin failures.

Dalbavancin is a novel lipoglycopeptide antimicrobial that received FDA label approval in 2014 for the treatment of acute bacterial skin and skin structure infection (ABSSSI). Because of its lengthy terminal half-life, dalbavancin is dosed at 1000 mg intravenously one time, followed by 500 mg intravenously one time on Day 8.

Dalbavancin was studied in a cohort of 31 patients scheduled for joint surgery. A onetime dose of dalbavancin 1000 mg was given before surgery. Patients had serial plasma pharmacokinetic samples collected up to 45 days postdose and one bone pharmacokinetic sample collected at 12, 24, 72, 168, 240, or 336 hours postdose. Samples were analyzed for dalbavancin in plasma, synovial fluid, skin, cartilage, and bone. The study found that concentrations of dalbavancin in bone were above the minimal bactericidal concentration for S. aureus at 14 days postdose. Adequate concentrations of dalbavancin were also detected in synovium and synovial fluid. Based on those results, dalbavancin may be a therapeutic option for the treatment of bone and joint infections; however, further clinical investigation is warranted (Baldassarre 2014).

Oritavancin is also a novel lipoglycopeptide that received label approval in 2014 for the treatment of ABSSSI. Oritavancin is dosed 1200 mg intravenously one time only. To date, there are no clinical data available regarding the use of oritavancin for the treatment of osteomyelitis.

Tigecycline

Tigecycline is a semisynthetic derivative of minocycline and has a broad spectrum of activity, including gram-positive, gram-negative, and anaerobic pathogens. Recent practice guidelines on the treatment of MRSA as well as PJI do not include tigecycline because of an FDA safety warning regarding increased mortality among patients treated with tigecycline versus comparator therapy (Osmon 2012, Liu 2003). In a phase 3 clinical trial, tigecycline did not meet noninferiority criteria when compared with ertapenem plus vancomycin (clinical cure rate 77.5% vs. 82.5% in the clinically evaluable group). In a subset of patients with confirmed osteomyelitis, tigecycline cure rates were higher than 36% (Lauf 2014). Tigecycline may need to be considered in infections caused by resistant gram-negative Enterobacteriaceae when other treatment options have been eliminated.

Ceftaroline

Ceftaroline is the first FDA-approved cephalosporin with activity against MRSA. It has label approval for treatment of ABSSSI and community-acquired bacterial pneumonia. It is well tolerated and normally dosed twice daily for those indications. In a rabbit model of MRSA acute osteomyelitis, ceftaroline and linezolid demonstrated better bactericidal activity in bone and marrow than did vancomycin. Ceftaroline also exhibited significant bactericidal activity against MRSA in joint infection (Jacqueline 2010).

Oral Antibiotic Options

Oral β-lactam antibiotics achieve serum concentrations less than 10% of parenteral equivalents and do not penetrate bone adequately enough to be reasonable oral options for the treatment of osteomyelitis in adults. Trimethoprim/sulfamethoxazole achieves bone concentrations higher than the MICs of susceptible organisms and has been studied extensively in the management of chronic osteomyelitis caused by staphylococcal infections. Because of concentration-dependent killing, high-dosing strategies such as 7–8 mg/kg/day of the trimethoprim component or 2 double-strength tablets twice daily are recommended (Spellberg 2012, Close 2002). Clindamycin reliably penetrates bone and is an option for the treatment of susceptible streptococcal and staphylococcal infections, including MRSA, in adults and children. Although it does have anaerobic activity, metronidazole achieves bone concentrations similar to its serum concentrations and is considered the drug of choice to cure anaerobic osteomyelitis.

Rifampin is recommended as an adjunctive therapy when biofilm is suspected to be present (e.g., when an infected prosthetic joint is retained). S. aureus can produce a multilayered biofilm that is a collection of microbial cells attached to a substrate or each other and embedded in a matrix of extracellular polymeric substance (Donlan 2002). Biofilm can develop on tissue, bone, or medically implanted devices and can act as a diffusion barrier that slows the penetration of antimicrobials. Inside the biofilm, bacteria can remain in a nonreplicating state and serve as a later cause of relapse (Brady 2008). Rifampin has excellent biofilm penetration and exhibits synergistic activity in combination with other antimicrobials (Zheng 2002). Rifampin should not be given as monotherapy or before surgical intervention because of the risk of rapid resistance development when a high bacterial inoculum size is present. For the bone penetration of highly bioavailable antimicrobials, see Table 3-3.

Fluoroquinolones have been used extensively for the treatment of chronic osteomyelitis. However, studies vary in size, design, use of debridement, and definition of clinical cure. Most studies report cure rates of 60%–80%, which were similar to cure rates for debridement. Failures were more likely when the infecting organism was *Pseudomonas* or *S. aureus*. Duration of therapy ranged from 12 to 16 weeks, and high doses were often used (e.g., ciprofloxacin 750 mg every 12 hours). No study has compared the use of higher doses with traditional dosing of fluoroquinolones for this indication.

A 2013 Cochrane review analyzed the effects of various antibiotic regimens for treating chronic osteomyelitis in adults. The review comprised eight trials with a total of 248 participants and complete data for review. Four trials compared highly bioavailable oral antimicrobials with parenteral therapy for the treatment of chronic osteomyelitis. No differences were found either in remission rate at 12 months or in the occurrence of adverse events of any severity. No trials compared duration of antimicrobials or stratified patients by type of organism causing the infection (Conterno 2013). Although fluoroquinolones are attractive options for the treatment of osteomyelitis because of their high oral bioavailability and relatively low cost, those advantages must be balanced against the risk of increased antimicrobial resistance from overuse.

Chronic Suppressive Therapy

Controversy exists regarding which patients should receive chronic suppressive therapy. Consideration for chronic suppressive therapy should be given in patients with debridement and joint retention, older or immunosuppressed patients, and patients with staphylococcal infections without the use of rifampin. Rifampin alone and linezolid should never be used for chronic suppression. Even in combination therapy, long-term rifampin is generally not recommended because of its toxicity. One study showed a 4-fold risk of treatment failure when chronic oral suppression was not used or was discontinued. That risk was greatest during the 4 months after discontinuation of antimicrobials. Most patients did not have treatment failures, so close monitoring may be sufficient without suppression (Byren 2009).

Outpatient Antimicrobial Therapy

The use of outpatient antimicrobial therapy (OPAT) can significantly reduce hospital stays when oral therapy is not an option. One retrospective review evaluated 454 patients treated with OPAT for osteomyelitis and an outpatient infectious diseases practice. Recurrences were noted in 31% of patients, and almost all occurred within 6 months (78%) or 1 year (95%). Peripheral vascular disease and diabetes were associated with risk of recurrence; age was not. When *S. aureus* was the causative pathogen, vancomycin was associated with a higher rate of recurrence compared with treatment with an antistaphylococcal penicillin. Cefazolin and ceftriaxone were not associated with higher risk of recurrence when compared with a penicillinase-resistant penicillin (Tice 2003).

For appropriate patients, OPAT is a reasonable treatment option. Considerations include the patient's ability to either travel to an outpatient infusion center or receive antimicrobial therapy at home, as well as the cost of therapy. Patients with recent histories of intravenous drug use are generally not considered candidates for OPAT. For patients who qualify, the use of OPAT can significantly increase quality of life, allowing them to participate in most normal daily activities while completing treatment. In situations in which a highly bioavailable oral antimicrobial can be given, OPAT would not be necessary. Patient education is also an important aspect. Because extended treatment duration is common, patients need to understand the importance of adherence to the selected treatment and monitoring plan, as well as the associated toxicities they should report to the health care team.

Conclusion

The aging population, in addition to advances in surgical options for prosthetic joint infections, has led to increases in the numbers of bone and joint infections in recent years. Management of those infections is usually complicated and requires interdisciplinary collaboration. Because of difficulties in diagnosis and treatment evaluation, few randomized controlled trials have been conducted. Increasing antimicrobial resistance requires close attention to pathogen-specific treatment. Pharmacists play an important role in appropriate antimicrobial selection, streamlining opportunities, and in patient monitoring and patient education

References

Baldassarre J, Van Wart S, Forrest A, et al. Pharmacokinetics of Dalbavancin (DAL) in Bone and Associated Tissues in Patients Undergoing Orthopedic Surgical Procedures. IDWeek Poster #398 (2014).

Birmingham MC, Rayner CR, Meager AK, et al. Linezolid for the treatment of multidrug resistant, gram-positive infections: experience from a compassionate-use program. Clin Infect Dis 2003;36:159-68.

Brady RA, Leid JG, Calhoun JH, et al. Osteomyelitis and the role of biofilms in chronic infection. FEMS Immunol Med Microbiol 2008;52:13-22.

Byren I, Bejon P, Atkins BL, et al. One hundred and twelve infected arthroplasties treated with "DAIR" (debridement, antibiotics and implant retention): antibiotic duration and outcome. J Antimicrob Chemother 2009;63:1264-71.

Byren I, Rege S, Campanaro E, et al. Randomized controlled trial of the safety and efficacy of daptomycin versus standard of care therapy for management of patients with osteomyelitis associated with prosthetic devices undergoing two-stage revision arthroplasty. Antimicrob Agents Chemother 2012;56:26-32.

Centers for Disease Control and Prevention (CDC). Cephalosporin susceptibility among Neisseria gonorrhoeae isolates—United States, 2000-2010. MMWR Morb Mortal Wkly Rep 2011;60:873-7.

Close SJ, McBurney CR, Garvin CG et al. Trimethoprim-sulfamethoxazole activity and pharmacodynamics against glycopeptide-intermediate *Staphylococcus aureus*. Pharmacotherapy 2002;22:983-9.

Conterno LO, Turchi MD. Antibiotics for treating chronic osteomyelitis in adults. Cochrane Database Syst Rev 2013(9)

Ernst AA, Weiss SJ, Tracy LA, et al. Usefulness of CRP and ESR in predicting septic joints. South Med J 2010;103:522.

Gallagher JC, Huntington JA, Culshaw D, et al. Daptomycin therapy for osteomyelitis: a retrospective study. BMC Infect Dis 2012;12:133.

Garrigos C., Murillo O, Euba G, et al. Efficacy of usual and high doses of daptomycin in combination with rifampin versus alternative therapies in experimental foreign-body infection by methicillin-resistant Staphylococcus aureus. Antimicrob Agents Chemother 2010;54:5251-6.

Hariharan P, Kabrhel C. Sensitivity of erythrocyte sedimentation rate and C-reactive protein for the exclusion of septic arthritis in emergency department patients. J Emerg Med 2011;40:428.

Holtom PD, Zalavras CG, Lamp KC, et al. Clinical experience with daptomycin treatment of foot or ankle osteomyelitis: a preliminary study. Clin Orthop Relat Res 2007;461:35-9.

Jacqueline C, Amandor G, Cailon J, et al. Efficacy of the new cephalosporin ceftaroline in the treatment of experimental methicillin-resistant *Staphylococcus aureus* acute osteomyelitis. J Antimicrob Chemother 2010;65:1749-52.

Karamanis EM, Matthaiou DK, Moraitis LI, et al. Fluoroquinolones versus β-lactam based regimens for the treatment of osteomyelitis: a meta-analysis of randomized controlled trials. Spine 2008;33:E297-304.

Lamp KC, Friedrich LV, Mendez-Vigo L, et al. Clinical experience with daptomycin for the treatment of patients with osteomyelitis. Am J Med 2007:120(10 Suppl 1):S13-20.

Lauf L, Ozvar Z, Mitha I et al. Phase 3 study comparing tigecycline and ertapenem in patients with diabetic foot infections with and without osteomyelitis. Diagn Microbiol Infect Dis. 2014 Apr;78(4):469-80.

Legout L, Valette M, Dezeque H, et al. Tolerability of prolonged linezolid therapy in bone and joint infection: protective effect of rifampicin on the occurrence of anaemia? J Antimicrob Chemother 2010;65:2224-30.

Liu C, Bayer A, Cosgrove S, et al. Clinical practice guidelines by the Infectious Diseases Society of America for the treatment of methicillin-resistant *Staphylococcus aureus* infections in adults and children. Clin Infect Dis 2011;52:e18-e55.

Lodise TP, Patel N, Lomaestro BM, et al. Relationship between initial vancomycin concentration –time profile and nephrotoxicity among hospitalized patients. Clin Infect Dis 2009;49:507-14.

Osmon DR, Berbari EF, Berendt AR, et al. Diagnosis and management of prosthetic joint infection: clinical practice guidelines by the Infectious Diseases Society of America. Clin Infect Dis 2013;56:1-25.

Parra-Ruiz J, Bravo-Molina A, Pena-Monje A, et al. Activity of linezolid and high-dose daptomycin, alone or in combination, in an in vitro model of Staphylococcus aureus biofilm. J Antimicrob Chemother 2012;2682-5.

Pea F, Viale P, Conjutti P, et al. Therapeutic drug monitoring may improve safety outcomes of long-term treatment with linezolid in adult patients. J Antimicrob Chemother 2012;67:2034-42.

Sharff KA, Graber CJ, Spindel SJ, et al. Ceftriaxone for methicillin-sensitive Staphylococcus aureus osteoarticular infections. Infect Dis Clin Pract 2014;22:132-40.

Sharff KA, Richards EP, Townes JM. Clinical management of septic arthritis. Curr Rheumatol Rep 2013;15:332-41.

Shmerling RH, Delbanco TL, Tosteson AN, et al. Synovial fluid tests. What should be ordered? JAMA 1990;264:1009.

Spellberg B, Lipsky BA. Systemic antibiotic therapy for chronic osteomyelitis in adults. Clin Infect Dis 2012;54:393-407.

Tice AD, Hoaglund PA, Shoultz DA. Outcomes of osteomyelitis among patients treated with outpatient parenteral antimicrobial therapy. Am J Med 2003;114:723-8.

Traunmuller F, Schintler MV, Metzler J, et al. Soft tissue and bone penetration abilities of daptomycin in diabetic patients with bacterial foot infections. J Antimicrob Chemother 2010;65:1252-7.

Wieland BW, Marcantoni JR, Bommarito KM, et al. A retrospective comparison of ceftriaxone versus oxacillin for osteoarticular infections due to methicillin-susceptible *Staphylococcus aureus*. Clin Infect Dis 2012;54:585-90.

Yin LY, Calhouon JH, Thomas TS, et al. Efficacy of telavancin in the treatment of methicillin-resistant *Staphylococcus aureus* osteomyelitis: studies with a rabbit model. J Antimicrob Chemother 2009;63:357-60.

Zheng Z, Stewart PS. Penetration of rifampin through Staphylococcus epidermidis biofilms. Antimicrob Agents Chemother 2002;46:900-3.

Zimmerli W, Widmer AF, Blatter M, et al. Role of rifampin for treatment of orthopedic implant-related staphylococcal infections: a randomized controlled trial. Foreign-Body Infection (FBI) Study Group. JAMA 1998;279:1537-41.

SELF-ASSESSMENT QUESTIONS

Questions 41 and 42 pertain to the following case.

G.P. is a 57-year-old man who has received a diagnosis of osteomyelitis of the tibia after a traumatic injury. The surgical bone culture reveals MRSA susceptible to all antimicrobials on the test panel (other than oxacillin). The vancomycin MIC is 2 mcg/mL. G.P. has no known drug allergies.

41. Which one of the following is best to recommend for G.P.?

    A. Daptomycin 4 mg/kg intravenous plus rifampin 300 mg orally twice daily x 8 weeks.
    B. Daptomycin 6 mg/kg intravenous x 8 weeks.
    C. Vancomycin 15 mg/kg intravenous q12 hours x 8 weeks.
    D. Linezolid 600 mg intravenous twice daily plus rifampin 300 mg orally twice daily x 8 weeks.

42. G.P. has completed 3 weeks of intravenous therapy and has experienced significant clinical improvement. He needs to return to work and cannot afford home health care because of a lack of prescription medication coverage. Which one of the following would be the best oral regimen for G.P. to complete his therapy?

    A. Trimethoprim/sulfamethoxazole DS 2 orally twice daily.
    B. Ciprofloxacin 500 mg orally twice daily.
    C. Levofloxacin 750 mg orally twice daily.
    D. Linezolid 600 mg orally twice daily.

Questions 43–45 pertain to the following case.

T.M. is a 25-year-old man who presents with septic arthritis of the knee. He has no known drug allergies and he has no history of trauma or injury. He does report upon further questioning that his girlfriend was treated for an infection last week.

43. Which one of the following is best to recommend for T.M.?

    A. Ceftriaxone 2 g intravenous every 24 hours.
    B. Vancomycin 15 mg/kg intravenous every 12 hours.
    C. Levofloxacin 500 mg intravenous every 24 hours.
    D. Levofloxacin 500 mg orally every 24 hours.

44. Synovial fluid is obtained from T.M.'s knee, and cultures return negative. However, a culture of his urethral discharge is positive for *N. gonorrhea*. He has received 4 days of intravenous ceftriaxone. Which one of the following is best to recommend for T.M.?

    A. Continue ceftriaxone 1 g intravenous daily plus azithromycin 1 g orally once.
    B. Levofloxacin 500 mg intravenous daily plus azithromycin 1 g orally once .
    C. Continue ceftriaxone 1 g intravenous daily.
    D. Cefixime 400 mg orally twice daily plus azithromycin 1 g orally once .

45. Which one of the following is the best duration of therapy for T.M.?

    A. 7 days.
    B. 10 days.
    C. 14 days.
    D. 21 days.

46. A patient who has MSSA septic arthritis is being treated with ceftriaxone 2 g intravenous q24 hours x 4 weeks in the outpatient infusion clinic. Which one of the following sets of laboratory parameters is best to monitor in this patient?

    A. Complete blood count (CBC), basic metabolic panel (BMP), creatinine phosphokinase (CPK).
    B. CBC, BMP, liver function test (LFT).
    C. CBC, CPK, erythrocyte sedimentation rate (ESR).
    D. CBC, BMP, ESR, C - reactive protein (CRP).

Questions 47–49 pertain to the following case.

N.C. is a 35-year-old woman who presents with a swollen painful knee x 3 weeks. Her boyfriend reports that she injects hydromorphone on a daily basis. N.C.'s ESR is elevated, as is her CRP.

47. Which one of the following would be best to initiate for N.C.?

    A. Vancomycin (pharmacy to dose).
    B. Linezolid 600 mg intravenous twice daily.
    C. Vancomycin (pharmacy to dose) plus ceftriaxone 2 g intravenous daily.
    D. Ceftriaxone 2 g intravenous daily.

48. N.C.'s synovial fluid culture is obtained and no organisms are seen on Gram stain. Final culture is negative. Which one of the following is best to recommend for N.C.?

    A. Discontinue antibiotics.
    B. Continue gram-positive and gram-negative coverage for 3 weeks.
    C. Continue gram-positive coverage for 3 weeks.
    D. Continue gram-negative coverage for 3 weeks.

49. After 6 days of the above therapy, N.C. is clinically improved and her physician wishes to discharge her. Which one of the following is best to recommend for N.C.?

A. Send to outpatient infusion center to complete 3 weeks of therapy.
B. Change to oral ciprofloxacin 500 mg twice daily.
C. Remain in the hospital for duration of antimicrobial therapy.
D. Discontinue antibiotics after 7 days and refer to support group.

Questions 50–52 pertain to the following case.

K.L. is a 65-year-old man (weight 80 kg) with a prosthetic hip infection with MRSA. Vancomycin MIC is 2 mcg/mL, but K.L. had worsening of infection on a prior course of vancomycin. His calculated CrCl is 35 mL/minute, and he is allergic to ceftriaxone (hives). The physician plans to initiate rifampin 300 mg orally twice daily.

50. K.L.'s physician asks you to recommend daptomycin dosing. Which one of the following daily intravenous daptomycin dosages is best to recommend for K.L.?

A. 320 mg every 24 hours.
B. 560 mg every 24 hours.
C. 800 mg every 24 hours.
D. 480 mg every 48 hours.

51. K.L.'s physician accepts your recommendation and orders therapy be continued for 6 weeks in the outpatient infusion clinic. Which of the following sets of laboratory parameters would be best to monitor in K.L.?

A. CBC, BMP, CPK
B. CBC, BMP, LFT
C. CBC, BMP, CRP, LFT
D. CBC, BMP, ESR, CRP

52. It is week 4 of therapy, and K.L. complains of muscle pain. All laboratory parameters are normal except for CPK, which is 3000 U/L. K.L.'s physician wishes to switch to an alternative therapy. Which one of the following is best to recommend for K.L.?

A. Vancomycin.
B. Continue daptomycin but decrease the dose.
C. Ceftaroline.
D. Telavancin.

Questions 53 and 54 pertain to the following case.

E.E. is a 45-year-old man who is started on empiric vancomycin for osteomyelitis of the radius after a traumatic injury. Five days later, E.E.'s culture grows MSSA.

53. Which one of the following is best to recommend for E.E.?

A. Continue vancomycin for duration of therapy.
B. Add rifampin to vancomycin for duration of therapy.
C. Change to cefazolin for duration of therapy.
D. Change to cefazolin and rifampin for duration of therapy.

54. E.E. has now completed 3 weeks of therapy. His physician wishes to change E.E. to oral therapy to complete the course. Which one of the following is best to recommend for E.E.?

A. Cephalexin 500 mg orally three times daily.
B. Ciprofloxacin 500 mg orally three times daily.
C. Ciprofloxacin 500 mg orally twice daily plus rifampin 300 mg orally twice daily.
D. Trimethoprim/sulfamethoxazole 2 orally twice daily.

Questions 55–57 pertain to the following case.

T.C. is a 53-year-old man with a history of diabetes mellitus, osteomyelitis with chronic foot wounds, hypertension, peripheral artery disease with bypass, and depression. Yesterday he had an MRI of the foot that is suggestive of ongoing osteomyelitis in the 5th metatarsal bone with probable abscess collection at the level of the 5th metatarsophalangeal joint, with a nonhealing wound along its plantar aspect and inflammatory changes extending into the 4th intertarsal space. T.C.'s previous bone culture after debridement (2 months ago) was positive for MRSA, and he received 4 weeks of oral linezolid. Today T.C. is afebrile and clinically stable.

55. Which one of the following is best to recommend for T.C.?

A. Start empiric vancomycin and piperacillin/tazobactam.
B. Schedule debridement of wound/abscess drainage and obtain cultures.
C. Resume linezolid therapy.
D. Repeat MRI in 3 days and then start antimicrobials if no improvement.

56. T.C. had surgery and is started on empiric vancomycin and piperacillin/tazobactam. The surgical culture grows moderate β streptococcus group C. Which one of the following is best to recommend for T.C.?

A. Continue vancomycin and piperacillin/tazobactam.
B. Continue vancomycin only.
C. Continue piperacillin/tazobactam only.
D. Change therapy to ceftriaxone.

57. His physician asks you whether T.C. is a candidate for outpatient antimicrobial therapy. Which one of the following would be the most important to assess to answer this question about T.C.?

    A. Payer source.
    B. Type of infection.
    C. Age of the patient.
    D. Renal function.

58. Which one of the following is the chief reason why fluoroquinolones should not be used as empiric therapy for pseudomonal osteomyelitis infection?

    A. Toxicity.
    B. Cost.
    C. Resistance.
    D. Drug interactions.

Questions 59 and 60 pertain to the following case.

W.V., a woman with post-traumatic osteomyelitis of the tibia, is referred to the outpatient infusion center. A culture is positive for *Enterobacter cloacae* sensitive to cefepime, ertapenem, meropenem, and tigecycline. Surgical debridement was performed this morning.

59. W.V.'s referring physician is not familiar with tigecycline and would like to know if it is a reasonable choice. Which one of the following is best to recommend regarding the use of tigecycline for W.V.?

    A. No, because it needs to be administered twice daily.
    B. No, because it has been associated with higher mortality rates when compared to other antimicrobials.
    C. Yes, because it provides good coverage of Enterobacter species and has low reported levels of resistance.
    D. Yes, because it is well tolerated in the outpatient setting.

60. W.V.'s physician decides to proceed with ertapenem because of once-daily administration. Which one of the following is best to recommend as length of treatment for W.V.?

    A. 2 weeks.
    B. 3 weeks.
    C. 6 weeks.
    D. 8 weeks.

Learner Chapter Evaluation: Bone and Joint Infections.

As you take the posttest for this chapter, also evaluate the material's quality and usefulness, as well as the achievement of learning objectives. Rate each item using this 5-point scale:

- Strongly agree
- Agree
- Neutral
- Disagree
- Strongly disagree

36. The content of the chapter met my educational needs.
37. The content of the chapter satisfied my expectations.
38. The author presented the chapter content effectively.
39. The content of the chapter was relevant to my practice and presented at the appropriate depth and scope.
40. The content of the chapter was objective and balanced.
41. The content of the chapter is free of bias, promotion, or advertisement of commercial products.
42. The content of the chapter was useful to me.
43. The teaching and learning methods used in the chapter were effective.
44. The active learning methods used in the chapter were effective.
45. The learning assessment activities used in the chapter were effective.
46. The chapter was effective overall.

Use the 5-point scale to indicate whether this chapter prepared you to accomplish the following learning objectives:

47. Design a treatment plan for a patient with bone and joint infection.
48. Evaluate the role of newer antimicrobials in the treatment of bone and joint infections.
49. Detect adverse effects related to antimicrobials used for treatment of bone and joint infections.
50. Develop a monitoring plan for antimicrobials used in the treatment of bone and joint infection.
51. Demonstrate an understanding of the role of outpatient antimicrobial therapy for patients with bone and joint infections.
52. Please provide any specific comments relating to any perceptions of bias, promotion, or advertisement of commercial products.
53. Please expand on any of your above responses, and/or provide any additional comments regarding this chapter:

Questions 54–56 apply to the entire Infectious Diseases I learning module.

54. How long did it take you to read the instructional materials in this module?
55. How long did it take you to read and answer the assessment questions in this module?
56. Please provide any additional comments you may have regarding this module:

INFECTIOUS DISEASES II PANEL

Series Editors:

John E. Murphy, Pharm.D., FCCP, FASHP
Professor of Pharmacy Practice and Science
Associate Dean for Academic Affairs and Assessment
University of Arizona College of Pharmacy
Tucson, Arizona

Mary Wun-Len Lee, Pharm.D., FCCP, BCPS
Vice President and Chief Academic Officer
Pharmacy and Health Sciences Education
Midwestern University
Professor of Pharmacy Practice
Midwestern University
Chicago College of Pharmacy
Downers Grove, Illinois

Faculty Panel Chair

Ian R. McNicholl, Pharm.D., FCCP,
BCPS (AQ-ID), AAHIVP
Associate Director, Medical Affairs
Gilead Sciences
Foster City, California

ANTIMICROBIAL RESISTANCE

Authors

Kristi M. Kuper, Pharm.D., BCPS
GSPC Clinical Pharmacy Manager
VHA Performance Services
Houston, Texas

Amy N. Schilling, Pharm.D., BCPS
Clinical Pharmacist – Infectious
Diseases/Internal Medicine
Department of Pharmacy
Memorial Hermann The Woodlands
The Woodlands, Texas

Reviewers

Jessica Cottreau, Pharm.D., BCPS
Associate Professor
Rosalind Franklin University of Medicine and Science
Chicago, Illinois

Kimberli M. Burgner, MS, Pharm.D., BCPS
Division Director, Clinical Pharmacy Services
Parallon
Richmond, Virginia

INVASIVE FUNGAL INFECTIONS

Authors

Russell E. Lewis, Pharm.D., FCCP, BCPS (AQ-ID)
Associate Professor of Medicine, Infectious Diseases
Department of Medical and Surgical Sciences
Infectious Diseases Unit, Policlinico
S.Orsola-Malpighi,
Alma Mater Studiorum Università di Bologna
Bologna, Italy

Reviewers

Douglas Slain, Pharm.D., FCCP, BCPS (AQ-ID)
Associate Professor and Infectious
Diseases Clinical Specialist
Department of Clinical Pharmacy
West Virginia University
Morgantown, West Virginia

Nancy E. Flentge, Pharm.D., BCPS
Patient Care Pharmacist
Department of Pharmacy
Baylor Scott & White Continuing Care Hospital
Temple, Texas

TUBERCULOSIS

Author

Alexandria Garavaglia Wilson, Pharm.D., BCPS (AQ-ID)
Assistant Professor, Pharmacy Practice
Division of Specialty Care Pharmacy
Department of Pharmacy Practice
St. Louis College of Pharmacy
Clinical Pharmacist, Infectious Diseases
Division of Infectious Diseases
Department of Medicine
Washington University School of Medicine
Saint Louis, Missouri

Reviewers

Ian R. McNicholl, Pharm.D., FCCP,
BCPS (AQ-ID), AAHIVP
Associate Director, Medical Affairs
Gilead Sciences
Foster City, California

Becky S. Linn, Pharm.D., BCPS
  Clinical Assistant Professor
  Department of Pharmacy Practice
  University of Wyoming School of Pharmacy
  Laramie, Wyoming

Matthew F. Ambury, Pharm.D., BCPS
  Assistant Director
  Pharmacy Department – Lemuel Shattuck Hospital
  Comprehensive Pharmacy Services
  Jamaica Plain, Massachusetts

The American College of Clinical Pharmacy and the authors thank the followinsg individuals for their careful review of the Infectious Diseases II chapters:

Ralph H. Raasch, Pharm.D., BCPS
  Associate Professor of Pharmacy (retired)
  Division of Practice Advancement
  and Clinical Education
  Eshelman School of Pharmacy
  The University of North Carolina at Chapel Hill
  Chapel Hill, North Carolina

Marisel Segarra-Newnham, Pharm.D., MPH, FCCP, BCPS
  Clinical Pharmacy Specialist, Infectious Diseases
  Pharmacy Service
  Veterans Affairs Medical Center
  West Palm Beach, Florida
  Clinical Assistant Professor of Pharmacy Practice
  University of Florida College of Pharmacy
  Gainesville, Florida

Antimicrobial Resistance

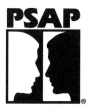

By Kristi M. Kuper, Pharm.D., BCPS; and Amy N. Schilling, Pharm.D., BCPS

Reviewed by Jessica Cottreau, Pharm.D., BCPS; and Kimberli M. Burgner, M.S., Pharm.D., BCPS

Learning Objectives

1. Demonstrate an understanding of common mechanisms of resistance in gram-positive and -negative organisms.
2. Distinguish between qualitative and quantitative testing methods for antimicrobial resistance detection.
3. Resolve discrepancies between in vitro and in vivo resistance testing results and treatment options.
4. Assess patients at risk of infection from multidrug-resistant organisms.
5. Devise a treatment plan for a patient who presents with an infection from a multidrug-resistant organism.
6. Demonstrate an understanding of the prevention and control of antimicrobial-resistant organisms.

Baseline Knowledge Statements

Readers of this chapter are presumed to be familiar with the following:
- Terminology associated with antimicrobial-resistant organisms prevalent in community and health care–associated infections
- Common infections caused by multidrug-resistant organisms
- Basic antimicrobial-susceptibility terminology and general familiarity with how microbiological break points are determined based on Clinical and Laboratory Standards Institute (CLSI) and U.S. Food and Drug Administration (FDA) guidelines
- The lack of new antimicrobials for the treatment of multidrug-resistant infections
- Basic infection prevention strategies applied in the health care setting

Additional Readings

The following free resources are available for readers wishing additional background information on this topic.
- U.S. Department of Health and Human Services. Centers for Disease Control and Prevention. Antibiotic resistance threats in the United States, 2013.
- World Health Organization. Antimicrobial resistance global report on surveillance, 2014.
- Liu C, Bayer A, Cosgrove SE, et al. Clinical practice guidelines by the Infectious
- Diseases Society of America for the treatment of methicillin-resistant Staphylococcus aureus infections in adults and children. Clin Infect Dis 2011;52:1-38.
- Kanj SS, Kanafani ZA. Current concepts in antimicrobial therapy against resistant gram-negative organisms: Extended-spectrum ß-lactamase-producing Enterobacteriaceae, carbapenem-resistant Enterobacteriaceae, and multidrug-resistant Pseudomonas aeruginosa. Mayo Clin Proc 2011;86:250-9.
- Centers for Disease Control and Prevention (CDC). Update to CDC's sexually transmitted diseases treatment guidelines, 2010: Oral cephalosporins no longer a recommended treatment for gonococcal infections. MMWR Morb Mortal Wkly Rep 2012;61:590-4.
- Dellit TH, Owens RC, McGowan JE, et al. Infectious Diseases Society of America and Society for Healthcare Epidemiology of America guidelines for developing an institutional program to enhance antimicrobial stewardship. Clin Infect Dis 2007;44:159-77.

INTRODUCTION

Bacteria have evolving defense mechanisms that enable them to continually change in order to evade death from antimicrobials. Shortly after the clinical use of penicillin began, penicillin-resistant staphylococci emerged. Similar trends were observed in later years with the introduction of methicillin in 1959 (methicillin-resistant *Staphylococcus aureus* in 1962), ceftazidime in 1985 (ceftazidime-resistant Enterobacteriaceae in 1987), and levofloxacin in 1996 (levofloxacin-resistant *Streptococcus pneumoniae* in the same year) (DHHS 2013). The CDC estimates that more than 2 million people are infected with antibiotic-resistant infections annually, resulting in 23,000 deaths. The yearly costs to the U.S. health system are estimated at $21 billion to $34 billion and an additional 8 million days in the hospital (WHO 2014). There is increasing concern in the health care community about the lack of antibiotics in the pipeline that would be effective against multidrug-resistant organisms. Currently, patients are becoming infected with organisms against which no antibiotic treatment is effective—a phenomenon not witnessed since the pre-antibiotic era.

Antibiotic resistance is defined as the ability of the bacteria to (1) grow in the presence of usually achievable concentrations of the antibiotic with normal doses and/or (2) have quantitative or qualitative interpretations that fall into the range where specific resistance mechanisms are likely and where efficacy has not been reliably shown in studies (CLSI 2014). Resistance is measured in vitro and may not reflect what occurs in vivo.

Antibiotic resistance may occur through either intrinsic or acquired mechanisms. Intrinsic resistance occurs in the genome of the species through gene mutation. Acquired resistance occurs through the receipt of new genetic material from another organism (Hollenbeck 2012). Plasmids, which are large segments of genetic material, can be transferred from one organism to another, and the resistance may transfer between two distinctly different organisms. Plasmids may cointegrate with transposons, which results in the acquisition of more than one resistance gene. Chromosomal elements within the organism may also transfer independently or may be mobilized by those plasmids. These mechanisms theoretically allow any portion of the microbial genome to modify on its own, resulting in an infinite number of ways that antibiotic resistance can occur (Rice 2012).

Gram-Positive Resistance
Drug-Resistant Streptococci

The *Streptococcus* genus can be subdivided into three primary groups (i.e., alpha, beta, or gamma) on the basis of hemolytic response to the organism growing on a blood agar plate (BAP). The BAP is a petri dish filled with agar containing red blood cells (usually from a sheep or horse) and nutrients to promote microbial growth. Streptococci that turn the red plate green or brown are classified as alpha hemolytic (or sometimes non–beta hemolytic). This indicates (1) partial lysing of the red cells and (2) the conversion of hemoglobin to methemoglobin by the organism (Todar 2014). Alpha hemolytic species include *Streptococcus pneumoniae* and viridans streptococci. Beta-hemolytic streptococci completely lyse red cells, resulting in a clear area on the BAP. Beta-hemolytic streptococci can be further classified into alphabetical Lancefield groupings. The types of beta-hemolytic streptococci that most commonly cause infections in humans include *S. pyogenes* (Group A) and *S. agalactiae* (Group B) (Facklam 2002). The third classification, gamma-hemolytic streptococci, produce no hemolysis and no plate color change; they are not covered in this review.

Antibiotic-resistance patterns among alpha-hemolytic streptococci vary widely within the category and compared with their beta-hemolytic counterparts. The viridans streptococci classification describes 26 different streptococcal species with similar phenotypes (Facklam 2002). They are often considered normal flora in the oropharynx and on the skin but can be pathogenic. Resistance rates among those organisms remain low for almost all categories of drugs except macrolides. Two primary mechanisms account for that resistance: chemical modification of the ribosomal target and active efflux pumps. Modification of the ribosomal target is mediated by a category of genes known as erythromycin ribosome methylase (or *erm*), resulting in cross-resistance to three different classes of drugs:

macrolides, lincosamides, and streptogramin B (referred to as MLS$_B$). In one study, of 264 isolates tested, penicillin susceptibility was 86.4% and clindamycin susceptibility was 87.5%, whereas erythromycin susceptibility was only 57.2%. Resistance was rarely identified among levofloxacin (94.7%), ceftriaxone (94.7%), and daptomycin (99.6%); resistance to tigecycline, linezolid, and vancomycin was not reported (Pfaller 2014).

Streptococcus pneumoniae

S. pneumoniae is one of the most virulent of the *Streptococcus* species; it is a common cause of upper and lower respiratory infections and the leading cause of bacterial disease in children and older people (Todar 2014). This species' multidrug resistance has increased steadily during the past decade. Penicillin resistance in *S. pneumoniae* is caused by alterations in penicillin-binding proteins (PBP) that may be naturally found in the bacteria or acquired through gene transfer from other species of streptococci (Couch 2014). The PBP is important for the production of peptidoglycan, a key component of the cell wall. Normally, ß-lactam antibiotics bind to the PBPs, disabling their ability to form a functional cell wall; the modifications prevent this from occurring.

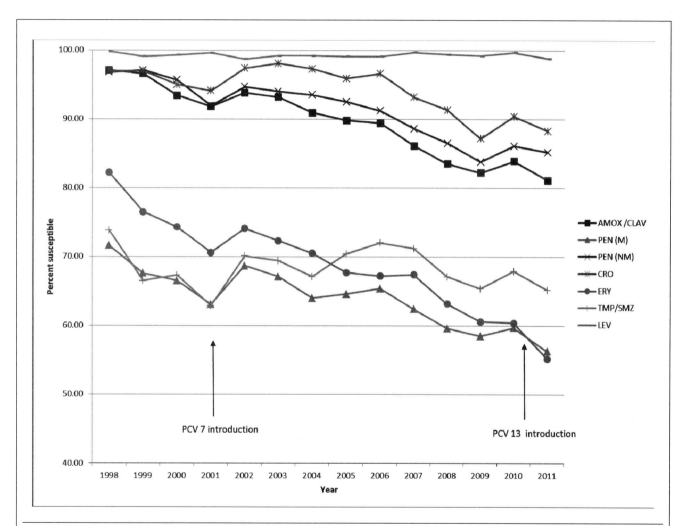

Figure 1-1. Susceptibility trends for six antimicrobial agents tested against 18,911 *S. pneumoniae* isolates from the United States; 1998-2011.

AMOX/CLAV = amoxicillin/clavulanate; CRO = ceftriaxone, ERY = erythromycin; TMP/SMZ = trimethoprim/sulfamethoxazole; LEV = levofloxacin; PEN (M) = penicillin (meningeal breakpoint ≤ 0.06 mcg/mL); PEN (NM) = penicillin (non-meningeal breakpoint ≤ 2 mcg/mL).

Information from Jones RN, Sader HS, Mendes RE, et al. Update on antimicrobial susceptibility trends among *Streptococcus pneumoniae* in the United States: report of ceftaroline activity from the SENTRY Antimicrobial Surveillance Program (1998-2011). Diag Microbiol Infect Dis 2013;75:107-9.

Penicillin-resistance patterns were reported in a 14-year longitudinal survey of 18,911 isolates collected from medical centers across the United States (Figure 1-1). Susceptibility to commonly used ß-lactam antibiotics such as penicillin, ceftriaxone, and amoxicillin/clavulanate decreased from 1998 to 2001 and later, from 2004 to 2009. An increase in susceptibility was seen from 2002 to 2003 because of the introduction of pneumococcal conjugate vaccine (PCV7), which resulted in a significant decline in invasive pneumococcal disease and resistance. However, the use of the vaccine resulted in clonal shifting of the multidrug-resistant (MDR) nonvaccine serotypes—specifically, 19A (Jones 2013). The newer strains replaced the serotypes covered by PCV7 as a cause of disease (Reinert 2009). A transient improvement in susceptibility was also observed among the ß-lactams upon the introduction of PCV13 in 2010, but the improvement did not persist into 2011.

Significant declines in susceptibilities have also persisted with non-ß-lactams such as erythromycin, clindamycin, tetracycline, and trimethoprim/sulfamethoxazole, as well as fluoroquinolones. The mechanisms of macrolide and clindamycin resistance are similar to those of viridans streptococci mentioned above (efflux and MLS_B). Almost 100% of macrolide-resistant *S. pneumoniae* found in the United States can be attributed to the MLS_B phenotype (Couch 2014). There is some variability of resistance rates within the fluoroquinolone class.

Resistance is driven primarily through the inhibition of DNA topoisomerases that the bacteria require to replicate. Efflux pumps may rarely have a role. Two key topoisomerases influence fluoroquinolone resistance: II and IV. Topoisomerase II, also known as DNA gyrase, is composed of two subunits: *gyrA* and *gyrB*; topoisomerase IV is composed of subunits *parC* and *parE*. When a mutation occurs in *S. pneumoniae*, it is most likely to occur at *parC* first, followed by a possible second mutation at *gyrA*. Mutations can occur at *parE* and *gyrB,* but they are not as common and are not associated with higher levels of resistance. A *parC* mutation results in reduced susceptibility to the respiratory quinolones (e.g., levofloxacin, moxifloxacin); the organism may still be reported as susceptible in standard laboratory testing (Couch 2014) but will have ciprofloxacin resistance. Typically, to cause complete resistance, the second *gyrB* mutation is required. Levofloxacin-resistant *S. pneumoniae* still remains uncommon (less than 1% of isolates). Ciprofloxacin resistance is more common, which explains why this drug is not first line for such infections as community-acquired bacterial pneumonia when *S. pneumoniae* is a predominant cause of disease.

Groups A and B Streptococci

Group A and Group B streptococci commonly cause infections in humans—specifically, in children and increasingly, in older and diabetic patients (Park 2014). *S. pyogenes*, also referred to as GAS (Group A streptococci), is commonly implicated as a cause of pharyngitis (i.e., strep throat) and impetigo, and it can cause severe disease. Its virulence comes from the production of a surface antigen that is protective against phagocytosis and improves survivability in the human host (Facklam 2002). *S. agalactiae*, or GBS (Group B streptococci), is often implicated in neonatal sepsis. Some pregnant women become colonized with GBS, which can be transferred to the neonate during vaginal delivery. Screening for GBS is a common practice in obstetric medicine and antibiotic prophylaxis iis administered during delivery to pregnant women who are positive.

Both GAS and GBS have retained excellent antibiotic susceptibility to narrow-spectrum antibiotics such as penicillin. In an analysis of 1082 isolates of GAS (n=579) and GBS (n=503) from patients across the United States from 2009 to 2011, all isolates tested were 100% susceptible to penicillin, ceftriaxone, tigecycline, linezolid, ceftaroline, vancomycin, and daptomycin. Both GAS and GBS were similarly matched in terms of levofloxacin resistance (0.5% and 0.8%, respectively) but had distinctly different rates of resistance to erythromycin, clindamycin, and tetracycline. Resistance to erythromycin, clindamycin, and tetracycline was more prevalent among GAS isolates (53.7%, 33%, and 85.1%, respectively) (Pfaller 2013). Only recently have the first case reports of two patients with vancomycin-resistant *S. agalactiae* emerged (Park 2014). Both strains tested positive for *vanG*, a gene found to cause vancomycin resistance in *E. faecalis*.

Drug-Resistant Staphylococci
Methicillin Resistance

Staphylococcus aureus is a gram-positive coccus that is the most common cause of health care–associated infections, according to surveillance data from the National Healthcare Safety Network (NHSN). Of the 3611 isolates reported to the NHSN, 54.6% were oxacillin resistant (NHSN 2013). *S. aureus* is a commensal organism that lives on the skin and in the nasopharynx (Boucher 2008); it is often implicated in bloodstream infections, pneumonia, and skin and soft tissue infections.

As stated above, penicillin resistance in *S. aureus* emerged quickly after drug discovery (Stryjewski 2014). By the 1950s, more than one-half of isolates were resistant; current resistance rates commonly exceed 90%. The mechanism of resistance is an inducible ß-lactamase (penicillinase) that inactivates the ß-lactam ring of penicillin, rendering it ineffective against the organism. Methicillin, a semisynthetic antibiotic stable to degradation effects was introduced in 1959. It offered a treatment alternative that could bypass the ß-lactamase and be used for the treatment of penicillin-resistant staphylococcal infections. Although methicillin is no longer available, the term methicillin-resistant *S. aureus*, or MRSA, has remained. Modern-day equivalents of methicillin include oxacillin, nafcillin, and dicloxacillin. The term MRSA may be used interchangeably with the more contemporary term oxacillin-resistant *S. aureus*.

The cell wall of *S. aureus* contains penicillin-binding proteins, which are transpeptidases that catalyze the cross-linking of peptidoglycan subunits. Those subunits are essential for the cell's structural integrity (Waxman 1983). When resistance is absent, the ß-lactam, a structural analog of the PBP substrate, will bind to the PBP. This disrupts the cell wall, which then leads to bacterial death. Methicillin-resistant *S. aureus* can bypass the effect of ß-lactams through the production of PBP2a. This transpeptidase is encoded by the gene *mecA*, which is located on a mobile piece on the bacterial genome known as the staphylococcal cassette chromosome (SCC). The term *SCCmecA* is commonly used to discuss the resistance mechanisms of MRSA. The PBP2a transpeptidase has a reduced affinity for ß-lactams and therefore is not inhibited by the ß-lactam antibiotics (Stryjewski 2014).

In the mid-1980s, MRSA became a common pathogen in hospitals. As medical interventions, device use, average patient age, and the number of patient comorbidities increased, so did the incidence of MRSA infections (Boucher 2008). Patients who had acquired MRSA were more likely to have established risk factors such as recent hospitalization or surgery, long-term care facility residence, history of injection drug use, or history of dialysis (Lowy 1998). Today MRSA is often resistant to multiple classes of antibiotics, including ß-lactams (penicillins, cephalosporins), macrolides, azalides (e.g., azithromycin), aminoglycosides, fluoroquinolones, and lincosamides (e.g., clindamycin) (Herman 2008). Clinicians must use antibiotics with more targeted activity against MRSA (e.g., vancomycin, linezolid, tedizolid, daptomycin, telavancin, oritavancin, dalbavancin).

The mid-1990s saw increasing reports of patients who had acquired MRSA in the absence of risk factors common in hospitalized patients. This strain of MRSA, deemed community-acquired MRSA (CA-MRSA), was unique from previously known strains because it appeared in patients with little or no health care exposure and no significant underlying risk factors (Box 1-1). In addition, the identified isolates were commonly susceptible to clindamycin, fluoroquinolones, and tetracyclines, as well as aminoglycosides; this had not been seen previously in hospital-associated strains (Naimi 2001). In one study of 1647 cases of CA-MRSA in three communities in Minnesota, Georgia, and Maryland, 77% involved skin and soft tissue infections; only 6% were considered invasive. Invasive infections included bacteremia, septic arthritis, and osteomyelitis (Fridkin 2005).

Many patients with CA-MRSA infections of the skin can be treated with drugs that are commonly available in oral form such as sulfamethoxazole/trimethoprim, doxycycline, minocycline, and clindamycin (Liu 2010). Oral linezolid and tedizolid are options but may be cost prohibitive.

Cutaneous abscesses can be treated by incision and drainage and may not require antibiotics. A randomized, double-blind trial enrolled 166 adults who presented to an outpatient clinic with surgically drainable abscesses. Diagnostic criteria for abscesses were (1) acute onset within 7 days before enrollment; (2) purulent aspirate or drainage; (3) erythema, tenderness, or induration of more than 2 cm in diameter; and (4) loculated fluid evident. Included were patients with underlying comorbidities, including immunocompromising conditions such as intravenous drug use, hepatitis (B and C), HIV, and diabetes, as well as febrile patients. All patients had their wounds drained by surgeons using standard procedures, and wound cultures were obtained for microbiological evaluation. After the procedure, the subjects were randomized to receive oral cephalexin 500 mg four times daily or placebo for a total of 7 days. Clinical cure rates were 90.5% in the placebo group versus 84.1% in the group that received cephalexin (p=0.25). *Staphylococcus aureus* was isolated from 114 of the 162 patients who had had cultures obtained. Ninety-nine of the 114 isolates were tested for antimicrobial susceptibility, and 87.8% were determined to be MRSA. The results of this study indicated that uncomplicated skin and soft tissue abscesses can be treated with surgical drainage alone even when caused by CA-MRSA (Rajendran 2007).

Glycopeptide Resistance

Vancomycin, a glycopeptide, received FDA label approval in 1958. Unlike resistance against penicillin and semisynthetic penicillins, resistance against vancomycin has been much slower to emerge (Stryjewski 2014). The

---

Box 1-1. Risk Factors for Community-Acquired MRSA

- Extremes of age (e.g., children younger than 2 years, adults 65 years and older)
- Situations that promote transmission from the skin of one person to another (e.g., athletes who participate in contact sports, men who have sex with men)
- Injection drug users
- Residence in close quarters such as in correctional facilities, residential homes, or shelters
- Military personnel
- Veterinarians, pet owners, and pig farmers
- African American
- Infections such as recent influenza-like illness, severe pneumonia, or concurrent skin and soft tissue infection
- History of colonization or recurrent infection with CA-MRSA including close contact or residence in same household with such a person

MRSA = methicillin-resistant *Staphylococcus aureus*.
Information from: Boucher HW, Corey GR. Epidemiology of methicillin-resistant *Staphylococcus aureus*. Clin Infect Dis 2008;46(suppl 5):S344-49; and Salgado CD, Farr BM, Calfee DP. Community-acquired methicillin resistant *Staphylococcus aureus*: a meta-analysis of prevalence and risk factors. Clin Infect Dis 2003;36:131-9.

first case of vancomycin-resistant *S. aureus* (VRSA) in the United States was identified in 2002. Since then, there have only been only 13 cases of VRSA reported in the United States and 33 worldwide (Askari 2012). Vancomycin resistance in *S. aureus* typically occurs because of transfer of the *vanA* gene cluster from vancomycin-resistant *Enterococcus* (usually copresent at the time of infection). In the United States, *E. faecium* is the most common *Enterococcus* species that is resistant to vancomycin. However, the VRSA cases reported were typically associated in a coinfection with species other than *E. faecium* (Limbago 2014).

Before 2006, the minimum inhibitory concentration (MIC) breakpoint to determine vancomycin susceptibility for *S. aureus* was 4 mcg/mL. That susceptibility breakpoint was lowered to 2 mcg/mL because microbiological and clinical evidence indicated that isolates with MICs of 4 mcg/mL or higher had failed to respond to vancomycin treatment and were associated with higher mortality rates than MRSA isolates with MICs of 2 mcg/mL or less (Tenover 2007).

Between the discrete breakpoints that define vancomycin susceptibility and resistance lie vancomycin-intermediate *Staphylococcus aureus* (VISA) and heterogeneous VISA (hVISA). Defined as *S. aureus* that has an MIC of 4 or 8 mcg/mL, VISA occurs when selection pressure is placed on a vancomycin-susceptible isolate, causing the organism to transform its cell wall and become less susceptible by "trapping" the vancomycin (van Hal 2011). The VISA is not clonal, and vancomycin susceptibility returns in vitro once the pressure of the antibiotic has been removed. Fortunately, the majority of VISA (>90%) are susceptible to minocycline, tigecycline, telavancin, and linezolid. A small number even retain susceptibility to methicillin (Stryjewski 2014). Although VISA strains have been identified, they are extremely rare (Richter 2014).

Slightly more common is hVISA, which is a resistant subpopulation of *S. aureus* that exists in a population of fully susceptible isolates; in published studies, this occurs at a rate of 1.3% (van Hal 2011). The hVISA is difficult to detect using commercial antimicrobial susceptibility testing systems, and an accurate and reproducible method to detect it is available only in a laboratory setting. The frequency of hVISA is vancomycin MIC dependent. In a study of 489 MRSA blood isolates collected in an 11-year span, no hVISAs were found when the vancomycin MIC was 1 mcg/mL or less, but they were present in 14%, 30%, and more than 80% of samples when the vancomycin MIC was 1.5, 2, and 3 mcg/mL, respectively (Musta 2009). The clinical implication of hVISA is that patients may not respond to vancomycin even when the infecting isolate is determined to be susceptible and the patient is receiving therapeutic doses of vancomycin. The hVISA is associated with high inoculum infections and persistent bacteremia, although the 30-day mortality rate is similar to that of vancomycin-susceptible *S. aureus* based on a pooled analysis of comparative studies (odds ratio, 1.18; 95% confidence interval, 0.81–1.74) (van Hal 2011).

Mupirocin Resistance

Mupirocin is a topical antibiotic with activity against streptococci and *S. aureus*, including MRSA. It is used for the local treatment of skin and soft tissue infections but is more commonly applied in the nares to reduce MSSA and/or MRSA colonization before elective surgery or in patients in intensive care units (ICUs) to reduce the incidence of MRSA infections (Huang 2013). Strains with low-level resistance (MIC 8–256 mcg/mL) can be eradicated effectively with mupirocin, but recolonization is seen more quickly than with fully susceptible isolates (Hetem 2013). Staphylococcal strains with high-level resistance (MIC $\geq$ 512 mcg/mL) have emerged but are difficult to detect because most hospital laboratories do not routinely test *S. aureus* for susceptibility against mupirocin. Most of the published data is reported from single centers or case reports (Richter 2014). In a study of 4131 clinical isolates from 43 U.S. medical centers tested, high-level mupirocin resistance was 3.2% in 2011, up from 2.2% in 2009 (p=0.006) (Richter 2014).

Coagulase-Negative Staphylococci

Organisms classified as coagulase-negative staphylococci (CoNS) get their name from the absence of the enzyme coagulase, which causes blood to clot. Unlike their coagulase-positive counterpart (e.g., *S. aureus*), CoNS are less virulent and usually considered contaminants rather than true pathogens (May 2014). The CoNS are classified as normal flora and typically reside on the skin and mucosa. The most common species is *S. epidermidis* (May 2014). However, they can be pathogenic, especially in immunocompromised hosts and neonates. Critically ill neonates are especially susceptible because their skin becomes immediately colonized with CoNS after birth, and the organisms can enter the bloodstream through breaks in the skin and by loss of mucosal integrity caused by the use of central venous catheters, ventilators, parenteral nutrition, and exposure to other invasive procedures (Marchant 2013). The majority of coagulase-negative staphylococci are resistant to oxacillin (about 80%), and resistance to other classes of antimicrobials is increasing.

Resistance trends of CoNS were assessed during a 13-year period (1999 to 2012), with a specific focus on *S. epidermidis*. Resistance to clindamycin increased from 43.4% to 48.5%. More pronounced was the increase in fluoroquinolone resistance. *S. epidermidis* resistance to ciprofloxacin increased steadily from 58.3% to 68.4% during the evaluation period, and levofloxacin resistance increased significantly from 57.1% in 1999, peaking at 78.6% in 2005 and then decreasing to 68.1% at the end of the evaluation period, in 2012. Multidrug-resistance trends (defined as resistant to levofloxacin, ciprofloxacin, oxacillin, and clindamycin) were similar to levofloxacin and strongly correlated with rates of retail pharmacy levofloxacin prescriptions (May 2014). This study not only provided one of the largest analyses of CoNS resistance over a multiyear period but also demonstrated the relationship between antibiotic use and the collateral damage incurred by human microbiological normal flora.

Because of the distinct resistance pattern of CoNS, vancomycin is usually used first line for treatment. Newer therapies such as daptomycin or linezolid may be considered for patients unable to tolerate vancomycin or for whom therapy has failed.

Drug-Resistant Enterococci

Enterococci are gram-positive cocci that are part of human normal flora but can also be colonizers or pathogens. Enterococci favor the environment of the gastrointestinal tract and are common causes of intra-abdominal infections, but they can also cause bacteremias, endocarditis, urinary tract infections, and wound infections. Enterococci were previously considered commensal organisms but now have emerged as common causes of health care–associated infections (Sievert 2013).

Vancomycin Resistance

Antibiotic exposure changes gut flora and facilitates colonization of the gastrointestinal tract by the vancomycin-resistant Enterococcus (VRE), which can lead to subsequent infection (Arias 2012). Vancomycin resistance is of great concern; it occurs when the MIC of vancomycin is 32 mcg/mL or more. The prevalence of vancomycin resistance is inversely proportional between E. faecalis and E. faecium, the two most common species of enterococci that infect humans. A survey of vancomycin resistance patterns in the United States in a 6-year period showed that the rate of vancomycin-resistant E. faecium was high (72.4%–80.9%), whereas the rate of vancomycin-resistant E. faecalis was low (not exceeding 6.2% in any year) (Sader 2014).

Vancomycin exerts its antimicrobial action on enterococci by binding to the D-ala-D-ala terminus of the peptidoglycan precursor, thus inhibiting synthesis of the cell wall. Resistance occurs when the organism modifies those precursors by replacing the terminal D-ala with D-lac or D-ser, resulting in a 1000-fold lower affinity of vancomycin binding (Hollenbeck 2012). There are six phenotypes of vancomycin resistance; the two most common are vanA and vanB. Those phenotypes are located on plasmids that allow the mechanism of vancomycin resistance to be transferred to other organisms such as S. aureus as previously mentioned (Rivera 2011). VanA and vanB resistance can be distinguished based on resistance to teicoplanin (available outside the United States), an antibiotic with resistant gram-positive activity. Organisms possessing the vanA phenotype are resistant to both vancomycin and teicoplanin; vanB phenotypes are resistant to vancomycin but susceptible to teicoplanin (Rivera 2011).

Treatment options for VRE can include linezolid, daptomycin, quinupristin/dalfopristin (E. faecium only), and tigecycline. Fosfomycin and nitrofurantoin can be considered for the treatment of VRE urinary tract infections (UTIs). Ampicillin plus gentamicin may be a useful option if the organism is susceptible, although this is not common. The choice of therapy depends on site of infection, duration of therapy required, and the patient's underlying risk factors for toxicities (e.g., myelosuppression with prolonged use of linezolid in patients with renal insufficiency) (Wu 2006).

Ampicillin Resistance

Enterococci have both intrinsic and acquired mechanisms of resistance that enable them to commonly be multidrug resistant. β-Lactam resistance in enterococci occurs because of lowered binding affinity of the penicillin-binding proteins of Enterococcus. The ß-lactam antibiotics (e.g., penicillins, cephalosporins) do not bind adequately to the PBP (with the possible exception of ampicillin) and therefore cannot inhibit cell wall synthesis (Hollenbeck 2012). Most E. faecalis strains are susceptible to ampicillin, but about 90% of hospital-associated E. faecium isolates are ampicillin resistant (Arias 2012). Susceptibility of enterococci to cephalosporins is rare, and patients receiving extended-spectrum cephalosporins may be predisposed to gastrointestinal colonization and subsequent infection by ampicillin-resistant E. faecium (Hollenbeck 2012).

Aminoglycoside Resistance

Aminoglycoside resistance in enterococci can be classified as low level (resulting from an intrinsic mechanism) or high level (acquired). Aminoglycoside resistance can occur through mechanisms such as reduced cell wall permeability, ribosomal mutation, and the presence of aminoglycoside-modifying enzymes. Each mechanism is distinct in its influence on aminoglycoside efficacy. For example, low cell wall permeability can cause low-level aminoglycoside resistance, but the synergistic effect of an aminoglycoside plus a ß-lactam antibiotic is preserved. Conversely, ribosomal mutation leads to high-level aminoglycoside resistance, rendering an aminoglycoside totally ineffective (Hollenbeck 2012). The Clinical and Laboratory Standards Institute provides guidelines for the detection of high-level resistance (CLSI 2014) using disk diffusion, broth microdilution, or agar dilution.

The presence of high-level aminoglycoside resistance indicates lack of synergistic effect of the drug when combined with a cell wall inhibitor. The method to screen for gentamicin resistance is different than the one for streptomycin. High-level gentamicin resistance implies resistance to other aminoglycosides (e.g., tobramycin, kanamycin, amikacin, netilmicin). Streptomycin resistance occurs through a separate mechanism, and hence both high-level gentamicin resistance and high-level streptomycin resistance should tested for and reported (Kuper 2009).

Emerging Resistance of Gram-Positive Organisms to Newer Agents

In the past 15 years, several new antibiotics with activity against MRSA and VRE have been approved (e.g., linezolid, tigecycline, ceftaroline, daptomycin, telavancin). Resistance has been reported in the literature (Table 1-1) but typically is found in patients with heavy preexposure to antibiotics, multiple comorbidities, or both. Linezolid was approved in 2000, and shortly thereafter, the first case of *S. aureus* resistance was reported in a patient who had received 1 month of linezolid therapy for dialysis-associated peritonitis. Resistance among *S. aureus* remains low, but of greater concern is the incidence of linezolid-resistant CoNS, which is 28 times more common (Gu 2013).

Staphylococci and enterococci remain highly susceptible to daptomycin and tigecycline. Both drugs are FDA approved for the treatment of vancomycin-susceptible *E. faecalis*, and they are commonly used off label for the treatment of vancomycin-resistant *E. faecium*. However, daptomycin nonsusceptible enterococci (DNSE) have been described in the literature. A retrospective case series of 25 patients during a 6-year period identified several risk factors for DNSE colonization and/or infection, including prior daptomycin exposure, concomitant gastrointestinal process, or immunosuppression. In those patients, higher doses or therapy with another drug may be warranted (Storm 2012).

Recently Approved Antimicrobials with Gram-Positive Activity

Oritavancin, approved by the FDA in August 2014, is a semisynthetic lipoglycopeptide analog of vancomycin. It is a single-dose intravenous antibiotic for acute bacterial skin and skin structure infections (ABSSSIs) caused by gram-positive bacteria (Corey 2014). Although oritavancin's mechanism of action resembles that of vancomycin (i.e., inhibiting peptidoglycan synthesis through inhibition of transglycosylation), it also has a secondary binding mechanism that accounts for its activity against vancomycin-resistant bacteria, as well as a third mechanism of cell membrane disruption (Zhanel 2012). Those properties contribute to the microbiological activity of the drug against methicillin-susceptible and -resistant *S. aureus*, *S. pneumoniae*, and enterococci, including VRE. In addition to its aerobic gram-positive activity, oritavancin has in vitro activity against *Clostridium difficile*, *C. perfringens*, and *Propionibacterium acnes* (Guskey 2010).

Dalbavancin is a second-generation lipoglycopeptide approved by the FDA in May 2014. In phase 3 clinical trials evaluating dalbavancin for ABSSSI caused by susceptible gram-positive bacteria, dalbavancin given as a one-time dose intravenously on days 1 and 8 was noninferior to twice-daily vancomycin followed by oral linezolid (Boucher 2014). Compared with oritavancin, dalbavancin has similar spectrum activity against staphylococci, streptococci, and vancomycin-susceptible enterococci, but it does not have clinically significant activity against vancomycin-resistant

enterococci containing *vanA* or *vanB* genes. It is also similar to oritavancin in its activity against anaerobes such as *C. difficile*, *C. perfringens*, or *Peptostreptococcus* and *Corynebacterium* spp. (Guskey 2010).

Tedizolid, a second-generation oxazolidinone, was approved in June 2014 for ABSSSIs including MRSA. Six days of tedizolid therapy in patients with ABSSSIs was noninferior to 10 days of linezolid therapy. Tedizolid has activity against MRSA, *S. pneumoniae*, and VRE, including certain linezolid-resistant *E. faecium* infections. Although adverse effects in clinical studies were similar to linezolid, tedizolid has not been shown to interact with serotonergic drugs. No significant thrombocytopenia was observed in phase 2 trials. The drug is available in once-daily intravenous and oral formulations (Kingsen 2014).

Gram-Negative Resistance
Extended-Spectrum β-Lactamases

Extended-spectrum ß-lactamases (ESBLs) emerged soon after the introduction of cephalosporins to clinical practice—most commonly in *Klebsiella pneumoniae* and *Escherichia coli*. Enterobacteriaceae are some of the most common pathogens that cause infection in humans. The incidence of ESBL-positive isolates varies based on local susceptibility patterns and type of bacteria. One study that evaluated isolates from intra-abdominal infections in 19 U.S. hospitals found the incidence of ESBL was highest in patients with *K. pneumoniae* (12.7%), with nearly 10% of *E. coli* producing ESBLs. Other bacteria producing ESBLs at lower rates were *Proteus mirabilis* (3.6%) and *K. oxytoca* (3.1%) (Hawser 2013).

Enterobacteriaceae are associated with infections ranging from simple cystitis to bacteremia and intra-abdominal infections. Patients most at risk of colonization and infection by ESBL-producing organisms are those who have had prolonged hospital stays and who have invasive medical devices (e.g., urinary catheters, endotracheal tubes, central venous lines). Because of their ability to confer resistance to extended-spectrum cephalosporins, they were termed ESBLs.

Two different classification systems exist for ß-lactamases: the Ambler molecular classification system and the Bush-Jacoby-Medeiros functional classification system. Generally, ESBLs are capable of conferring resistance by hydrolysis of all penicillins; of first-, second-, and third-generation cephalosporins; and of aztreonam (Paterson 2005). The AmpC ß-lactamases are in Ambler structural classification class C and in Bush-Jacoby-Medeiros functional classification group 1 (Jacoby 2009). Because of their ability to hydrolyze a broad range of ß-lactams, ESBL-producing organisms have limited treatment options (Table 1-2). Carbapenems have the most-consistent activity against these bacteria.

ß-Lactam/ß-lactamase combinations—specifically, high-dose piperacillin/tazobactam—can be active against ESBL-producing bacteria; and this option is susceptible to the inoculum effect, wherein higher MICs and treatment failures occur in infections with high colony-forming units per mL, such as pneumonias (Peterson 2008). Although carbapenems remain first line, one study found that piperacillin/tazobactam may be a viable treatment option for ESBL-producing *E. coli* when the source was either urinary or biliary (Rodríguez-Baño 2012).

Although cefepime has activity against ESBL-producing bacteria, the MICs for cefepime rise significantly when the inoculum of the treated infection increases. Because of the effect of higher inoculum, cefepime is not a first-line choice for ESBL-producing bacteria. If cefepime is considered as a treatment option, it should be used at a higher dose (e.g., 2 g every 8 hours). Fosfomycin retains activity

Table 1-1. Incidence of Resistance to Newer Therapies Among *Staphylococcus aureus* and Enterococci in the United States

Drug Name	FDA approved breakpoint susceptibility (mcg/mL)	Frequency of non-susceptibility (Year)	Mechanism of resistance	Reference
Staphylococcus aureus				
Ceftaroline	≤ 1 [a]	0.6% (2011)	Decreased PBP2a binding affinity Alterations in PBP2a	Richter 2014 Mendes 2012
Daptomycin	≤ 1 [a]	0.1% (2011)	Decreased diffusion due to thickened cell wall Genetic mutations responsible for membrane charge regulation	Richter 2014 van Hal 2011
Linezolid	≤ 4	0.1% (2011)	Mutations in ribosomal binding site (23S rRNA) Mutation in ribosomal proteins Acquisition of ribosomal gene (*cfr*)	Gu 2013 Richter 2014
Telavancin	≤ 1 [a]	0% (2012)	Genetic mutation resulting in thickened cell wall Altered membrane fluidity	FDA Advisory 2012
Tigecycline	≤ 0.5	0.4% (2011)	Unknown	Richter 2014
Enterococci				
Ceftaroline	NA			
Daptomycin	≤ 4 [b]	0.25% (2011)	Genetic mutation in membrane proteins Resulting in reduced cell wall depolarization	Arias 2012 Sader 2014
Linezolid	≤ 2	0.34% (2011)	Mutant ribosomal RNA genes	Rice 2009 Mendes 2014
Tigecycline	≤ 0.25 [b]	0.5% (2011)	Unknown	Sader 2014

[a]Includes MRSA

[b]*Enterococcus faecalis*, vancomycin susceptible isolates only

FDA = U.S. Food and Drug Administration; MRSA = methicillin-resistant *Staphylococcus aureus*; NA = not applicable; NR = not reported; PBP2a = penicillin binding protein 2a; PI = package insert.

Information from: Arias CA, Murray BE. The rise of the Enterococcus: beyond vancomycin resistance. Nat Rev Microbiol 2012;10:266-78; U.S. Food and Drug Administration. Transcript of the Anti-Infective Drugs Advisory Committee (AIDAC) Meeting, November 29, 2012; Gu B, Kelesidis T, Tsiodras, et al. The emerging problem of linezolid-resistant *Staphylococcus*. J Antimicrob Chemother 2013;68:4-11; Mendes R, Tsakris A, Sader HS, et al. Characterization of methicillin-resistant *Staphylococcus aureus* displaying increased MICs of ceftaroline. J Antimicrob Chemother 2012;67:1321-4; Mendes RE, Flamm RK, Hogan P, et al. Summary of linezolid activity and resistance mechanisms detected during the 2012 LEADER surveillance program for the United States. Antimicrob Agents Chemother 2014;58:1243; Rice LB. The clinical consequences of antimicrobial resistance. Curr Opin Microbiol 2009;12:476-81; Richter S, Diekema DJ, Heilmann DP, et al. Activities of vancomycin, ceftaroline, and mupirocin against *Staphylococcus aureus* isolates collected in a 2011 national surveillance study in the United States. Antimicrob Agents Chemother 2014;58;740-5. Sader HS, Farrell DJ, Flamm RK, et al. Daptomycin activity tested against 164,457 bacterial isolates from hospitalised patients: summary of 8 years of a worldwide surveillance programme (2005–2012). Inter J Antimicro Agents 2014;43:l465-9; and van Hal SJ, Paterson DL, Gosbell IB. Emergence of daptomycin resistance following vancomycin-unresponsive *Staphylococcus aureus* bacteraemia in a daptomycin-naïve patient—a review of the literature. Eur J Clin Microbiol Infect Dis 2011;30:603-10.

against ESBL-producing organisms, and although available in a parenteral formulation outside the United States, it is available only in an oral formulation in the United States. Fosfomycin remains a therapeutic option for urinary tract infections caused by ESBL-producing organisms.

Carbapenem-Resistant Enterobacteriaceae

Because of the broad-spectrum antibiotic use of carbapenems for ESBL infections, carbapenem-resistant Enterobacteriaceae (CRE) have emerged as serious threats (Schwaber 2008). Enterobacteriaceae are gram-negative bacteria normally found in the human gastrointestinal tract. Despite more than 70 genera in this family, the most commonly reported to be associated with infection are the *Escherichia coli, Klebsiella pneumoniae,* and *Enterobacter* spp. (CDC 2013). Uncommon in the United States before 2000, CRE are implicated in more than 9000 health care–associated infections annually (CDC 2013; DHHS 2013).

According to the CDC National Healthcare Safety Network surveillance system data, the percentage of total Enterobacteriaceae that were carbapenem resistant has increased to 4.2% from 1.2% in 2001 (CDC 2013). Invasive infections with CRE are associated with mortality rates of 40% or higher (Patel 2008). Such carbapenem resistance is related primarily to hydrolyzing enzymes, or carbapenemases. The primary carbapenemases are ß-lactamase *Klebsiella pneumoniae* carbapenemase (KPC) and Verona integrin-encoded metallo-ß-lactamase (VIM). The KPC confers resistance to all cephalosporins, aztreonam, and ß-lactamase inhibitors, including clavulanic and tazobactam. Although KPC was initially detected in *K. pneumoniae* isolate, that resistance has been detected in other Enterobacteriaceae (e.g., *E. coli, K. oxytoca, Enterobacter, Serratia*). That resistance mechanism is highly mobile, transferring between bacteria by way of plasmids (Nordmann 2009).

Table 1-2. Treatment Options Based on Classification of Beta-Lactamase Enzymes

Ambler Class	Bush-Jacoby-Medeiros group	Enzyme type	Common organisms	Treatment
A	2b, 2be, 2br, 2c, 2e, 2f	ESBL (TEM, SHV, CTX-M)	*E. coli, Klebsiella* spp., *Proteus mirabilis*	Carbapenems
		Carbapenemases (KPC, IMI)	Enterobacteriaceae, *P. aeruginosa*	Colistin, polymyxin B, tigecycline
B	3	Carbapenemases (VIM, IMP, NDM)	*Acinetobacter baumannii,* Enterobacteriaceae, *P. aeruginosa*	Colistin, polymyxin B, tigecycline
C	1	AmpC ß-lactamases (AmpC)	*Enterobacter* spp., *Citrobacter* spp., *Morganella morganii, P. aeruginosa, Serratia marcescens*	Cefepime, carbapenems
D	2d	AmpC ß-lactamases (CMY, FOX, DHA, ACC)	*Klebsiella* spp., *Salmonella* spp., *C. freundi., E. aerogenes, P. mirabilis, E. coli*	Cefepime, carbapenems
		Broad-spectrum ß-lactamases including carbapenemases (OXA)	*Acinetobacter baumannii,* Enterobacteriaceae, *P. aeruginosa*	Colistin, polymyxin B, tigecycline

ESBL = Extended-spectrum-beta-lactamase; KPC = *Klebsiella pneumoniae* carbapenemase.

Information from: Kanj SS, Kanafani ZA. Current concepts in antimicrobial therapy against resistant gram-negative organisms: extended-spectrum ß-lactamase-producing Enterobacteriaceae, carbapenem-resistant Enterobacteriaceae, and multidrug-resistant *Pseudomonas aeruginosa.* Mayo Clin Proc 2011;86:250-9; and Thomson KS. ESBL, AmpC, and carbapenemase issues. J Clin Microbiol 2010;48:1019-25.

Treatment options for KPC- and VIM-producing organisms include the polymyxins, tigecycline, and aminoglycosides, depending on susceptibility results. Two recent studies reviewed combination therapy with colistin-polymyxin B or tigecycline with a carbapenem and found lower mortality when compared with monotherapy of colistin-polymyxin B or tigecycline for the treatment of KPC-producing *K. pneumoniae* bacteremia (Qureshi 2012; Tumbarello 2012).

New Delhi Metallo-ß-Lactamase

The New Delhi metallo-ß-lactamase (NDM) was first characterized in 2009 from a *K. pneumoniae* urine isolate in a Swedish patient of Indian origin (Yong 2009). The name is attributed to its origins in India, but it has now spread because of international travel. The first U.S. cases were reported in 2009 (Rasheed 2013; Gupta 2011). The NDM-1 is present in more than one bacterial species and can be transmissible between species on genetic elements that encode multiple resistance genes. The NDM was initially isolated from a strain of *Klebsiella*; since then, other Enterobacteriaceae—including *E. coli* and *Enterobacter cloacae*—have acquired the genetic elements and have been discovered worldwide. From April 2009 to March 2011, 9 NDM-producing Enterobacteriaceae were isolated (5 *K. pneumoniae*, 2 *E. coli*, 1 *Enterobacter cloacae*, and 1 *Salmonella enterica*). Those isolates were resistant to all ß-lactams, including aztreonam, as well as commonly used aminoglycosides and fluoroquinolones (Rasheed 2013).

Since 2011, additional isolates have been reported in the United States, including an outbreak of NDM-producing *K. pneumoniae*, which was described in an acute-care hospital in Denver. Eight patients were identified in the outbreak, but only three required treatment for the NDM-producing *K. pneumoniae*, which pinpointed the risk of the spread of those organisms without active infection (MMWR 2012). Those isolates are often susceptible only to the polymyxins and tigecycline (Kumarasamy 2010; Moellering 2010).

Multidrug-Resistant Acinetobacter baumannii

Multidrug-resistant *Acinetobacter baumannii* (MDR AB) is associated with hospital-acquired infections—most commonly pneumonia but also central-line-associated bloodstream infections, UTIs, and surgical-site infections. Typically, MDR isolates of *A. baumannii* are defined as resistant to three or more classes of antibiotics (Manchanda 2010). *A. baumannii* has both the ability to survive for prolonged periods under dry conditions and an innate ability to upregulate mechanisms of resistance and acquire mechanisms transferred from other organisms. The mechanisms of resistance in MDR AB include efflux pumps, porin modification, target site modification, and antibiotic-inactivating enzymes. Multidrug-resistant *Acinetobacter baumannii* can be resistant to many or, in some cases, all commercially available classes of antibiotics, including carbapenems, thereby leading to the need for more unconventional treatment combinations and more research into therapeutic options for those infections (Kim 2009).

One study described carbapenem- and ampicillin/sulbactam-resistant (CASR) *A. baumannii* bloodstream infections at a single medical center from January 2006 to April 2009. There were 274 patients with bloodstream infections; 25% were caused by CASR *A. baumannii*. Of those patients with CASR *A. baumannii* bloodstream infections, 43% died in the hospital compared with 20% of those with non-CASR *A. baumannii*; but this was not significant after adjustment by multivariate analysis for severity of illness (Chopra 2013).

The mainstays of therapy for MDR AB include polymyxins—primarily colistin—or tigecycline. Aminoglycosides can also be considered depending on isolate susceptibility. Because of the lack of treatment options for MDR AB infections, data are limited; but some treatment options include ampicillin/sulbactam, when susceptible. Synergy with colistin has been reported in combination with many agents, including carbapenems, sulbactam, and rifampin. In particular, the colistin-with-rifampin combination showed promising results, although the only statistically significant finding was time to microbiological clearance with combination therapy based on the small number of patients involved (Pogue 2013).

Multidrug-Resistant Pseudomonas aeruginosa

Pseudomonas aeruginosa is an aerobic gram-negative bacterium associated with both community-acquired and hospital-acquired infections. Nosocomial infections caused by *P. aeruginosa* include UTIs, bloodstream infections, pneumonias, surgical site infections, and burn injury infections. Such infections are common in the hospital setting and associated with high morbidity and mortality. For patients with cystic fibrosis, *P. aeruginosa* is a common and recurrent cause of infections found in more than half of respiratory cultures from those patients.

Multidrug-resistant *P. aeruginosa* is increasingly being cultured from patients in ICUs. One study reviewed the isolates cultured from patients hospitalized in the United States who had pneumonia or bacteremia. The MDR *P. aeruginosa* was defined as resistant to three or more drug classes. From 2000 to 2009, the overall proportion of MDR *P. aeruginosa* isolates from the total isolated *P. aeruginosa* (205,526 isolates) increased from 10.7% to 13.5% in bloodstream infections and from 19.2% to 21.7% in pneumonia (Zilberberg 2013). The MDR isolates were more often isolated from ICU than from non-ICU populations.

The MDR *P. aeruginosa* arises from a variety of mechanisms of resistance, including chromosomally mediated resistance mechanisms against quinolones with DNA gyrase mutations or aminoglycoside-modifying enzymes leading to aminoglycoside resistance or increased

Patient Care Scenario

A 72-year-old woman (height 62", weight 72 kg) is admitted from a nursing facility for acute abdominal pain after a recent open cholecystectomy. Her WBC count is 15.2 x 10³ cells/mm³, heart rate is 112 beats/minute, blood pressure is 90/58 mm Hg, and her temperature is 38.1°C. She has a history of heart failure, hypertension, chronic kidney disease (CKD; SCr 2.8 mg/dL) and ulcerative colitis. One month ago, she was admitted to the hospital and found to have acute cholecystitis. During that admission, she was taken to the OR with plans for a laparoscopic cholecystectomy. According to the operative note, due to adhesions, the procedure had to be converted to an open cholecystectomy. After her surgery, she was transferred to a long-term acute care facility to complete 14 days of intravenous ertapenem. While all cultures during the hospitalization were negative she did have elevated white blood cells and a fever in the first 3–4 days after her surgery. Her surgeon wanted the patient to complete 14 days of intravenous antibiotic therapy. While at the nursing facility, she completed her intravenous antibiotics and was progressing nicely in her rehabilitation. Her home drugs before this admission include aspirin 81 mg orally daily, furosemide 20 mg orally twice daily, carvedilol 12.5 mg orally twice daily, and pravastatin 20 mg nightly.

The patient is admitted from the ED with signs of sepsis. The emergency room gave her one dose of piperacillin/tazobactam and vancomycin. They have begun intravenous fluids and norepinephrine. She is taken back to the OR and intra-abdominal fluid cultures are sent from OR. She is transferred to the ICU after surgery and continued on piperacillin/tazobactam and vancomycin. Two days later, the patient is transferred to a regular nursing unit and the culture results reveal the following susceptibilities:

Enterobacter cloacae		
Antibiotic	**MIC**	**Interpretation**
Amikacin	≤ 16	S
Ampicillin	≥ 32	R
Ampicillin/sulbactam	≥ 32/16	R
Ceftriaxone	≥ 32	R
Cefepime	≥ 16	R
Gentamicin	≥ 16	R
Levofloxacin	≥ 8	R
Meropenem	≥ 8	R
Piperacillin/tazobactam	≥ 128/4	R
Tetracycline	≥ 16	R
Trimethoprim/sulfamethoxazole	≥ 4/76	R
Tobramycin	≥ 16	R
Additional susceptibility testing in progress		

The surgeon has asked you to review the case and recommend antibiotics.

Answer

The surgeon poses a difficult question in this case. The patient's recent exposure to broad-spectrum antibiotics and recent residence at a LTAC facility puts this patient at increased risk of multidrug-resistant bacteria. This is a carbapenem-resistant *Enterobacteriaceae* (CRE). These isolates are typically susceptible to colistin and tigecycline. This isolate is also susceptible to amikacin. This patient has CKD and her SCr is 2.8 mg/dL. Amikacin and colistin are both nephrotoxic agents. This patient has stabilized is on the regular nursing unit. The only remaining option would be tigecycline. The susceptibility to tigecycline would need to be verified by the microbiology lab, but with the patient's elevated SCr, the risk likely outweighs the benefit of colistin or amikacin. Tigecycline is a non-nephrotoxic treatment option.

1. Kanj SS, Kanafani ZA. Current concepts in antimicrobial therapy against resistant Gram-negative organisms: extended-spectrum beta-lactamase-producing Enterobacteriaceae, carbapenem-resistant Enterobacteriaceae, and multidrug-resistant Pseudomonas aeruginosa. Mayo Clin Proc 2011;86:250-9.
2. Perez F, van Duin D. Carbapenem-resistant Enterobacteriaceae: a menace to our most vulnerable patients. Cleve Clin J Med 2013;80:225-33.
3. Van Duin D, Kaye KS, Neuner EA, et al. Carbapenem-resistant *Enterobacteriaceae*: a review of treatment and outcomes. Diagn Microbiol Infect Dis 2013;75:115-20.

production of a chromosomally mediated AmpC ß-lactamase. Decreasing porins or increasing efflux pumps can modify outer-membrane permeability to decrease antibiotic entry into the cell. *P. aeruginosa* can also import resistance mechanisms for extended-spectrum ß-lactamases and carbapenemases, including metallo-ß-lactamases (Lister 2009).

Initial treatment with a combination of agents may increase the rate of appropriate initial empirical therapy. *P. aeruginosa* has demonstrated synergistic killing with ß-lactam combinations in vitro. Such combinations have included antipseudomonal ß-lactams with aminoglycosides. Clinical studies of combination therapy have shown conflicting results. Based on additional studies, initial empirical treatment with two antipseudomonal agents and with de-escalation to monotherapy when susceptibilities are available is reasonable. Monotherapy with an aminoglycoside has shown poor clinical outcomes and should not be considered for de-escalation. Optimal dosing regimens are crucial to prevent resistance and treat the infection. Because of the increase in MDR *P. aeruginosa* and other resistant gram-negative bacteria, polymyxin B and polymyxin E (colistin) are more commonly used empirically if resistance is suspected based on the local antibiogram (Kanj 2011).

Antibiotic-Resistant *Neisseria gonorrhoeae*

Antibiotic-resistant *Neisseria gonorrhoeae* is an increasing problem in the United States because the primary method of controlling infection is treatment with antibiotics. In the early 1990s, the recommended treatment options included either ciprofloxacin or a cephalosporin. Because of increased fluoroquinolone resistance in all regions of the United States, the CDC in 2007 modified treatment recommendations to ceftriaxone or cefixime only (Chesson 2014). More recently, the CDC changed recommendations to include combination therapy consisting of a single intramuscular dose of ceftriaxone 250 mg with either azithromycin 1 g by mouth once daily or doxycycline 100 mg by mouth twice daily for 7 days. The rationale is that combination therapy will improve treatment efficacy and delay development of resistance, with azithromycin as the preferred second agent. Because of continued increase in cefixime MICs, the CDC no longer recommends this agent as a treatment option (CDC 2012).

Recent clinical trials of intravenous gentamicin plus oral azithromycin and of gemifloxacin plus oral azithromycin have shown promise, with nearly 100% clinical cure. The increased use of non-culture-based technology makes traditional susceptibility results more difficult to obtain, which makes surveillance of this increasingly resistant *N. gonorrhoeae* complicated to monitor.

Enterics

The incidence of resistance in foodborne outbreaks is of increasing concern. The most common causes of foodborne illnesses include *Salmonella, Shigella,* and *Campylobacter* (Scallan 2011). *Salmonella* foodborne illness is associated with diarrhea, fever, and abdominal cramps lasting 4–7 days. *Salmonella* was recently associated with eight outbreaks linked to live poultry (CDC 2012). Most patients recover without treatment, but severe cases of diarrhea can require hospitalization. If bacteria spread to the bloodstream, antibiotics are required. Some populations are more susceptible to severe disease (e.g., older patients, infants, patients with immunocompromise). Treatment options for severe infections include fluoroquinolones, third-generation cephalosporins, and ampicillin.

Many *Salmonella* serotypes have been identified. The most common include Enteritidis, Typhimurium, and Newport. *Salmonella* Typhimurium is commonly resistant to many different antimicrobial agents, and *Salmonella* Newport strains have been identified that are resistant to 7 antimicrobial agents. A recent outbreak was associated with *Salmonella* Heidelberg from a poultry farm. Of 10 isolates submitted to the CDC's National Antimicrobial Resistance Monitoring System for Enteric Bacteria laboratory, 9 were resistant to at least one antibiotic and 3 were found to be multidrug resistant.

Shigella outbreaks occur that can be food- or water-borne. Because of the small inoculum required for infection, *Shigella* is easily spread by the fecal-to-oral route, especially in areas where hygiene is poor. *Shigella sonnei* is the most common species in the United States. Although decreasing in incidence since 1995, outbreaks continue to occur, with increasing resistance to first-line options such as ampicillin and trimethoprim/sulfamethoxazole. Alternative treatments such as fluoroquinolones, ceftriaxone, and azithromycin should be considered.

Campylobacter is one of the most common causes of diarrhea in the United States. Human diarrhea is caused primarily by *Campylobacter jejuni*. Antibiotic therapy is recommended in severe cases, but supportive care often is effective. Most cases are isolated and associated with eating raw or undercooked poultry, but infection can also occur by drinking contaminated water or by contact with an infected dog or cat. The primary treatment options are azithromycin or fluoroquinolones (e.g., ciprofloxacin). The percentage of human isolates resistant to ciprofloxacin increased from 12% to 24% between 1997 and 2011. That resistance is thought to be related to the use of fluoroquinolones in poultry flocks for food production, although that practice was discontinued in 2005 (Nelson 2007). The resistant strain continues to circulate in the poultry population as well as among travelers from foreign countries.

Anaerobe Resistance

Anaerobes are organisms that by definition do not need oxygen to grow. They constitute a large part of the intestinal flora and are colonizers of the oral and upper respiratory airways and the female genital tract (Boente 2010). Organisms that commonly infect humans include *Bacteroides fragilis, Prevotella, Actinomyces,* and gram-positive, spore-forming rods such as *Clostridium perfringens* and *C. difficile.* These organisms are challenging to identify in the hospital because of (1) the difficulty involved in correctly performing the collection, transport, and manipulation of isolates to get accurate culture and susceptibility results; and (2) the lack of uniform adoption of interpretive breakpoints (Schuetz 2014). Therefore, most of the therapy used for treating suspected anaerobic infection is empiric.

Epidemiologic studies have identified increasing resistance among those organisms. Factors influencing resistance include the species, the organism's ribotype, geographic location, antibiotic consumption, and specimen type (Boyanova 2014). *Bacteroides fragilis* is the most common organism in the *Bacteroides* group, which is a collection of 24 different species. It is highly resistant to penicillin and ampicillin (97%), and cephalosporin resistance is increasing (Schuetz 2014).

Resistance to ß-lactams is caused primarily by the production of ß-lactamases and less often caused by the expression of altered penicillin-binding proteins. Increasing resistance has been reported with other drugs such as cefoxitin, cefotetan, clindamycin, and moxifloxacin. Because of that resistance, cefotetan and clindamycin were removed from the Infectious Diseases Society of America (IDSA) guidelines for the treatment of complicated intra-abdominal infections. Fortunately, susceptibility of *B. fragilis* to extended-spectrum ß-lactam/ß-lactamase inhibitors (piperacillin/tazobactam) and carbapenems has remained above 90% and 98.5%, respectively, thereby eliminating the need for duplicate anaerobic coverage. Resistance to metronidazole is rare. Susceptibility of other *Bacteroides* in the *B. fragilis* group can vary. A survey of 6574 *B. fragilis* group isolates showed that *B. ovatus* was resistant to carbapenems, and *B. vulgaris* was more resistant to piperacillin/tazobactam and moxifloxacin (Schuetz 2014).

Similar to *B. fragilis*, *Prevotella*, an anaerobic gram-negative rod, is highly resistant to penicillin, ampicillin, and tetracycline but has retained 90% susceptibility to moxifloxacin, metronidazole, carbapenems, and amoxicillin/clavulanate (Boyanova 2014). A study comparing *Prevotella* isolates from two separate decades showed that clindamycin susceptibility went from 91% in 1993–94 to 69% in 2012, making clindamycin a less-useful drug for treatment (Schuetz 2014).

Anaerobes that have the most visibility in the hospital setting are the gram-positive spore-forming rods in the *Clostridium* group. Although *C. perfringens* and *C. difficile* can be identified easily, susceptibility testing is rarely performed. Conversely to *B. fragilis*, *C. perfringens* has excellent susceptibility to penicillin. However, like *B. fragilis*, clindamycin resistance is increasing (Schuetz 2014). Susceptibility of *C. difficile*, a highly pathogenic organism that can be acquired in both the health care and community settings, varies with ribotype. In a recent study of 508 stool samples collected from May 2011 to April 2013, 29 different ribotypes were identified. The most common, ribotype 027, made up 28.1% of isolates. Collectively, 36% of isolates were resistant to clindamycin or moxifloxacin, with ribotype 027 being most resistant to moxifloxacin (92.3%). Decreased susceptibility to vancomycin was detected in 13.2% of all isolates but was almost 3-fold higher with ribotype 027 (39.1%). Metronidazole resistance was not identified in any of the 508 isolates, although the authors noted that the method of testing used in this study to assess resistance (E test) may not be optimal (Tickler 2014).

Methods for Detecting Mechanisms of Resistance

Five different interpretive categories exist in microbiology to define the relationship between bacteria and antibiotics: susceptible, susceptible-dose dependent, intermediate, resistant, and nonsusceptible (Table 1-3). The category is determined based on breakpoints, which are numerical measurements of the ability of an antibacterial to kill a target organism. Breakpoints can be determined in many ways. A *microbiological* breakpoint refers to the MIC for an antibiotic against wild-type bacteria as compared with organisms of the same species that possess either acquired or selected resistance mechanisms. Large numbers of in vitro MIC tests are required to obtain this information. A *clinical* breakpoint is based on organisms obtained from clinical infections in prospective clinical trials. The use of clinical isolates facilitates comparison of antimicrobial activity between (1) organisms known to cause infection and (2) organisms grown in a controlled laboratory setting. Clinical isolates can also help determine whether a breakpoint should be adjusted based on the site of infection (e.g., urinary tract, cerebrospinal fluid). A *pharmacokinetic-pharmacodynamic* breakpoint is derived from human and/or animal data and is modeled by using mathematical or statistical models such as Monte Carlo simulation. Monte Carlo simulation is a statistical model that uses actual data to simulate thousands of scenarios and then predict the probabilities of reaching select values when large numbers of patients are treated with the antibiotic regimen being examined (Turnridge 2007).

Qualitative
Disk Diffusion
Tests used to detect antimicrobial susceptibility can be divided into qualitative and quantitative. Qualitative tests will provide the interpretation of susceptible, intermediate, susceptible-dose dependent, or resistant, but they do not provide the MIC. The most common qualitative-testing method was described by Kirby and Bauer in 1965 and involved using a disk impregnated with a predetermined concentration of a single antibiotic. Once an organism is grown on an agar plate, subcolonies are sampled and then reconstituted into a standard solution (0.5 McFarland standard or 1×10^8 colony-forming units/mL) using broth or saline. The concentration of the solution is important because too-concentrated inoculum can result in false resistance, and low concentration of solution can result in false susceptibility. One or more different antibiotic disks are placed at least 24 mm apart and typically incubated for 16 to 24 hours depending on the organism and laboratory testing procedures. During incubation, antibiotic molecules diffuse out from the disk onto the agar, which creates an antibiotic concentration gradient. If the concentration of the antibiotic is high enough to eliminate the organism, then no growth will be seen. Eventually, the concentration is not sufficient enough to inhibit growth, thereby creating a zone of growth inhibition edge. That edge is where no obvious visible growth can be seen by the naked eye unless specified in testing procedures. If the lawn of growth is satisfactory, the microbiologist uses calipers or an automated plate reader to measure the diameter of the zone of inhibition around the disk. The zone diameter is measured in millimeters, and the diameter is compared with interpretive

breakpoints that define whether the bacteria are susceptible, intermediate, or resistant to the antibiotic in the specific disk (Kuper 2009).

A commonly used disk diffusion test is the D test. A D test is performed on isolates of MRSA that have a characteristic resistance to erythromycin but susceptibility to clindamycin upon initial testing. That resistance occurs through a transferable resistance mechanism (MLS$_B$) (Herman 2008). In a D test, *S. aureus* isolates that have the characteristic erythromycin-resistant/clindamycin-susceptible pattern are subcultured on an agar plate, and then disks with the respective antibiotics are placed onto the agar plate per a CLSI procedure (CLSI 2014). After incubation, if resistance is not present, the zone of inhibition around the clindamycin disk will be a concentric circle. If the transferable resistance mechanism is present, the edge of the zone closest to the erythromycin disk will be flattened, which appears as a *D* shape. A positive D test indicates that resistance to clindamycin is likely to occur during clindamycin therapy for *S. aureus*.

Quantitative

Quantitative tests in microbiology are valuable when an MIC is needed for therapy guidance and to determine antibiotic dosing, especially in critical infections (e.g., endocarditis, bacteremia). Common examples of quantitative tests include broth microdilution (e.g., theoretical test tubes) and the E test. In broth microdilution, each well or test tube contains a different fixed concentration of antibiotic. The solution is inoculated with a standard concentration of the organism to be tested and is then incubated. The MIC result is determined as the lowest concentration from the first well where there is no visible growth (Jorgensen 2009).

The E test is done with a test strip that has a predefined gradient of antibiotic that goes from highest to lowest concentration when moving from the top of the strip down. The concentration is calibrated across a wide range of doubling dilutions. When applied to an agar plate that contains bacteria, the antibiotic from the strip transfers onto the plate, creating a parabolic-shaped zone of inhibition.

Table 1-3. Interpretive Categories in Antimicrobial Susceptibility Testing with Examples

Category	Definition	Example
Susceptible	Growth of isolates is inhibited by specific concentrations of antibiotics that are achieved when recommended doses for the site of infection are used	*K. pneumoniae* with a cefepime MIC ≤ 2 mcg/mL based on a dose of 1 g every 12 hours
Susceptible dose dependent (SDD)	Susceptibility may exist but is dependent on the use of a higher dose, more frequent doses, or both.	*K. pneumoniae* with a cefepime MIC of 4 mcg/mL based on a dose of 1 g every 8 hours or 2 g every 12 hours
Intermediate	Isolates with antibacterial MICs that are achievable in blood and tissue but may have suboptimal response compared to fully susceptible isolates. Clinical efficacy in body sites is implied because it is reflective of where the drugs are physically concentrated or when a higher dose of an antibiotic can be used	*E. coli* with a levofloxacin MIC of 4 mcg/mL
Resistant	Isolates are not inhibited by the usual achievable concentrations of the antibiotic with normal doses and/or have MICs or zone diameters that fall in the range where specific resistance mechanisms are likely and efficacy has not been reliably shown in studies	*Pseudomonas aeruginosa* with a piperacillin/tazobactam MIC of $\geq$ 128/4 mcg/mL
Non susceptible	Used for isolates that only have a susceptibility classification because of the absence or rare occurrence of resistant strains.	*Enterococcus* species with a daptomycin MIC above 4 mcg/mL

Information from: Clinical and Laboratory Standards Institute, Performance Standards for Antimicrobial Susceptibility Testing: Twenty-Fourth Informational Supplement. CLSI document M-100 S24 (Electronic). Clinical and Laboratory Standards Institute, Wayne, Pennsylvania, 2014.

The MIC is determined by reading the number on the calibrated strip at the narrow end of the parabola (Biomerieux 2014) (Figure 1-2).

Automation

Modern laboratories generally use a combination of qualitative and quantitative manual testing methods with the use of an automated susceptibility-testing system that eliminates the microbiologist's hands-on time. The systems use commercially available panels that contain several antimicrobials and, usually, growth factors that enhance microbial growth rate. They may use a series of expert algorithms to determine more quickly the type of organism and its susceptibility pattern. Major advantages of an automated system are that it reduces technician time and produces more consistently reproducible results. A major disadvantage is that the systems can interpret the results within a plus-or-minus 1 (2-fold) dilution, which can lead to inaccurate reporting of the true MIC. For example, an *E. coli* isolate with an MIC of 2 mcg/mL to ciprofloxacin by broth microdilution (defined as intermediate by FDA breakpoint) might be interpreted as having an MIC of 1 mcg/mL by the automated system. This is defined as a minor error. In this case, the interpretation by the automated system would actually be considered acceptable for reporting on a culture-and-sensitivity report. The FDA has specific guidance on error types and acceptability rates.

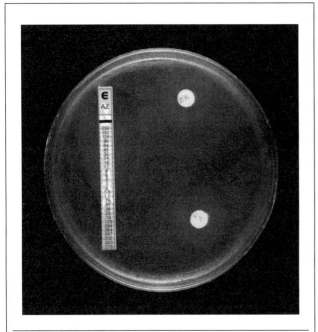

Figure 1-2. Testing antibiotic susceptibility on a plate growing S. agalactiae. The long strip on the left (E test) contains azithromycin. The top round disk is tetracycline, and the bottom disk is erythromycin.

Image courtesy of Dr. Richard Facklam, CDC. Public Health Image Library #10852.

Clinical Translation and Discrepancy Resolution

One caveat of antimicrobial susceptibility testing is that it represents the activity of the antimicrobial against the organism only at a certain point in time and in a controlled environment outside the host. The susceptibility or resistance determination does not fully represent either (1) how the organism acts in vivo or (2) the effect of antimicrobial pressure that is exerted on the organism over time. Those factors can lead to a disparity between the testing result reported by the microbiology laboratory and the efficacy of the drug in eradicating infections. For example, ESBL-producing organisms may be reported as susceptible to cefotetan or cefepime, but some studies show that those drugs are associated with a worse outcome when compared with the use of carbapenems. Other common examples of in vitro/in vivo discrepancies are clindamycin susceptibility against MRSA as discussed above, aminoglycoside monotherapy for systemic infections, and the induction of AmpC ß-lactamases by *Enterobacter*, which are expressed in the presence of third-generation cephalosporins (Kanj 2011). In those three cases, organisms interpreted as susceptible can later become resistant during therapy.

Another common case of in vitro/in vivo disconnect is the discrepancy between piperacillin/tazobactam susceptibility and outcome in patients infected with *P. aeruginosa*. One team performed a retrospective cohort study of patients infected with pseudomonal bacteremia over a 4-year period. A total of 34 bacteremia episodes were identified in which the isolates had an MIC of 32 mcg/mL or 64 mcg/mL to piperacillin/tazobactam. Both MICs by definition were considered to be susceptible based on the antimicrobial-testing standards in place at the time. Of the 34 cases, 7 patients were treated with piperacillin/tazobactam compared with 27 patients in the control arm of the study (received a non-piperacillin/tazobactam therapy). Thirty-day mortality was 85.7% in the piperacillin/tazobactam group versus 22.2% in the control group (p=0.004). Time to hospital mortality was shorter in the piperacillin/tazobactam group (p<0.001). Those data, in conjunction with other published studies, led the CLSI to lower the susceptibility breakpoint from 64/4 mcg/mL to 16/4 mcg/mL (CLSI 2014; Tam 2008).

Despite that reduction, many hospital antimicrobial susceptibility testing systems may not use that lower breakpoint until it is approved by the FDA or is internally validated at the local facility. It is important that the clinician recognize those discrepancies so as to avoid selection of an antibiotic that could result in clinical failure during therapy.

Risk Factors

Antibiotic therapy is becoming increasingly challenging because of increasingly drug-resistant bacteria, and therefore, identification of risk factors becomes crucial. Delay in initiation of effective antimicrobial therapy has been associated with increased morbidity and mortality (Garnacho-Montero 2003). Current guidelines for the treatment of hospital-acquired pneumonia—published by the American Thoracic Society (ATS) and IDSA—have set forth risk factors for multidrug-resistant pathogens, including antimicrobial therapy in the previous 90 days, more than 5 days of current hospitalization, high rates of resistant bacteria in the community or the specific care unit, and any risk factors for health care–associated pneumonia or immunosuppression therapy (ATS 2005). One study sought to identify patients with increased risk of antibiotic-resistant bloodstream infections from the community. The most commonly identified organism was *Staphylococcus aureus* (41.2%) followed by enterococcal species (24.3%) and *P. aeruginosa* (20.2%). Other, less commonly identified organisms were *Streptococcus pneumoniae* (16.6%), *A. baumannii* (10%), and *Klebsiella pneumoniae* (9.9%). The most significant predictors of resistance in those bloodstream infections were prior residence in a skilled nursing facility, advanced age, presence of malignancy, and prior hospitalization (Wolfe 2014).

Patients with diabetes are at increased risk of resistant bacteria because of poor glycemic control and increased exposure to antibiotics (Boyanoya 2013). Such patients are at increased risk of UTIs, lower respiratory tract infections, cellulitis, osteomyelitis, peritonitis, and sepsis (Knapp 2013; Koh 2012). Diabetes has also been associated with invasive MRSA infections with vancomycin MICs higher than 2 mg/L and increased risk of VRE colonization and infection. Gram-negative isolates from diabetes patients are more often resistant when compared with patients without diabetes. The first report of NDM-1 was in a patient with diabetes. Whether related to previous antibiotic use in a patient with uncontrolled diabetes or as an independent risk factor, glycemic control remains important to prevent and effectively help manage these infections.

Since the 1950s, antibiotics have been used in livestock and poultry, with larger farms housing higher numbers of animals requiring improved disease control (Mathew 2004). Although the evidence is limited, it is clear that antibiotic use in this circumstance over time can result in resistant bacteria. The bacteria can be transmitted from animals to humans. The bacteria most commonly affected are *Salmonella* and *Campylobacter*, but emerging resistance has also been associated with *E. coli*, enterococci, and others. The risk those resistant bacteria pose to humans is not well studied but could include increases in duration of illness, severity of illness, and infections that may have not have otherwise occurred. Strategies for maintaining the health of both humans and animals—without increasing the levels of antibiotic resistance—must continue to be explored (Angulo 2004).

Preventing the Spread of Antibiotic Resistance

In addition to identifying patients with risk factors for multidrug-resistant bacteria, it is crucial to take actions that prevent the spread of infection—especially in health care settings, where this issue is often encountered.

Environmental factors that can be modified include strict hand hygiene adherence for prevention of all types of infections. Environmental infection control by means of stringent cleaning and disinfection processes is crucial because some multidrug-resistant organisms can survive for prolonged periods on hospital surfaces (Sandora 2012). Invasive devices used in the hospital setting to provide patient care are associated with most of the infections in the ICU.

Specific steps can be taken to mitigate risk factors for ventilator-associated pneumonia, central venous catheter–related bloodstream infections, and catheter-associated urinary tract infections (Peleg 2010). The antimicrobial stewardship team should include an infectious disease physician, a pharmacist with training in infectious diseases, a clinical microbiologist, an infection preventionist, and an information technologist. Such programs result in decreases in antimicrobial use and improved patient care (Dellit 2007).

New and Emerging Antimicrobial Therapies

On July 9, 2012, the Generating Antibiotics Incentives Now (GAIN) Act was signed into law to correct the lack of safe and effective treatment options for antibiotic resistant infections. This legislation, which promotes the development of new antibiotics, designated certain new antibiotics as qualified infectious disease products (QIDPs). Many of the antibiotics currently under development and discussed below are designated QIDPs.

As mentioned above, tedizolid is a second-generation oxazolidinone approved by the FDA for ABSSSI, including MRSA. Phase 2 trials are now under way for hospital-acquired and ventilator-associated bacterial pneumonia. Radezolid, the first biaryl oxazolidinone, maintains activity against linezolid-resistant bacteria. This agent has completed phase 2 trials for ABSSSIs and community-acquired bacterial pneumonia.

Ceftolozane (CXA-201) with tazobactam is under development; this novel, intravenous, antipseudomonal cephalosporin is being examined in combination with the familiar ß-lactamase inhibitor tazobactam in a 2:1 ratio of ceftolozane to tazobactam. The New Drug Application has been submitted to the FDA for approval for complicated urinary tract infections (cUTIs) and complicated intra-abdominal infections (cIAIs). Phase 3 trials are under way for its use in hospital-acquired bacterial pneumonia and ventilator-associated bacterial pneumonia.

Avibactam (NXL-104) is a novel intravenous ß-lactamase inhibitor. It was initially researched in combination with both ceftaroline and ceftazidime, although ceftaroline/avibactam is no longer under development. Ceftazidime/avibactam, currently in clinical trials, has activity against ESBLs and some carbapenem-resistant Enterobacteriaceae. Although effective against AmpC-producing *Pseudomonas*, ceftazidime/avibactam does not retain activity against metallo-ß-lactamase producers. Phase 3 trials are under way to evaluate use in patients with cIAIs (in combination with metronidazole) and cUTIs.

Carbavance is an investigational agent that is a combination of a novel ß-lactamase inhibitor (RPX7009) with a carbapenem (RPX2014) for intravenous treatment of hospitalized patients with serious infections, including those caused by KPC-producing bacteria. Carbavance has completed early pharmacokinetic and safety studies and enrollment has begun in phase 3 clinical trials for the treatment of CRE and in patients with complicated UTIs

Two fluoroquinolones in late-stage development are delafloxacin and finafloxacin. Delafloxacin is undergoing phase 3 trials for ABSSSI, including MRSA, and also for infection caused by *N. gonorrhoeae*. The intravenous formulation is being studied, with the oral formulation to be studied in the future. Finafloxacin is enrolling patients for phase 2 clinical trials for treatment of cUTI and/or acute pyelonephritis. Finafloxacin is available in intravenous and oral formulations and also maintains activity against MRSA. An oral, nonfluorinated quinolone, nemonoxacin, has activity against MRSA and vancomycin-resistant pathogens. Phase 2 trials are complete for community-acquired bacterial pneumonia and diabetic foot infections.

A tetracycline derivative, omadacycline, is being studied as an intravenous and oral formulation for ABSSSI, UTI, and community-acquired bacterial pneumonia. Solithromycin is a fluoroketolide undergoing phase 3 trials for community-acquired bacterial pneumonia.

Fusidic acid has been widely used throughout the world but is currently under development in the United States as an oral agent for ABSSSI and prosthetic joint infection caused by gram-positive bacteria, including MRSA (Moellering 2011; Howden 2006).

Other commonly used antibiotics that target gram-negative bacteria are being studied in novel formulations for improved drug delivery to the site of infection. Liposomal amikacin is currently in late-stage clinical trials. The liposomal formulation for inhalation is thought to improve penetration of the antibiotic into mucus and biofilm, and the local instillation leads to increased local concentrations of antibiotics. Liposomal tobramycin was previously under orphan drug status but is no longer under development. Lastly, ciprofloxacin inhaled powder is under investigation in a study recruiting patients with cystic fibrosis and non–cystic fibrosis bronchiectasis.

CONCLUSION

Antibiotic resistance remains a challenge in health care and results in increased morbidity and mortality. New antibiotics are under development, but the threat of resistance persists because of the continually modifiable genetic mechanisms that bacteria evolve. Identification of risk factors and prevention of infection are important to reduce the rate of antibiotic resistance. The consistent application of proven and newer diagnostic techniques in the microbiology laboratory will enable those organisms to be identified and treated early in the infection, resulting in improved outcomes.

REFERENCES

American Thoracic Society and Infectious Diseases Society of America. Guidelines for the management of adults with hospital-acquired, ventilator-associated, and healthcare-associated pneumonia. Am J Resp Crit Care Med 2005;171:388-416.

Angulo FJ, Nargund VN, Chiller TC. Evidence of an association between use of anti-microbial agents in food animals and anti-microbial resistance among bacteria isolated from humans and the human health consequences of such resistance. J Vet Med B Infect Dis Vet Public Health 2004;51:374-9.

Arias CA, Murray BE. The rise of the Enterococcus: beyond vancomycin resistance. Nat Rev Microbiol 2012;10:266-78.

Askari E, Tabatabal S, Arianpoor A, et al. VanA-positive vancomycin–resistant *Staphylococcus aureus*: systematic search and review of reported cases. Infect Dis Clin Prac 2012;21:91-3..

Practice Points

When addressing the identification and treatment of antibiotic resistant organisms, practitioners should consider the following:

- *Streptococcus pneumoniae*, an alpha hemolytic streptococci, is commonly resistant to several classes of antimicrobials but susceptibility to fluoroquinolones remains high.
- Uncomplicated cutaneous abscesses caused by MRSA can often be treated with incision and drainage alone. There are several treatment options if an antimicrobial is required.
- Carbapenems are first line for the treatment of systemic (e.g., non urinary) infections caused by extended-spectrum ß-lactamase (ESBLs) producing bacteria.
- Treatment options for carbapenem-resistant Enterobacteriaceae (CREs) are limited but may include aminoglycosides, polymyxins, and/or tigecycline. The addition of a carbapenem to one or more of these therapies may have benefit despite in vitro resistance.
- *Pseudomonas aeruginosa* and *Acinetobacter baumannii* are commonly multi-drug resistant and are implicated in infections in patients with previous health care exposure and multiple comorbidities. They are often multi-drug resistant and may require combination therapy empirically until antibiotic susceptibilities are known.
- Antibiotic monotherapy is no longer recommended to treat gonorrheal infections because of antibiotic resistance. First-line therapy includes a combination of a single intramuscular dose of ceftriaxone with either azithromycin once or doxycycline for 7 days.
- Antibiotic susceptibility testing represents the susceptibility of an organism at a certain point in time and does not consider biologic factors. There are some discrepancies and inherent errors that clinicians should be aware of to avoid the selection of antibiotics that will be rendered in effective in vivo.

Biomerieux E test technical brochure. BioMerieux Inc.

Boente RF, Ferreira LQ, Falcão LS, et al. Detection of resistance genes and susceptibility patterns in Bacteroides and Parabacteroides strains. Anaerobe 2010;16:190-4.

Boucher HW, Corey GR. Epidemiology of methicillin-resistant Staphylococcus aureus. Clin Infect Dis 2008;46(suppl 5):S344-49.

Boucher HW, Wilcox M, Talbot GH, et al. Once-weekly dalbavancin versus daily conventional therapy for skin infections. N Engl J Med 2014;370:2169-79.

Boyanova L, Kolarov R, Mitov I, et al. Recent evolution of antibiotic resistance in the anaerobes as compared to previous decades. Anaerobe 2014;10.1016/j.anaerobe.2014.05.004.

Boyanova L, Mitoy I. Antibiotic resistance rates in causative agents of infections in diabetic patients: rising concerns. Expert Rev Anti Infect Ther 2013;11:411-20.

Centers for Disease Control and Prevention (CDC). Diagnosis and treatment of Salmonella.

Centers for Disease Control and Prevention (CDC). Update to CDC's sexually transmitted diseases treatment guidelines, 2010: oral cephalosporins no longer a recommended treatment for gonococcal infections. MMWR Morb Mortal Wkly Rep 2012;61:590-4.

Centers for Disease Control and Prevention (CDC). Incidence and trends of infection with pathogens transmitted commonly through food - Foodborne Diseases Active Surveillance Network, 10 U.S. sites, 1996-2012. MMWR Morb Mortal Wkly Rep 2013;62:283-7.

Centers for Disease Control and Prevention (CDC). Notes from the field: hospital outbreak of carbapenem-resistant Klebsiella pneumonia producing new Delhi metallo-beta-lactamase—Denver, Colorado, 2012. Morb Mortal Wkly Rep 2013;6:108.

Centers for Disease Control and Prevention (CDC). Vital signs: carbapenem-resistant Enterobacteriaceae. MMWR Morb Mortal Wkly Rep 2013;62:165-70.

Centers for Disease Control and Prevention (CDC). Two new promising treatment options for gonorrhea. [Press Release]

Chesson HW, Kirkcaldy RD, Gift TL, et al. Ciprofloxacin resistance and gonorrhea incidence rates in 17 Cities, United States, 1991–2006. Emerg Infect Dis 2014;20:612-9.

Clinical and Laboratory Standards Institute, Performance Standards for Antimicrobial Susceptibility Testing: Twenty-Fourth Informational Supplement. CLSI document M-100 S24 (Electronic). Clinical and Laboratory Standards Institute, Wayne, Pennsylvania 2014.

Chopra T, Marchaim D, Awali RA, et al. Epidemiology of bloodstream infections caused by Acinetobacter baumannii

and impact of drug resistance to both carbapenems and ampicillin-sulbactam on clinical outcomes. Antimicrob Agents Chemother 2013;57:6270-5.

Corey GR, Kabler H, Mehra P, et al. Single-dose oritavancin in the treatment of acute bacterial skin infections. N Engl J Med 2014;370:2180-90.

Couch KA, Geide T. ASHP therapeutic position statement on strategies for identifying and preventing pneumococcal resistance. Am J Health Sys Pharm 2014;71:417-24.

Dellit TH, Owens RC, McGowan JE, et al. Infectious Diseases Society of America and the Society for Healthcare Epidemiology of America guidelines for developing an institutional program to enhance antimicrobial stewardship. Clin Infect Dis 2007;44:159-77.

Facklam R. What happened to the streptococci: Overview of taxonomic and nomenclature changes. Clin Microbiol Rev 2002;15:613-30.

Fridkin SK, Hageman JC, Morrison M, et al. Methicillin-resistant Staphylococcus aureus disease in three communities. N Engl J Med 2005;352:1436-44.

Garnacho-Montero J, Garcia-Garmenda JL, Barrero-Almodovar A, et al. Impact of adequate empirical antibiotic therapy on the outcome of patients admitted with sepsis. Crit Care Med 2003;31:2742-51.

Guskey MT, Tsuji BT. A comparative review of the lipoglycopeptides: oritavancin, dalbavancin, and telavancin. Pharmacotherapy 2010;30:80-94.

Gu B, Kelesidis T, Tsiodras, et al. The emerging problem of linezolid-resistant Staphylococcus. J Antimicrob Chemother 2013;68:4-11.

Gupta N, Limbago BM, Patel JB, et al. Carbapenem-resistant Enterobacteriaceae: epidemiology and prevention. Clin Infect Dis 2011;53:60-7.

Hawser SP, Badal RE, Bouchillon SK, et al. Monitoring the global in vitro activity of ertapenem against Escherichia coli from intra-abdominal infections. SMART 2002-2010. Int J Antimicrob Agents 2013; 41:224-8.

Herman RA, Kee VR, Moores KG, et al. Etiology and treatment of community-associated methicillin-resistant Staphylococcus aureus. Am J Health Syst Pharm 2008;65:219-25.

Hetem DJ, Bonten M. Clinical relevance of mupirocin resistance in Staphylococcus aureus. J Hosp Infect 2013; 5:249-56.

Hollenbeck BL, Rice LB. Intrinsic and acquired resistance mechanisms in enterococcus. Virulence 2012;3:421–33.

Howden BP, Grayson ML. Dumb and dumber – the potential waste of a useful antistaphylococcal agent: emerging fusidic acid resistance in Staphylococcus aureus. Clin Infect Dis 2006;42:394-400.

Huang SS, Septimus E, Kleinman K, et al. Targeted versus universal decolonization to prevent ICU infection. New Engl J Med 2013;368:2255-65.

Jacoby GA. AmpC beta-lactamases. Clin Micro Rev 2009;22:161-82.

Jones RN, Sader HS, Mendes RE, Flamm RK. Update on antimicrobial susceptibility trends among Streptococcus pneumoniae in the United States: report of ceftaroline activity from the SENTRY Antimicrobial Surveillance Program (1998-2011). Diag Microbiol Infect Dis 2013;75:107-109.

Jorgensen J, Ferrarro MJ. Antimicrobial susceptibility testing: A review of general principles and contemporary practices. Clin Infect Dis 2009;49:1749-55.

Kanj SS, Kanafani ZA. Current concepts in antimicrobial therapy against resistant gram-negative organisms: extended-spectrum beta-lactamase-producing Enterobacteriaceae, carbapenem-resistant Enterobacteriaceae, and multidrug-resistant Pseudomonas aeruginosa. Mayo Clin Proc 2011;86:250-9.

Kim BN, Peleg AY, Lodise TP, et al. Management of meningitis due to antibiotic-resistant Acinetobacter species. Lancet Infect Dis 2009;9:245-55.

Kisgen JJ, Mansour H, Unger NR, Childs LM. Tedizolid: A new oxazolidinone antimicrobial. Am J Health Syst Pharm 2014;71:621-33.

Knapp S. Diabetes and infection: is there a link? A mini-review. Gerontology 2013;59:99-104.

Koh GC, Peacock SJ, van der Poll T, et al. The impact of diabetes on the pathogenesis of sepsis. Eur J Clin Microbiol Infect Dis. 2012;31:379-88.

Kumarasamy KK, Toleman MA, Walsh TR, et al. Emergence of a new antibiotic resistance mechanism in India, Pakistan, and the UK: a molecular, biological, and epidemiological study. Lancet Infect Dis 2010;10:597-602.

Kuper KM, Boles DM, Mohr JF, Wanger A. Antimicrobial susceptibility testing: a primer for clinicians. Pharmacotherapy 2009;29:1326-43.

Limbago BM, Kallen AJ, Zhu W, et al. Report of the 13th vancomycin resistant Staphylococcus aureuseus isolate from the United States. J Clin Microbiol 2014;52:998-1002.

Lister PD, Wolter DJ, Hanson ND. Antibacterial-resistant Pseudomonas aeruginosa: clinical impact and complex regulation of chromosomally encoded resistance mechanisms. Clin Micro Rev 2009;22:582-610.

Liu C, Bayer A, Cosgrove SE, et al. Clinical practice guidelines by the Infectious Diseases Society of America for the treatment of methicillin-resistant Staphylococcus aureus infections in adults and children. Clin Infect Dis 2011;52:e18-55.

Lowy FD. Staphylococcus aureus infections. N Engl J Med 1998; 339:520–32.

Manchanda V, Sanchaita S, Singh NP. Multidrug resistant Acinetobacter. J Glob Infect Dis. 2010;2:291–304.

Marchant EA, Boyce GK, Sadarangani M, et al. Neonatal sepsis due to coagulase-negative staphylococci. Clin Dev Immunol. 2013.

Mathew AG, Cissell R, Liamthong S. Antibiotic resistance in bacteria associated with food animals: A United States perspective of livestock production. Foodborne Pathog Dis 2004;7:115-33.

May L, Klein EY, Rothman R, et al. Trends in antibiotic resistance in coagulase-negative staphylococci in the United States, 1999 to 2012. Antimicrob Agents Chemo 2014;58:1404-9.

Moellering RC. NDM-1: a cause for worldwide concern. N Engl J Med 2010;363:2377-9.

Musta AC, Riederer K, Shemes S, et al. Vancomycin MIC plus heteroresistance and outcome of methicillin-resistant Staphylococcus aureus bacteremia: Trends over 11 years. J Clin Microbiol 2009;47;1640-4.

Moellering RC, Grayson ML. Introduction: fusidic acid enters the United States. Clin Infect Dis 2011;52:S467-8.

Naimi TS, LeDell KH, Boxrud DJ, et al. Epidemiology and clonality of community-acquired methicillin-resistant Staphylococcus aureus in Minnesota, 1996–1998. Clin Infect Dis 2001;33:990–6.

Nelson, JM, Chiller TM, Powers JH, et al. Fluoroquinolone-resistant Campylobacter species and the withdrawal of fluoroquinolones from use in poultry: A public health success story. Clin Infect Dis 2007;44:977-80.

Nordmann P, Cuzon G, Naas T. The real threat of Klebsiella pneumoniae carbapenemase-producing bacteria. Lancet Infect Dis 2009;9:228-36.

Park C, Nichols M, Schrag SJ. Two cases of invasive vancomycin-resistant Group B streptococcus infection. New Engl J Med 2014;370;885-6.

Patel G, Huprikar S, Factor SH, et al. Outcomes of carbapenem-resistant Klebsiella pneumoniae infection and the impact of antimicrobial and adjunctive therapies. Infect Control Hosp Epidemiol 2008;29:1099-106.

Patel JB, Gorwitz RJ, Jernigan JA. Mupirocin resistance. Clin Infect Dis 2009;49:935-41.

Paterson DL, Bonomo RA. Extended-spectrum beta-lactamases: a clinical update. Clin Micro Rev 2005;18:657-86.

Peleg AY, Hooper DY. Hospital-acquired infections due to Gram-negative bacteria. N Engl J Med 2010;362:1804-13.

Peterson LR. Antibiotic policy and prescribing strategies for therapy of extended-spectrum beta-lactamase-producing Enterobacteriaceae: the role of piperacillin-tazobactam. Clin Microbiol Infect 2008;14:181-4.

Pfaller MA, Flamm RK, Sader HS, et al. Ceftaroline activity against bacterial organisms isolated from acute bacterial skin and skin structure infections in United States medical centers (2009–2011). Diag Microbiol and Infect Dis 2014;78:422–8.

Jones RN, Sader, HS, Mendes RE, et al. Update on antimicrobial susceptibility trends among Streptococcus pneumoniae in the United States: report of ceftaroline activity from the SENTRY Antimicrobial Surveillance Program (1998–2011). Diag Microbiol and Infect Dis 2013;75:107–9.

Pogue JM, Mann T, Barber KE, et al. Carbapenem-resistant Acinetobacter baumannii: epidemiology, surveillance and management. Expert Rev of Anti-infect Ther 2013;11:383-93.

Qureshi ZA, Paterson DL, Potoski BA, et al. Treatment outcome of bacteremia due to KPC-producing Klebsiella pneumoniae: superiority of combination antimicrobial regimens. Antimicrob Agents Chemother 2012;56:2108-13.

Rajendran PM, Young D, Maurer T, et al. Randomized, double-blind, placebo controlled trial of cephalexin for treatment of uncomplicated skin abscesses in a population at risk for community-acquired methicillin-resistant Staphylococcus aureus infection. Antimicrob Agents and Chemo 2007;51:4044-8.

Rasheed JK, Kitchel B, Zhu W, et al. New Delhi metallo-β-lactamase–producing Enterobacteriaceae, United States. Emerg Infect Dis 2013;19:870-8.

Rice LB. Mechanisms of resistance and clinical relevance of resistance to beta-lactams, glycopeptides, and fluoroquinolones. Mayo Clin Proc 2012;87:198-208.

Richter S, Diekema DJ, Heilmann DP, et al. Activities of vancomycin, ceftaroline, and mupirocin against Staphylococcus aureus isolates collected in a 2011 national surveillance study in the United States. Antimicrob Agents Chemother 2014;58;740-5.

Rivera AM, Boucher HW. Current concepts in antimicrobial therapy against select Gram-Positive organisms: Methicillin-resistant Staphylococcus aureus, penicillin-resistant pneumococci, and vancomycin-resistant enterococci. Mayo Clin Proc 2011;86:1230-42.

Rodríguez-Baño J, Navarro MD, Retamar P, et al. β-Lactam/β-lactam inhibitor combinations for the treatment of bacteremia due to extended-spectrum β-lactamase-producing Escherichia coli: a post hoc analysis of prospective cohorts. Clin Infect Dis 2012;54:167-74.

Sader HS, Farrell DJ, Flamm RK, et al. Variation in Potency and Spectrum of Tigecycline Activity against Bacterial Strains from U.S. Medical Centers since its approval for clinical use (2006-2012). Antimicrob Agents Chemother 2014;58:2274-80.

Sievert DM, Ricks P, Edwards JR, et al. Antimicrobial-Resistant Pathogens Associated with Healthcare-Associated Infections: Summary of Data Reported to the National Healthcare Safety Network at the Centers for Disease Control and Prevention, 2009–2010. Infect Control Hosp Epidemiol 2013;34:1-14.

Sandora TJ, Goldmann DA. Preventing lethal hospital outbreaks of antibiotic-resistant bacteria. N Engl J Med 2012;367:2168-70.

Scallan E, Hoekstra RM, Angulo FJ, et al. Foodborne illness acquired in the United States - major pathogens. Emerg Infect Dis 2011;17:7-15.

Schwaber MJ, Carmeli Y. Carbapenem-resistant Enterobacteriaceae: a potential threat. JAMA 2008;300:2911-3.

Schuetz AN. Antimicrobial Resistance and Susceptibility Testing of Anaerobic Bacteria. Clin Infect Dis 2014;59:698-705.

Sievert DM, Ricks P, Edwards JR, et al. Antimicrobial-resistant pathogens associated with Healthcare-Associated Infections: Summary of data reported to the National Healthcare Safety Network at the Centers for Disease Control and Prevention, 2009–2010. Infect Control Hosp Epidemiol 2013;34:1-14.

Stryjewski ME, Corey GR. Methicillin-resistant Staphylococcus aureus: an evolving pathogen. Clin Infect Dis 2014;58(S1):S10-9.

Storm JC, Diekema DJ, Kroeger JS, et al. Daptomycin exposure precedes infection and/or colonization with daptomycin non-susceptible Enterococcus. Antimicrob Resistance and Infection Control 2012;1:19.

Tam VH, Gamez EA, Weston JS, et al. Outcomes of bacteremia due to Pseudomonas aeruginosa with reduced susceptibility to piperacillin-tazobactam: implications on the appropriateness of the resistance breakpoint. Clin Infect Dis 2008:46:862-7.

Tenover FC, Moellering RC. The rationale for revising the Clinical and Laboratory Standards Institute vancomycin minimal inhibitory concentration interpretive criteria for Staphylococcus aureus. Clin Infect Dis 2007;44:1208-15.

Tickler IA, Goering RV, Whitmore JD, et al. Strain types and antimicrobial resistance patterns of Clostridium difficile isolates from the United States: 2011-2013. Antimicrob Agents and Chemo 2014;58:4214-8.

Todar's Online Textbook of Bacteriology.

Tumbarello M, Viale P, Viscoli C, et al. Predictors of mortality in bloodstream infections caused by *Klebsiella pneumoniae* carbapenemase-producing K. pneumoniae: importance of combination therapy. Clin Infect Dis 2012;55:943-50.

Turnidge J, Paterson DL. Setting and revising antibacterial susceptibility breakpoints. Clin Microbiol Rev 2007;20:391-408.

U.S. Department of Health and Human Services (US DHHS). Centers for Disease Control and Prevention. Antibiotic resistance threats in the United States, 2013.

van Hal S, Paterson DL. Systematic review and meta-analysis of the significance of heterogeneous vancomycin-intermediate *Staphylococcus aureus* isolates. Antimicrob agents Chemother 2011;55:405-10.

Waxman DJ, Strominger JL. Penicillin-binding proteins and the mechanism of action of b-lactam antibiotics. Annu Rev Biochem 1983;52:825-69.

Wolfe CM, Cohen B, Larson E. Prevalence and risk factors for antibiotic-resistant community-associated bloodstream infections. J Infect Public Health 2014;7:224-32.

World Health Organization. Antimicrobial resistance global report on surveillance 2014.

Wu V, Wang Y, Wang C, et al. High frequency of linezolid-associated thrombocytopenia and anemia among patients with end-stage renal disease. Clin Infect Dis 2006;42:66-72.

Yong D, Toleman MA, Giske CG, et al. Characterization of a new metallo-beta-lactamase gene, bla NDM-1, and a novel erythromycin esterase gene carried on a unique genetic structure in Klebsiella pneumoniae sequence type 14 from India. Antimicrob Agents Chemother 2009;53:5046-54.

Zhanel GG, Schweizer F, Karlowsky JA. Oritavancin: mechanism of action. Clin Infect Dis 2012:54;S214-9.

Zilberberg MD, Shorr AF. Prevalence of multidrug-resistant *Pseudomonas aeruginosa* and carbapenem-resistant Enterobacteriaceae among specimens from hospitalized patients with pneumonia and bloodstream infections in the United States from 2000 to 2009. J Hosp Med 2013;8:559-63.

SELF-ASSESSMENT QUESTIONS

Questions 1 and 2 pertain to the following case.

L.S. is a 68-year-old woman who is receiving hemodialysis for end-stage kidney disease secondary to poorly controlled diabetes mellitus, which is now managed with insulin. Her current drugs include insulin glargine, insulin aspart, paroxetine, and metoprolol. She presents for one of her three weekly dialysis sessions and complains of fever, chills, and loss of appetite over the past 2 days. Examination results are: temperature 39°C (102.2°F), respiratory rate 21 breaths/minute, heart rate 103 beats/minute, and blood pressure 96/52 mm Hg. Upon auscultation, a grade 3/ 6 systolic murmur is detected. L.S. is transferred to the hospital and admitted with suspected sepsis. Therapy is initiated with vancomycin and ceftriaxone. Multiple blood cultures drawn on admission later reveal *Enterococcus faecium* with an MIC to vancomycin of 32 mcg/mL.

1. Which one of the following would best treat L.S.'s infection after the culture and susceptibility results are known?

    A. Ceftaroline
    B. Linezolid.
    C. Daptomycin.
    D. Meropenem

2. On day 1, L.S. has transthoracic echocardiography, which reveals a 0.7-cm vegetation on her tricuspid valve. The hospitalist is also reviewing the culture and susceptibility report and notices that the *E. faecium* culture report indicates an MIC of ≥ 500 mcg/mL to gentamicin and ≥ 2000 mcg/mL for streptomycin. Which one of the following is best to recommend for L.S.?

    A. Continue the antibiotic selected above with no changes.
    B. Add gentamicin to the regimen for synergy.
    C. Add streptomycin to the regimen for synergy.
    D. Discontinue the above regimen and start imipenem/cilastatin.

3. An 86-year-old woman is admitted from a long-term care facility with a non-healing sacral decubitus ulcer that has not responded to levofloxacin. Which one of the following is mostly likely the cause of this patient's infection?

    A. Methicillin resistant *S. epidermidis.*
    B. Vancomycin-resistant *S. aureus.*
    C. Levofloxacin-resistant *S. pneumoniae.*
    D. Methicillin-resistant *S. aureus.*

Questions 4 and 5 pertain to the following case.

H.S. is a 27-year-old Hispanic man who has just returned from a 5-month tour of duty on a naval submarine. He presents to the military health clinic complaining of lower quadrant pain and three episodes of vomiting in the past 12 hours. His temperature is 38.2°C (100.8°F), WBC count is 18 x 10^3 cells/mm^3, heart rate is 92 beats/minute, and blood pressure is 100/78 mm Hg. H.S. is transported to the nearest emergency room where a CT with contrast indicates a ruptured appendix. He is taken quickly to the OR for an emergency appendectomy.

4. Which one of the following would be best to recommend for H.S.?

    A. Piperacillin/tazobactam and metronidazole.
    B. Piperacillin/tazobactam and clindamycin .
    C. Cefotetan plus metronidazole.
    D. Ceftriaxone plus metronidazole.

5. After the appendectomy, H.S. is transferred to the surgical floor for monitoring. The following morning, the surgical resident conducts a physical examination of H.S. and notices a 5-cm boil on the inside of his left thigh. Upon interview, he notes that it was getting larger despite 5 days of applying a triple antibiotic topical ointment that he was given by the medical assistant aboard the submarine. How many risk factors does H.S. have for community-acquired MRSA?

    A. 0
    B. 1
    C. 2
    D. 3

Questions 6 and 7 pertain to the following case.

G.F. is an 88-year-old man with a history of diabetes. He is admitted with increased swelling and redness around an ulcer on the second toe of his left foot. Five days ago, G.F. saw his primary care physician who initiated trimethoprim/sulfamethoxazole twice daily. G.F. is sent for MRI, which does not show osteomyelitis of left second metatarsal. He is taken to surgery for irrigation and debridement of the ulcer. Initial Gram stain shows gram-positive cocci.

6. Which one of the following is most likely causing G.F.'s symptoms?

    A. Coagulase-negative staphylococci.
    B. Methicillin-resistant *S. aureus.*
    C. Group A Streptococcus.
    D. Group B Streptococcus.

7. Based on the most likely culture result from GF's ulcer, which one of the following is best to recommend for G.F.?

   A. Linezolid.
   B. Amoxicillin/clavulanate.
   C. Azithromycin.
   D. Ceftriaxone.

Questions 8 and 9 pertain to the following case.

K.P. is a 33-year-old man; he has been a quadriplegic since receiving a gunshot wound at the age of 18. K.P. has no known drug allergies. He reports foul odor from a sacral wound upon dressing changes and overall feeling unwell. Vitals on admission included temperature 38.5°C, heart rate 111 beats/minute, blood pressure 95/62 mm Hg; laboratory tests results include WBC 18.1 x 10³ cells/mm³. Physical examination reveals a large foul-smelling sacral decubitus ulcer. Chart review reveals K.P. has a history of ESBL-producing *Enterobacter aerogenes* and MRSA from the wound.

8. Which one of the following combination regimens is best to recommend for K.P.?

   A. Ceftriaxone and daptomycin.
   B. Piperacillin/tazobactam and vancomycin.
   C. Meropenem and daptomycin.
   D. Ciprofloxacin and minocycline.

9. K.P. is taken to the surgery for immediate debridement. Culture results return on postoperative Day 2.

4+ *Acinetobacter baumannii*		
Antibiotic	**MIC**	**Interpretation**
Ampicillin/sulbactam	≥ 32/16	R
Ceftazidime	≥ 32	R
Ceftriaxone	≥ 64	R
Cefepime	≥ 32	R
Gentamicin	≥ 16	R
Levofloxacin	≥ 8	R
Meropenem	4	I
Piperacillin/ tazobactam	≥ 128/4	R
Tetracycline	≥ 16	R
Trimethoprim/ sulfamethoxazole	≥ 4/76	R
Tobramycin	≥ 16	R
Additional susceptibility testing in progress		

Which one of the following is best to recommend for K.P. until additional susceptibility results are available?

   A. Meropenem
   B. Rifampin.
   C. Colistin.
   D. Amikacin.

10. A 52-year-old woman with diabetes presents on a Saturday morning with right lower extremity erythema and swelling that has been worsening over the last 2 days. Her laboratory test results include WBC 12.5 x 10³ cells/mm³ and temperature in ER was 37.1°C. Her heart rate was 81 beats/minute and blood pressure 131/89 mm Hg. She just started a new job so she can't take time away from work. She needs to be discharged to go to work Monday morning. She agrees to follow up with her primary care provider to ensure cellulitis is improving. Which one of the following drug regimens is most appropriate for this patient?

   A. Oritavancin.
   B. Daptomycin.
   C. Ceftaroline.
   D. Fusidic acid.

11. Drug X is a promising new agent for the management of MRSA pneumonia. Because it is unethical to compare Drug X to placebo, which one of the following trial designs would best show this agent's efficacy for MRSA pneumonia to obtain FDA approval?

   A. Noninferiority trial.
   B. Randomized, crossover.
   C. Case series.
   D. Retrospective, cohort.

12. A 21-year-old woman has a medical history significant for cystic fibrosis. She reports being increasingly short of breath and increased productive cough with green sputum over the last couple days. She is noticeably wheezing on physical examination. Her home drugs include tobramycin by nebulization for management of chronic *Pseudomonas aeruginosa* colonization with the susceptibility pattern below from a previous admission.

Pseudomonas aeruginosa		
Antibiotic	**MIC**	**Interpretation**
Amikacin	4	S
Cefepime	16	I
Ciprofloxacin	≥4	R
Gentamicin	≥16	R
Levofloxacin	≥8	R
Meropenem	1	S
Piperacillin/tazobactam	≥128/4	R
Tobramycin	4	S

Her pulse oximeter shows 89% O₂ saturation, blood pressure 125/81 mm Hg, heart rate 125 beats/minute. Her laboratory test results show SCr 0.9 mg/dL and WBC 15.3 x 10³ cells/mm³. Which one of the following empiric combination regimens is best to recommend for this patient?

A. Ceftriaxone, gentamicin, vancomycin.
B. Meropenem, tobramycin, vancomycin.
C. Meropenem, amikacin, vancomycin.
D. Piperacillin/tazobactam, tobramycin, daptomycin.

Questions 13 and 14 pertain to the following case.

J.R. is a 23-year-old man who presents to the emergency department (ED) with burning with urination and discharge from his penis. He reports two recent episodes of unprotected sex with two different women he met at a bar. He has never had an sexually transmitted infection but knows nothing about the sexual history of his partners. The ED physician orders a swab of the urethral discharge to be sent to the lab, and he would like to treat for *Neisseria gonorrhea* and *Chlamydia trachomatis*.

13. Which one of the following is best to recommend for J.R.?

    A. Cefixime plus azithromycin.
    B. Ciprofloxacin.
    C. Ceftriaxone plus azithromycin.
    D. Doxycycline.

14. Seven days later, J.R. presents again to the ED. He initially had partial relief of his signs and symptoms but now the discharge from his penis has started again. The ED calls the microbiology lab and confirms that the patient did test positive for *N. gonorrhea*. Which one of the following is best to recommend for J.R.?

    A. Treat once again with the initial regimen.
    B. Send the isolate to a reference lab for susceptibility testing.
    C. Treat with cefixime plus azithromycin.
    D. Consider gemifloxacin monotherapy. **?**

Questions 15 and 16 pertain to the following case.

R.G. is a 75-year-old man who resides in a long-term care facility. He presents with bilateral hip pain after falling today. He usually uses a walker but headed to the restroom without it today, lost his balance, and fell. R.G. denies loss of consciousness but was unable to ambulate after his fall. Per family, he had radiography which showed a slight fracture in one lumbar vertebrae. R.G. is currently on clopidogrel and being treated empirically for the last 5 days with trimethoprim/sulfamethoxazole for a suspected UTI. His temperature on admission is 37.5°C, heart rate 106 beats/minute, blood pressure 90/65 mm Hg. Urinalysis shows nitrite positive, leukocyte esterase positive, WBC greater than 182 per HPF, RBC greater than 182 per HPF, and a new urine culture is pending. Laboratory tests reveal WBC 16.2 x 10³ cells/mm³ and SCr 2.5 mg/dL.

15. Which one of the following is best to recommend for R.G.?

    A. Stop therapy.
    B. Continue trimethoprim/sulfamethoxazole.
    C. Initiate intravenous cefepime.
    D. Change therapy to nitrofurantoin.

16. R.G.'s WBC and body temperature have been improving. He has been working with physical therapy routinely in preparation for discharge in the next 24 hours. R.G.'s urine culture reveals the following:

Klebsiella pneumoniae		
Antibiotic	**MIC (mcg/mL)**	**Interpretation**
Ampicillin	≥32	R
Ampicillin/sulbactam	≥32/16	R
Cefazolin	≥16	R
Ceftriaxone	≥16	R
Cefepime	8	S-DD
Ciprofloxacin	0.03	S
Colistin	0.25	S
Gentamicin	≥8	R
Levofloxacin	0.12	S
Nitrofurantoin	≥256	R
Piperacillin/tazobactam	≥128/4	R
Meropenem	≥8	R
Tetracycline	≥8	R
Tigecycline	0.5	S

Which one of the following is best to recommend for R.G.?

    A. Tigecycline.
    B. Colistin.
    C. Cefepime.
    D. Ciprofloxacin.

17. An 8-year-old unvaccinated boy is admitted with lethargy, nausea, vomiting, and a current temperature of 103.1°F. A cerebrospinal fluid culture was obtained and vancomycin and ceftriaxone were initiated. Culture results reveal *Streptococcus pneumoniae*. Which of the following would best guide antimicrobial therapy based on minimum inhibitory concentrations in this patient?

    A. D-test.
    B. Disk diffusion.
    C. Gram stain.
    D. E-test.

Questions 18 and 19 pertain to the following case.

V.Y. is a 64-year-old woman (height 5'2", weight 65 kg) who is admitted to a rehabilitation facility. She was hospitalized for 2 weeks after a fall resulted in a C7 fracture and spinal cord injury with dysphagia, neurogenic bowel and bladder, sacral pressure ulcer s/p flap, and spasm of muscle. V.Y. has no known drug allergies. Her Tmax over last 24 hours is 100.6°F, heart rate 78 beats/minute, blood pressure 130/74 mm Hg, and respiratory rate 16 breaths/minute. She has a solitary kidney, SCr 0.8 mg/dL, and a neurogenic bladder requiring intermittent straight catheterization. Urinalysis showed 50 WBCs, positive for nitrites and leukocyte esterase with many bacteria. V.Y. has history of urinary tract infections caused by ESBL + *E. coli*. She was last treated for a UTI 5 months ago.

18. Which one of the following would be the best empiric treatment for V.Y.?

    A. Ampicillin.
    B. Levofloxacin.
    C. Bactrim.
    D. Ertapenem.

19. Which one of the following puts V.Y. at greatest risk of multidrug-resistant pathogens?

    A. Recent hospitalization.
    B. Immunosuppressive therapy.
    C. Spinal cord injury.
    D. Prior antimicrobial therapy.

20. A 45-year-old woman presents to the ED with nausea, vomiting, diarrhea, fever, and abdominal cramping for the last 4 days. Her vitals include heart rate 90 beats/minute, blood pressure 105/63 mm Hg, and temperature 100.3°F. She reports discovering yesterday that the chia seeds she daily consumes were part of a national recall due to *Salmonella* contamination. The patient is admitted for intravenous hydration and antibiotics. Which one of the following is best to recommend for this patient?

    A. Ciprofloxacin.
    B. Cefazolin.
    C. Azithromycin.
    D. Trimethoprim/sulfamethoxazole.

Learner Chapter Evaluation: Antimicrobial Resistance.

As you take the posttest for this chapter, also evaluate the material's quality and usefulness, as well as the achievement of learning objectives. Rate each item using this 5-point scale:

- Strongly agree
- Agree
- Neutral
- Disagree
- Strongly disagree

1. The content of the chapter met my educational needs.
2. The content of the chapter satisfied my expectations.
3. The author presented the chapter content effectively.
4. The content of the chapter was relevant to my practice and presented at the appropriate depth and scope.
5. The content of the chapter was objective and balanced.
6. The content of the chapter is free of bias, promotion, or advertisement of commercial products.
7. The content of the chapter was useful to me.
8. The teaching and learning methods used in the chapter were effective.
9. The active learning methods used in the chapter were effective.
10. The learning assessment activities used in the chapter were effective.
11. The chapter was effective overall.

Use the 5-point scale to indicate whether this chapter prepared you to accomplish the following learning objectives:

12. Demonstrate an understanding of the common mechanism of resistance of gram-positive and -negative organisms.
13. Distinguish between qualitative and quantitative testing methods for antimicrobial resistance detection.
14. Resolve discrepancies between in vitro and in vivo resistance testing results and treatment options.
15. Assess patients at risk of infection from multidrug-resistant organisms.
16. Devise a treatment plan for a patient who presents with an infection from a multidrug-resistant organism.
17. Demonstrate an understanding of the prevention and control of antimicrobial-resistant organisms.
18. Please provide any specific comments relating to any perceptions of bias, promotion, or advertisement of commercial products.
19. Please expand on any of your above responses, and/or provide any additional comments regarding this chapter:

INVASIVE FUNGAL INFECTIONS

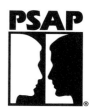

By RUSSELL E. LEWIS, PHARM.D., FCCP, BCPS (AQ-ID)

Reviewed by Douglas Slain, Pharm.D., FCCP, BCPS (AQ-ID); and Nancy E. Flentge, Pharm.D., BCPS

LEARNING OBJECTIVES

1. Detect epidemiologic risk factors associated with recent invasive fungal infection outbreaks in patients without immunocompromise.
2. Judge whether current evidence supports a prophylactic versus preemptive antifungal therapeutic approach for managing invasive candidiasis in non-neutropenic patients.
3. Justify the frontline use of combination therapy for cryptococcal meningitis and invasive aspergillosis.
4. Develop an algorithm for therapeutic drug monitoring of antifungals.
5. Analyze the advantages of newer triazole antifungals and formulations.

INTRODUCTION

Fungal infections have an enormous impact on human health. Superficial fungal infections of the skin and nails are among the most common human afflictions, affecting one-quarter of the world's population (around 1.8 billion people) (Havlickova 2008). Some 50%–75% of women of childbearing age will develop at least one episode of vulvovaginal candidiasis, with 4%–8% experiencing more than four infections per year (Sobel 2007). Infection with HIV/AIDS is associated with an additional 10 million cases of oropharyngeal candidiasis and 2 million cases of esophageal candidiasis yearly; this infection is especially prevalent in developing countries with limited health care resources. Even in developed countries, oral thrush is a common problem in neonates, denture wearers, users of inhaled corticosteroids, and those with immunocompromise.

In contrast to superficial fungal infections, invasive fungal infections are much less common but of greater medical concern because of their disproportionately high rates of mortality. One study team estimated that 1.5 million people die each year from the 10 most common invasive fungal diseases (Table 2-1), which is higher than World Health Organization mortality estimates for tuberculosis (1.4 million) and malaria (1.2 million) (Brown 2012). However, in all probability, those numbers

---

BASELINE KNOWLEDGE STATEMENTS

Readers of this chapter are presumed to be familiar with the following:
- Basic microbiology of invasive fungal pathogens
- Pharmacology of systemic antifungal agents
- Pathophysiology and common risk factors for common invasive fungal infections
- General treatment principles of invasive candidiasis, cryptococcal meningitis, and invasive aspergillosis

ADDITIONAL READINGS

The following free resources are available for readers wishing additional background information on this topic. Infectious Diseases Society of America treatment guidelines for:
- Aspergillosis
- Blastomycosis
- Cryptococcosis
- Coccidiodomycosis
- Candidiasis
- Histoplasmosis

underestimate the true mortality burden of invasive fungal disease, considering that the four most common infections (i.e., cryptococcosis, invasive candidiasis, invasive aspergillosis, and *Pneumocystis jiroveci* pneumonia) are often underdiagnosed and are not reportable to public health agencies.

Recent unprecedented outbreaks of fungal disease in immunocompetent patient populations have also raised public awareness. In 2012, a Massachusetts pharmacy compounded methylprednisolone contaminated with dematiaceous mold *Exserohilum rostratum*, which was responsible for one of the largest health care–associated infection outbreaks in U.S. history. A total of 751 patients in 20 states developed fungal infections of the central nervous system (CNS) or joints after epidural or articular injections with the contaminated steroid. For reasons that are not clear, smaller regional outbreaks of histoplasmosis, blastomycosis, and coccidioidomycosis are also being reported with greater frequency in immunocompetent populations.

This chapter reviews recent changes in the epidemiology of invasive fungal infections and key studies published in the past 3 years regarding the treatment of invasive candidiasis, cryptococcosis, and invasive aspergillosis. New data are presented concerning the role of therapeutic drug monitoring in antifungal use, emerging toxicities from long-term antifungal use, and newer triazole antifungal formulations and drugs.

EPIDEMIOLOGY

U.S. Multistate Fungal Meningitis Outbreak

In September 2012, the Tennessee Department of Health received a report of fungal meningitis in a patient in his 50s who had a history of degenerative lumbar disc and joint disease but was not immunocompromised

Table 2-1. Top 10 Invasive Fungal Pathogens

Disease (most common species)	Location	Estimated number of life-threatening infections/year	Mortality rates (% in infected population)
Opportunistic invasive mycoses			
Cryptococcosis	Worldwide	> 1,000,000	30-95
Pneumocystis	Worldwide	> 400,000	46-75
Candidiasis	Worldwide	> 400,000	20-70
Aspergillosis	Worldwide	> 200,000	30-90
Mucormycosis	Worldwide	> 10,000	20-80
Endemic dimorphic mycoses[a]			
Blastomycosis (*Blastomyces dermatitidis*)	Midwestern and Atlantic United States	~ 3000	< 2-68
Coccidioidomycosis (*Coccidioides immitis/ Coccidioides posadasii*)	Southwestern United States	~ 25,000	< 1-70
Histoplasmosis (*Histoplasma capsulatum*)	Midwestern United States	~ 25,000	28-50
Paracoccidioidomycosis (*Paracoccidioides brasiliensis*)	Brazil	~ 4000	5-27
Penicilliosis (*Penicillium marneffei*)	Southwest Asia	> 8000	2-75

[a]Endemic dimorphic fungal data estimated were limited to U.S. regions where reporting was considered accurate; however these infections can occur at many locations throughout the world.

Information from: Brown GD, Denning DW, Gow NAR, et al. Hidden killers: human fungal infections. Sci Transl Med 2012;4:165rv13.

(Pettit 2012). Four weeks before admission, the patient had received the last in a series of epidural injections of methylprednisolone for low back pain. The patient presented with an 8-day history of headache and neck pain of progressing severity associated with malaise, nausea, fever, and chills. The patient initially improved on antibiotic therapy and was discharged home, but he was soon readmitted with worsening symptoms. A culture of cerebrospinal fluid from the first admission showed *Aspergillus fumigatus*, and the fluid was also positive for the *Aspergillus* galactomannan antigen. Despite treatment with voriconazole and liposomal amphotericin B, the patient developed multiple cerebral and cerebellar infarcts and died 22 days after admission. At autopsy, multiple areas of fungal hyphal invasion were found in the brain and in the area of the lumbar spinal leptomeninges compatible with direct inoculation of fungal spores into the epidural space. Within 1 week, seven additional meningitis cases following epidural injections were identified in patients treated at the same clinic, and a common source was identified: compounded, preservative-free methylprednisolone from the New England Compounding Center (NECC) in Framingham, Massachusetts (Kainer 2012).

Once the source was identified, the Centers for Disease Control and Prevention (CDC) and state health departments mobilized to contact 13,534 potentially exposed patients and prescribers in 23 states who may have received or administered contaminated methylprednisolone purchased from NECC. Unlike the index patient, subsequent cases were positive for *E. rostratum*, a dematiaceous mold rarely associated with human infections. *E. rostratum* was subsequently cultured from unopened, compounded methylprednisolone vials at NECC. The CDC quickly developed a diagnostic polymerase chain reaction (PCR) assay for cerebrospinal fluid, standardized case definitions for infection, and drafted provisional diagnostic and treatment recommendations for this rare mold despite virtually no published human data.

Voriconazole was proposed to be the preferred treatment for *E. rostratum* meningitis based on the agent's excellent penetration into the CNS and cerebrospinal fluid compared with other triazoles (e.g., posaconazole) despite minimum inhibitory concentrations (MICs) relatively higher than *Aspergillus* spp. (i.e., 1–4 mcg/mL) (Pappas 2013). Consequently, the initial CDC recommendation for patients with suspected infection was to administer high doses of intravenous voriconazole (6 mg/kg every 12 hours), with verification of serum drug trough concentrations of at least 2–5 mcg/mL weekly for the first 6 weeks of therapy. De-escalation of voriconazole dosages to 4 mg/kg every 12 hours was recommended if patients were later confirmed not to have involvement of the spine. In patients with more severe clinical presentation (e.g., overt meningitis, hemorrhagic stroke), initial recommendations included the addition of high-dose liposomal amphotericin B (7.5 mg/kg daily) to the voriconazole regimen.

Subsequent recommendations advised a lower dose (5–6 mg/kg/day) secondary to high rates of nephrotoxicity in the predominantly older population afflicted by the outbreak (Pappas 2013).

With the intensive outreach on the parts of the CDC and public health departments, patients were identified earlier and treated before progressing to overt meningitis with hemorrhagic or ischemic stroke. During the second half of the outbreak, exposed patients were more likely to present with indolent forms of the infection, including epidural abscess, phlegmon, discitis, or vertebral osteomyelitis. Nevertheless, those infections created a diagnostic predicament because of the long latency period after injections with the contaminated steroid (up to 8 months) and symptoms that overlapped the patients' previous chronic back or joint pain. Clinical management was further complicated by the limited sensitivity of laboratory diagnosis for this unusual pathogen (only 30% of cases were positive for PCR, culture, or histopathology). As a result, many asymptomatic exposed patients were subjected to repeated lumbar punctures and MRI of the spine over the following months, whereas other patients opted to receive months of empiric voriconazole therapy.

Eventually, 751 fungal infection cases in 20 states were linked to the *E. rostratum*–contaminated methylprednisolone, resulting in an attack rate of 5% and 64 deaths (8.5%). Perhaps the most important lesson learned from that outbreak was the importance of coordination between local, state, and national public health agencies for rapid response to uncommon infection outbreaks (Bell 2013). In the absence of clinical data, real-time diagnostic algorithms and treatment strategies also had to be developed; these strategies used expert input for a rare pathogen causing infection in unusual sites because virtually no data existed to define optimal treatment or length of therapy (Pappas 2013).

Clinicians also learned about the tolerability of high-dose systemic antifungal therapy. High dosages of liposomal amphotericin B (7.5 mg/kg/daily) were associated with unacceptable nephrotoxicity rates in this mostly older population. High-dose voriconazole was associated with significantly increased rates (65%) of severe CNS adverse effects and hallucinations (distinct from visual disturbances) versus what had been reported with standard doses (2%–6%). One-third of patients developed significant increases in serum transaminases, with many more patients complaining of cognitive difficulties, memory loss, and indecisiveness. Patients commonly reported nausea, vomiting, and extreme fatigue along with cheilitis, alopecia, and skin and nail changes. Voriconazole-associated periostitis (caused by excessive fluoride levels) and severe phototoxic reactions were also reported with high-dose therapy (discussed in the following).

Finally, the 2012 outbreak exposed inadequacies in the U.S. Food and Drug Administration (FDA) and state

91

oversight of the compounding pharmacies that manufacture and distribute sterile products. In response, the Drug Quality and Security Act, aimed at regulating compounding pharmacies and establishing a track-and-trace pedigree system for compounded drugs, was signed into law in 2013. Because many aspects of the law are voluntary and will be phased in over a decade (Outterson 2013), it is unclear whether sufficient safeguards are now in place to prevent future rare fungal pathogen outbreaks of a similar scope.

Endemic Mycosis Outbreaks

Histoplasmosis, blastomycosis, and coccidioidomycosis are invasive fungal infections caused by inhalation of thermally dimorphic conidia (spores) of *Histoplasma capsulatum*, *Blastomyces dermatitidis*, and *Coccidioides immitis*/*Coccidioides posadasii*. Depending on the inoculum exposure and immune function of the host, those fungi can produce disease ranging from self-limited mild pneumonia to lethal disseminated disease, especially in patients with suppressed cell-mediated immunity (e.g., patients with AIDS, patients taking high-dose corticosteroids, patients on tumor-necrosis-factor-α inhibitor therapy, or patients with transplants and receiving immunosuppressive therapy). Although those mycoses are found worldwide, the majority of reported infections are endemic to certain regions of the United States: the Ohio and Mississippi River Valleys for histoplasmosis; the Great Lakes region and southeastern and south-central states bordering the Mississippi and Ohio River basins for blastomycosis, and southern Arizona, West Texas, and the southern and central valleys of California and southwestern New Mexico for coccidioidomycosis (Table 2-2).

Outbreaks of histoplasmosis were recently described in healthy children and adults who participated in cave exploration, who were near camp bonfires whose wood was taken from large bird roosts, and who were involved volunteer work at campsites. All of those activities presumably result in aerosolization of soil heavily contaminated with bird or bat droppings, which enhances *H. capsulatum* growth.

In June 2012, 32 counselors at a city-sponsored day camp in Omaha developed acute respiratory illness after a pre-camp cleanup week which included activities such as raking leaves, cleaning picnic tables, and digging fire pits without wearing personal protective equipment. Bat excrement was present throughout the campsite and in many

Table 2-2. Risk Factors for Invasive Fungal Infections in Immunocompetent Patients

Mycoses	Risk factors
Histoplasmosis	• Midwestern states along Ohio and Mississippi river valleys • Exposure to bat guano (cave exploration, campsites) or other large bird roosts, demolition or construction
Blastomycosis	• Southeastern and Midwestern states along Ohio and Mississippi river valleys, and Great Lakes region • Outdoor activities near waterways in great lakes region
Coccidioidomycosis	• Residence in Southern Arizona, Southern California, Southwest New Mexico or West Texas
Aspergillosis	• Preexisting lung cavities (e.g., tuberculosis) • Chronic obstructive pulmonary disease receiving inhaled corticosteroids • Cystic fibrosis
Mucormycosis	• Penetrating injuries from natural disasters (tornadoes, tsunamis, hurricane, volcanic eruptions) • Penetrating injuries from combat • Contamination of medical supplies (bandages, adhesive tape, wood tongue depressors, needles) • Contamination of bedding, hospital linens
Phaeohyphomycosis (*Exserohilum rostratum*)	• Injection with contaminated compounded preservative-free methylprednisolone
Fusariosis	Contaminated contact lens solution

camp shelters. Of the 32 counselors, 19 (59%) met a CDC-established case definition for histoplasmosis, with 10 (31%) requiring systemic antifungal therapy for their infections. Fortunately, no hospitalizations or deaths occurred.

Blastomycosis is endemic in Wisconsin, and previous outbreaks have been associated with recreational activities near waterways in the state. However, in 2009–2010, a large outbreak of blastomycosis cases (n=55) was reported in north-central Wisconsin clustered among Asian persons of Hmong ethnicity (Roy 2013). A majority of patients (70%) required hospitalization for antifungal therapy, and 2 deaths (5%) ensued. Unlike previous outbreaks, no outdoor activity or exposure linked the documented infections, which was suggestive of an unidentified, dispersed environmental source. Reasons for the predominance of cases among the Hmong population were perplexing but may have involved a yet-undefined genetic predisposition for infection in that population.

The incidence of coccidioidomycosis, also known as valley fever, has increased during the past decade, possibly because of the improved sensitivity of serologic diagnostic tests, changing weather patterns, and continued population growth in endemically affected areas. In American states where coccidioidomycosis is a reportable disease, incidence increased from 5.3 cases per 100,000 persons in 1998 to 42.6 cases per 100,000 persons in 2011. About 20,000 cases are reported annually in the United States, with more than 60% of them in Arizona. Concentrated outbreaks of coccidioidomycosis required the closure of two state prisons in the San Joaquin Valley in California because of exceedingly high attack rates in the inmate populations.

Although most people exposed to coccidioidomycosis do not become ill, about 160 exposed individuals die from coccidioidomycosis annually, with thousands more patients facing years of disability and surgery. About 9% of infected patients contract severe pneumonia, and 1% potentially develop CNS infections that are incurable with current systemic antifungals.

Newer triazoles (voriconazole, posaconazole, and, in the future, isavuconazole) have good activity against endemic fungi, but clinical experience with those agents is limited. Therefore, current treatment guidelines still largely recommend itraconazole, fluconazole (select cases of coccidioidomycosis), and amphotericin B as the main treatments for endemic mycoses.

Most patients with histoplasmosis do not require antifungal therapy unless they have either moderate to severe pulmonary disease lasting more than 4 weeks or chronic cavitary disease. Itraconazole remains the preferred agent (loading doses of 200 mg three times daily and then 200 mg twice daily) with therapy continued for at least 6–12 weeks. Serum trough levels of itraconazole should be monitored periodically to ensure levels greater than 0.5 mcg/mL. In patients with severe pulmonary complications (e.g., hypoxemia, respiratory distress), treatment may be initiated with liposomal amphotericin

B (3 mg/kg/day) plus intravenous methylprednisolone 0.5–1 mg/kg/day to reduce pulmonary inflammation. After 1–2 weeks of therapy, patients can be transitioned to oral itraconazole if they have improved clinically.

Unlike acute histoplasmosis, most patients with blastomycosis require antifungal therapy. Treatment is initiated with itraconazole 200 mg three times daily for 3 days, followed by 200 mg twice daily for 6–12 months. Liposomal amphotericin 3–5 mg/kg/day is recommended as initial therapy for patients with severe disease or CNS involvement or in immunocompromised patients, and continued for 4–6 weeks, followed by itraconazole for at least 12 months.

Most immunocompetent patients with coccidioidomycosis do not initially require treatment but are monitored for evidence of progressing disease for at least 1 year. Alternatively, patients who are immunosuppressed, are pregnant, or have severe symptoms (e.g., greater than 10% loss in body weight, 3 weeks of fever, extensive pneumonia, anti-coccidioidal titers more than 1:16, disability, or symptoms persisting more than 2 months) require immediate treatment, typically with at least 400 mg/day of fluconazole or itraconazole. Although amphotericin B formulations are recommended in pregnant patients because of the teratogenic effects of triazoles, a recent Danish registration study did not find evidence of birth defects in the neonates of women who took itraconazole during their first trimester (Molgaard-Nielsen 2013). However, the majority of women analyzed in that registry received low cumulative doses of triazoles for thrush. Therefore, azoles should preferably be restricted until after the second trimester and then used only in desperate cases when amphotericin B therapy is not feasible.

Mucormycosis After Natural Disasters

Mucormycosis is a rare but aggressive mold infection that causes sinopulmonary or disseminated infections in patients with diabetic ketoacidosis, prolonged neutropenia, or severe immunosuppression after solid organ or hematopoietic stem cell transplantation. Outbreaks of skin and soft tissue mucormycosis are occasionally reported in less-immunocompromised or nonimmunocompromised patients after penetrating trauma with damp or soil-contaminated debris is sustained during a natural disaster (e.g., volcanic eruption, tsunami), combat explosions, or motor vehicle crash. Nosocomial outbreaks of mucormycosis have been linked to contaminated bandages, adhesive tape, wooden tongue depressors, ostomy bags, and even bed linens.

On May 22, 2011, a tornado with winds of more than 200 miles per hour struck Joplin, Missouri, resulting in 1000 injuries and 160 deaths. On June 3, a local physician notified public health services that 2 patients hospitalized with injuries sustained from the tornado had developed necrotizing fungal soft tissue infections. During the investigation, a total of 13 cases of soft tissue mucormycosis were identified, with 5 deaths (38%) (Neblett Fanfair 2012). All of the patients had tornado-related wounds, including fractures (85%), blunt trauma (69%), and penetrating trauma (38%). The CDC identified *Apophysomyces trapeziformis* as the causative Mucorales by DNA sequencing of infected tissue samples. In multivariate analysis, the risk of soft tissue mucormycosis was found to be linked to the number of penetrating wounds sustained. Most patients were initially treated with antibiotic therapy or antifungals without anti-Mucorales activity but were switched to lipid amphotericin B formulations once the diagnosis was suspected. No infections were reported among emergency personnel or first responders to the disaster. Nevertheless, this report highlights the importance of the environmental Mucorales fungus as a cause of necrotizing soft tissue infection after natural disaster or severe injury, and it should prompt early consideration of empiric lipid amphotericin B until the infection can be ruled out.

Antifungal Resistance Update

Antifungal resistance can be classified into microbiologic resistance, clinical resistance, or a combination of the two. Microbiologic resistance occurs when growth of the infecting organism occurs at antifungal concentrations higher than what suppresses growth of wild-type organisms that do not harbor acquired resistance mutations. Alternatively, clinical resistance occurs when antifungal concentrations required for growth inhibition in the laboratory exceed what can be safely achieved in patients (Pfaller 2012). Clinical break point (CBP) values define which MIC cutoff the clinicians treating the patient should consider nonsusceptible or resistant (i.e., which MIC ranges correspond to S, I, and R on the susceptibility report). Typically, CBPs are set by using (1) statistical analysis of MIC epidemiologic data (MIC population distributions), (2) genetic analysis of resistance mechanisms, (3) pharmacokinetic and pharmacodynamic studies, and (4) clinical outcome data from patients (Pfaller 2012).

Recently, the Clinical and Laboratory Standards Institute has lowered triazole and echinocandin CBPs for some *Candida* species in an attempt to improve the sensitivity of testing methods for detecting microbiologic-resistant subpopulations. As a result, *C. glabrata* resistance rates have increased for some triazoles and echinocandins—specifically, for micafungin (n=354 isolates tested; 0.8%–7.6%), anidulafungin (n=110 isolates tested; 0.9%–7.3%), and voriconazole (n=593 isolates tested; 0.1%–18.4%). Rates of fluconazole resistance among *C. albicans* (n=1196 isolates tested) also increased from 2.1%–5.7% (Fothergill 2014). Those changing CBPs have contributed in part to increasing rates of antifungal resistance in recent years. However, new patterns of emerging multidrug resistance, especially among *C. glabrata* and *A. fumigatus*, are becoming major concerns (Alexander 2013; Verweij 2007).

Echinocandin and Triazole Multidrug Resistance in *C. glabrata*

Echinocandins are among the preferred antifungal treatment regimens for invasive candidiasis, especially in critically ill patients, because of excellent safety and potency, including fluconazole-resistant strains (Pappas 2009). Echinocandins inhibit β-(1,3)-D-glucan synthase in susceptible fungi by targeting *FKS* catalytic subunits of the enzyme, which are encoded by three genes: *FKS1*, *FKS2*, and *FKS3*. Mutations in those *FKS* genes result in an increase in the MICs for all three echinocandins. Several case series have suggested a correlation between clinical failure of echinocandin therapy and presence of *FKS* mutations in *C. glabrata* (Shields 2012).

In the past, *FKS*-resistance mutations were rarely detected in epidemiologic studies, confirming the widely held belief that echinocandin resistance was rare. Widespread use of echinocandins in the past decade, however, has brought selective pressure in many institutions for the emergence of echinocandin-resistant strains. For example, one team reported a significant increase in echinocandin resistance at Duke University Medical Center during 2001–10 (Alexander 2013). In an analysis of 293 episodes (313 isolates) of *C. glabrata* bloodstream infection, resistance increased from 4.9% to 12.3% among echinocandins (with 10.3% resistant to all three echinocandins) and from 18% to 30% with fluconazole. Among 78 fluconazole-resistant isolates, 14% were resistant to one or more echinocandins. Risk factors for isolation of *FKS* mutant strains included solid-organ transplantation, multiple episodes of *C. glabrata* bloodstream infection, and prior echinocandin therapy. Although those data are derived from a single institution and may not reflect susceptibility trends at other institutions, they underscore the importance of both rapid identification of *Candida* to the species level and antifungal susceptibility testing to detect such clinically important resistance trends. Most patients with echinocandin-resistant strains were treated successfully with lipid amphotericin B formulations or triazole-echinocandin combinations.

A more recent, population-based analysis of echinocandin resistance performed by the CDC in four U.S. cities (Atlanta, Baltimore, Knoxville, and Portland) reported that 3.1%–3.8% of *C. glabrata* isolates (n=1032 isolates tested) are resistant to multiple echinocandins (Pham 2014).

Triazole Resistance in *Aspergillus* spp.

The 2008 Infectious Diseases Society of America guidelines for invasive aspergillosis marginally recommended antifungal-susceptibility testing for triazole resistance in patients who had positive cultures—especially in the context of prior azole therapy—although it was recognized that there were very limited clinical data to support that recommendation (Walsh 2008). Since the publication of those guidelines, reports of multi-triazole and multi-drug resistance in *Aspergillus* spp. have increased. In 2007, a

Patient Care Scenario

A 52-year-old man with relapsed acute myeloid leukemia (AML) presents with cough and fever 2 months after starting salvage chemotherapy with a current absolute neutrophil count (ANC) of 200 cells/mm^3. He is not currently taking antibacterial or antifungal prophylaxis. The patient was admitted to the hospital and treated with vancomycin and cefepime for a small lobar infiltrate observed on chest radiography. On the third day of treatment, the patient had persistent fever and experienced a seizure that lasted for 30 minutes despite administration of lorazepam and phenytoin. The patient required intubation and was transferred to the intensive care unit for further management. High-resolution computer tomography revealed multiple hypodense lesions in the brain and lung.

Answer

Although survival rates with invasive aspergillosis have improved over the last decade with earlier diagnosis and new treatment options, patients with advanced hematological malignancies can still present with disseminated infection associated with high mortality. Clearly, a patient with relapsing AML and disseminated infection involving the brain has a poor prognosis that in the past was 100% fatal. In the voriconazole era, average survival rates have improved to 30%–40% and may be as high as 60% if patients are diagnosed early and have not previously received antifungals. Nevertheless, there are other issues to consider in this patient that may have contributed to voriconazole failure. First, despite receiving a relatively high-dose voriconazole therapy (6 mg/kg every 12 hours) the patient had relatively low serum trough concentrations on the fifth day of therapy. This

The patient was started on 6 mg/kg of voriconazole every 12 hours. A serum galactomannan was positive at an index of 2.8. The patient underwent bronchoscopy, which subsequently revealed positive cultures for *Aspergillus fumigatus*. Serum trough concentrations of voriconazole on the fifth day of therapy were 0.5 mcg/mL. Unfortunately, fever persisted and a repeat CT scan demonstrated progression of the brain and lung lesions. The patient was switched to liposomal amphotericin B 5 mg/kg/daily plus caspofungin 50 mg per day. Unfortunately, the patient continued to deteriorate on the combination regimen and later died. What are the most likely reasons for the failure of antifungal therapy in this patient?

could be the result of a drug interaction, particularly if the patient was still receiving phenytoin, which is an inducer of cytochrome P450 enzymes.

Another possibility is that the isolate is resistant to voriconazole. *Aspergillus fumigatus* isolates are not routinely subjected to susceptibility testing in many hospitals because resistance has been previously considered to be a rare phenomenon. Nevertheless, in a case similar to the one described above, investigators in the Netherlands noticed that isolates recovered from the lungs of patients who failed voriconazole frequently exhibited elevated MICs (> 2 mcg/mL) to voriconazole and other triazoles, and these isolates were untreatable with triazole monotherapy when tested in animal infection models.

1. Schwartz S, Ruhnke M, Ribaud P, et al. Improved outcome in central nervous system aspergillosis, using voriconazole treatment. Blood 2005;106:2641-5.
2. Pascual A, Csajka C, Buclin T, et al. Challenging recommended oral and intravenous voriconazole doses for improved efficacy and safety: Population pharmacokinetics–based analysis of adult patients with invasive fungal infections. Clin Infect Dis 2012;55:381-90.
3. Verweij PE, Mellado E, Melchers WJG. Multiple-triazole–resistant aspergillosis. N Engl J Med 2007;356:1481-3.

new mechanism of resistance in *A. fumigatus*—associated with amino acid substitutions in the *cyp51a* gene that encodes 14-alpha demethylase target inhibited by triazoles and an upstream gene promoter (TL/L98H)—was identified among 13 isolates cultured from 9 patients in the Netherlands. Two of the 9 patients died while receiving voriconazole or posaconazole therapy. Isolates with that mutation exhibit elevated and possibly untreatable MICs (> 2 mcg/mL) to voriconazole, itraconazole, and, often posaconazole (MICs > 0.5 mcg/mL). Surprisingly, 4 of the 9 patients (44%) had not received prior azole therapy, suggesting a possible environmental source.

In a follow-up analysis conducted by the same researchers, the same dominant resistance mechanism (TL/L98H) was identified in environmental cultures of the hospital and surrounding community, suggesting patients were colonized with the resistant isolates before admission to the hospital (Rijs 2009). Notably, azole fungicides are widely used in the Netherlands to prevent pre- and

postharvest spoilage in grain. Azoles are also used for preservation of materials such as paints, coatings, and wallpaper pastes and are routinely applied to mattresses to prevent fungal growth.

Azole-resistant *A. fumigatus* has been reported in China, Canada, the United States, and several European countries, with especially high levels in the Netherlands and the United Kingdom. Other *cyp51a* mutations have also been identified that can confer varying degrees of resistance to voriconazole and posaconazole. In the United Kingdom, a national referral center for fungal diseases in Manchester reported that triazole resistance rates among *Aspergillus* climbed from 0% in 1997–98 to 5% in 2004–05, 17% in 2007, and 20% in 2009 among the 230 isolates tested (Bueid 2010). During 2008–09, 78% of triazole resistant-strains were reistant to multiple agents, but 43% of isolates did not have the previously identified *cyp51a* mutations, suggesting that azole-resistant strains of *A. fumigatus* are not only increasing but also evolving new resistance mechanisms (Pfaller 2012).

Optimal treatment regimens for triazole-resistant *A. fumigatus* infections are still not well defined. Experimental infections induced with the resistant strains in animal models responded to treatment with either combination regimens consisting of lipid amphotericin B formulations and echinocandins or higher dosages of triazoles (i.e., individualized dosing to maintain troughs of 2–5 mg/L) in combination with echinocandins.

Similar to *Candida* spp., those trends point to the growing need for routine susceptibility testing of *Aspergillus* spp. in both clinical and, possibly, environmental isolates. Clearly, centers that do not perform susceptibility testing for *Aspergillus* spp. will not find evidence of resistance, perhaps leading to a false sense of security. Testing also requires isolation of *Aspergillus* spp. in pure culture, which is becoming less common because patients are getting diagnosed earlier by means of high-resolution computed tomography (CT) and the serum galactomannan antigen test. Therefore, nonculture PCR-based assays may ultimately be required to detect those resistance mutations. Nevertheless, the emerging resistance patterns could have enormous therapeutic consequences for the future use of the triazole antifungals in the prevention and treatment of invasive aspergillosis.

MANAGEMENT OF INVASIVE FUNGAL INFECTIONS

New Diagnostic Approaches for Invasive Candidiasis

Invasive candidiasis remains a common infection in neutropenic and nonneutropenic critically ill patients, with crude mortality rates of 30%–40% despite antifungal therapy. It has become increasingly evident that difficulty in early diagnosis of the infection remains a major challenge in reducing the mortality associated with the infection. Invasive candidiasis encompasses several infectious syndromes broadly categorized as candidemia or deep-seated infections (infections of tissue sites beneath mucosal surfaces). About one-third of all patients with invasive candidiasis fall into one of three groups at the time of diagnosis: (1) patients with candidemia in the absence of deep-seated candidiasis, (2) candidemia associated with deep-seated candidiasis, and (3) deep-seated candidiasis without candidemia (Clancy 2013).

Invasive candidiasis is most commonly diagnosed by blood culture, which probably identifies (1) the majority of patients with candidemia alone, (2) fewer patients with a combination of deep-seated disease and intermittent candidemia, and (3) virtually no patients who have infection limited to deep tissues at the time of culture. As a result, one-half of all episodes of invasive candidiasis are missed by blood cultures. Therefore, the development of new

diagnostic tools that do not rely exclusively on microbiologic isolation of *Candida* has become a priority (Clancy 2013).

Several non–culture-based diagnostic tests have shown promise for early diagnosis of invasive candidiasis and ar being increasingly used in some hospitals during routine patient care. β-D-glucan (BDG) is a cell wall constituent of *Candida* species and several other fungi that can be detected in as little as 1 hour by using a modification of a common bacterial endotoxin assay. Generally, patients at risk are tested twice weekly and two consecutive positive results greater than 60 pg/mL are considered positive. In a recent meta-analysis of 11 diagnostic studies, the sensitivity of the BDG test for detecting invasive candidiasis was 75%, with a specificity of 56%–96%. Specifically, false-positive results are observed more often in patients in intensive care units (ICUs) who have gram-positive or gram-negative bacteremia and are receiving antibiotics or human blood products, patients with wounds covered with surgical gauze or dressings (which can contain glucan), patients undergoing hemodialysis, and patients with chemotherapy-associated mucositis (Karageorgopoulos 2012). Limited clinical experience also suggests that decreasing BDG levels correlates with treatment response to echinocandin antifungals.

Antibody-detection strategies based on detection of the *Candida* cell wall polysaccharide, mannan, or IgG antimannan antibodies have shown some promise for the diagnosis of candidemia and deep-seated candidiasis, with reported sensitivity and specificity rates of 83% and 87%, respectively. Notably, the performance of the assay is not consistent across all *Candida* species with limited detection of *C. parapsilosis* and *C. guilliermondii*. It is also unclear how antifungal therapy and severe immunosuppression may influence test performance.

Finally, a number of PCR-based diagnostic platforms for invasive candidiasis have been studied; these offer the advantages of higher sensitivity (including deep-seated infections) and faster diagnosis, often preceding positive blood cultures by 1–28 days. In a meta-analysis of those assays, the pooled sensitivity and specificity estimates of PCR-based tests were reported at 95% and 92%, respectively. However, lower specificity may be observed in patients colonized with *Candida*, which is common in patients in ICUs (Avni 2010). Nucleic-acid-based techniques are also useful for shortening the time it takes for definitive identification of yeast cultures to the species level (i.e., species-specific PNA FISH probe for rapid identification of *C. glabrata*). Other techniques such as matrix-assisted laser desorption/ionization time of flight (MALDI-TOF) and magnetic-resonance-based technologies have shown promise for identifying *Candida* species in whole blood specimens in as little as 3 hours, which could shorten the time to earlier diagnosis.

Understanding the potential clinical utility of such tests requires consideration of the overall prevalence of inasive candidiasis in the ICU, which averages in many centers from 1% to 3%. Specifically, would a positive BDG test alone in an ICU patient justify preemptively starting antifungal therapy even if the patient is afebrile? If a post-test probability of infection of more than 20% would justify starting antifungal therapy, then a positive BDG test alone may not warrant starting antifungal therapy in asymptomatic ICU patients because these patients would be predicted to have a probability of infection of only 10% with a positive test (Figure 2-1). This is especially true considering the likelihood of false-positive results. However, two consecutive negative BDG tests could rule out infection by lowering the patient's post-test probability of infection to less than 1%. If a higher-prevalence subpopulation (e.g., 20%) could be identified a priori by using a validated risk model or score (Ostrosky-Zeichner 2011), then BDG screening of a this population might improve the clinical utility of the test for diagnosing occult invasive candidiasis (40%), thereby justifying preemptive antifungal use. The latter example of identifying a high-risk subgroup for screening with a non-culture-based diagnostic test is the basis of preemptive diagnostic-driven approaches for using antifungal therapy rather than an empiric or symptom- or fever-driven strategy when the patient already has active infection. The possibility of preemptive therapy was a major consideration in a recent National Institute of Allergy and Infectious Diseases Mycoses Study Group (NIAID/MSG) trial of caspofungin prophylaxis for invasive candidiasis in the ICU.

Echinocandin Prophylaxis for Invasive Candidiasis in the ICU

Given the excess mortality associated with invasive candidiasis in the ICU, antifungal prophylaxis may be warranted in high-risk populations (e.g., patients undergoing liver transplantation). Nevertheless, routine use of antifungal prophylaxis is associated with increased risk of resistance, increased toxicity, and increased cost. An alternative approach would be to treat high-risk ICU patients preemptively before evidence of infection as seen from screening by using a non-culture-based diagnostic test such as BDG as described above. Yet no large or multicenter studies have examined the efficacy and safety of either invasive candidiasis prophylaxis or a preemptive-treatment approach.

In 2014, the NIAID/MSG completed a randomized, double-blind, placebo-controlled trial of caspofungin prophylaxis followed by preemptive therapy for invasive candidiasis among patients at high risk in the ICU setting (Ostrosky-Zeichner 2014). The study used a validated invasive candidiasis risk-prediction score that identified

---

Pivotal Study That May Change Practice

MSG-01: A randomized, double-blind placebo-controlled trial of caspofungin prophylaxis followed by preemptive therapy for invasive candidiasis in high-risk adults in the critical care setting. Clin Infect Dis 2014;58:12-26.

Setting: Invasive candidiasis is the third most common bloodstream infection in the intensive care unit associated with excess mortality, but antifungal prophylaxis or preemptive treatment strategies utilizing infection biomarkers had not been examined in prospective, multicenter clinical trials.

Design: Multicenter, randomized, double-blinded, placebo controlled trial of caspofungin as antifungal prophylaxis in 222 adults with risk-score predicted incidence of invasive candidiasis of at least 20% in the placebo arm (ICU for at least 3 days, receiving mechanical ventilation, antibiotic therapy, central venous catheter, and one additional risk factor (parenteral nutrition, dialysis, surgery, pancreatitis, systemic steroids or other immunosuppressant therapy). Subjects had their serum β-D-glucan measured twice weekly. The primary end point was the incidence of proven or probable candidiasis by EORTC/MSG criteria in patients who did not have infection at baseline. Patients with proven or probable invasive candidiasis (most frequently diagnosed by BDG) were unblinded and allowed to receive caspofungin (preemptive treatment), including patients found to have a positive BDG or culture at baseline.

Outcomes: The incidence of proven or probable invasive candidiasis in the placebo and caspofungin arms was 16.7% vs. 9.8% for prophylaxis (p=0.14) and 30.4% vs. 18.8% for the preemptive approach (p=0.04). No significant differences were found between caspofungin and placebo in mortality, safety outcomes, additional antifungal use or length of ICU stay within 7 days.

Impact: This is the first multicenter clinical trial to compare echinocandin prophylaxis versus placebo for invasive candidiasis in the ICU. In the end, the trial did not have sufficient power to demonstrate a significant reduction in the incidence of invasive candidiasis with echinocandin prophylaxis. Although the incidence of invasive candidiasis was predicted to be 20% in the placebo arm and less than 5% in the caspofungin arm, the actual incidence rates were 16.7% and 9.8%, respectively. Nevertheless, preemptive administration of an echinocandin was associated with lower rates of proven or probable invasive candidiasis, even though this analysis included some patients with candidemia at the time of enrollment (Muldoon and Denning 2014). Therefore a pure preemptive strategy (i.e. BDG or PCR screening of non-neutropenic ICU patients) requires further study before it can be recommended as a treatment approach for ICU patients.

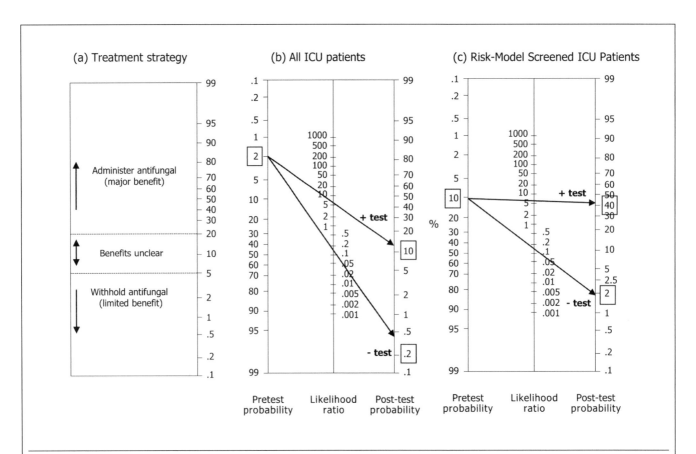

Figure 2-1. Possible impact of β-D-glucan assay on pre-and post-test probability of invasive candidiasis. Estimates were generated using recently published predictive performance data published for the β-D-glucan assay as an example (positive likelihood ratio 6.03 [95% CI 4.25-8.57], negative likelihood ratio 0.15 [95% CI 0.07-0.29]) (Held 2013). The pretest probability of invasive candidiasis is estimated based on a (b) general ICU population-2%; or a risk-score identified subpopulation (c) 10%. Likelihood ratios were convert pre-test and to post-test probability using the Bayes theorem algorithms presented above.

18% of patients admitted to the ICU with a predicted invasive candidiasis incidence rate of more than 10%.

In the end, no benefit was found with caspofungin prophylaxis in terms of reducing the incidence of proven or probable invasive candidiasis or patient mortality. Therefore, prophylaxis among nonneutropenic patients should be restricted to patient populations with proven benefit: post-gastrointestinal perforation, severe pancreatitis, liver/pancreas or small-bowel transplant recipients, and extremely-low-birth-weight neonates in units with high rates of invasive candidiasis (Pappas 2009). Nevertheless, the study provided some evidence that a preemptive approach using BDG might be feasible and could significantly reduce the incidence of invasive candidiasis among selected patients at high risk.

Impact of Treatment Outcomes on Invasive Candidiasis

The number of antifungal agents for invasive candidiasis has increased in the past 2 decades, yet the optimal treatment strategy is still largely unknown because non-inferiority registration trials do not typically have the power to demonstrate significant reductions in all-cause mortality. One team performed patient-level reviews of seven randomized trials of invasive candidiasis published in the past 2 decades to identify the treatment variables associated with 30-day crude mortality (Andes 2012). The authors' database contained 1915 patients with a crude 30-day mortality rate of 31.4% and an antifungal treatment success rate of 67.4%. On one hand, the authors found that increasing age, APACHE II score, use of immunosuppressive therapy, and infection with *C. tropicalis* were independent predictors of patient mortality. On the other hand, removal of central venous catheters and treatment with an echinocandin were associated with decreased mortality.

Although this paper is best viewed as a type of hybrid meta-analysis, it does support most of the invasive candidiasis treatment guidelines endorsed by the Infectious Diseases Society of America (Pappas 2009). Morover, that study confirmed that echinocandins should be considered first-line treatment for invasive candidiasis, even in less critically ill patients with lower APACHE II scores (Clancy 2012). Certain experts have questioned the findings related specifically to improved mortality among patients who had catheter removal, because that variable was not well standardized across clinical trials (i.e., a possible bias toward earlier removal in less-ill patients cannot be excluded). In addition, the studies used in the analysis did not specifically compare responses for deep-tissue candidiasis, especially at anatomic sites where echinocandin penetration is poor (e.g., meninges, endophthalmitis, urosepsis) (Felton 2014).

In an editorial accompanying that analysis, the author emphasized that the majority of independent risk factors for mortality identified suggest that underlying host illness is the major driver of outcomes. Therefore, further improvements in survival will require development and validation of early intervention strategies such as nonculture diagnostics and preemptive therapy (Clancy 2012).

Combination Therapy for Cryptococcal Meningitis

Increased access to antiretroviral therapy has dramatically improved survival of patients with HIV infection who live in resource-limited areas. Nevertheless, diagnosis of HIV in such regions often occurs later, when many patients present with opportunistic infections. About 1 million cases of cryptococcal meningitis develop annually and are associated with 625,000 deaths, which exceeds the number of deaths attributed to tuberculosis (Park 2009).

The case fatality rate of cryptococcal meningitis in sub-Saharan Africa ranges from 35% to 65%, which is significantly higher than the rate in most developed countries (10%–20%). Reasons for the higher mortality include delayed diagnosis, limited ability to manage life-threatening complications (e.g., elevated intracranial pressure) because of insufficient access to resources, and scarce availability of first-line antifungal treatments amphotericin B and flucytosine.

Amphotericin B (0.7–1.0 mg/kg/day) plus flucytosine (100 mg/kg day) is recommended as standard 2-week induction therapy for cryptococcal meningitis (Perfect 2010). This regimen has long been known to produce faster sterilization of the cerebrospinal fluid and lower risk of relapse. Yet that regimen has not been proved to increase survival over amphotericin B monotherapy. Access to flucytosine is limited in many areas where the burden of cryptococcal meningitis is highest. Fluconazole is widely available and less toxic but it is also associated with higher failure rates when used as monotherapy. Therefore, a key question is whether flucytosine is actually needed as part of combination therapy for cryptococcal meningitis, or if fluconazole could be administered with amphotericin B as an equivalent induction regimen.

This question was addressed in a landmark study—a randomized, three-group, open-label trial of induction antifungal therapy for cryptococcal meningitis. Patients (n=229) were randomized to receive either amphotericin B 1 mg/kg/day for 4 weeks; or a 2-week induction regimen of amphotericin B 1 mg/kg/day plus flucytosine (100 mg/

kg/day) or amphotericin B 1 mg/kg/day plus fluconazole (400 mg twice daily). Induction therapy was followed by a maintenance regimen of fluconazole 400 mg daily for 6 weeks. At 70 days after randomization, significantly

---

Pivotal Study That May Change Practice

Marr K, Schlamm H, Rottinghaus S, et al. A randomised, double-blind study of combination antifungal therapy with voriconazole and anidulafungin versus voriconazole monotherapy for primary treatment of invasive aspergillosis.

Setting: Invasive aspergillosis remains a common infectious complication of the treatment of hematological malignancies and hematopoietic stem cell transplantation. Voriconazole and echinocandins may be synergistic against *Aspergillus* species and have shown benefit in preclinical and small clinical studies, but evidence from a prospective clinical trial is lacking.

Design: Multicenter, randomized, placebo-controlled blinded, study in 93 sites, 24 countries. Patients (n=429) with hematological malignancies or recent allogeneic hematopoietic stem cell transplantation were randomized to receive intravenous voriconazole 6 mg/kg loading dose every 12 hours for 2 days followed by 4 mg/kg twice daily plus intravenous anidulafungin 200 mg loading dose on day 1, then 100 mg anidulafungin daily or voriconazole alone plus placebo. Patients remained on the combination for at least 2 weeks, which could be continued up to 4 weeks. After the first week of therapy, voriconazole could be transitioned to oral (300 mg twice daily) therapy. The primary end point of the trial was 6-week all- cause mortality, with secondary end points of safety and a global treatment response assessed by a blinded data review committee (DRC).

Outcomes: Most patients (79%) entered into the trial had a diagnosis of invasive aspergillosis based on radiographic findings and positive galactomannan antigen alone. In the modified intent to treat (mITT) population (i.e. treated patients with DRC-confirmed diagnosis of proven or probable aspergillosis), 6-week mortality was 19.3% for the combination and 27.5% for monotherapy, P=0.09. Other secondary end points favored combination therapy with no safety differences, however, DRC-assessments of treatment response actually favored patients randomized to voriconazole monotherapy, but were confounded by a high proportion of non-evaluable cases (i.e. patients did not have follow-up radiographic examination).

Impact: This is the first large, multicenter clinical trial to prospectively compare monotherapy versus combination therapy for invasive aspergillosis. In the end, the trial only had only moderate statistical power to detect a treatment effect, therefore only a trend towards improved survival with the combination was found compared to voriconazole. However, a greater benefit with combination therapy was observed in patients with earlier-diagnosed aspergillosis.

---

fewer deaths had occurred among patients receiving amphotericin B plus flucytosine versus patients receiving amphotericin B alone (hazard ratio 0.61; 95% confidence interval [CI], 0.39–0.97; p=0.04). Combination therapy with fluconazole had no significant impact on survival over amphotericin B monotherapy. Notably, the amphotericin B–flucytosine combination was associated with more-rapid clearance of yeast from the cerebrospinal fluid versus clearance by other regimens. Rates of adverse effects were similar in all groups, even though neutropenia was slightly more common in patients receiving amphotericin B–flucytosine or amphotericin B–fluconazole combinations versus amphotericin B monotherapy (34% and 32% vs. 19%, p=0.04). Notably, flucytosine levels were not monitored in patients (Day 2013).

The findings of this study are significant for two reasons. First, it was one of very few studies in infectious diseases (outside of highly active antiretroviral therapy for HIV and, possibly, tuberculosis treatment) in which a combination regimen that produces rapid clearance of pathogens at the site of infection was shown to significantly improve survival (Perfect 2013). Second, the study underscored an urgent need to improve (1) access to flucytosine availability in developing countries where the mortality burden of cryptococcosis is highest and (2) resources for early diagnosis and safe administration of amphotericin B.

Combination Therapy for Invasive Aspergillosis

Invasive aspergillosis remains a common infectious complication in patients with hematologic malignancies and in recipients of hematopoietic stem cell transplantation. Based on the results of a randomized trial in which voriconazole was associated with improved survival compared with amphotericin B deoxycholate followed by other FDA-approved antifungal therapy, voriconazole is currently recommended for treatment of invasive aspergillosis. Voriconazole blocks the synthesis of ergosterol, an essential structural component of the fungal cell membrane. As discussed above, anidulafungin, caspofungin, and micafungin are three similar echinocandin antifungals that block the synthesis of branched β-glucan in the fungal cell wall. Multiple studies in vitro and in animal models, as well as small clinical studies, have suggested that administration of an echinocandin with voriconazole may be synergistic and improve survival. Until recently, prospective clinical studies have been lacking.

Results were recently published from a multicenter, randomized clinical trial comparing voriconazole-anidulafungin combination therapy with voriconazole monotherapy. This trial enrolled patients at 93 sites in 26 countries from July 2008 to May 2011. In a unique departure from previous studies of invasive aspergillosis, the primary end point of the study was all-cause mortality at 6 weeks after randomization—a period identified in previous clinical trials as representing the period of highest risk of death attributable to mold infection.

After enrollment of 454 patients, 277 met the criteria for proven or probable aspergillosis (135 patients for combination therapy, 142 voriconazole monotherapy). Most of the patients (218/277, or 79%) were diagnosed by CT findings and a positive serum or bronchoalveolar lavage galactomannan antigen; only a minority (11%) of patients were diagnosed by culture of histopathology. When the study was unblinded, 6-week mortality was found to be lower in modified-intent-to-treat patients randomized to receive the combination versus voriconazole monotherapy (19.3% vs. 27.5%; p=0.09; 95% CI, -19.0 to 1.5%). The mortality difference between combination therapy versus monotherapy was even greater among a subpopulation of patients with diagnoses based solely on galactomannan antigen (17/108 or 15.7% vs. 30/110 or 27.3%; p=0.04; 95% CI, -22.7 to-0.4%). Interestingly, assessment of overall treatment response by a blinded data review committee actually favored patients randomized to the monotherapy arm (43% vs. 32.6%). However, the committee's analysis was confounded by a high proportion of patients who were nonevaluable after treatment (e.g., did not have follow-up chest CT scans), which may have been more common in patients with good clinical response on combination therapy.

Statistically, this trial fell short of demonstrating a significant survival benefit with combination therapy. The statistical assumptions underlying the trial design required combination therapy to be associated with 10% better survival rates—rates not reached in the primary study population (8.2% difference) but achieved in patients with galactomannan-diagnosed infection (11.2% difference). For clinicians, the question that remains is whether an 8%–11% improvement in survival is clinically significant even if it is not statistically significant in the context of this trial. For comparison, a landmark trial of posaconazole prophylaxis for patients with acute myeloid leukemia/myelodysplastic syndrome reported a 7% absolute risk reduction in all-cause mortality (number needed to treat [NNT] 14 patients to save 1 life). Therefore, a similar if not better survival benefit could be argued for combination therapy overall (NNT=12 patients) or for patients with galactomannan antigen–diagnosed disease (NNT= 9 patients).

Antifungal Therapeutic Drug Monitoring

Despite a lack of definitive data from large clinical trials, therapeutic drug monitoring (TDM) is becoming increasingly recognized as a useful tool for optimizing the efficacy and safety of certain antifungal agents. Generally, an antifungal must meet three criteria for antifungal TDM to be clinically useful. First, a sensitive assay must be available in the clinical laboratory or, possibly, in a reference laboratory that will report results back in a timely fashion. Otherwise, the monitoring's impact on clinical decisions will be limited. Second, the antifungal must have a well-established therapeutic range, such that a higher probability of treatment success and either acceptable or lower toxicity risk is shown if patients are dosed to maintain concentrations within that therapeutic window. Finally, the drug must have significant intra- or interpatient pharmacokinetic variability, such that likely variations in drug exposure with standard dosages could jeopardize the effectiveness of therapy using standard dosing guidelines. Currently, four antifungals (flucytosine, itraconazole, voriconazole, and posaconazole oral solution) are considered to meet those criteria and have established indications or guidelines for TDM (Ashbee 2013; Andes 2009).

The question of whether TDM should be performed routinely in all patients versus only in select situations depends on clinical scenario, severity of infection, cost, and local availability of the assay. A growing consensus from clinical experience and case reports suggests several circumstances in which TDM can be helpful, and when those situations arise, more-intensive monitoring may be justified. Table 2-3 gives an overview of those clinical scenarios.

The therapeutic ranges for voriconazole and posaconazole have been defined primarily from single-center, retrospective studies and can be considered only general guides for dosing (Ashbee 2013). Moreover, it should be acknowledged that all of the systemic antifungal agents currently in clinical use are typically prescribed and dose-adjusted without resorting to TDM. Nevertheless, in a recent prospective, randomized, blinded, single-center trial of TDM during voriconazole therapy in 100 patients, the proportion of voriconazole discontinuations because of adverse events was significantly lower in the TDM group than in the non-TDM group (4% vs. 17%; $p=0.02$) (Park 2012). More important, higher rates of either complete or partial response were observed in patients managed with TDM versus those without (81% vs. 57%; $p=0.04$). That study and several others suggest that antifungal TDM may reduce drug discontinuation because of adverse events and improve the treatment response in invasive fungal infections. Figure 2-2 gives a sample algorithm for antifungal TDM in clinical practice.

Table 2-3. Therapeutic Drug Monitoring in the Prevention or Treatment of Invasive Fungal Infections

Clinical scenario	Examples, comment
Populations with increased pharmacokinetic variability	Impaired GI function; hepatic (voriconazole, posaconazole, itraconazole) or renal (flucytosine) dysfunction; pediatric patients, elderly patients, obese patients, critically-ill patients
Changing pharmacokinetics	Intravenous to oral switch, changing GI function, changing hepatic or renal function, physiological-instability
Interacting medications	Patient receiving medication that induce CYP3A4, antacids, proton-pump inhibitors (itraconazole capsules, posaconazole suspension), antiretroviral medications
Poor prognosis disease	Extensive or bulky infection, lesions contiguous with critical structures, CNS infection, multifocal or disseminated infection
Compliance	Important issue with prolonged outpatient therapy or secondary prophylaxis
Suspected breakthrough fungal infection	TDM can establish whether fungal disease progression occurred in the setting of inadequate antifungal exposure
Suspected drug toxicity, especially neurotoxicity (voriconazole) or hematological toxicity (flucytosine)	Although exposure-response relationships are described for other toxicities (e.g., hepatotoxicity), the utility of TDM to prevent their occurrence is less well established

Information from: Andes D, Pascual A, Marchetti O. Antifungal therapeutic drug monitoring: Established and emerging indications. Antimicrob Agents Chemother 2009;53:24-34; and Ashbee HR, Barnes RA, Johnson EM, et al. Therapeutic drug monitoring (TDM) of antifungal agents: guidelines from the British Society for Medical Mycology. J Antimicrob Chemother 2014;69:1162-76.

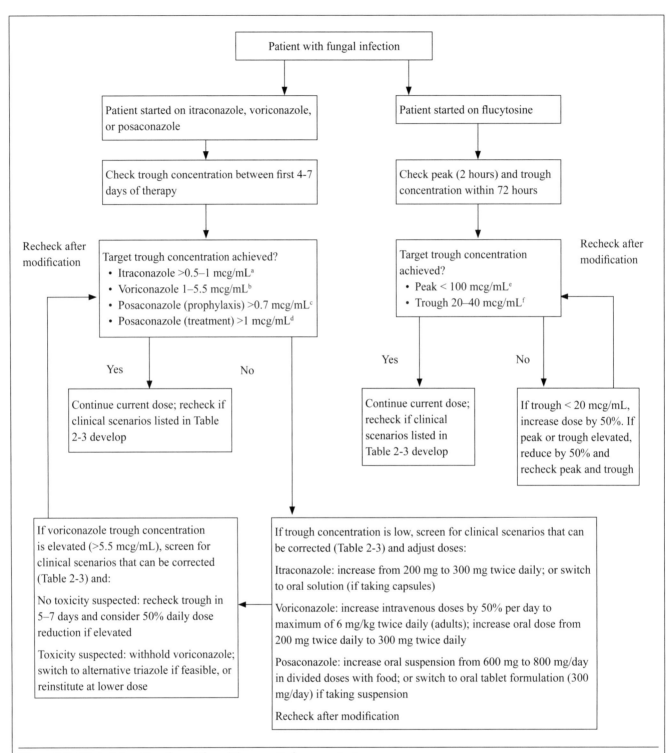

Figure 2-2. Clinical algorithm for antifungal therapeutic drug monitoring.

[a]Itraconazole serum troughs associated with efficacy, 0.5–1 mcg/mL; limited retrospective data have associated troughs of > 3 mcg/mL with increased adverse effects.

[b]Voriconazole troughs >1 mcg/mL are associated with a higher probability of clinical response; troughs > 5.5 mcg/mL are associated with higher incidence of CNS adverse effects.

[c]Posaconazole troughs of < 0.7 mcg/mL are associated with higher incidence of breakthrough fungal infections during prophylaxis.

[d]Posaconazole troughs > 1.0 mcg/mL were associated with higher probability of treatment response for invasive aspergillosis. Currently, no recommended trough threshold has been defined for toxicity.

[e]Flucytosine peak concentrations > 100 mcg/mL associated with increased risk of myelotoxicity.

[f]Flucytosine trough concentration of 20–40 mcg/mL recommended to prevent the rapid selection of resistance in yeast.

Emerging Chronic Antifungal Toxicities

Antifungal therapy can be associated with a number of potential adverse effects. The most common acute adverse effects are (1) infusion-related reactions with conventional and lipid amphotericin B formulations and echinocandins and (2) nephrotoxicity with amphotericin B therapy. Liver injury can occur with any antifungal, typically presenting as asymptomatic increases in serum aminotransferases and, less commonly, alkaline phosphatase or total bilirubin. Management of hepatic injury from antifungals is largely empiric and without clear recommendations. Although mild increases in serum transaminases (i.e., less than three times the upper limit of normal) often resolve spontaneously even with continued therapy, most clinicians switch to alternative antifungals if liver injury markers remain elevated or continue to increase over several days. Typically, patients may be switched from one class of antifungal to another (e.g., triazole to lipid amphotericin B) or to another drug in the same class (e.g., voriconazole to posaconazole) depending on clinical situation, infection status, and risk of toxicities or drug interactions with the alternative therapy. The incidence of liver injury reported in clinical trials is probably highest with itraconazole and voriconazole, followed by amphotericin B formulations, posaconazole, and the echinocandins/fluconazole (Wang 2010).

Oral antifungal formulations—particularly, itraconazole solution and posaconazole suspension—can cause gastrointestinal distress, especially in patients already experiencing chemotherapy-associated nausea and vomiting. Voriconazole is also associated with several unique adverse effects such as transient visual disturbance, changes in color perception (photopsia), and less commonly, hallucinations, which are more common in patients with elevated trough concentrations (Pascual 2012).

Drug interactions are major recurring problems with all antifungals, but especially triazole antifungals, which are inhibitors of cytochrome P450 (CYP) 3A4. More than 200 important interactions have been documented pharmacokinetically in humans taking triazole antifungals, but the number of theoretical pharmacokinetic drug-drug interactions probably exceeds 2000 (Bruggemann 2009). Some of those interactions can lead to undetectable blood levels of triazole antifungals or, conversely, dangerous overdosing with (1) immunosuppressive agents used after transplantation, (2) anesthetic agents, (3) medications affecting cardiac conduction, or (4) cancer chemotherapy. Consequently, all patients receiving triazole antifungal agents should have their drug regimens carefully screened, preferably with an electronic medication database that is either commercial (e.g., Lexi-Interact, Micromedex) or noncommercial (e.g., www.aspergillus.org.uk).

Prolonged use of triazole antifungals can be associated with toxicities that often get misdiagnosed or attributed to the patient's underlying diseases or infection. Peripheral neuropathy has been reported as an acute complication of pharmacokinetic interactions between triazoles and vincristine, but can also develop in up to 10% of patients after prolonged (> 4 months) therapy with a triazole. In a single-center retrospective cohort analysis from 2007–10, peripheral neuropathy was reported in 17% of patients taking itraconazole, 9% taking voriconazole, and 3% taking posaconazole (Baxter 2011). Nearly all of the peripheral neuropathy episodes presented as numbness or tingling in the extremities, whereas four episodes presented as predominant leg weakness. The majority of cases were axonal, length-dependent neuropathies in patients who recovered after triazole medication was discontinued. The authors concluded that patients on long-term triazole therapy should be monitored for neurologic symptoms, and if peripheral neuropathy is suspected, diagnosis should include (1) nerve conduction studies, (2) exclusion of other causes, and (3) consideration of dose reduction or cessation of therapy.

Dermatologic reactions are recurring problems with all antimicrobial agents, including antifungals. The most common reactions are rash and photosensitivity reactions. Occasionally, serious immune cutaneous reactions, including Stevens-Johnson syndrome, toxic epidermal necrolysis, and erythema multiforme have been reported during treatment, but the risk of such rare reactions does not appear to be statistically higher for triazoles than for other antimicrobial agents.

More recently, an association between phototoxic skin reactions and progression to squamous cell carcinoma was identified in several case series with voriconazole. Risk factors included prolonged treatment (typically, longer than 6 months), strong sun exposure, ongoing immunosuppression or post-transplant phase, advanced age, and light-colored skin. Patients may progress in stages from an initial phototoxic reaction to the development of actinic keratosis, followed by squamous cell carcinoma within 1–3 years depending on concomitant risk factors (Epaulard 2013). Therefore, all patients who develop a phototoxic reaction during the first 6 months of voriconazole therapy should be routinely evaluated by a dermatologist and potentially switched to alternative agents if antifungal therapy must be continued.

The mechanism underlying severe phototoxic reactions to voriconazole may involve the chromophore properties of voriconazole metabolites acting as photosensitizing agents in the skin. Although voriconazole itself does not absorb UVA/B spectrum rays, principal metabolite voriconazole N-oxide does absorb radiation in the UVA/UVB spectrum. Therefore, the phototoxicity risk may have a CYP2C19 pharmacogenetic component, or it could be influenced by concomitant drugs that alter the metabolism of voriconazole.

Prolonged voriconazole therapy has been associated with the development of diffuse, painful periostitis (Wermers 2011). Because voriconazole contains fluorine, the mechanism of toxicity is hypothesized to result from fluoride excess. Patients often complain of nonspecific pain in the hands, finger swelling, fatigue, and diffuse musculoskeletal pain. Skeletal imaging often reveals evidence of osteosclerosis, hyperostotic periostitis, periarticular changes, and ligamentous calcifications. In the initial phases, bony lesions form on the fingers, forearms, and femurs that eventually regress during an osteoclastic phase, leaving residual periosteal bone growth. Serum fluoride concentrations are often elevated (normal, 1–4 mol/L) and occasionally toxic (>15 mol/L). Therefore, fluoride toxicity should be suspected in any patient on long-term voriconazole therapy who presents with those symptoms. Cessation of voriconazole or switching to other antifungal agents has been associated with reversal of the syndrome.

New Triazole Antifungals and Formulations

New Posaconazole Formulations

Broader-spectrum triazole antifungals often display less-favorable pharmaceutical properties, especially with respect to reliable dissolution and absorption in the human gastrointestinal tract. To overcome those limitations, triazoles are often formulated with cyclodextrin, which circumvents solubility problems but causes gastrointestinal adverse effects of a drug when taken orally. In the case of posaconazole, a micronized suspension was developed to improve the surface area available for dissolution without the aid of cyclodextrin. However, clinical experience has confirmed that the absorption of posaconazole suspension is still erratic in many populations and greatly affected by food intake, gastric pH, and intestinal motility. Systemic bioavailability can be improved if the posaconazole suspension is administered in divided daily doses to be taken with high-fat meals, nutritional supplements, or acidic beverages. Nevertheless, such measures may still result in inadequate blood levels among many high-risk populations.

New delayed-release and intravenous formulations of posaconazole have been developed that are capable of predictably achieving higher serum posaconazole levels than the older suspension formulation. The 100-mg tablet formulation releases the entire dose of posaconazole in the small intestine by using pH-sensitive polymers to maximize absorption (Percival 2014). Consequently, dosing is different from that of the conventional oral suspension, which is administered at 600–800 mg/day in divided doses. With the tablet formulation, a loading dose of 300 mg (three 100-mg tablets) is taken twice daily on the first day, followed by a 300-mg daily maintenance dose on the second day and thereafter. Average steady-state posaconazole serum concentrations with the tablet formulation were significantly higher than those achieved with the highest absorbable dose of the oral posaconazole suspension (1.1 mcg/mL vs. 0.52 mcg/mL) (Duarte 2012; Ezzet 2005). Notably, the average concentrations achieved with the tablet are above the target serum levels proposed for prophylaxis and treatment of invasive fungal infections (>700 ng/mL and 1000 ng/mL, respectively).

In a second dose-escalation study of the new tablet formulation, average steady-state concentrations (after 7 days of daily dosing) from 200 mg once daily, 200 mg twice daily, and 400 mg daily for the delayed-release tablets were 1310 ng/mL, 2550 ng/mL, and 2360 ng/mL, respectively, after two doses of posaconazole tablets each on day 1 (Krishna 2012). However, pharmacokinetic modeling suggested that the concentrations achieved from 400 mg of delayed-release tablets administered twice daily may exceed safe limits and lead to increased risk of hepatic injury. To date, adverse events with the tablet have been mild and similar to those that occur with the suspension, consisting most commonly of headaches, nausea, and abnormalities in liver function tests (Krishna 2012).

Posaconazole tablets cannot be chewed or crushed, which may limit use of the oral formulation in critically ill patients. Therefore, the recent approval of a cyclodextrin-solubilized intravenous formulation (18 mg/mL) could improve the utility of this agent in those populations. In a phase 3 study of patients with acute myeloid leukemia/myelodysplastic syndrome or postallogeneic hematopoietic stem cell transplantation, intravenous posaconazole was administered 300 mg twice daily on day 1 (loading dose) followed by 300 mg daily on subsequent days. Patients who could tolerate the oral suspension were allowed to switch to 300 mg three times daily after at least 4 days of intravenous therapy, which resulted in somewhat lower exposures (0.95 mcg/mL with 300 mg three times daily orally) compared with patients who remained on 300-mg intravenous therapy daily (1.30 mcg/mL) (Cornely 2013). Adverse effects with the intravenous infusion were similar to those of the oral suspension, although thrombophlebitis is common if the drug is administered through a peripheral catheter; therefore, the drug should be administered over 90 minutes through a central line..

Isavuconazole

Isavuconazole represents an alternative strategy for developing a broader-spectrum triazole antifungal without the pharmacokinetic drawbacks of older agents. Isavuconazole is a triazole antifungal with a spectrum of activity similar to that of posaconazole, including most *Candida* spp., *Aspergillus* spp., and some Mucorales and endemic fungi (Falci 2013). It is unknown whether isavuconazole is active against multi-triazole–resistant *A. fumigatus,* although strains harboring the TR/L98H mutation often exhibited elevated isavuconazole MICs (>8 mcg/mL), suggesting cross-resistance is still a concern.

Isavuconazole is unique from other triazoles because it is administered as a prodrug, isavuconazonium, which is rapidly cleaved in vivo to the active drug, isavuconazole, and an inactive prodrug cleavage product: BAL8728. Consequently, isavuconazole does not require cyclodextrin for solubilization and is available in both cyclodextrin-free intravenous formulations and a hard gelatin capsule. Isavuconazole also displays a relatively long elimination half-life (56–77 hours after oral administration, 76–104 hours after intravenous administration) and is cleared through hepatic metabolism, with possibly fewer drug interactions than voriconazole and itraconazole. However, like other triazoles, isavuconazole is an inhibitor of CYP3A4 and can interfere with the pharmacokinetics of drugs metabolized through this pathway.

Recently, a pivotal phase 3 randomized, double-blind, multicenter trial compared isavuconazole with voriconazole for the primary treatment of invasive mold infections in patients with hematologic malignancy caused by *Aspergillus* spp. or other filamentous fungi (Maertens 2004). Patients with probable or proven invasive mold infection (European Organisation for Research and Treatment of Cancer /MSG definitions) were randomized to receive either intravenous isavuconazole 200 mg three times daily or voriconazole 6 mg/kg intravenously every 12 hours on day 1 and then 4 mg/kg every 12 hours, with an option for oral isavuconazole 200 mg every 12 hours or oral voriconazole 200 mg every 12 hours thereafter. The primary end points of all-cause mortality through day 42 in the intent-to-treat population (n=516 patients) were 19% in the isavuconazole group and 20% in the voriconazole group. Overall responses (a composite of clinical, mycologic, and radiologic responses) at end of therapy, as assessed by the independent data review committee, were 35% for isavuconazole versus 36% for voriconazole.

Adverse events caused by isavuconazole were statistically fewer relative to voriconazole, including hepatobiliary (9% vs. 16%), skin (34% vs. 43%), and eye disorders (15% vs. 27%). In addition, isavuconazole showed statistically fewer study drug-related adverse events relative to voriconazole (42% vs. 60%). Therefore, isavuconazole appears to be a promising alternative to voriconazole for the treatment of invasive aspergillosis.

Conclusion

Pharmacists play key roles on multidisciplinary teams that care for patients with invasive fungal infections. Because antifungal therapies have multiple limitations in terms of spectrum (resistance), pharmacokinetics, toxicities, and cost, no single antifungal agent is appropriate for all patients, and treatment must be individualized and frequently modified for optimal outcomes. The pharmacist is generally the health care team member most qualified to screen for and interpret potential drug interactions, recommend potential drug or dosage changes based on susceptibility testing and therapeutic drug monitoring results. Familiarity with and application of those skills can substantially improve the probability of successful treatment with fewer drug-related toxicities in patients with life-threatening, invasive fungal infections.

Invasive fungal infections continue to be associated with disproportionately high morbidity and mortality, with a growing impact even in populations not classically considered to have immunocompromise. Although new antifungal therapies and diagnostic approaches have improved outcomes for some mycoses, those therapeutic gains may be threatened in the not-too-distant future by the growing prevalence of multidrug resistance among *C. glabrata* and *Aspergillus* spp. Therefore, antifungal susceptibility testing will likely play a greater role in the management of such infections if isolates are available for testing. The importance of amphotericin B–flucytosine combination therapy for improving survival from cryptococcal meningitis has now been proved, yet a similar survival benefit for combination therapy in patients with invasive aspergillosis is less certain. Therapeutic-drug monitoring of triazole antifungals and flucytosine is now considered a standard of care, although the monitoring strategies are still debated and will likely evolve with new antifungals and new formulations that have improved pharmacokinetics. Finally, as patients remain on antifungals for progressively longer periods, new toxicities are emerging that may require treatment alterations or reconsiderations of the risks and benefits of continued therapy.

References

Alexander BD, Johnson MD, Pfeiffer CD, et al. Increasing echinocandin resistance in Candida glabrata: clinical failure correlates with presence of FKS mutations and elevated minimum inhibitory concentrations. Clin Infect Dis 2013;56:1724-32.

Andes D, Pascual A, Marchetti O. Antifungal therapeutic drug monitoring: Established and emerging indications. Antimicrob Agents Chemother 2009;53:24-34.

Andes DR, Safdar N, Baddley JW, et al. Impact of treatment strategy on outcomes in patients with candidemia and other forms of invasive candidiasis: a patient-level quantitative review of randomized trials. Clin Infect Dis 2012;54:1110-22.

Ashbee HR, Barnes RA, Johnson EM, et al. Therapeutic drug monitoring (TDM) of antifungal agents: guidelines from the British Society for Medical Mycology. J Antimicrob Chemother 2014;69:1162-76.

Avni T, Leibovici L, Paul M. PCR diagnosis of invasive candidiasis: systematic review and meta-analysis. J Clin Microbiol 2010;49:665-70.
\Baxter CG, Marshall A, Roberts M, et al. Peripheral neuropathy in patients on long-term triazole antifungal therapy. J Antimicrob Chemother 2011:2136-39.

Bell BP, Khabbaz RF. Responding to the outbreak of invasive fungal infections: the value of public health to Americans. JAMA 2013;309:883-84.

Brown GD, Denning DW, Gow NAR, Levitz SM, Netea MG, White TC. Hidden killers: human fungal infections. Sci Transl Med 2012;4:165rv13.

Brüggemann RJ, Alffenaar JW, Blijlevens N, et al. Clinical relevance of pharmacokinetic interactions of azole antifungal drugs with coadministered agents. Clin Infect Dis 2009;48:1441-58.

Bueid A, Howard SJ, Moore CB, et al. Azole antifungal resistance in Aspergillus fumigatus: 2008 and 2009. J Antimicrob Chemother 2010;65:2116-18.

Clancy CJ, Nguyen MH. The end of an era in defining the optimal treatment of invasive candidiasis. Clin Infect Dis 2012;54:1123-5.

Clancy CJ, Nguyen MH. Finding the "Missing 50%" of invasive candidiasis: How nonculture diagnostics will improve understanding of disease spectrum and transform patient care. Clin Infect Dis 2013;56:1284-92.

Cornely OA, Haider S, Grigg A, et al. Phase 3 pharmacokinetic and safety study of posaconazole IV in patients at risk for invasive fungal infection. Interscience Conference on Antimicrobial Agents and Chemotherapy. Denver, Colorado: ASM; 2013.

Day JN, Chau TTH, Wolbers M, et al. Combination antifungal therapy for cryptococcal meningitis. N Engl J Med 2013;368:1291-302.

Duarte RF, Lopez J, Cornely AO, et al. Phase 1b study of new posaconazole tablet for prevention of invasive fungal infections in high-risk patients with neutropenia. Antimicrob Agent Chemother 2014;58:5758-65.

Epaulard O, Villier C, Ravaud P, et al. A multistep voriconazole-related phototoxic pathway may lead to skin carcinoma: results from a French nationwide study. Clin Infect Dis 2013;57:e182-88.

Ezzet F, Wexler MD, Courtney R, et al. Oral bioavailability of posaconazole in fasted healthy subjects: comparison between three regiments and basis for clinical dosage recommendations. Clin Pharmacokinet 2005;44:211-20.

Falci DR, Pasqualotto AC. Profile of isavuconazole and its potential in the treatment of severe invasive fungal infections. Infect Drug Resist 2013;6:163-74.

Felton T, Troke PF, Hope WW. Tissue penetration of antifungal agents. Clin Microbiol Rev 2014;27:68-88.

Fothergill AW, Sutton DA, McCarthy DI, Wiederhold NP. The Impact of new antifungal breakpoints on antifungal resistance in Candida Species. J Clin Microbiol 2014;52:994-97.

Havlickova B, Czaika VA, Friedrich M. Epidemiological trends in skin mycoses worldwide. Mycoses. 2008;51 Suppl 4:2-15.

Held J, Kohlberger I, Rappold E, et al. Comparison of (1->3)-β-D-glucan, mannan/anti-mannan antibodies, and Cand-Tec Candida antigen as serum biomarkers for candidemia. J Clin Microbiol 2013;51:1158-64.

Kainer MA, Reagan DR, Nguyen DB, et al. Fungal infections associated with contaminated methylprednisolone in Tennessee. N Engl J Med 2012;367:2194-203.

Karageorgopoulos DE, Vouloumanou EK, Ntziora F, et al. β-D-glucan assay for the diagnosis of invasive fungal infections: a meta-analysis. Clin Infect Dis 2011;52:750-70.

Krishna G, Ma L, Martinho M, et al. A new solid oral tablet formulation of posaconazole: a randomized clinical trial to investigate rising single-and multiple-dose pharmacokinetics and safety in healthy volunteers. J Antimicrob Chemother 2012;67:2725-30.

Maertens J, Patterson T, Rahav G, et al. A phase 3 randomized, double-blind trial evaluating isavuconazole versus voriconazole for the primary treatment of invasive fungal infections caused by Aspergillus spp. and other filamentous fungi. European Congress of Clinical Microbiology and Infectious Diseases (ECCMID). European Society of Clinical Microbiology and Infectious Diseases; 2004. Abstract O23Oa.

Marr K, Schlamm H, Rottinghaus S, et al. A randomised, double-blind study of combination antifungal therapy with voriconazole and anidulafungin versus voriconazole monotherapy for primary treatment of invasive aspergillosis. Annals Interm Med 2014 In press

Muldoon EG, Denning DW. Editorial commentary: prophylactic echinocandin: is there a subgroup of intensive care unit patients who benefit? Clin Infect Dis 2014;58:1227-29.

Mølgaard-Nielsen D, Pasternak B, Hviid A. Use of oral fluconazole during pregnancy and the risk of birth defects. N Engl J Med 2013;369:830-39.

Neblett Fanfair R, Benedict K, Bos J, et al. Necrotizing cutaneous mucormycosis after a tornado in Joplin, Missouri, in 2011. N Engl J Med 2012;367:2214-25.

Ostrosky-Zeichner L, Pappas PG, Shoham S, et al. Improvement of a clinical prediction rule for clinical trials on prophylaxis for invasive candidiasis in the intensive care unit. Mycoses 2011;54:46-51.

Ostrosky-Zeichner L, Shoham S, Vazquez J, et al. MSG-01: A randomized, double-blind, placebo-controlled trial of caspofungin prophylaxis followed by preemptive therapy for invasive candidiasis in high-risk adults in the critical care setting. Clin Infect Dis 2014;58:1219-26.
Outterson K. The Drug Quality and Security Act--mind the gaps. N Engl J Med 2013;370:97-99.

Pappas PG, Kauffman CA, Andes D, et al. Clinical Practice Guidelines for the Management Candidiasis: 2009 Update by the Infectious Diseases Society of America. Clin Infect Dis 2009;48:503-35.

Pappas PG, Kontoyiannis DP, Perfect JR, Chiller TM. Real-time treatment guidelines: considerations during the Exserohilum rostratum outbreak in the United States. Antimicrob Agents Chemother 2013;57:1573-76.

Park BJ, Wannemuehler KA, Marston BJ, et al. Estimation of the current global burden of cryptococcal meningitis among persons living with HIV/AIDS. AIDS 2009;23:525-30.

Park WB, Kim N-H, Kim K-H, et al. The effect of therapeutic drug monitoring on safety and efficacy of voriconazole in invasive fungal infections: a randomized controlled trial. Clin Infect Dis 2012;55:1080-87.

Pascual A, Csajka C, Buclin T, et al. Challenging recommended oral and intravenous voriconazole doses for improved efficacy and safety: Population pharmacokinetics-based analysis of adult patients with invasive fungal infections. Clin Infect Dis 2012;55:381-90.

Percival KM, Bergman SJ. Update on Posaconazole Pharmacokinetics: Comparison of old and new formulations. Curr Fungal Infect Rep 2014;8:139-45.

Perfect JR. Efficiently killing a sugar-coated yeast. N Engl J Med 2013;368:1354-56.

Perfect JR, Dismukes WE, Dromer F, et al. Clinical practice guidelines for the management of cryptococcal disease: 2010 update by the infectious diseases society of america. Clin Infect Dis 2010;50:291-322
.

Pettit AC, Kropski JA, Castilho JL, et al. The index case for the fungal meningitis outbreak in the United States. N Engl J Med 2012;367:2119-25.

Pfaller MA. Antifungal drug resistance: mechanisms, epidemiology, and consequences for treatment. Am J Med 2012;125(1 Suppl):S3-13.

Pham CD, Iqbal N, Bolden CB, et al. Role of FKS mutations in C. glabrata: MIC values, echinocandin resistance and multidrug resistance. Antimicrob Agents Chemother 2014;58:4690-96.

Roy M, Benedict K, Deak E, et al. A large community outbreak of blastomycosis in Wisconsin with geographic and ethnic clustering. Clin Infect Dis 2013;57:655-62.

Shields RK, Nguyen MH, Press EG, et al. The presence of an FKS mutation rather than MIC is an independent risk factor for failure of echinocandin therapy among patients with invasive candidiasis due to Candida glabrata. Antimicrob Agent Chemother 2012;56:4862-69.

Snelders E, Veld RAG, Rijs AJM, Kema GHJ, Melchers WMJ, Verweij PE. Possible environmental origin of resistance of Aspergillus fumigatus to medical triazoles. Appl. Environ Microbiol 2009;75:4053-4057.

Sobel JD. Vulvovaginal candidosis. Lancet 2007;369:1961-71.

Verweij PE, Mellado E, Melchers WJ. Multiple-triazole-resistant aspergillosis. N Engl J Med 2007;356:1481-3.

Walsh TJ, Anaissie EJ, Denning DW, et al. Treatment of aspergillosis: Clinical practice guidelines of the Infectious Diseases Society of America. Clin Infect Dis 2008;46:327-60.

Wang J-L, Chang C-H, Young-Xu Y, Arnold Chan K. Systematic review and meta-analysis of the tolerability and hepatotoxicity of antifungal use in empirical and definitive therapy for invasive fungal infection. Antimicrob Agents Chemother 2010;54:2409-19.

Wermers RA, Cooper K, Razonable RR, et al. Fluoride excess and periostitis in transplant patients receiving long-term voriconazole therapy. Clin Infect Dis 2011;52:604-11.

SELF-ASSESSMENT QUESTIONS

21. A 34-year-old man suffered penetrating abdominal trauma, multiple lacerations, and fractures during a motor vehicle crash. He underwent emergency splenectomy and repair of his right femur. On post-operative day 5, he remains in the surgical intensive care unit (ICU) receiving mechanical ventilation and on piperacillin/tazobactam and daptomycin. However, over the last 48 hours on antibiotic therapy he has developed a rapidly progressing, soft tissue infection with necrosis surrounding one of his puncture wounds. Which one of the following regimens is best to recommend for this patient?

    A. Caspofungin 70-mg loading dose, then 50 mg daily.
    B. Fluconazole 800-mg loading dose, then 400 mg daily.
    C. Liposomal amphotericin B 5 mg/kg/daily.
    D. Voriconazole 6 mg/kg every 12 hours plus anidulafungin 200-mg loading dose then 100 mg daily.

22. A 66-year-old woman is referred to your hospital with a complaints of recurrent fevers, night sweats, 15-lb weight loss, and poor appetite over the last 4 months. She has received 2-week courses of azithromycin, levofloxacin, amoxicillin/clavulanate, and is currently finishing doxycycline. Her medical history is otherwise unremarkable. Her social history is notable for a recent retirement 6 months ago from a job as an elementary school teacher in Indianapolis, Indiana with relocation to a town near Phoenix, Arizona to be closer to her sister. She reports no unusual outdoor activities or exposures, tick or animal bites, and has not been traveling. Her only other reported symptoms are an erythematous rash around her neck and shoulders that appeared when her fever started. Chest radiography taken 2 weeks ago was negative. Assuming the patient has an endemic fungal infection, which one of the following recommendations would be most appropriate?

    A. Withhold antifungal therapy, and follow the patient with serological studies.
    B. Itraconazole capsules 200 mg three times daily x 3 days then 200 mg twice daily. *Blasto*
    C. Fluconazole tablet 200 mg daily.
    D. Admit the patient to the hospital and administer liposomal amphotericin B 3 mg/kg plus methylprednisolone 1 mg/kg.

Questions 23–25 pertain to the following case.

T.P. is a 67-year-old man with *Exserohilum rostratum* epidural abscess that developed after an injection with contaminated methylprednisolone. He has been taking oral voriconazole

350 mg twice daily for 4 months but presents to the clinic with complaints of pain in his shoulders and hands that is getting progressively worse. He also complains of difficulty concentrating and chapped lips. His other drugs include chlorthalidone 25 mg daily and rosuvastatin 10 mg daily. T.P.'s laboratory values were notable for elevated ALP (150 mcg/L).

23. Which one of the following voriconazole toxicities is most consistent with T.P.'s shoulder and hand pain?

    A. Voriconazole-associated periostitis (fluoride toxicity).
    B. Voriconazole-associated hepatotoxicity.
    C. Myopathy resulting from pharmacokinetic drug-drug interactions between voriconazole and rosuvastatin.
    D. Voriconazole-associated peripheral neuropathy.

24. Because of the adverse effects above, voriconazole is discontinued and T.P. is switched to posaconazole delayed-release tablets 300 mg once daily. What is the major limitation of using posaconazole versus voriconazole in T.P.?

    A. Increased hepatotoxicity of posaconazole versus voriconazole.
    B. Increased risk of drug interactions versus voriconazole.
    C. Higher resistance (MICs) of *E. rostratum* to posaconazole versus voriconazole.
    D. Less predictable cerebrospinal fluid or brain concentrations of posaconazole versus voriconazole.

25. Two months later, T.P. returns to clinic reporting improvement in his joint pain but with a severe sunburn on his scalp that developed after a very short time (< 20 minutes) in direct sunlight. His trough posaconazole level is 1.5 mcg/mL. Which one of the following would be best to recommend for T.P.?

    A. Reduce the posaconazole dose to 100 mg twice daily.
    B. Immediately discontinue posaconazole.
    C. Continue the posaconazole dose and advise the patient to limit sun exposure.
    D. Switch the patient back to voriconazole.

26. Based on your knowledge of the diagnostic performance characteristics of the β-D-glucan (BDG) test, which approach would be the most justifiable use of this test in support of stewardship initiatives to reduce unnecessary antifungal use in the ICU?

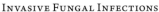

A. Perform twice-weekly screening of serum BDG in all febrile ICU patients; allow antifungals to be started only in patients with two positive tests.

B. Perform twice-weekly screening of serum BDG in all asymptomatic ICU patients; administer prophylaxis if the patient has a positive test.

C. Perform BDG test in conjunction with blood cultures in patients with suspected candidemia and 72 hours later, discontinue empiric antifungal therapy if BDG test and cultures are negative.

D. Administer echinocandin prophylaxis to patients with high *Candida* risk scores (> 10% incidence); start antifungals in lower-risk patients only if BDG or cultures are positive

Questions 27 and 28 pertain to the following case.

R.C. is a 63-year-old man admitted 2 weeks ago for partial colectomy. He was doing well postoperatively until day +3 when he developed fever, increasing WBC count, and respiratory distress. Chest radiography showed a right lower-lobe infiltrate. He was transferred to the surgical ICU where he was intubated, a central venous catheter was placed, and he was started on piperacillin/tazobactam plus levofloxacin. R.C. initially improved, but after 4 days in the ICU his fever recurred. Daptomycin was added to cover a possible catheter infection, which has not been changed. Repeat chest radiography shows improvement, but R.C.'s urine and sputum cultures are growing yeast. Blood cultures are pending.

27. Assuming R.C. has invasive candidiasis, which one of the interventions below would best improve his chances of survival?

    A. Start antifungal treatment with an echinocandin.
    B. Start treatment with a combination of an echinocandin and triazole antifungal.
    C. Remove the central venous catheter and replace with a peripherally-inserted catheter.
    D. Perform abdominal CT of the gut to identify possible source of *Candida* infection for early drainage.

28. Forty-eight hours later, R.C.'s blood cultures are positive for yeast identified as *Candida glabrata*. You are asked what is the probability of resistance to echinocandins, and if the isolate should be submitted for antifungal susceptibility testing. Which of the following statements is the most accurate response?

    A. Echinocandin resistance is uncommon; therefore, testing is not indicated.
    B. Echinocandin resistance rates are high enough to justify MIC testing.
    C. There are no data correlating echinocandin resistance detected in the laboratory with treatment outcome in patients.

D. Echinocandin resistance is primarily reported in *C. albicans*, rarely in *C. glabrata*.

29. A 57-year-old man has undergone an allogeneic, hematopoietic stem cell transplantation for acute myeloid leukemia. His post-transplant course was complicated by multiple bacterial infections, cytomegalovirus reactivation, and acute graft-versus-host disease. At 110 days after transplantation, he developed an episode of fever with a nodular infiltrate on chest CT, despite oral voriconazole prophylaxis 300 twice daily (most recent trough level on admission is 1.2 mcg/mL). Bronchoscopy is performed and is positive for *Aspergillus* galactomannan antigen and a mold is growing in culture. Which one of the following is best to recommend for this patient?

    A. Discontinue voriconazole, start liposomal amphotericin B 5 mg/kg/daily, and submit the isolate for susceptibility testing.
    B. Discontinue voriconazole, start liposomal amphotericin B 5 mg/kg/daily.
    C. Add caspofungin 70-mg loading dose, then 50 mg daily.
    D. Switch the patient to posaconazole tablet 300 mg twice daily day 1, then 300 mg daily thereafter.

30. You are asked to help revise treatment guidelines for opportunistic infections for immunocompromised patients in your hospital. It has been recommended that combination amphotericin B plus fluconazole should be listed as an alternative to the standard amphotericin B + flucytosine induction regimen for cryptococcal meningitis, because fluconazole is associated with fewer adverse effects and does not require routine therapeutic drug monitoring. Which of the following responses is best regarding fluconazole plus amphotericin B combinations for cryptococcal meningitis?

    A. Amphotericin B-fluconazole induction therapy is not recommended because this combination is antagonistic versus amphotericin B monotherapy.
    B. Amphotericin B-fluconazole induction therapy is not associated with a survival advantage versus amphotericin B monotherapy.
    C. Amphotericin B-fluconazole combination therapy is associated with lower risk of anemia compared with amphotericin B-flucytosine.
    D. Amphotericin B-fluconazole is an acceptable alternative given the excellent cerebrospinal fluid penetration of fluconazole.

31. Your institutional pharmacy and therapeutics committee is developing guidelines for the use of combination antifungal regimens in the hematology

population. There is some difference of opinion among the committee members as to whether combination therapy may be justified for the initial treatment of invasive aspergillosis or should be reserved only for patients with breakthrough infection that has failed monotherapy. Which one of the following statements best describes the current evidence of voriconazole plus anidulafungin versus voriconazole monotherapy for invasive aspergillosis?

A. The greatest survival improvement was re ported among patients with disease diagnosed by CT imaging and *Aspergillus galactomannan.*

B. The greatest survival benefit was observed in patients with culture-diagnosed infection.

C. The only statistically significant benefit over monotherapy was found in patients with breakthrough infection.

D. No survival benefit was found with combination therapy, even in subgroup analysis.

Questions 32 and 33 pertain to the following case.

P.T. is a 56-year-old man undergoing initial remission-induction chemotherapy for acute myeloid leukemia. After completion of his chemotherapy, he is started on posaconazole oral suspension 200 mg three times daily for prophylaxis.

32. P.T.'s physician asks you to make a recommendation for therapeutic drug monitoring (TDM). Which one of the following is best to recommend for P.T.?

A. Check a posaconazole peak concentration (2 hours after dose) with the third dose to ensure levels are greater than 1 mcg/mL.

B. Check a trough level at 4–7 days to ensure levels are greater than 0.7 mcg/mL.

C. Check a trough level at 4–7 days to ensure levels are less than 5.5 mcg/mL to avoid hepatotoxicity.

D. There is no evidence that posaconazole serum levels correlate with clinical outcome.

33. P.T.'s trough level returns as "undetectable" (< 0.2 mcg/mL) and he has poor appetite. Which one of the following modifications would have the greatest impact on increasing P.T.'s blood concentrations?

A. Switch to posaconazole delayed release tablet, 300-mg twice daily loading dose on day 1, then 300 mg daily.

B. Increase the suspension dose to 400 mg three times daily.

C. Administer the posaconazole suspension with an acidic beverage.

D. Instruct the patient to take the posaconazole suspension with ice cream.

34. You are asked by the analytical laboratory of your hospital to review how voriconazole trough therapeutic ranges will be reported to clinicians. Which one of the following reports is most consistent with current TDM evidence for voriconazole?

A. Efficacy > 0.5 mcg/mL; hepatotoxicity > 6 mcg/mL.

B. Prophylaxis efficacy > 0.7 mcg/mL; treatment efficacy > 5 mcg/mL.

C. Efficacy > 0.5 mcg/mL, visual changes > 5 mcg/mL.

D. Efficacy > 1.0 mcg/mL; central nervous system (CNS) toxicity > 5.5 mcg/mL.

35. A 42-year-old woman with Hodgkin's lymphoma is started on BEACOPP (bleomycin, etoposide, doxorubicin, cyclophosphamide, vincristine, procarbazine, and prednisone) and has developed severe weakness in the arms and legs during the last 48 hours. She is immediately transferred to the ICU. Her only other medications are valacyclovir 500 mg twice daily, posaconazole suspension 400 mg twice daily, and levofloxacin 500 mg daily. Which one of the following best explais this patient's acute-onset limb weakness?

A. CNS viral infection.

B. Intracranial bleed.

C. Procarbazine-posaconazole drug interaction.

D. Vincristine-posaconazole drug interaction.

Questions 36 and 37 pertain to the following case.

J.Z. is a 9-year-old boy with acute lymphoblastic leukemia in remission who received a cord-blood allogeneic hematopoietic stem cell transplant. He engrafted after 42 days without acute graft-versus-host disease. He is currently weaning off cyclosporine but continues to take valacyclovir, voriconazole, and trimethoprim/sulfamethoxazole. During his clinic visit at Day +90, J.Z. is noted to have erythema of the cheeks and nose, cheilitis, and small blisters on the nose and lips. He also has small patchy areas of erythema on sun-exposed parts of his arms. Otherwise he has no complains, fever, or other skin lesions. He denies excessive sun exposure (only rides his bike in front of the house in mornings) and applies sunscreen before going outside. He reports no unusual exposures, no pets, or other sick contacts.

36. Which one of the following reasons is the most likely explanation for J.Z.'s skin changes?

A. Chronic graft versus host disease.

B. Viral exanthem.

C. Voriconazole-associated phototoxicity.

D. Trimethoprim/sulfamethoxazole hypersensitivity.

37. Which one of the following is best to consider with repect to voriconazole therapy in J.Z.?

A. No changes because trimethoprim/sulfamethoxazole is the most likely cause of rash.
B. Voriconazole can be continued, but the patient should avoid any sunlight.
C. Reduce the voriconazole dose by 50% and confirm serum trough levels to be less than 5.5 mcg/mL.
D. Discontinue voriconazole; if antifungal prophylaxis is still required, initiate posaconazole.

A. Switch the patient to posaconazole delayed release tablet 300 mg daily after loading dose.
B. Discontinue voriconazole, start liposomal amphotericin B 7.5 mg/kg day. ✗
C. Reduce the voriconazole dose to 200 mg twice daily. ✗
D. Continue current therapy as aminotransferase levels will likely return to normal on therapy. ✗

38. A 48-year-old man with a history of severe chronic obstructive pulmonary disease had emergency abdominal surgery 1 week ago. He remains mechanically ventilated in the ICU and is receiving continuous tube feeds by nasogastric tube. A recent tracheal aspirate was positive for _Aspergillus_, so he was started on posaconazole suspension 200 mg four times daily with tube feeds. His last trough posaconazole concentration was less than 0.2 mcg/mL. Which one of the following is best to recommend for this patient?

A. Increase posaconazole dose to 300 mg four times daily.
B. Administer crushed posaconazole tablets, 300 mg daily.
C. Discontinue any acid suppression therapy, continue the same dose.
D. Switch the patient to intravenous voriconazole.

39. Which one of the following statements best describes the advantages of isavuconazole versus voriconazole?

A. Available in both intravenous and oral formulations. ✓
B. Improved activity against _Aspergillus fumigatus_ harboring TR/L98H mutation. ✗
C. Fewer hepatobiliary, skin, or eye adverse effects.
D. Lack of cytochrome drug-drug interactions involving cytochrome P450. ✗

40. A 78-year-old man with Philadelphia chromosome positive-chronic lymphocytic leukemia is receiving antifungal treatment for biopsy confirmed _Aspergillus_ sinusitis. Because of low voriconazole blood levels, his dose was steadily increased to 350 mg twice daily to maintain a trough concentrations of 1.5–2 mcg/mL. Comedication consisted of imatinib (100 mg once a day), pregabalin (150 mg twice a day) and methadone (20 mg three times a day), and fentanyl patches (200 mcg), and oxycodone (10 mg) on demand. During the next month of therapy, serum alanine (ALT) and aspartate (AST) transaminases gradually increased to values of 10 times the upper level of normal (ULN). His voriconazole trough levels have been consistently of 1-2 mcg/mL on his current dose. Which one of the following recommendations would best manage this patient's antifungal therapy?

LEARNER CHAPTER EVALUATION: INVASIVE FUNGAL INFECTIONS.

As you take the posttest for this chapter, also evaluate the material's quality and usefulness, as well as the achievement of learning objectives. Rate each item using this 5-point scale:

- Strongly agree
- Agree
- Neutral
- Disagree
- Strongly disagree

20. The content of the chapter met my educational needs.
21. The content of the chapter satisfied my expectations.
22. The author presented the chapter content effectively.
23. The content of the chapter was relevant to my practice and presented at the appropriate depth and scope.
24. The content of the chapter was objective and balanced.
25. The content of the chapter is free of bias, promotion, or advertisement of commercial products.
26. The content of the chapter was useful to me.
27. The teaching and learning methods used in the chapter were effective.
28. The active learning methods used in the chapter were effective.
29. The learning assessment activities used in the chapter were effective.
30. The chapter was effective overall.

Use the 5-point scale to indicate whether this chapter prepared you to accomplish the following learning objectives :

31. Detect epidemiologic risk factors associated with recent invasive fungal infection outbreaks in patients without immunocompromise.
32. Judge whether current evidence supports a prophylactic versus preemptive antifungal therapeutic approach for managing invasive candidiasis in non-neutropenic patients.
33. Justify the frontline use of combination therapy for cryptococcal meningitis and invasive aspergillosis.
34. Develop an algorithm for therapeutic drug monitoring of antifungals.
35. Analyze the advantages of newer triazole antifungals and formulations.
36. Please provide any specific comments relating to any perceptions of bias, promotion, or advertisement of commercial products.
37. Please expand on any of your above responses, and/ or provide any additional comments regarding this chapter:

TUBERCULOSIS

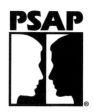

By Alexandria Garavaglia Wilson, Pharm.D., BCPS (AQ-ID)

Reviewed by Ian R. McNicholl, Pharm.D., FCCP, BCPS (AQ-ID), AAHIVP; Becky S. Linn, Pharm.D., BCPS; and Matthew F. Ambury, Pharm.D., BCPS

LEARNING OBJECTIVES

1. Develop a treatment plan for a patient with active tuberculosis.
2. Develop a treatment plan for a patient with latent tuberculosis.
3. Devise a management plan for drug interactions with tuberculosis treatment.
4. Devise a management plan for adverse drug reactions with tuberculosis treatment.

INTRODUCTION

Tuberculosis (TB) is caused by *Mycobacterium tuberculosis* (MTB). There are 2 different forms of TB: latent TB infection (LTBI) and active TB disease. The treatments of LTBI and of active TB disease require different medication therapies and durations. Untreated LTBI may progress to active TB. In addition to being potentially deadly, active disease is highly infectious and therefore a public health concern.

Epidemiology

According to the Centers for Disease Control and Prevention (CDC), about one-third of the world's population is infected with TB. In 2012, around 9 million people became sick with TB, leading to about 1.3 million TB-related deaths. Those statistics make TB the number one cause of infectious-disease-related deaths. Worldwide, 13% of the people who developed TB in 2012 were also infected with human immunodeficiency virus (HIV). Because of the attention given TB, the number of new cases of TB in the world is declining by about 2% per year. Compared with 1990, the TB mortality rate in 2012 had decreased by 45%, with the largest number of cases having occurred in Southeast Asia, Africa, and Western Pacific regions (WHO 2013).

In the United States, there were 3.2 cases of TB per 100,000 persons in 2012, representing a 5.9% decline in case rate from the previous year. Ten states and the District of Columbia had incidences of TB higher than the national average in 2012, with California, Florida, New York, and Texas accounting for 50% of the total number of cases

---

BASELINE KNOWLEDGE STATEMENTS

Readers of this chapter are presumed to be familiar with the following:
- Basic pathophysiology of tuberculosis
- Mechanism of action of antimycobacterial medications
- Potential adverse drug reactions of first-line antimycobacterial medications
- Potential drug-drug interactions associated with first-line antimycobacterial medications
- Treatment of active tuberculosis disease as outlined by American Thoracic Society guidelines
- Treatment of latent tuberculosis infection as outlined by Centers for Disease Control and Prevention guidelines

ADDITIONAL READINGS

The following free resources are available for readers wishing additional background information on this topic.
- American Thoracic Society, Centers for Disease Control and Prevention, and Infectious Diseases Society of America. Treatment of tuberculosis. MMWR 2003;52(RR11):1-77.
- American Thoracic Society and Centers for Disease Control and Prevention. Targeted tuberculin testing and treatment of latent tuberculosis infection. MMWR 2000;(RR06):1-54.
- Centers for Disease Control and Prevention. Treatment for latent TB infection [home page on the Internet].

Abbreviations in This Chapter

IGRA	Interferon gamma release assay
LTBI	Latent tuberculosis infection
MDRTB	Multidrug-resistant tuberculosis
MTB	*Mycobacterium tuberculosis*
XDRTB	Extensively drug-resistant tuberculosis

nationally. Foreign-born cases of TB account for 63% of national cases; this statistic has been increasing since 1993. In the United States from 2007 to 2012, the top five home countries of foreign-born people with TB were China, India, Mexico, the Philippines, and Vietnam; 7% of foreign-born patients with TB were HIV infected (CDC 2012).

Risk Factors

Tuberculosis may spread from person to person when infectious droplet nuclei become aerosolized through coughing, sneezing, or speaking. The risk of exposure to infection is determined by degree of intimacy, duration of contact, the environment, and degree of infectiousness. The risk of infection that progresses to active disease depends on an infected individual's immune system and function of cell-mediated immunity. When the immune system cannot respond to the bacilli, active disease will occur.

There are two types of active disease: primary disease and reactivation. Primary disease is the continued progression to active disease after infection. Reactivation can occur many years after infection, and immunosuppression increases the risk of reactivation. Active disease is infectious and most commonly occurs in the lungs. Because MTB may disseminate throughout the body, infection may occur outside the lungs. Extrapulmonary disease may or may not be infectious depending on the site of the infection.

Primary TB disease after infection is possible in any patient but is most common among children in the first few years of life and among immunocompromised individuals. In primary disease, a patient acquires the organism, and infection continues to progress into active disease. Reactivation of disease occurs more commonly than does primary infection. The lifetime risk of infection that progresses to disease is 10%, with around 5% risk in the first 18 months (Andrews 2012). That risk is much higher in patients infected with HIV because of suppression of cellular immunity, which results in a 10% annual risk of progression. One test used to assess for the presence of LTBI is the tuberculin skin test (TST). The criterion for positivity of the skin test is determined by the presence or absence of an individual's risk factors (Table 3-1). The other type of testing for TB infection—interferon gamma release assay (IGRA)—does not depend on the presence or absence of risk factors for interpretation of the results.

One patient population not included in Table 3-1, although at risk of TB infection that progresses to active disease, is recipients of tumor necrosis factor (TNF) antagonist therapy. The rates of active TB in patients receiving TNF antagonists are 10- to 100-fold higher than in the general population. An assessment for LTBI is recommended before a patient begins treatment with one of these agents. If a positive test result confirms the presence of TB infection, the patient should begin LTBI therapy. The TNF antagonist therapy may begin 1–2 months after the initiation of therapy for LTBI. If a TB skin test is performed, a result of 5 mm or greater is considered positive (Cush 2010, Solovic 2010).

Pathophysiology

Patients with active pulmonary TB disperse droplet nuclei containing MTB into the air, where they may remain for several hours. These nuclei are inhaled by others and eventually some of the organisms settle in the alveoli of the lungs of an exposed person and begin to replicate. Released bacilli may spread throughout the body by means of the lymphatic system or bloodstream, and in 2 to 8 weeks, macrophages will ingest the bacilli. Upon presentation to white blood cells, an immune response is triggered; the bacillus becomes engulfed by white blood cells and a granuloma is formed to contain it. However, if the immune system is unable to contain the bacilli, then the organism will begin to multiply.

The body's response to MTB depends on the host's cell-mediated immune function. T lymphocytes, mainly CD4$^+$ cells or T helper cells, activate macrophages and destroy immature macrophages that contain, but do not kill, bacilli. Those cells also produce cytokines (e.g., interferon gamma and interleukins) as part of the immune response.

After the entry of MTB into a host, tuberculosis can take several different forms: latent infection, primary disease, reactivated disease, and/or extrapulmonary disease. In 90% of cases of TB infection, MTB is contained as asymptomatic latent infection that is not infectious (Zumla 2013).

Clinical Presentation and Diagnosis

Latent Infection

Patients with LTBI are usually asymptomatic. Targeted tuberculin testing is performed to identify patients at high risk of developing active TB disease and to treat individuals found to be infected with MTB. The one exception to that is the testing of people at low risk who could potentially be exposed in the future. In any individuals found to have LTBI, a normal chest radiograph is required to exclude active pulmonary disease.

There are two types of tests available to determine TB infection: TSTs and IGRAs. The TSTs consist of placing purified protein derivative intradermally and assessing for a delayed hypersensitivity reaction in 48–72 hours as a response to the tuberculous antigens. There are several concerns with the use of TSTs, including the need for patient follow-up, reliance on injection technique and test interpretation, and the influence of prior bacillus Calmette-Guérin (BCG) vaccine administration and impaired cell-mediated immunity. In particular, recipients of BCG vaccine typically test positive, leaving it unknown whether the positive result is caused by the vaccine or by true infection. There is also a risk that patients with impaired cellular immunity may not be able to mount a response to the skin test, potentially producing a false-negative result (Schluger 2013). The criteria for interpreting a purified protein derivative result depends on patient-related risk factors (see Table 3-1).

Newer IGRA tests eliminate the concerns surrounding the use of TSTs. The IGRAs are blood tests in which a patient's blood is mixed with mycobacterial antigens, and the amount of interferon gamma is measured. If a patient is infected, T cells will produce interferon gamma when antigen-presenting cells show mycobacterial antigens. There are currently two U.S. Food and Drug Administration (FDA)–approved IGRAs in use: QuantiFERON-TB Gold and T-SPOT. Although the assays are slightly different in the ways they measure the amount of interferon gamma,

they are considered equally reliable. The benefits of the IGRAs include (1) no need for a second patient follow-up visit for the test reading and (2) no need for reliance on injection technique and subjective interpretation of the result. In additional, IGRAs distinguish between past receipt of BCG vaccine and TB infection and do not rely on immune function for host response. In general, IGRAs are more sensitive and more specific than TSTs, although one potential consideration is the higher cost of performing an IGRA compared with a TST (Schluger 2013).

When a TST is indicated, the CDC recommends that either a TST or an IGRA be used. An IGRA is preferred over a TST for recipients of BCG vaccine and for patients with low likelihood of follow-up. A TST is preferred for children younger than 5 years. In general, a TST and an IGRA are not recommended to be performed together. Either test may be used for a recent close contact or annual screening (CDC 2010).

Active Disease

Most patients with active TB have pulmonary disease. Before the HIV epidemic, 80% of TB cases were pulmonary disease. Common symptoms of pulmonary disease include productive cough, weight loss, fatigue, fever,

Table 3-1. Tuberculosis: Criteria for Positivity of PPD, by Risk Group

≥ 5 mm Induration	≥ 10 mm Induration	≥ 15 mm Induration
HIV	Recent immigrants (within past 5 years) from high prevalence countries	Persons with no risk factors for TB
Recent contacts of TB patients	IVDA	
Fibrotic changes on chest radiography consistent with prior TB	Residents and employees of the following high risk congregate settings: prisons and jails, nursing homes and other long-term care facilities for the elderly, hospitals, and other health care facilities, residential facilities for patients with AIDS, and homeless shelters	
Organ transplant recipients and other immunosuppressed patients (receiving the equivalent of > 15 mg/day of prednisone > 1 month)	Mycobacteriology laboratory personnel	
Also Pt's receiving + NF antagonist See pg 114 upper ↙PP	Persons with the following clinical conditions that place them at high risk: silicosis, DM, CRF, some hematologic disorders (e.g., leukemias and lymphomas), other specific malignancies (e.g., carcinoma of head or neck and lung), weight loss of > 10% IBW, gastrectomy, and jejunoileal bypass	
	Children younger than 4 years or infants, children, and adolescents exposed to adults at high risk	

AIDS = acquired immunodeficiency syndrome; CRF = chronic renal failure; DM = diabetes mellitus; HIV = human immunodeficiency virus; IBW = ideal body weight; IVDA = intravenous drug abuse; PPD = purified protein derivative.
Adapted from American Thoracic Society and Centers for Disease Control and Prevention. Targeted tuberculin testing and treatment of latent tuberculosis infection. MMWR 2000;(RR-6):1-54.

night sweats, and hemoptysis. Extrapulmonary TB may also occur, and symptoms depend on the site of infection. Possible forms of extrapulmonary disease include meningitis, genitourinary, lymph node, pleural, skeletal, gastrointestinal, pericardial, and miliary or disseminated. Extrapulmonary TB is more common in patients with HIV infection and may account for up to two-thirds of TB disease in that patient population.

The physical examination of a patient with active TB disease may be nonspecific. Laboratory findings may suggest normochromic, normocytic anemia and/or hypo-albuminemia. For pulmonary disease, chest radiography, chest computed tomography, or magnetic resonance imaging may reveal cavitations in the lungs.

Culture remains the gold standard for diagnosis and is required for drug-susceptibility testing; however, nucleic acid amplification tests may detect MTB earlier, with results in 24–48 hours instead of weeks. The CDC recommends nucleic acid amplification testing on at least one respiratory specimen from a patient with active signs or symptoms of pulmonary TB when the diagnosis is being considered. Nucleic acid amplification testing is also recommended when the result may influence management or control activities (CDC 2009a).

American Thoracic Society (ATS) guidelines recommend three consecutive sputum collections 8 to 24 hours apart for acid-fast bacilli staining and culture. Induced sputum collection or bronchoscopy may be necessary. Testing for susceptibility to isoniazid, rifampin, and ethambutol should be performed on all positive initial cultures. Second-line drug susceptibility testing is required only in patients who have been treated previously, in patients who have been in contact with an individual with known drug resistance, for isolates with resistance to rifampin or two first-line medications (i.e., isoniazid, rifampin, pyrazinamide, ethambutol), and for positive cultures after a patient has been on therapy for more than 3 months.

TREATMENT

Latent infection

Isoniazid administered daily for 9 months is the preferred therapy for all patients with LTBI. Twice-weekly administration for the same duration may be considered in patients with adherence problems. For patients unable to take isoniazid, rifampin administered daily for 4 months may be used. The treatment regimens for LTBI are summarized in Table 3-2 and Figure 3-1. Because of the relatively lengthy course of therapy for the treatment of LTBI, recent studies have assessed shorter courses of therapy for MTB infection (CDC 2012, 2011). In December 2012, the CDC updated its treatment regimens for LTBI to include a new, 12-week treatment using isoniazid and rifapentine. Three published studies have examined the use of that treatment regimen for LTBI.

In a phase II study on TB household contacts in Brazil, patients were randomized to receive rifapentine 900 mg plus isoniazid 900 mg by mouth daily for 12 weeks (n=206) or rifampin 450–600 mg plus pyrazinamide 750–1500 mg by mouth daily for 8 weeks (n=193). The study enrolled 399 patients, and a 2-year follow-up was planned; however, the study was stopped early because of significantly more hepatotoxicity in the rifampin-plus-pyrazinamide arm. At that time, there were 3 active cases of TB in the rifapentine-plus-isoniazid arm and 1 in the rifampin-plus-pyrazinamide arm (Schechter 2006).

An open-label, randomized, noninferiority trial in the United States, Canada, Brazil, and Spain compared rifapentine 900 mg plus isoniazid 900 mg by mouth weekly for 3 months by way of directly observed therapy (DOT) with isoniazid 300 mg orally daily for 9 months by way of self-administration. The study had nearly 4000 participants and a follow-up of 33 months. Modified intention-to-treat analysis revealed similar efficacy rates between the two arms, significantly greater rates of completion of therapy in the isoniazid-plus-rifapentine arm, and higher levels of hepatotoxicity and discontinuations secondary to adverse drug reactions in the isoniazid-only arm (Sterling 2011).

A randomized study in South Africa involved 1100 patients infected with HIV and with mean CD4$^+$ counts of 484/mm^3 for the treatment of LTBI. The four study arms included rifapentine 900 mg and isoniazid 900 mg by mouth weekly for 12 weeks; rates per 100 person-years of active TB or death were similar to those of the control arm of isoniazid 300 mg by mouth daily for 6 months (Martinson 2011).

In summary, isoniazid 900 mg plus rifapentine 900 mg by mouth weekly for 12 weeks is as effective as daily isoniazid therapy for LTBI and with greater completion rates and fewer safety concerns. As a result, the CDC recommends isoniazid and rifapentine for individuals with LTBI who are at least 12 years of age. Because of its weekly administration, this regimen should be administered by DOT. Daily self-administered isoniazid regimens have completion rates of 60% or less in typical settings. A potential advantage of the new regimen is a decrease in administration time, which leads to increased therapy completion rates. It should be considered in patients unlikely to complete 9 months of therapy. Because of lack of data the regimen is not recommended for children younger than 2 years, patients with HIV infection who are receiving antiretrovirals, pregnant women, or patients who became infected after exposure to an individual with active TB disease that is resistant to isoniazid or rifampin.

Although 9 months of isoniazid remains the preferred regimen based on the strongest evidence, that new regimen was added to the list of alternative therapies alongside isoniazid for 6 months and, when isoniazid cannot be used, rifampin for 4 months. If patient follow-up and a lengthier treatment duration are concerns, 12 weeks of weekly isoniazid and rifapentine is the preferred treatment regimen.

Table 3-2. LTBI Treatment

Drug	Adult Dose (Oral)	Pediatric Dose (Oral)	Frequency of Administration	Duration	Minimal Doses	Comments
Preferred						
Isoniazid	5 mg/kg (300 mg)	10–20 mg/kg (300 mg)	Daily	9 months	270	
Preferred DOT						
Isoniazid	15 mg/kg (900 mg)	20–40 mg/kg (900 mg)	Twice weekly	9 months	76	DOT
Alternatives						
Isoniazid	5 mg/kg (300 mg)		Daily	6 months	180	Avoid if patient infected with HIV, fibrotic lesions on chest radiography, or child
Isoniazid	15 mg/kg (900 mg)		Twice weekly	6 months	52	DOT
Isoniazid + rifapentine	Isoniazid: 15 mg/kg, max 900 mg Rifapentine: > 50 kg, 900 mg		Weekly	12 weeks	12	DOT
Rifampin	10 mg/kg (600 mg)		Daily	4 months	120	If intolerant of isoniazid or isoniazid-resistant

DOT = directly observed therapy; LTBI = latent tuberculosis infection.

Information from: American Thoracic Society and Centers for Disease Control and Prevention. Targeted tuberculin testing and treatment of latent tuberculosis infection. MMWR 2000;(RR-6):1-54; and Centers for Disease Control and Prevention. Recommendations for use of an isoniazid-rifapentine regimen with direct observation to treat latent Mycobacterium tuberculosis infection. MMWR 2011;60:1650-3.

Because of the incidence of severe liver injuries and death, the CDC no longer recommends rifampin plus pyrazinamide for the treatment of LTBI. With the new regimen, the CDC recommends baseline hepatic-chemistry blood tests for patients with HIV infection, patients with liver disorders, women within 3 months of delivery of a child, and patients who drink alcohol regularly (CDC 2012, 2011). Box 3-1 outlines the dosing of the isoniazid-plus-rifapentine regimen.

Active Disease
First-Line Agents

Four first-line drugs are available for the treatment of active TB disease: isoniazid, rifampin (or rifabutin or rifapentine), pyrazinamide, and ethambutol. In general, rifabutin and rifapentine are used as alternative rifamycins when the use of rifampin is precluded. Mycobacteria may exist in three forms: extracellular dividing organisms, dormant organisms present in macrophages, and semidormant organisms with some metabolic activity

---

Box 3-1. Isoniazid plus Rifapentine Dosing for LTBI Treatment

Isoniazid[a]
   15 mg/kg rounded up to the nearest 50 or 100 mg; 900 mg maximum orally

Rifapentine[b]
   10–14 kg: 300 mg orally
   14.1–25 kg: 450 mg orally
   25.2–32 kg: 600 mg orally
   32.1–49.9 kg: 750 mg orally
   > 50 kg: 900 mg maximum orally

[a]Formulated as 100- and 300-mg tablets
[b]Formulated as 150-mg tablets that should be kept sealed in packaged blister packs until used.
Information from Centers for Disease Control and Prevention. Recommendations for use of an isoniazid-rifapentine regimen with direct observation to treat latent *Mycobacterium tuberculosis* infection. MMWR 2011;60:1650-3.

present in granulomas. Both isoniazid and rifampin possess bactericidal activity and work on actively replicating cells. Isoniazid disrupts the cell wall of the organism by inhibiting the synthesis of mycolic acid. Rifampin works by inhibiting RNA synthesis. Isoniazid and rifampin may also have activity against dormant and semidormant populations. Pyrazinamide has bacteriostatic or bactericidal activity and works against dormant and semidormant organisms by converting to pyrazinoic acid in mycobacteria. Ethambutol is bacteriostatic, and it works by inhibiting arabinosyl transferase to impair the synthesis of the mycobacterial cell wall.

Isoniazid, rifampin, pyrazinamide, and ethambutol are used in combination for the first 8 weeks, followed by isoniazid and rifampin (provided the isolate is susceptible) for 18 weeks more. In general, the drugs are administered daily. However, for patients with adherence problems, twice-weekly dosing may be the preferred option. Such alternative dosing begins after the completion of 2 weeks of daily therapy. Any therapy administered at any frequency other than daily must be administered by DOT. Table 3-3 outlines regimens for the treatment of active TB disease. Table 3-4, Table 3-5, and Table 3-6 outline the dosing of first-line agents. The WHO guideline treatment recommendations differ slightly and include three times weekly dosing and a slightly lower dose of isoniazid (10 mg/kg/dose versus 15 mg/kg/dose) (ATS 2003).

Isoniazid

Of the potential adverse drug reactions secondary to isoniazid, the two most significant are hepatotoxicity and peripheral neuropathy. Effects on the liver range from asymptomatic transaminitis to fatal hepatitis. The risk of clinical hepatitis is increased in patients of greater age, patients with underlying liver dysfunction caused by heavy alcohol consumption, and patients in the postpartum period. The guidelines do not recommend routine monitoring for all patients but do recommend monthly liver function tests (1) for patients with preexisting liver disease, (2) for patients who develop abnormal liver function, and (3) whenever symptoms of hepatotoxicity occur. There is an increased risk of peripheral neuropathy in patients with diabetes, HIV infection, kidney failure, alcoholism, and

---

Patient Care Scenario

A 34-year-old woman (height 67 inches, weight 65 kg) presents to the infectious disease clinic after the placement of a PPD skin test 2 days ago. The area of induration measures 16 mm. She has no comorbidities and is not currently pregnant. Her vaccine history includes receipt of the BCG vaccine. Her home drugs include ethinyl estradiol 0.03 mg/levonorgestrel 0.15 mg orally daily. She has no known drug allergies. At her visit, she has no complaints and denies the presence of a cough. On physical examination, she is afebrile and her pulmonary examination is within normal limits. Her kidney and liver function are normal. Chest radiography is ordered and returns with no abnormalities. A T-spot is ordered and returns positive. The patient recently moved back to the United States from China, where she has taught English to elementary students for the last several years. She is currently staying with family but plans to move out of state to look for a teaching position in around 6 months. What is the most appropriate recommendation for this patient's TB therapy?

Answer

This patient's diagnosis is LTBI. The PPD is positive based on a PPD reading of at least 15 mm for an otherwise healthy individual with no criteria that lower the cutoff for PPD positivity to 5 or 10 mm. The tests for TB infection, the PPD and T-spot, are both positive. Although receipt of the BCG vaccine may result in a positive PPD, it will not result in a positive IGRA such as a T-spot. However, before therapy for LTBI can be initiated, active TB must be ruled out. Initiation of LBTI with one or two, rather than four medications, may result in the development of drug resistance. At the visit, the patient is asymptomatic and normal chest radiography rules out active pulmonary TB. There are two preferred treatment regimens for the treatment of LTBI, isoniazid for 9 months or isoniazid plus rifapentine for 12 weeks. The regimens work equally well, but because of the patient's impending move out-of-state and potential lack of follow-up, the shorter regimen is preferred. Isoniazid 900 mg (15 mg/kg to a maximal dose of 900 mg) by mouth and rifapentine 900 mg (weight greater than 50 kg) by mouth weekly for 12 weeks. As a weekly regimen, the drugs should be administered by DOT. Pyridoxine 25–50 mg by mouth daily should be considered to prevent potential peripheral neuropathy secondary to isoniazid. As a strong inducer of cytochrome P450, the rifapentine will reduce the serum concentration of ethinyl estradiol, making it an unreliable form of contraception. The patient should be educated on this risk and encouraged to use a second form of birth control that is nonhormonal and, therefore, without drug-drug interactions, for the time that she remains on rifapentine.

---

1. American Thoracic Society, Centers for Disease Control and Prevention and the Infectious Disease Society of America. Treatment of tuberculosis. MMWR 2003;52(RR-11):1-77.
2/ CDC, NIH, IDSA. Guidelines for the prevention and treatment of opportunistic infections in HIV-infected adults and adolescents: recommendations from the Centers for Disease Control and Prevention, the National Institutes of Health, and the HIV Medicine Association of the Infectious Diseases Society of America. 2014

other comorbidities associated with neuropathy and in pregnant and breast-feeding women. To help prevent the potential adverse reaction of peripheral neuropathy, the treatment guidelines recommend pyridoxine 25 mg by mouth daily for patients with risk factors (ATS 2003).

As a major 2E1 substrate and a strong 2C19 inhibitor, isoniazid has interactions with cytochrome P450 (CYP). It also has moderate inhibition of CYP 1A2, CYP 2D6, and CYP 2E1. Two notable drug-drug interactions with isoniazid are phenytoin and carbamazepine.

Rifamycins

Rifampin is the preferred rifamycin. However, rifabutin and rifapentine may also be considered first line in certain circumstances. Rifabutin may substitute for rifampin when warranted by drug interactions.

The rifamycins may cause hepatotoxicity, especially when given in combination with other hepatotoxic drugs such as isoniazid. The rifamycins cause red-orange discoloration of body secretions (e.g., urine, sweat, tears) and soft contact lenses may become permanently stained. Rifabutin may also cause uveitis, which is a dose-related adverse effect. The treatment guidelines do not recommend routine monitoring of the rifamycins (ATS 2003).

Rifampin is a potent CYP3A4 inducer. Rifabutin is also an inducer but is not as potent as rifampin. Rifabutin is usually a safer alternative, but dosing adjustments and close monitoring may become necessary. Any drug that is a major substrate of CYP 3A4 will be affected by rifampin, including many of the antiretrovirals. In additional, rifabutin is a CYP 3A4 substrate, and it could be affected by other strong inhibitors or inducers. Those drug interactions are summarized in Table 3-7.

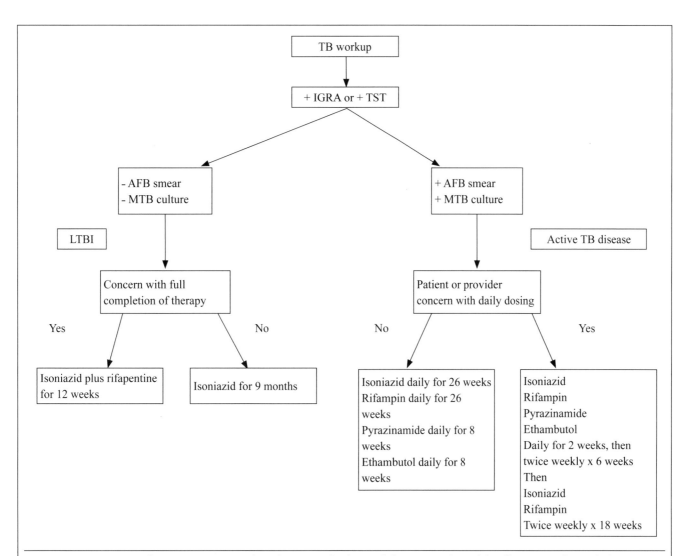

Figure 3-1. Active versus latent TB treatment algorithm. Directly observed therapy is indicated for all regimens that include medications dosed at frequencies less than once daily.

AFB = acid-fast bacillus; IGRA = interferon gamma release assay; LTBI = latent tuberculosis infection; MTB = *Mycobacterium tuberculosis*; PPD = purified protein derivative; TB = tuberculosis

Table 3-3. Active Tuberculosis Treatment

Regimen	Meds	Initial phase Interval and Dosing (Oral)	Regimen	Meds	Continuation phase Interval and Dosing (Oral)	Total doses (minimal duration)
1	INH RIF PZA ETH	7 days/wk for 56 doses (8 weeks) OR 5 days/week for 40 doses (8 weeks)	a	INH RIF	7 days/week for 126 doses (18 weeks) OR 5 days/week for 90 doses (18 weeks)	182–130 (26 weeks)
			b	INH RIF(not if patient infected with HIV and CD4$^+$ <100 cells/mm^3)	2x/week for 36 doses (18 weeks)	92–76 (26 weeks)
			c	INH Rifapentine (not if patient infected with HIV)	1x/week for 18 doses (18 weeks)	74–58 (26 weeks)
2	INH RIF PZA ETH	7 days/week for 14 doses (2 weeks), then 2x/week for 12 doses (6 weeks) OR 5 days/week for 10 doses (2 weeks), then 2x/week for 12 doses (6 weeks)	a	INH RIF (not if patient infected with HIV and CD4$^+$ <100 cells/mm^3)	2x/week for 36 doses (18 weeks)	62–58 (26 weeks)
			b	INH Rifapentine (not if patient infected with HIV)	1x/week for 18 doses (18 weeks)	44–40 (26 weeks)
3	INH RIF PZA ETH	3x/week for 24 doses (8 weeks)	a	INH RIF	3x/week for 54 doses (18 weeks)	78 (26 weeks)
4	INH RIF ETH	7 days/week for 56 doses (8 wk) OR 5 days/week for 40 doses (8 weeks)	a	INH RIF	7 days/week for 217 doses (31 weeks) OR 5 days/week for 155 doses (31 weeks)	273–195 (39 weeks)
			b	INH RIF	2x/week for 62 doses (31 weeks)	118–102 (39 weeks)

ETH = ethambutol; HIV = human immunodeficiency virus; INH = isoniazid; PZA = pyrazinamide; RIF = rifampin.

Adapted from American Thoracic Society, Centers for Disease Control and Prevention and the Infectious Disease Society of America. Treatment of tuberculosis. MMWR 2003;52(RR-11):1-77. This document was published in January 2015. Certain aspects of this document may be out of date, and caution should be used when applying the information in clinical practice and other usages.

Pyrazinamide

Pyrazinamide has the potential to cause hepatotoxicity. It may also cause polyarthralgias, which respond to aspirin or nonsteroidal anti-inflammatory agents (ATS 2003) and asymptomatic hyperuricemia. Because of its potential to rarely cause acute gouty arthritis, the use of pyrazinamide is a precaution for patients with a preexisting diagnosis of gout and a contraindication in the presence of acute gout (ATS 2003).

Ethambutol

Ethambutol may cause retrobulbar neuritis, which may present as decreased visual acuity or decreased red-green color discrimination. The adverse reaction is dose related and therefore occurs at a higher incidence in patients with renal insufficiency and patients receiving more than 30 mg/kg/day. To monitor, the guidelines recommend baseline visual acuity and color discrimination testing in all patients, as well as a monthly assessment of visual disturbances. However, monthly visual acuity and color discrimination testing is recommended only for patients taking more than 15–25 mg/kg/day, patients receiving the drug for more than 2 months, and patients with renal insufficiency (ATS 2003). Any change in vision warrants discontinuation of ethambutol.

Table 3-4. Isoniazid and Rifamycins for Active Tuberculosis

Usual daily dose	2x/week dose	3x/week dose	Maximal dose	Adverse drug reactions	Routine monitoring
Isoniazid[a]					
5 mg/kg (300 mg)	15 mg/kg (900 mg)	15 mg/kg (900 mg)	900 mg	Asymptomatic transaminases Clinical hepatitis Fatal hepatitis Peripheral neurotoxicity CNS effects Lupus-like syndrome Hypersensitivity reaction Monoamine poisoning Diarrhea	LFTs monthly for patients with preexisting liver disease or those who develop abnormal liver function LFTs and development of symptoms
Rifampin[a]					
10 mg/kg (600 mg)	10 mg/kg (600 mg)	10 mg/kg (600 mg)	600 mg	Cutaneous reactions Gastrointestinal reactions Flu-like syndrome Hepatotoxicity Severe immunologic reactions Orange discoloration of bodily fluids	
Rifabutin[a]					
5 mg/kg (300 mg)	5 mg/kg (300 mg)	5 mg/kg (300 mg)	300 mg	Hematologic toxicity Uveitis Gastrointestinal symptoms Polyarthralgias Hepatotoxicity Pseudojaundice Rash Flu-like syndrome Orange discoloration of bodily fluids	
Rifapentine[a]					
Other dosing: weekly					
15 mg/kg (900 mg)				See rifampin	

Note: Isoniazid available as 50-, 100-, and 300-mg tabs; rifampin available as 150- and 300-mg caps; rifabutin available as 150 mg; rifapentine available as 150 mg.

[a]No dosing change in renal insufficiency (CrCl <30 mL/minute or hemodialysis)

LFT = liver function tests.

Adapted from American Thoracic Society, Centers for Disease Control and Prevention and the Infectious Disease Society of America. Treatment of tuberculosis. MMWR 2003;52(RR-11):1-77. This document was published in January 2015. Certain aspects of this document may be out of date, and caution should be used when applying the information in clinical practice and other usages.

Table 3-5. Pyrazinamide for Active Tuberculosis

Interval	40–55 kg	56–75 kg	76-90 kg	Dosing in renal insufficiency (CrCl <30 mL/minute or hemodialysis)	Adverse drug reactions	Routine monitoring
Daily	1000 mg (18.2–25 mg/kg)	1500 mg (20–26.8 mg/kg)	2000 mg (22.2–26.3 mg/kg)	25–35 mg/kg/dose 3x/week (instead of daily)	Hepatotoxicity Gastrointestinal symptoms Non-gouty polyarthralgia Asymptomatic hyperuricemia Acute gouty arthritis Transient morbilliform rash Dermatitis	Liver function tests in patients with underlying liver disease
3x/week	1500 mg (27.3–37.5 mg/kg)	2500 mg (33.3–44.6 mg/kg)	3000 mg (33.3–39.5 mg/kg)			
2x/week	2000 mg (36.4–50 mg/kg)	3000 mg (40–53.6 mg/kg)	4000 mg (44.4–52.6 mg/kg)			

Pyrazinamide available as 500 mg tab (scored).

Adapted from American Thoracic Society, Centers for Disease Control and Prevention and the Infectious Disease Society of America. Treatment of tuberculosis. MMWR 2003;52(RR-11):1-77. This document was published in January 2015. Certain aspects of this document may be out of date, and caution should be used when applying the information in clinical practice and other usages.

Second-Line Agents

In general, second-line drugs are reserved for resistant MTB (Table 3-8). Second-line agents are less effective and have greater potential for causing toxicities. They may also be injectable drugs and therefore more challenging from an administration standpoint.

Drug-resistant TB

Antimicrobial resistance of TB can be either primary or acquired and is of increasing concern. Multidrug-resistant TB (MDRTB) is defined as TB that is resistant to isoniazid and rifampin. Extensively drug-resistant TB (XDRTB) is defined as MDRTB plus resistance to any fluoroquinolone and any second-line injectable agent.

In the United States, about 1% of cases are MDRTB; 2 cases of XDRTB were reported in 2012. Only 1% of TB cases were primary multidrug resistant. However, because of potential barriers in developing countries, the percentage of drug-resistant TB is much higher worldwide. In 2012, 3.6% of new TB cases were MDRTB and 9.6% were XDRTB. There are issues with treating TB with second-line agents, and only 48% of MDRTB cases were treated successfully (WHO 2013; CDC 2012). One potential barrier to successful treatment is the lack of resources for diagnosis and therapy (Chan 2013). In general, the treatment of MDRTB is relatively longer and more expensive and has more safety concerns when compared with the treatment of susceptible TB.

For MDRTB, WHO recommends that regimens include at least pyrazinamide, a fluoroquinolone, a parenteral agent, ethionamide (or prothionamide), and either cycloserine or p-aminosalicylic acid if cycloserine cannot be used. The recommended durations of treatment for MDRTB is 8 months of an intensive treatment phase and a total of 20 months for most patients. In 2013, bedaquiline became available as an alternative agent for the treatment of drug-resistant TB. Bedaquiline is in the new class of antibiotics called diarylquinolines. Agents in this class inhibit mycobacterial ATP synthase—leading to MTB's inability to generate energy, which is essential to MTB growth and reproduction (Chahine 2013). Bedaquiline is bactericidal and active against both actively replicating and dormant organisms (Chan 2013).

In light of the need for agents to treat drug-resistant TB—despite the lack of phase 3 studies—the FDA approved the labeling of bedaquiline for use in adult patients with pulmonary MDRTB (resistance to rifampicin and isoniazid). The December 2012 approval was based on phase 2 studies, with the time to sputum culture conversion as an indicator of efficacy. A single study on bedaquiline has been published along with a 2-year follow-up study. Study C208 (n=47) was a double-blind, randomized, placebo-controlled superiority study in patients with new-onset MDRTB (Diacon 2012, 2009). Treatment arms included a background regimen administered for 18–24 weeks with and without bedaquiline for the initial 8 weeks of treatment. Patients in the bedaquiline arm received 400 mg by mouth daily for 14 days and then 200 mg by mouth three times per week. Patients who received bedaquiline plus a background regimen had a faster median time to sputum culture conversion, which was the primary end point. At 8 weeks, the hazard ratio was 11.8 (95% confidence interval [CI], 2.3–61.3, p=0.003), and the difference remained significant in favor of bedaquiline at 24 weeks. At week 8, the secondary end point of sputum culture conversion rate was greater in the bedaquiline arm (difference 38.9%; 95% CI, 12.3%, 63.1%; p=0.004). Adverse drug reactions occurred more often in the bedaquiline arms than the placebo arm and included nausea, arthralgia, and headache; however, only nausea was significantly greater at 8 weeks (26% vs. 4%, p=0.04). Although not significant, there was a greater increase in mean corrected QT interval in the bedaquiline arm. There were no adverse events of corrected QT greater than 500 msec.

Dosing

The recommended dosing of bedaquiline is 400 mg by mouth once daily for 2 weeks, followed by 200 mg by mouth three times weekly (with at least 48 hours between doses) for 22 weeks, given with food. It should be administered by DOT. There is no dosing adjustment for patients with mild to moderate kidney or liver impairment. However, bedaquiline should be used with caution in patients with severe renal or hepatic impairment. Bedaquiline is available as a 100-mg tablet.

Pharmacokinetics

Bedaquiline is a major substrate of CYP3A4. As a result, its use is not recommended in combination with strong 3A4 inducers. In combination with strong CYP3A4 inhibitors, bedaquiline should be limited to 14 consecutive days unless the benefit outweighs the risk.

Safety

Bedaquiline has two boxed warnings: QT prolongation and increased risk of death. The prescribing information recommends frequent monitoring by electrocardiography (baseline and at least at 2, 12, and 24 weeks). In additional, serum potassium, calcium, and magnesium should be monitored and corrected as necessary. More frequent electrocardiography is indicated if bedaquiline is used in combination with other drugs with QT prolongation potential. If there is development of a clinically significant ventricular arrhythmia or QTcF interval greater than 500 msec confirmed by repeat electrocardiography, then bedaquiline should be discontinued.

Baseline, monthly, and as-needed liver tests (ALT, AST, ALF, and bilirubin) should be obtained. Bedaquiline should be discontinued if aminotransferases increase more than 2 times the upper limit of normal with elevated total bilirubin, if aminotransferases increase higher than 8 times the upper limit of normal, or if aminotransferase elevations continue beyond 2 weeks. Elevations should be confirmed within 48 hours. Because of the lack of data,

Table 3-6. Ethambutol for Active Tuberculosis

Interval	40–55 kg	56–75 kg	76–90 kg	Dosing in renal insufficiency (CrCl<30 mL/minute or hemodialysis)	Adverse drug reactions	Routine Monitoring
Daily mg	800 mg (14.5–20 mg/kg)	1200 mg (16–21.4 mg/kg)	1600 mg (17.8–21.1 mg/kg)	15–25 mg/kg/dose 3x/week (instead of daily)	Retrobulbar neuritis Peripheral neuritis Cutaneous reactions	Baseline and monthly visual acuity and color discrimination testing Visual disturbances monthly Monthly visual acuity and color discrimination testing for doses greater than 15-25 mg/kg, patients receiving ethambutol for more than 2 months, and any patient with renal insufficiency
3x/week mg	1200 mg (21.8–30 mg/kg)	2000 mg (26.7–35.7 mg/kg)	2400 mg (26.7–31.6 mg/kg)			
2x/week	2000 mg (36.4–50 mg/kg)	2800 mg (37.3–50 mg/kg)	4000 mg (44.4–52.6 mg/kg)			

Ethambutol available as 100- and 400-mg tabs.
Adapted from American Thoracic Society, Centers for Disease Control and Prevention and the Infectious Disease Society of America. Treatment of tuberculosis. MMWR 2003;52(RR-11):1-77. This document was published in January 2015. Certain aspects of this document may be out of date, and caution should be used when applying the information in clinical practice and other usages.

Table 3-7. Rifamycins and Antiretroviral Drug Interactions

NNRTI

Rifamycin	Antiretroviral	Effect	Recommendation
Rifabutin	Efavirenz	Rifabutin: AUC ↓ 38%	Rifabutin 450-600 mg once daily or 600 mg 3x/week if not co-administered with a PI
	Etravirine	Rifabutin and metabolite: AUC ↓ 17% Etravirine: AUC ↓ 37%, Cmin ↓ 35%	Do not co-administer if using with a ritonavir boosted PI. Rifabutin 300 mg once daily
	Rilpivirine	Rilpivirine: AUC ↓ 46%	Contraindicated. Do not co-administer.
Rifampin	Efavirenz	Efavirenz: AUC ↓ 26%	Monitor virologic response. Consider efavirenz TDM. Some clinicians suggest efavirenz 800 mg if > 60 kg.
	Etravirine	Etravirine: Significant ↓ possible	Do not co-administer.
	Rilpivirine	Rilpivirine: AUC ↓ 80%	Contraindicated. Do not co-administer.
Rifapentine	Efavirenz Etravirine Rilpivirine	NNRTI: ↓ expected	Do not co-administer.

PIs

Rifamycin	Antiretroviral	Effect	Recommendation
Rifabutin	Boosted atazanavir	Rifabutin: AUC ↑ 110% and metabolite AUC ↑ 2101% (rifabutin 150 mg once daily with PI compared with rifabutin 300 mg once daily alone)	Rifabutin 150 mg once daily or 300 mg 3x/week. Monitoring antimycobacterial activity and consider rifabutin TDM. This PK data is from healthy volunteers. Lower rifabutin exposure has been reported in HIV infected patients.
	Boosted darunavir	Rifabutin: metabolite AUC ↑ 881% (rifabutin 150 mg every other day with PI compared with rifabutin 300 mg once daily alone)	
	Boosted lopinavir	Rifabutin: rifabutin and metabolite AUC ↑ 473% (rifabutin 150 mg once daily with PI compared with rifabutin 300 mg daily alone)	
Rifampin	All PIs	PI: ↓ concentration > 75%	Do not co-administer.
Rifapentine	All PIs	PI: ↓ expected	Do not co-administer.

INSTIs

Rifamycin	Antiretroviral	Effect	Recommendation
Rifabutin	Boosted elvitegravir (with cobicistat)	Rifabutin: active metabolite AUC ↑ 625% (rifabutin 150 mg every other day with boosted elvitegravir compared to rifabutin 300 mg once daily alone) Elvitegravir: AUC ↓ 21%, Cmin ↓ 67%	Do not co-administer.
	Dolutegravir	Dolutegravir: Cmin ↓ 30% (rifabutin 300 mg daily)	No adjustment
	Raltegravir	Raltegravir: AUC ↑ 19%, Cmax ↑ 39%, Cmin ↓ 20%	No adjustment
Rifampin	Boosted elvitegravir (with cobicistat)	Elvitegravir and cobicistat: significant ↓ expected	Do not co-administer.

Table 3-7. Rifamycins and Antiretroviral Drug Interactions *(continued)*

	Dolutegravir	Dolutegravir: AUC ↓ 54%, Cmin ↓ 72% (dolutegravir 50 mg twice daily compared to dolutegravir alone) Dolutegravir: AUC ↑ 33%, Cmin ↑ 22% (dolutegravir 50 mg twice daily compared to 50 mg daily plus rifampin)	Dolutegravir 50 mg twice daily Avoid dolutegravir if documented or suspected integrase inhibitor mutations. Consider rifabutin
	Raltegravir	Raltegravir: AUC ↓ 40% and Cmin ↓ 61% (raltegravir 400 mg) Raltegravir: AUC ↑ 27% and Cmin ↓ 53% (raltegravir 800 mg twice daily with rifampin compared to raltegravir 400 mg twice daily alone)	Raltegravir 800 mg twice daily Monitor virologic response. Consider rifabutin as alternative
Rifapentine	Boosted elvitegravir (with cobicistat)	Elvitegravir and cobicistat: significant ↓ expected	Do not co-administer
CCR5 antagonists			
Rifabutin	Maraviroc	Maraviroc: ↓ possible	With strong CYP3A4 inhibitor: maraviroc 150 mg twice daily Without a strong CYP3A4 inducer or inhibitor: maraviroc 300 mg twice daily
Rifampin	Maraviroc	Maraviroc: AUC ↓ 64%	Co-administration is not recommended Maraviroc 600 mg twice daily Maraviroc 300 mg twice daily if using with a strong CYP3A4 inhibitor
Rifapentine	Maraviroc	Maraviroc: ↓ expected	Do not co-administer

AUC = area under the curve; CCR5 = chemokine receptor type 5; Cmax = maximum concentration; Cmin = minimum concentration; INSTI = integrase strand transferase inhibitor; NNRTI = nonnucleoside reverse transcriptase inhibitor; PI = protease inhibitor.

Adapted from: DHHS. Panel on Antiretroviral Guidelines for Adults and Adolescents. Guidelines for the use of antiretroviral agents in HIV-1-infected adults and adolescents; and CDC, NIH, IDSA. Guidelines for the prevention and treatment of opportunistic infections in HIV-infected adults and adolescents: recommendations from the Centers for Disease Control and Prevention, the National Institutes of Health, and the HIV Medicine Association of the Infectious Diseases Society of America. 2014

bedaquiline should be avoided in children and pregnant or nursing women.

The WHO and the CDC have published interim guidelines on the use of bedaquiline (CDC 2013). According to CDC provisional guidelines for its use, bedaquiline may be used for the treatment of pulmonary MDRTB with resistance to both isoniazid and rifampin—in combination with at least three other active drugs when an effective treatment regimen cannot otherwise be provided. The use of bedaquiline may be considered on a case-by-case basis for the following patient populations: children, patients with HIV infection, pregnant women, patients with extrapulmonary MDRTB, and patients with comorbidities on concomitant drugs. Bedaquiline use beyond 24 weeks may also be considered on a case-by-case basis. It should be administered by DOT for 24 weeks, with the continuation of other antituberculosis drugs for an additional 4–5 months because of its long half-life. If a dose of bedaquiline is missed during the first 2 weeks, the patient should skip that missed dose. If a dose is missed during or after week 3 of therapy, it should be taken as soon as possible and the scheduled regimen resumed. Monitoring of symptoms should be performed weekly, and culture monitoring should follow the standard of care for patients with MDRTB in the United States (i.e., monthly throughout and at the completion of therapy, even following conversion to a negative culture). Precautions and recommended monitoring for hepatotoxicity and QT prolongation are consistent with bedaquiline prescribing information (CDC 2013).

According to the CDC, the manufacturer of bedaquiline is developing a registry to track all patients who receive the drug. The registry will be maintained through

Table 3-8. Second-line Agents for Treatment of Tuberculosis

Group	Description	Agent
2	Injectable agents	Kanamycin Amikacin Capreomycin
3	Fluoroquinolones	Levofloxacin Moxifloxacin Ofloxacin
4	Less effective second-line agents	Ethionamide Prothionamide Cycloserine Terizidone p-aminosalicylic acid
5	Less effective with minimal clinical data	Clofazimine Linezolid Amoxicillin/clavulanate Thiacetazone Clarithromycin Imipenem

Information from Daley CL, Caminero JA. Management of multidrug resistant tuberculosis. Semin Respir Crit Care Med 2013;34:44-59.

Table 3-9. Potential TB Drugs in Clinical Development

Phase I	Phase II	Phase III
	AZD5847	Delamanid (OPC-67683)
	Bedaquiline (TMC-207)	Gatifloxacin
	Linezolid	Moxifloxacin
	Novel regimens	Rifapentine
	PA-824	
	Rifapentine	
	SQ-109	
	Sutezolid (PNU-100480)	

Information from Working Group on New TB Drugs [homepage on the Internet].

December 2018 and a final report will be issued in August 2019. The manufacturer is also required to conduct a multicenter, double-blind, placebo-controlled phase 3 randomized trial in patients with MDRTB as part of the conditions associated with accelerated approval.

According to WHO, bedaquiline may be added to a regimen to treat pulmonary MDRTB in adult patients provided the principles of designing a second-line regimen are followed (WHO 2013). Other requirements include close monitoring for safety, proper management of adverse drug reactions and drug-drug interactions, and the obtaining of patients' informed consent.

Other Agents

Other drugs with potential roles in the treatment of active TB (both drug susceptible and drug resistant) include the fluoroquinolones, especially levofloxacin and moxifloxacin; oxazolidinones (linezolid and sutezolid); nitroimidazoles (delamanid and PA-824); clofazimine; meropenem plus clavulanate; SQ109; and the benzothiazinone BTZ043. Those agents have been found to have activity against MTB. There are also studies on shortening the duration of therapy. In the current WHO guidelines, moxifloxacin and levofloxacin are recommended for the treatment of MDRTB (Kwon 2014). Table 3-9 lists drugs under study for the treatment of tuberculosis.

Special Populations

HIV Infection

When compared with the general population, patients infected with HIV have a relatively higher risk of TB progression to active disease as well as a higher mortality rate. In addition to disease progression, concerns about drug interactions and immune reconstitution inflammatory syndrome (IRIS) remain particularly relevant for this patient population. Because of the potential for many drug interactions with most classes of antiretrovirals, interactions with rifamycins are significant and may affect the treatment of LTBI and active TB disease (see Table 3-7). About 10% of patients with HIV infection who initiate therapy for active TB disease develop IRIS (Zumla 2013). This syndrome may be paradoxical or unmasking. Paradoxical TB IRIS may result when TB therapy is initiated before combination antiretroviral therapy (cART). Inflammation, either local or systemic, may occur within 1–4 weeks of starting cART and typically lasts 2–3 months. Risk factors include a low CD4$^+$ count, extrapulmonary TB, and the initiation of cART within 2 months of the initiation of TB treatment. The unmasking of TB IRIS occurs within the first weeks of ART and results from an unrecognized TB infection. Symptoms have a rapid onset, and to minimize the potential for that reaction, the guidelines recommend that initiation of these drugs be spaced in an untreated patient and that all coinfected patients receive ART. If the patient is cART naive and has a CD4$^+$ less than 50 cells/mm^3, then

Table 3-10. Pharmacokinetic Parameters of First-Line Antimycobacterial Drugs

Agent	Usual adult dosage	Usual Cmax (mcg/mL)	Usual tmax (hours)	Normal half life (hours)
Isoniazid	300 mg daily 900 mg twice weekly	3–6 9–18	0.75–2	Polymorphic - Fast: 1.5 - Slow: 4
Rifampin	600 mg daily	8–24	2	3
Rifabutin	300 mg daily	0.3–0.9	3–4	25
Rifapentine	600 mg daily	8–30	5	15
Pyrazinamide	25 mg/kg daily 50 mg/kg twice weekly	20–50 40–100	12	9
Ethambutol	25 mg/kg daily 50 mg/kg twice weekly	2–6 4–12	2–3	Biphasic: - A: 2-4 - B: 12-14

Cmax = maximum concentration; tmax = time to maximum absorption.
Adapted from Peloquin CA. Therapeutic drug monitoring in the treatment of tuberculosis. Drugs 2002;62:2169-83.

ART should be initiated within 2 weeks of TB therapy. For $CD4^+$ greater than 50 cells/mm³, ART should be initiated by 8 to 12 weeks after TB therapy (CDC 2014).

Pregnancy

Because of the risks of disease to a pregnant woman and fetus, active TB disease should be treated. With the exception of pyrazinamide, the first-line antimycobacterial agents (isoniazid, rifampin, and ethambutol) may be used safely in pregnancy. The use of pyrazinamide is controversial, and the guidelines differ. The ATS guidelines recommend against the use of pyrazinamide in pregnant women because of lack of available safety data; WHO recommends its use. Without pyrazinamide, the total duration of therapy should be at least 9 months (ATS 2003). Pyridoxine should be administered to prevent peripheral neuropathy secondary to isoniazid. To avoid exposing the fetus to medication, the treatment of LTBI in a pregnant woman may be delayed until delivery, provided there is low risk of progression to active TB disease.

Renal Insufficiency

Renal dosing of first-line antimycobacterial medications requires an increase in the dosing interval rather than a reduction in dose to avoid compromising the achievable peak serum concentration (see Table 3-4 and Table 3-5). To avoid potential removal—especially removal of pyrazinamide—patients on hemodialysis should receive drugs after a dialysis session. There are no data involving the use of these agents in peritoneal dialysis.

Extrapulmonary TB

Some forms of extrapulmonary TB differ in treatment durations and indication for the use of corticosteroids compared with the standard treatment of pulmonary TB. In general, treatment duration is 6–9 months, with the exception of tuberculosis meningitis, whose treatment duration is 9–12 months, according to the treatment guidelines. All treatment regimens remain the same as those used for treating pulmonary TB, except that the once-weekly combination of isoniazid and rifapentine is not recommended because of lack of experience. Corticosteroids may be adjunct therapies for treating TB meningitis and pericarditis (ATS 2003).

Pediatrics

For the treatment of a pediatric patient with active TB disease, isoniazid, rifampin, and pyrazinamide should be first-line therapy. Ethambutol should be avoided because of the difficulty in monitoring for ophthalmologic adverse reactions in this patient population. Directly observed therapy must be used for all children. The recommended frequency of antimycobacterial medication dosing is either daily or twice weekly.

MONITORING

According to treatment guidelines, there are three key efficacy-monitoring parameters for pulmonary TB. Firstly, sputum acid-fast bacilli smears should be performed early to determine response to therapy and noninfectiousness. Smears may be performed every 2 weeks until two consecutive samples are negative. Monthly sputum cultures should be performed until two consecutive negative results are obtained. Secondly, the patient should undergo monthly clinical evaluations that assess for adverse drug reactions and adherence. Finally, chest radiography should be performed after 2 months of therapy and possibly at the end of therapy to establish a new baseline. The monitoring of extrapulmonary TB depends on the site of the infection.

For potential adverse drug reactions and their respective monitoring parameters, see Table 3-4, Table 3-5, and Table 3-6. The active TB treatment guidelines provide recommendations for the management of adverse drug reactions.

Because of the predictable pharmacokinetics and the proven efficacy of standard doses (Table 3-10), routine therapeutic drug monitoring (TDM) of first-line MTB medications is not recommended by the active TB disease treatment guidelines (ATS 2003). Instead, TDM is recommended in the setting of treatment failure caused by nonadherence or resistance, medical conditions that alter drug pharmacokinetics, or MDRTB with second-line medications. Despite their being recommended in some situations, there are no validated therapeutic ranges for these drugs. Besides the relationships between (1) ethambutol and ocular toxicity and (2) pyrazinamide and hepatotoxicity, much of the relationship between drug dose and serum concentration and toxicity remains unknown. Other disadvantages of TDM include time and expense. Therapeutic drug monitoring of antimycobacterial medications involves the monitoring of peak serum concentrations because trough serum concentrations are typically below the limit of detection for the assays, thereby making them of no value. Because of some variation in time to absorption, serum concentrations may be best measured at 6 hours postdose (ATS 2003; Peloquin 2002).

CONCLUSION

The clinical presentations and management of active TB disease and LTBI differ greatly. One similarity between active disease and latent infection is the relatively lengthy period of treatment with potentially toxic agents. Adherence, monitoring and managing potential adverse drug reactions, and managing potential drug-drug interactions are critical components of the treatment plan.

REFERENCES

American Thoracic Society, Centers for Disease Control and Prevention and the Infectious Disease Society of America. Treatment of tuberculosis. Am J Respir Crit Care Med 2003;167:603-62.

American Thoracic Society and Centers for Disease Control and Prevention. Targeted tuberculin testing and treatment of latent tuberculosis infection. MMWR 2000;(RR-6):1-51.

Andrews JR, Noubary F, Walensky RP et al.. Risk of progression to active tuberculosis following reinfection with Mycobacterium tuberculosis. Clin Infect Dis 2012;54:784-91.

Centers for Disease Control and Prevention. Provisional CDC guidelines for the use and safety monitoring of bedaquiline fumarate (Sirturo) for the treatment of multidrug-resistant tuberculosis. MMWR 2013;62:1-12.

Centers for Disease Control and Prevention. Recommendations for use of an isoniazid-rifapentine regimen with direct observation to treat latent Mycobacterium tuberculosis infection. MMWR 2011;60:1650-3.

Centers for Disease Control and Prevention. Updated guidelines for using interferon gamma release assays to detect Mycobacterium tuberculosis infection – United States, 2010. MMWR. 2010;59(RR-5):1-25.

Centers for Disease Control and Prevention. Updated guidelines for the use of nucleic acid amplification tests in the diagnosis of tuberculosis. MMWR 2009;58:7-10.

Centers for Disease Control and Prevention (CDC). Plan to combat extensively drug-resistant tuberculosis. Recommendations of the federal tuberculosis task force. MMWR 2009;58(RR-3).

Centers for Disease Control and Prevention (CDC). Reported Tuberculosis in the United States, 2012.

Centers for Disease Control and Prevention (CDC). Treatment for Latent TB Infection. Centers for Disease Control and Prevention.

Chahine EB, Karaoui LR, Mansour H. Bedaquiline: a novel diarylquinoline for multi-drug resistant tuberculosis. Ann Pharmacother 2014;48:107-15.

Chan B, Khadem TM, Brown J. A review of tuberculosis: focus on bedaquiline. Am J Health-Syst Pharm 2013;70:1984-94.

Cush JJ, Winthrop K, Dao K et al. Screening for Mycobacterium tuberculosis: questions and answers for clinical practice. Drug Safety Quarterly June 2010:1-2.

Diacon AH, Donald PR, Grobusch et al. Randomized pilot trial of eight weeks of bedaquiline (TMC 207) treatment for multidrug resistant tuberculosis: long-term outcome, tolerability, and effect on emergence of drug resistance. Antimicrob Agents Chemother 2012;56:3271-6.

Diacon AH, Pym A, Grobusch M et al. The diarylquinoline TMC207 for multidrug-resistant tuberculosis. N Eng J Med 2009;360:2397-405.

Kwon YS, Jeong BH, Koh WJ. Tuberculosis: clinical trials and new drug regimens. Curr Opin Pulm Med 2014;20:280-6.

Martinson NA, Barnes GL, Moulton LH, et al. New regimens to prevent tuberculosis in adults with HIV infection. N Engl J Med 2011;365:11-20.

Peloquin CA. Therapeutic drug monitoring in the treatment of tuberculosis. Drugs 2002; 62:2169-83.

Schechter MS, Zajdenverg R, Falco G et al. Weekly rifapentine/isoniazid or daily rifampin/pyrazinamide for latent tuberculosis in household contacts. Am J Respir Crit Care Med 2006;173:922-6.

Schluger NW. Advances in the diagnosis of latent tuberculosis infection. Semin Respir Crit Care Med 2013;34:60-6.

Sirturo Clinical Trials. Janssen. Last updated December 4 2013.

Solovic I, Seser M, Gomez-Reino JJ et al. The risk of tuberculosis related to tumour necrosis factor antagonist therapies: a TBNET consensus statement. Eur Respir J 2010;36:925-49.

Sterling TR, Villarino E, Borisov AS, et al. Three months of rifapentine and isoniazid for latent tuberculosis infection. N Engl J Med 2011:365:2155-66.

World Health Organization. Guidelines for the programmatic management of drug-resistant tuberculosis. 2011 update.

World Health Organization. The use of bedaquiline for the treatment of multidrug-resistant tuberculosis. Interim policy guideline.

World Health Organization. Global TB Report 2013 executive summary. World Health Organization.

Zumla A, Raviglione M, Hafner R et al. Tuberculosis. N Engl J Med 2013;368:745-55.

SELF-ASSESSMENT QUESTIONS

41. A 36-year-old patient with HIV infection presents to the clinic after a positive T-spot. The patient is currently on antiretroviral therapy (ART) consisting of tenofovir, emtricitabine and lopinavir/ritonavir with an undetectable HIV RNA and CD4$^+$ count of 610 cells/mm^3. At today's visit, the patient endorses a cough and a chest radiography reveals a cavitary lesion. Sputum smears are pending. What is the most appropriate medication to add to isoniazid, ethambutol, and pyrazinamide for the treatment of pulmonary tuberculosis (TB) in this patient?

    A. Rifampin 600 mg by mouth daily.
    B. Rifabutin 150 mg by mouth every other day.
    C. Rifabutin 150 mg by mouth daily.
    D. Rifapentine 900 mg by mouth weekly.

42. A 40-year-old man with HIV infection presents to the clinic for follow-up. Currently, the patient has a CD4$^+$ count of 510 cells/mm^3 and is not taking antiretrovirals because of his poor adherence to clinic appointments. At a visit last year, the patient had a positive Quantiferon Gold test. Records indicate that attempts to contact the patient have been unsuccessful and, therefore, the patient has not been treated. The patient's chest radiography is normal. Through discussion about starting ART at today's visit, the patient shares that he will be leaving the country for a few weeks in 5 months and does not wish to take any medications with him. Therefore, he will not be starting ART at this time. Which one of the following would best treat latent tuberculosis infection (LTBI) in this patient?

    A. Rifampin 400 mg by mouth daily for 4 months.
    B. Isoniazid 300 mg by mouth daily for 6 months.
    C. Isoniazid 900 mg by mouth weekly plus rifapentine 900 mg by mouth weekly for 12 weeks.
    D. Isoniazid 300 mg by mouth daily plus rifampin 600 mg by mouth daily for 8 weeks.

43. A 32-year-old man (height 67 inches, weight 78 kg) with HIV infection presents to the clinic for follow-up 2 days after placement of his purified protein derivative (PPD) skin test. The area of induration measures 7 mm. The patient denies symptoms of pulmonary TB and a chest radiography is read as normal. The patient is currently taking tenofovir/emtricitabine and raltegravir and labs include a CD4$^+$ count of 496 cells/mm^3 and HIV-1 RNA of 6231 copies/mL. Which one of the following is best to recommend for this patient?

    A. No treatment is indicated at this time.
    B. Isoniazid 900 mg by mouth once daily for 6 months.
    C. Isoniazid 900 mg by mouth once daily for 9 months.
    D. Isoniazid 900 mg and rifapentine 900 mg by mouth once daily for 3 months.

44. A new patient is referred to your clinic with a positive PPD at 7 mm. The patient received the BCG vaccine years ago. The patient denies fever, chills, night sweats, and cough. The Quantiferon Gold is negative. Which one of the following is best to recommend for this patient?

    A. No therapy is indicated.
    B. Repeat the PPD.
    C. Isoniazid, rifampin, pyrazinamide, and ethambutol.
    D. Isoniazid.

45. A 49-year-old medical assistant (height 68 inches, weight 100 kg) reports new symptoms of cough and night sweats to the occupational health department. Her previous annual PPDs have been negative. A T-spot and a chest radiography reveals an upper lobe infiltrate consistent with TB. The patient has no comorbidities. Her home drugs include a daily multivitamin and calcium. Laboratory test results include SCr 0.9 mg/dL and ALT 20 IU/L. Which one of the following is best to recommend for this patient's initial therapy?

    A. Isoniazid 300 mg, rifampin 600 mg, pyrazinamide 2500 mg, ethambutol 1600 mg daily for 8 weeks.
    B. Isoniazid 300 mg, rifampin 600 mg, pyrazinamide 1500 mg, ethambutol 1200 mg daily for 8 weeks.
    C. Isoniazid 900 mg, rifampin 600 mg, pyrazinamide 2000 mg, ethambutol 1600 mg daily for 2 weeks, then twice weekly for 6 weeks.
    D. Isoniazid 300 mg, rifampin 600 mg, pyrazinamide 1500 mg, ethambutol 1200 mg daily for 2 weeks, then twice weekly for 6 weeks.

46. A 40-year-old woman is referred to the infectious disease clinic for an evaluation before the initiation of infliximab by her rheumatologist. A PPD test is placed and the result is 9 mm. Which one of the following is best to recommend for this patient?

A. Isoniazid 300 mg daily for 6 months and start infliximab in 1 month.
B. Isoniazid 300 mg daily for 9 months and start infliximab now.
C. Isoniazid 300 mg daily for 9 months and start infliximab in 1 month.
D. Isoniazid 300 mg daily and start infliximab after completion of isoniazid.

47. A 56-year-old man (height 70 inches, weight 62 kg) on hemodialysis is initiating therapy for active TB. Which one of the following is best to recommend for this patient?

A. Isoniazid 300 mg, rifampin 600 mg, pyrazinamide 1500 mg, and ethambutol 1200 mg daily.
B. Isoniazid 300 mg and rifampin 600 mg daily, and pyrazinamide 1500 mg and ethambutol 1200 mg three times weekly.
C. Isoniazid 300 mg, rifampin 600 mg, pyrazinamide 1500 mg, and ethambutol 1200 mg three times weekly.
D. Isoniazid 900 mg, rifampin 900 mg, pyrazinamide 1500 mg, and ethambutol 1200 mg three times weekly.

48. A 40-year-old patient on itraconazole for histoplasmosis plans to initiate an active TB regimen including bedaquiline. His laboratory test results are SCr 1.5 mg/dL and ALT 16 IU/L. Which one of the following bedaquiline regimens is best for this patient?

A. 400 mg by mouth daily for 2 weeks.
B. 200 mg by mouth daily for 8 weeks.
C. 200 mg by mouth three times weekly for 16 weeks.
D. 400 mg by mouth daily 24 weeks.

49. A 46 year-old man is diagnosed with pulmonary multidrug resistant TB. The isolate is susceptible to all second-line agents. The patient's comorbidities include seizures and chronic renal insufficiency. Baseline labs reveal SCr 1.5 mg/dL, ALT 20 IU/L, and hematocrit 31%. Baseline electrocardiography reveals QTc 450 msec. His home drugs include valproic acid. Which one of the following is best to recommend for this patient?

A. Isoniazid, ethambutol, and bedaquiline.
B. Rifampin, pyrazinamide, and bedaquiline.
C. Ethambutol, amikacin, pyrazinamide, and bedaquiline.
D. Ciprofloxacin, rifabutin, amikacin, and bedaquiline.

Questions 50–52 pertain to the following case.

K.C. is a 48-year-old man (height 72 inches, weight 68 kg) who presents to the emergency room with cough. After an extensive workup, he receives a diagnosis of HIV infection and active pulmonary TB. His CD4$^+$ count is 210/mm^3 and HIV-1 RNA is 580,000 copies/mL. Other laboratory test results include SCr 1.1 mg/dL and ALT 11 IU/L . K.C. is not currently taking any medications. The patient expresses concern with the need to take daily medications.

50. Which one of the following is best to recommend for K.C.?

A. Start ART and antituberculosis therapy today.
B. Start antituberculosis therapy today and ART in 2 weeks.
C. Start antituberculosis therapy today and ART in 2 months.
D. Start antituberculosis therapy today and ART in 4 months.

51. Which one of the following is the best antituberculosis regimen for K.C.?

A. Isoniazid 900 mg, rifampin 600 mg, pyrazinamide 1500 mg, and ethambutol 1200 mg once daily for 2 weeks, then twice weekly for 6 weeks followed by isoniazid 900 mg and rifampin 600 mg twice weekly for 18 weeks.
B. Isoniazid 900 mg, rifabutin 300, pyrazinamide 1500 mg, and ethambutol 1200 mg once daily. for 8 weeks followed by isoniazid 900 mg and rifabutin 300 mg twice weekly for 18 weeks.
C. Isoniazid 300 mg, rifampin 300 mg, pyrazinamide 2000 mg, and ethambutol 1600 mg once daily x 2 weeks, then isoniazid 900 mg, rifampin 300 mg, pyrazinamide 4000 mg, and ethambutol 4000 mg twice weekly for 6 weeks followed by isoniazid 300 mg and rifampin 300 mg twice weekly.
D. Isoniazid 300 mg, rifabutin 300 mg, pyrazinamide 1500 mg, and ethambutol 1200 mg once daily x 2 weeks, then isoniazid 900 mg, rifabutin 300 mg, pyrazinamide 3000 mg, and ethambutol 2800 mg twice weekly for 6 weeks followed by isoniazid 900 mg and rifabutin 300 mg twice weekly.

52. At his follow-up visit, K.C. reports taking isoniazid, rifabutin 300 mg, pyrazinamide, and ethambutol with 100% adherence. The plan is to initiate tenofovir, emtricitabine, and efavirenz for HIV. Which one of the following adjustments would be best to make to K.C.'s antituberculosis regimen?

A. Change rifabutin to rifampin 300 mg by mouth once daily.
B. Change rifabutin to 450 mg by mouth once daily.
C. Change rifabutin to 150 mg by mouth once daily.
D. Decrease efavirenz to 300 mg by mouth once daily.

Questions 53–55 pertain to the following case.

L.B. is a 33-year-old woman who has a positive PPD and a cavitation on chest radiography. She presents to the clinic to start TB therapy. L.B.'s laboratory results include SCr 1 mg/dL, ALT 15 IU/L, hematocrit 33%, and urine human chorionic gonadotropin (hCG) (+).

53. Which one of the following is best to initiate for L.B.?

    A. Isoniazid, rifampin, pyrazinamide, and ethambutol.
    B. Isoniazid, rifampin, and ethambutol.
    C. Isoniazid, rifampin, ethambutol, and moxifloxacin.
    D. Isoniazid and rifampin.

54. At her 2-month visit, L.B. reports 100% adherence and denies any missed doses. She does inquire about reducing her pill burden. Which one of the following would be the most critical objective parameter to obtain at this time for L.B.?

    A. SCr.
    B. ALT.
    C. Monofilament test.
    D. Eye examination.

55. At the time that appropriate therapy is initiated, LB is at highest risk of developing which one of the following adverse drug reactions?

    A. Optic neuritis.
    B. Hepatotoxicity.
    C. Gout.
    D. Peripheral neuropathy.

56. Which one of the following patients has the highest risk of optic neuritis?

    A. A 48-year-old woman (height 68 inches, weight 70 kg) with a CrCl of 30 mL/minute who is taking ethambutol 1600 mg by mouth three times weekly.
    B. A 56-year-old man (height 68 inches, weight 90 kg) with a CrCl of 30 mL/minute who is taking ethambutol 1600 mg by mouth once daily.
    C. A 40-year-old man (height 68 inches, weight 70 kg) with a CrCl of 60 mL/minute who is taking ethambutol 1600 mg by mouth three times weekly.
    D. A 35-year-old woman (height 68 inches, weight 90 kg) with a CrCl of 50 mL/minute who is taking ethambutol 1600 mg by mouth once daily.

Questions 57–59 pertain to the following case.

T.M. is a 45-year-old man (height 68 inches, weight 73 kg) who received a diagnosis of TB meningitis and HIV infection around 6 weeks ago. At that time, he was started on isoniazid 300 mg by mouth once daily, rifabutin 300 mg

by mouth once daily, ethambutol 1200 mg by mouth once daily, and pyrazinamide 1500 mg by mouth once daily administered DOT by the health department. Two weeks ago, T.M. was started on antiretrovirals of tenofovir/emtricitabine by mouth once daily, raltegravir 400 mg by mouth twice daily, darunavir 800 mg by mouth once daily, and ritonavir 100 mg by mouth once daily. At the time that antiretrovirals were initiated, his rifabutin was changed to 150 mg by mouth every other day. No other changes were made to T.M.'s medications.

57. Which one of the following is the most likely clinically significant outcome to expect after the initiation of antiretroviral medications for T.M.?

    A. Decreased tenofovir.
    B. Increased raltegravir.
    C. Decreased rifabutin.
    D. Increased rifabutin.

58. At today's visit, T.M. states 100% adherence to all drugs. His laboratory test results are within normal limits, including SCr 1.01 mg/dL and ALT 14 IU/L. His CD4$^+$ is 150 cells/mm^3 and HIV-1 RNA is less than 20 copies/mL. Peak and trough serum concentrations are ordered for the antimycobacterial drugs. Serum concentrations of antimycobacterial medications are ordered for 6 hours after the last administered dose with the following results:

Isoniazid 5.5 mcg/mL
Rifabutin 0.1 mcg/mL
Ethambutol 4.6 mcg/mL
Pyrazinamide 29.7 mcg/mL

Serum trough concentrations of antimycobacterial medications are ordered immediately before the next dose with the following results:

Isoniazid 0.5 mcg/mL
Rifabutin 0.1 mcg/mL
Ethambutol 1.6 mcg/mL
Pyrazinamide 9.3 mcg/mL

Which one of the following agents in T.M.'s regimen most requires an adjustment?

    A. Isoniazid.
    B. Rifabutin.
    C. Ethambutol.
    D. Pyrazinamide.

59. Which one of the following is best to recommend for T.M.?

    A. Increase rifabutin to 150 mg by mouth once daily.
    B. Change rifabutin to rifampin 600 mg by mouth once daily.

C. Increase darunavir to 1200 mg by mouth once daily.

D. Change darunavir to 600 mg by mouth twice daily.

60. A woman (height 66 inches, weight 70 kg) is beginning the continuation phase of active TB disease. Because the patient has had adherence issues in the past, the medications will be administered by DOT. Which one of the following is the most appropriate regimen for this patient?

A. Isoniazid 300 mg, rifampin 600 mg, ethambutol 1200 mg, pyrazinamide 1500 mg once daily for 8 weeks.

B. Isoniazid 600 mg and rifampin 300 mg by mouth once daily for 26 weeks.

C. Isoniazid 900 mg and rifampin 600 mg by mouth twice weekly for 18 weeks.

D. Isoniazid 900 mg and rifapentine 900 mg by mouth once weekly for 26 weeks.

LEARNER CHAPTER EVALUATION: TUBERCULOSIS.

As you take the posttest for this chapter, also evaluate the material's quality and usefulness, as well as the achievement of learning objectives. Rate each item using this 5-point scale:

- Strongly agree
- Agree
- Neutral
- Disagree
- Strongly disagree

38. The content of the chapter met my educational needs.
39. The content of the chapter satisfied my expectations.
40. The author presented the chapter content effectively.
41. The content of the chapter was relevant to my practice and presented at the appropriate depth and scope.
42. The content of the chapter was objective and balanced.
43. The content of the chapter is free of bias, promotion, or advertisement of commercial products.
44. The content of the chapter was useful to me.
45. The teaching and learning methods used in the chapter were effective.
46. The active learning methods used in the chapter were effective.
47. The learning assessment activities used in the chapter were effective.
48. The chapter was effective overall.

Use the 5-point scale to indicate whether this chapter prepared you to accomplish the following learning objectives:

49. Develop a treatment plan for a patient with active tuberculosis.
50. Develop a treatment plan for a patient with latent tuberculosis.
51. Devise a management plan for drug interactions with tuberculosis treatment.
52. Devise a management plan for adverse drug reactions with tuberculosis treatment.
53. Please provide any specific comments relating to any perceptions of bias, promotion, or advertisement of commercial products.
54. Please expand on any of your above responses, and/or provide any additional comments regarding this chapter:

Questions 55–57 apply to the entire Infectious Diseases II learning module.

55. How long did it take you to read the instructional materials in this module?
56. How long did it take you to read and answer the assessment questions in this module?
57. Please provide any additional comments you may have regarding this module:

INFECTIOUS DISEASES III PANEL

Series Editors:

John E. Murphy, Pharm.D., FCCP, FASHP
Professor of Pharmacy Practice and Science
Associate Dean for Academic and Professional Affairs
University of Arizona College of Pharmacy
Tucson, Arizona

Mary Wun-Len Lee, Pharm.D., FCCP, BCPS
Vice President and Chief Academic Officer
Pharmacy and Health Sciences Education
Midwestern University
Professor of Pharmacy Practice
Midwestern University
Chicago College of Pharmacy
Downers Grove, Illinois

Faculty Panel Chair

Ian R. McNicholl, Pharm.D., FCCP,
BCPS (AQ-ID), AAHIVP
Associate Director, Medical Affairs
Gilead Sciences
Foster City, California

INFECTIONS IN PATIENTS WITH MALIGNANCIES

Author

Melissa Badowski, Pharm.D., BCPS
Clinical Assistant Professor
Department of Pharmacy Practice, Section
of Infectious Diseases Pharmacotherapy
University of Illinois at Chicago, College of Pharmacy
Chicago, Illinois

Reviewers

Shellee A. Grim, Pharm.D., MS-CTS, BCPS
*Clinical Pharmacist, Transplant Infectious Diseases
Department of*
Loyola University Health System
Maywood, Illinois
Adjunct Clinical Associate Professor
Department of Pharmacy Practice
University of Illinois at Chicago
Chicago, Illinois

Inna S. Tsuker, Pharm.D., BCPS
Pharmacy Clinical Coordinator
Department of Pharmacy
Cancer Treatment Centers of America,
Eastern Regional Medical Center
Philadelphia, Pennsylvania

HEPATITIS C

Authors

Michelle T. Martin, Pharm.D., BCPS, BCACP
Clinical Pharmacist
University of Illinois Hospital and
Health Sciences System
Assistant Professor
Department of Pharmacy Practice
University of Illinois at Chicago College of Pharmacy
Chicago, Illinois

Ian R. McNicholl, Pharm.D., FCCP,
BCPS (AQ-ID), AAHIVP
Associate Director, Medical Affairs
Gilead Sciences
Foster City, California

Reviewers

Paulina Deming, Pharm.D.
Clinical Associate Professor of Pharmacy
College of Pharmacy
Project ECHO
University of New Mexico Health Sciences Center
Albuquerque, New Mexico

Carolyn Orendorff, Pharm.D., BCPS
Clinical Pharmacy Coordinator
Department of Pharmacy
Virtua Health
Voorhees, New Jersey

Quynh-Chi Duong, Pharm.D., BCPS
Chief Pharmacist
Department of Warm Springs Pharmacy
USPHS/IHS/Warm Springs Health
and Wellness Center
Warm Springs, Oregon

HIV Infection

Authors

Craig R. Ballard, Pharm.D., AAHIVP
Pharmacist Specialist-HIV
Internal Medicine-Owen Clinic
University of California San Diego Health System
Health Sciences Associate Clinical Professor
Department of Pharmacy
University of California San Diego Skaggs School
of Pharmacy and Pharmaceutical Sciences
San Diego, California

Lucas Hill, Pharm.D., AAHIVP
Clinical Pharmacist
University of California San Diego
San Diego, California

Reviewers

Taylor K. Gill, Pharm.D., BCPS, AAHIVP
Clinical Pharmacy Specialist – Internal Medicine
Department of Pharmacy
Via Christi Hospitals Wichita, Inc.
Wichita, Kansas

Thomas J. Kleyn, Pharm.D., BCPS, AAHIVP
Assistant Professor
Department of Pharmacy Practice and Administration
Western University of Health Sciences
Pomona, California

The American College of Clinical Pharmacy and the authors thank the following individuals for their careful review of the Infectious Diseases III chapters:

Emilie L. Karpiuk, Pharm.D., BCPS, BCOP
Oncology Pharmacist
Department of Pharmacy
Froedtert Hospital
Milwaukee, Wisconsin

Mary Wun-Len Lee, Pharm.D., FCCP, BCPS
Vice President and Chief Academic Officer
Pharmacy and Health Sciences Education
Midwestern University
Professor of Pharmacy Practice
Midwestern University
Chicago College of Pharmacy
Downers Grove, Illinois

Marianne McCollum, Ph.D., BSPharm, BCPS
Assistant Dean for Assessment
School of Pharmacy
Rueckert-Hartman College for Health Professions
Regis University
Denver, Colorado

Infections in Patients with Malignancies

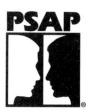

By Melissa Badowski, Pharm.D., BCPS

Reviewed by Shellee A. Grim, Pharm.D., MS-CTS, BCPS; and Inna S. Tsuker, Pharm.D., BCPS

Learning Objectives

1. Demonstrate an understanding of the risk factors and causes of bacterial, viral, and fungal infections in those with hematologic or solid-tumor malignancies.

2. Distinguish between patients at high risk, moderate risk, and low risk for febrile neutropenia.

3. Develop an infectious diseases pharmacotherapeutic plan for treatment and prophylaxis of antibacterial, antifungal, and antiviral infections in a patient with malignancy (solid and hematologic).

4. Assess the safety profiles of anti-infective drugs used to manage and prevent antibacterial, antifungal, and antiviral infections.

5. Evaluate drug therapy for the presence of drug-drug interactions in those receiving treatment or prophylaxis for febrile neutropenia.

6. Evaluate the role of hematopoietic growth factors in the prevention of febrile neutropenia.

Introduction

It is estimated that 1.6 million Americans annually will receive a new cancer diagnosis (ACS 2014). For many, chemotherapy is an essential component of treatment; however, it causes significant neutropenia, which may lead to infectious morbidity and mortality. About 10% of those receiving chemotherapy experience infectious complications requiring hospitalization (CDC 2013). Each episode of febrile neutropenia (FN) can cost on average $19,110 (Kuderer 2006). Infectious complications are sources of inpatient mortality in up to 9.5% of those with a malignancy (Kuderer 2006). Infections may be consequences of chemotherapy, surgery to remove a tumor or its burden, hematopoietic cell transplantation (HCT), the use of indwelling devices, and/or repeated exposure to the health care setting.

Baseline Knowledge Statements

Readers of this chapter are presumed to be familiar with the following:
- Physiology of hematopoiesis
- Consequences of neutropenia
- Common chemotherapy regimens causing neutropenia
- Common infections associated with neutropenia
- General drug knowledge of anti-infectives

Additional Readings

The following free resources are available for readers wishing additional background information on this topic.
- Flowers CR, Seidenfeld J, Bow EJ, et al. Antimicrobial prophylaxis and outpatient management of fever and neutropenia in adults treated for malignancy: American Society of Clinical Oncology clinical practice guideline. J Clin Oncol 2013;31:794-810.
- Freifeld AG, Bow EJ, Sepkowitz KA, et al. Clinical practice guideline for the use of antimicrobial agents in neutropenic patients with cancer: 2010 update by the Infectious Diseases Society of America. Clin Infect Dis 2011;52:e56-e93.
- Tomblyn M, Chiller T, Einsele H, et al. Guidelines for preventing infectious complications among hematopoietic cell transplantation recipients: a global perspective. Biol Blood Marrow Transplant 2009;15:1143-38.

Risk Factors

Immunodeficiency

Patients with malignancies are at increased risk of infection caused by deficiencies in cell-mediated and humoral immunity. Those with cell-mediated deficiencies such as hematologic malignancies as seen in acute and chronic leukemia, non-Hodgkin and Hodgkin lymphomas, and myelodysplastic syndrome experience dysfunction in T-lymphocyte and macrophage functions. In addition, advanced or refractory hematologic malignancy may be caused by bone marrow failure because of the malignancy or by several rounds of cytotoxic or immunosuppressive therapies. Increased risk of opportunistic infections caused by bacteria, fungi, and viruses occurs in individuals undergoing allogeneic HCT for up to 2 years post-transplantation (Marr 2002; Wald 1997).

Patients with multiple myeloma and chronic lymphocytic leukemia experience hypogammaglobulinemia, which causes B-cell dysfunction from impaired humoral immunity. In addition, patients receiving steroids and/or chemotherapy, or patients who have undergone splenectomy (in this case, to diagnose Hodgkin disease) are at particularly high risk of developing infection caused by *Streptococcus pneumoniae*.

Disruption of Mucosal Barriers

Disruption of skin and mucosal linings secondary to surgery, diagnostic procedures, indwelling-device placement, venous puncture, catheterization, and radiation impairs the first line of defense against local flora. Disruptions of normal skin flora result in bacterial infections caused by *Streptococcus aureus*, *Streptococcus epidermidis*, or streptococci. Chemotherapy-induced gastrointestinal (GI) mucositis may cause a disruption of mucosal barriers; this may lead to herpes simplex virus (HSV) reactivation, which manifests as oral ulcers.

Environmental and Health Care

Patients with immunocompromise are susceptible to infections caused either by pathogens with which the host is colonized or pathogens acquired from environmental exposure. Without strict adherence to infection control guidelines, hospital personnel can transfer pathogens to through improper hand sanitation or by contaminated medical equipment. Most infections in patient populations are caused by a patient's own skin or gut flora. The use of broad-spectrum antibiotics, chemotherapeutic agents, and acid suppressants may alter GI flora and integrity and thus increase the risk of infection.

Food safety is important for patients undergoing or recovering from cancer treatments. Raw or unpasteurized products, lunch meats, and unwashed fruits and vegetables can cause foodborne illnesses such as *Escherichia coli*, *Campylobacter*, *Listeria*, *Norovirus*, *Salmonella*, *Toxoplasma*, or *Vibrio* (FDA 2014).

Water is another source of bacteria for the patient with immunocompromise. Tap water from a city water supply is relatively safe. For patients using well water, the water should be boiled for at least 1 minute before drinking and should be stored in a clean, covered container in the refrigerator for up to 72 hours (NCI 2011). Water filtration will not remove harmful organisms from well water and should not replace boiling the water. Bottled water should be distilled or go through reverse osmosis filtration to remove organisms responsible for stomach or intestinal infections (NCI 2011). Water filtration systems are not safe to use unless chlorine has been added to them. Water filters must be able to remove coliforms and *Cryptosporidium*. In addition, portable water systems filter out chemicals but not bacteria (NCI 2011).

It is recommended that people with pets should consider giving up their pets to avoid exposure to additional infectious organisms. Patients on high-dose steroids and those undergoing treatment for lymphoma and leukemia should strongly consider avoiding pets during this time (NIH 2014). Patients should wash their hands thoroughly after handling a pet or disposing of pet feces. It is recommended that patients with cats should have someone else clean the litter box to avoid exposure to *Toxoplasma*. If the patient must change cat litter, rubber gloves and a face mask should be worn.

Neutropenia

Neutropenia is defined as an absolute neutrophil count (ANC) of less than 500 cells/mm^3 or an ANC that is expected to fall below 500 cells/mm^3 in the next 48 hours. When profound neutropenia occurs (ANC below 100 cells/mm^3), the risk of acquiring a potentially life-threatening bacteremia is as high as 20% (Freifeld 2011; Schimpff 1986).

The risk of neutropenia, including degree and duration as well as development of febrile neutropenia, is modulated by type of chemotherapy (Table 1-1). Alkylating agents, antimetabolites, anthracyclines, topoisomerase inhibitors, taxanes, and vinca alkaloids increase the risk of chemotherapy-induced neutropenia. In patients receiving treatment for advanced acute and chronic leukemia, certain tyrosine kinase inhibitors (e.g., bosutinib, dasatinib, imatinib, nilotinib) can also cause neutropenia. Advanced age, prior or concurrent chemotherapy or radiation, poor nutrition, and end-organ dysfunction all are risk factors for chemotherapy-induced neutropenia (Fausel 2010). Concomitant immunodeficiency, advanced malignancy, high doses, and lengthy duration of chemotherapy may dull signs of infection and fever.

Lymphopenia

Lymphopenia refers to a lymphocyte count of less than 1000 cells/mm^3 and can lead to infections with bacteria, viruses, fungi, and parasites (NIH 2013). High-dose corticosteroids used concomitantly with chemotherapy have a profound impact on neutrophils and lymphocytes. In addition, certain chemotherapy agents used most commonly for the management of leukemia and lymphoma have been known to cause lymphopenia (see Table 1-1).

Noninfectious Fever

As many as 25% of individuals with cancer may experience fever before diagnosis (Brusch 1988). Those with fevers of more than 38.3°C (100.9°F) on several occasions for more than a 3-week period should receive a workup for malignancy, assuming that infections, connective tissue disorders, and drug reactions have been ruled out. Various antimicrobials, antineoplastic, cardiovascular, immunosuppressant, nonsteroidal anti-inflammatory, anticonvulsant, antidepressant, and other agents may be responsible for drug fevers (Patel 2010). Individuals with advanced lymphoma, leukemia, renal cell carcinoma, and hepatocellular carcinoma and those with metastatic hepatocellular carcinoma typically present with fevers for a prolonged time. Fevers may occur because of tumor release of cytokines and inflammatory markers, tumor necrosis or inflammation, tumor obstruction, venous thromboembolism, or altered thermoregulation secondary to hypothalamic metastases.

FEBRILE NEUTROPENIA

Febrile neutropenia refers to those with neutropenia and fevers (defined as higher than 38.3°C [101°F] or higher than 38.0°C [100.4°F] for a 1-hour period). As many as 50% of those with solid tumors and more than 80% of those with hematologic malignancy will develop

Table 1-1. Chemotherapy-Induced Febrile Neutropenia, Neutropenia, and Lymphopenia: Risk Stratification of Agents by Incidence

	High Risk (Incidence >20%)	Intermediate Risk (Incidence 10%–20%)	Low Risk (Incidence <10%)
Febrile Neutropenia	Clofarabine	Azacitidine	Aflibercept
	Decitabine	Gemtuzumab	Arsenic
	Ponatinib	Omacetaxine	Bendamustine
	Vincristine (liposomal)	Pertuzumab	Bevacizumab
		Rituximab	Bosutinib
		Topotecan	Brentuximab
		Vinorelbine	Cabazitaxel
			Cyclophosphamide
			Dactinomycin
			Dasatinib
			Docetaxel
			Epirubicin
			Eribulin
			Gemcitabine
			Imatinib
			Irinotecan
			Ixabepilone
			Lenalidomide
			Nelarabine
			Nilotinib
			Paclitaxel (nanoparticle)
			Pemetrexed
			Pomalidomide
			Pralatrexate
			Trastuzumab

Table 1-1. Chemotherapy-Induced Febrile Neutropenia, Neutropenia, and Lymphopenia: Risk Stratification of Agents by Incidence (*continued*)

	High Risk (Incidence >20%)	Intermediate Risk (Incidence 10%–20%)	Low Risk (Incidence <10%)
Neutropenia	Aflibercept Azacitidine Bendamustine Bevacizumab Bosutinib Busulfan Cabazitaxel Carboplatin Cetuximab Clofarabine Dasatinib Decitabine Docetaxel Epirubicin Eribulin Etoposide Fludarabine Ibritumomab Ibrutinib Imatinib Irinotecan Ixabepilone Lenalidomide Nelarabine Nilotinib Obinutuzumab Ofatumumab Omacetaxine Paclitaxel Paclitaxel (nanoparticle) Pertuzumab Pomalidomide Ponatinib Recombinant Interferon Alfa-2b Rituximab Romidepsin Topotecan Vinorelbine	Arsenic Bexarotene Bortezomib Brentuximab Carfilzomib Crizotinib Daunorubicin Doxorubicin Pralatrexate Sunitinib Temozolomide Trametinib Trastuzumab Vincristine (liposomal)	Ado-trastuzumab Aldesleukin[a] Cabozantinib Capecitabine Chlorambucil[a] Cyclophosphamide[a] Dabrafenib Dactinomycin[a] Doxorubicin (Liposomal) Enzalutamide Everolimus Gefitinib Lapatinib Methotrexate[a] Pazopanib Pemetrexed Radium-223 Ramucirumab Regorafenib Sorafenib Temsirolimus Vandetanib Vorinostat
Lymphopenia	Bendamustine Clofarabine Gemtuzumab Obinutuzumab Temozolomide Ponatinib Rituximab Romidepsin Trametinib	Cabozantinib Capecitabine Carfilzomib Everolimus Exemestane Ibritumomab Omacetaxine Radium-223 Sorafenib Sunitinib Temsirolimus	Abiraterone Axitinib Chlorambucil Crizotinib Dabrafenib Imatinib Lenalidomide Mechlorethamine Nilotinib Pazopanib Pomalidomide Regorafenib

[a]Incidence not reported.
Risk categories based on Grade 3–4 adverse events from package insert data.

FN, yet only 20%–30% will develop clinical infections (Klastersky 2004). Infection risk stratification in those with neutropenia (Table 1-2) is based on type or treatment of malignancy, anticipated duration of neutropenia, and Multinational Association of Supportive Care in Cancer (MASCC) risk index score (Klastersky 2000). The MASCC score is calculated by burden of disease (asymptomatic/mild symptoms = 5 points, moderate symptoms = 3 points), lack of hypotension (systolic blood pressure > 90 mm Hg = 5 points), lack of chronic obstructive pulmonary disease (4 points), solid tumor or no previous invasive fungal infection (4 points), outpatient status (3 points), no dehydration (3 points), and age less than 60 years (2 points) (Klastersky 2000). A score of 21 or more identifies patients at low risk of serious complications of febrile neutropenia.

Patients who experience fever in the setting of neutropenia should be carefully evaluated for underlying infection: the usual signs and symptoms may be absent because of decreased lymphocytes and failure to mount an inflammatory response at the site of infection. Pain at the site of infection may be the only symptom the patient reports. During periods of neutropenia, it is essential to continually assess the patient for infection. At least two sets of blood cultures should be obtained in all patients on initial assessment. If fever persists while the patient is receiving empirical antibiotics, it is recommended to repeat daily blood cultures for 2 days. For patients without metastatic disease but with suspected infection, cultures should be guided by signs and symptoms of infection.

Empiric Antibiotic Therapy (Patients at Low Risk)

For patients deemed low risk of infection in the setting of FN (Figure 1-1), outpatient management with ciprofloxacin and amoxicillin/clavulanate is recommended for empiric management; ciprofloxacin monotherapy or a combination of ciprofloxacin and clindamycin may be used as second-line options (Freifeld 2011). Monotherapy with ciprofloxacin is considered inadequate because of inadequate coverage of gram-positive organisms. Monotherapy with oral levofloxacin 750 mg or moxifloxacin 400 mg daily may be an alternative, but there are not enough clinical data to support that practice (Freifeld 2011). Recently, a double-blind, multicenter study performed in Europe demonstrated that once-daily oral moxifloxacin 400 mg was as effective and safe as oral ciprofloxacin 750 mg twice daily plus amoxicillin/clavulanate 1000 mg twice daily (Kern 2013). For those unable to tolerate oral drugs, who experience nausea or vomiting, or who have previously taken fluoroquinolone prophylaxis, it may be warranted to use intravenous antibiotics at home, in the clinic, or in the inpatient setting. For those patients improving while on intravenous antibiotics and able to take them orally, transition to and observation of oral therapy can be done outside the health care setting. For those who defervesce on therapy, antibiotics should continue until ANC is more

than 500 cells/mm³ and rising. If the patient is still experiencing persistent fever or is clinically unstable after 2–4 days of empiric antibiotic therapy, the patient should be hospitalized for administration of broad-spectrum intravenous antibiotics. Antibiotics may need to be modified based on culture results and/or infection site. For those with documented infections, Table 1-3 lists agents that may be added to empiric management, and Table 1-4 describes duration of treatment.

Empiric Antibiotic Therapy (Patients at High Risk)

Prevention of morbidity and mortality caused by bacterial pathogens is the goal of initiating empiric antibiotic therapy in patients with FN. It is estimated that 23% of FN cases resulted in bacteremia; of these, around 57% are infected with gram-positive organisms, 34% with gram-negative organisms, and 9% with polymicrobial infections (Klastersky 2007). Recent data suggest a shift to a higher incidence of gram-negative infections in this population; this shift is also associated with a greater risk of mortality (Trecarichi 2014). Unfortunately, in many cases, blood culture results return negative, and empiric antibiotic therapy should continue until the ANC is more than 500 cells/mm³ and increasing. In those patients who are still neutropenic after completing treatment courses for documented infections, fluoroquinolone prophylaxis should be restarted until the neutropenia resolves (Freifeld 2011). Empiric antibiotic selection should be based on infection risk assessment, local antimicrobial susceptibilities to suspected pathogens, infection site, suspected pathogens, clinical instability, recent antibiotic use, and drug allergy or tolerability.

For high-risk patients (see Table 1-2), the risk of infection is greater than 20%; therefore, inpatient management with broad-spectrum intravenous antibiotics that have coverage against *Pseudomonas aeruginosa* and other serious gram-negative pathogens should be initiated (Figure 1-2). It is estimated that around 20% of gram-negative infections in those with FN are secondary to *P. aeruginosa*, although *Acinetobacter* spp., *Stenotrophomonas maltophilia*, and multidrug-resistant gram-negative infections are more common in this population (Trecarichi 2014). Recommended first-line monotherapy is with an antipseudomonal β-lactam agent (cefepime), carbapenem (imipenem/cilastatin or meropenem), or penicillin/β-lactamase inhibitor combination (piperacillin/tazobactam). Monotherapy with those recommended agents has been found to be as effective as combination therapy and with fewer adverse events. Although not studied directly in patients with FN, no mortality benefit was found in those receiving combination therapy for *P. aeruginosa* compared with monotherapy (Bowers 2013; Hu 2013; Vardakas 2013). Combination therapy may be considered in complicated or resistant cases based on local susceptibility data.

Concern about empiric cefepime initiation in neutropenic patients arose when a meta-analysis of 19 randomized

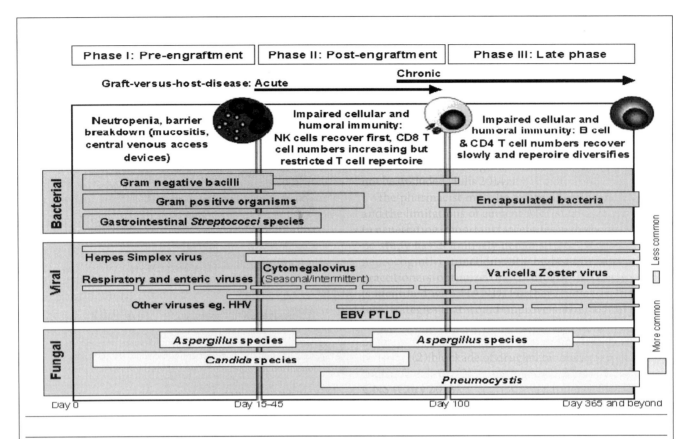

Figure 1-1. Timeline of infectious diseases in hematopoietic cell transplant recipients.

Reprinted with permission from Tomblyn M, Chiller T, Einsele H, et al. Guidelines for preventing infectious complications among hematopoietic cell transplantation recipients: a global perspective. Biol Blood Marrow Transplant 2009;15:1143-238

controlled trials demonstrated increased risk of 30-day mortality compared with other β-lactams (risk ratio [RR] 1.41; 95% confidence interval [CI], 1.08–1.84) (Yahav 2007). Subsequently, an analysis of all-cause mortality associated with cefepime failed to demonstrate increased risk (Nguyen 2009). The U.S. Food and Drug Administration (FDA) evaluated trial and patient data in another meta-analysis and failed to find increased risk of 30-day mortality associated with cefepime (RR, 1.20; 95% CI, 0.82–1.76). Therefore, cefepime is still recommended as a first-line empiric antibiotic for FN (FDA 2009).

Extended spectrum β-lactamases, carbapenem-resistant Enterobacteriaceae, and various multidrug-resistant pathogens are emerging as causes of severe gram-negative infections in this population, which is constantly exposed to the health care setting and/or receiving prophylactic or empiric courses of antibiotics. It is important to consider multidrug-resistant organisms in patients with immunocompromise and follow local epidemiology and susceptibility patterns.

Empiric initiation of vancomycin should not be considered without the presence of clinically suspected, serious intravenous catheter-related infection, positive blood cultures indicating gram-positive bacteria (before known identification and susceptibility), hemodynamic instability, sepsis, known colonization with penicillin- or cephalosporin-resistant pneumococci or methicillin-resistant *Staphylococcus aureus* (MRSA), soft tissue infection, or radiographic documentation of pneumonia. Initiation of vancomycin should be judicious because of the emergence of vancomycin-resistant enterococci and the potential development of vancomycin-intermediate and vancomycin-resistant *S. aureus* in this population. Empiric initiation of vancomycin was not routinely associated with improved mortality or duration of fever, yet may increase the risk of nephrotoxicity (Paul 2005). In addition, although coagulase-negative staphylococci are routinely isolated in neutropenic patients with bacteremia, there is no urgent need to treat a single positive culture with vancomycin because this is routinely a contaminant. If vancomycin is initiated based on clinical presentation or suspicion of a severe gram-positive infection, therapy should be reassessed after 2 to 3 days and discontinued if a resistant gram-positive pathogen is not identified. Furthermore, ceftaroline, daptomycin, linezolid, quinupristin/dalfopristin, telavancin, and tigecycline are not indicated in empiric management of high-risk febrile neutropenia.

A 61-year-old woman (height 68", weight 68 kg) with stage IV breast cancer was admitted to the intensive care unit for suspected sepsis from a skilled nursing facility. The nursing staff reported that the patient was found unresponsive in her bed. Her other medical history consisted of coronary artery disease, depression, diabetes, hypertension, and peripheral neuropathy. She has no known drug allergies. Her drugs on admission included aspirin 81 mg daily, atorvastatin 20 mg orally nightly, duloxetine 40 mg orally daily, lisinopril 40 mg orally daily, metformin 1000 mg orally twice daily, metoprolol succinate 100 mg orally daily, and vinorelbine

36.6 mg/m². Her vital signs upon admission were blood pressure: 80/50 mm Hg; heart rate: 121 beats/minute; respiratory rate: 29 breaths/minute; and temperature: 95.9 °F. The patient received 1 L of fluids and two sets of blood cultures and a urine culture were drawn. The intensivist wants to start empiric therapy for *Pseudomonas aeruginosa* because more cases of multi-drug resistant infections have been identified. You are consulted by the intensive care team on whether to initiate monotherapy or combination therapy for empiric coverage. What would be best to recommend for this patient's antibacterial therapy?

	Admission labs
SCr (mg/dL)	1.3
White blood cells (x 103 cells/mm³)	1.0
Bands (%)	20
Neutrophils (%)	25
Urine culture	pending
Blood culture	pending

Answer

This scenario describes a very difficult and controversial patient case to approach. The patient's immunosuppressed status and skilled nursing facility stay increases her risk of *P. aeruginosa* infection. In addition, this region is experiencing an increase in pseudomonal infections. Although not studied directly in patients with febrile neutropenia, no mortality benefit was found in patients receiving combination therapy. This patient may benefit from combination therapy because of the complicated case, treatment with

vinorelbine, and the presence of multi-drug resistance in the region. Empiric therapy with an anti-pseudomonal β-lactam antibiotic (piperacillin/tazobactam, cefepime, imipenem/cilastatin, or meropenem) plus an aminoglycoside (gentamicin, tobramycin, or amikacin) or fluoroquinolone (ciprofloxacin or levofloxacin) should be recommended in this patient. Based on blood culture results, empiric therapy should be modified or narrowed based on speciation and susceptibility data.

1. Bowers DR, Liew YX, Lye DC, et al. Outcomes of appropriate empiric combination versus monotherapy for *Pseudomonas aeruginosa* bacteremia. Antimicrob Agents Chemother 2013;57:1270-4.
2. Freifeld AG, Bow EJ, Sepkowitz KA, et al. Clinical practice guideline for the use of antimicrobial agents in neutropenic patients with cancer: 2010 update by the Infectious Diseases Society of America. Clin Infect Dis 2011;52:e56-e93.
3. Hu Y, Li L, Li W, et al. Combination antibiotic therapy versus monotherapy for Pseudomonas aeruginosa bacteraemia: a meta-analysis of retrospective and prospective studies. Int J Antimicrob Agents 2013;42:492-6.
4. Vardakas KZ, Tansarli GS, Bliziotis IA, et al. β-Lactam plus aminoglycoside or fluoroquinolone combination versus β-lactam monotherapy for Pseudomonas aeruginosa infections: a meta-analysis. Int J Antimicrob Agents 2013;41:301-10.

For patients who have defervesced and have negative cultures, empiric antibiotics should be continued until ANC is more than 500 cells/mm³ and rising. For those with documented infections, antibiotics should be modified, if necessary, and antibiotics continued for 7–14 days based on microbiologic data. In addition, antibiotics may be continued beyond 14 days until ANC is more than 500 cells/mm³ and rising. Alternatively, outpatient quinolone prophylaxis is sometimes resumed if a patient is afebrile with no documented infection. If the patient has persistent fever but is clinically stable, empiric antibiotics should be continued and then assessed for infection site. If fever persists beyond 4–7 days despite broad-spectrum antibiotics in high-risk patients with anticipated neutropenia lasting longer than 10

days and with no identified source of infection, initiation of empiric antifungal therapy should be considered.

Empiric Antifungal Therapy

Invasive fungal infections remain a significant cause of morbidity and mortality in patients with immunocompromise who are receiving treatment for their underlying malignancies (Auberger 2008). Fungal etiology is usually considered when a patient who is receiving empiric antibiotics for 4 or more days still experiences FN or has recurrent fever (Freifeld 2011). Intensive cytotoxic chemotherapy increases the risk of invasive fungal infections. Because *Candida* colonizes on mucosal surfaces, it may enter the bloodstream through mucosal barrier breakdown, resulting in a bloodstream infection. Although the use of azole prophylaxis, commonly with fluconazole, has minimized the incidence of invasive fungal infections in patients at high risk of infection, there is a risk of azole-resistant pathogens. For patients not receiving fluconazole for prophylaxis, fluconazole may be initiated as empiric therapy. Infections caused by *Candida krusei*, *Candida glabrata*, and molds should be considered in those already receiving fluconazole prophylaxis because its spectrum of activity is limited.

Individuals considered high risk of invasive mold infections (e.g., aspergillosis, zygomycosis [mucormycosis], fusariosis) include patients with profound neutropenia of 10–15 days, recipients of allogeneic HCT, or those receiving high-dose steroids. Empiric antimold antifungal initiation should occur after 4 days of empiric antibiotic therapy in patients who remain febrile or have recrudescent fever, unless the patients are receiving appropriate prophylaxis. On study identified that the onset of *Aspergillus* infections was bimodal and peaked at days 16 and 96 post-transplantation (Wald 1997). For patients receiving antifungal prophylaxis, switching to a different class of anti-mold antifungal agent should be considered. Amphotericin B, itraconazole, voriconazole, posaconazole, or an echinocandin can be considered as an alternative to fluconazole. The use of itraconazole is limited by its erratic bioavailability and absorption. In one study, voriconazole prevented 26% of invasive fungal infections compared with 31% with liposomal amphotericin B. In addition, voriconazole was associated with fewer breakthrough infections compared with liposomal amphotericin B (1.9% vs. 5.0%, p=0.02), but noninferiority was not demonstrated with voriconazole compared with liposomal amphotericin B (Walsh 2002). Therefore, liposomal amphotericin B remains the preferred therapy in those at high risk of invasive mold infection, yet voriconazole is a reasonable alternative.

Echinocandins have activity against *Candida* and *Aspergillus* species. A comparative analysis between caspofungin and liposomal amphotericin B as empiric therapy for invasive fungal infections in persistent FN showed similar success, breakthrough fungal infections, and resolution of FN. Caspofungin was associated with a higher success rate (52% vs. 26%, p=0.04) and lower mortality (11% vs. 44%) in those with baseline invasive fungal infections compared with those receiving liposomal amphotericin. Furthermore, caspofungin was associated with fewer adverse events (Walsh 2004). It is expected that not only caspofungin but also micafungin and anidulafungin are appropriate empiric agents for treatment of presumed fungal infections in FN; however, clinicians must keep in mind the limited echinocandins' antimold activity.

Antifungal therapy may be withheld from patients with FN who are clinically stable and have no systemic recovery of fungi or evidence of chest or sinus fungal infection on computed tomography. For those at low risk of fungal infection, empiric antifungal therapy is not warranted (Freifeld 2011).

Pneumocystis jiroveci

Allogeneic HCT recipients, patients receiving treatment for acute lymphocytic leukemia, and recipients of alemtuzumab, high-dose steroids, or rituximab have the highest risk of *Pneumocystis jiroveci* infection (Martin-Garrido 2013; Bollée 2007). In addition, those receiving purine analog therapy, T-cell depleting agents, prolonged corticosteroid therapy (prednisone equivalent of 20 mg or greater for at least 4 weeks), temozolomide plus radiation, or autologous HCT should be considered at intermediate risk of *P. jiroveci* pneumonia (PJP). Although rare because of effective prophylaxis, PJP should be in the differential diagnosis for patients presenting with diffuse pulmonary infiltrates and who were not receiving PJP prophylaxis in the presence of impaired cell immunity. Therapy for PJP consists of trimethoprim/sulfamethoxazole 5 mg/kg every 8 hours. In those unable to tolerate or with an allergy to trimethoprim/sulfamethoxazole and who have mild to moderate disease, atovaquone, clindamycin plus primaquine (assuming glucose-6-phosphate dehydrogenase (G6PD) negative), or trimethoprim plus dapsone (assuming G6PD negative) may be used as alternative therapy. In patients with severe disease and for whom trimethoprim/sulfamethoxazole is contraindicated, pentamidine intravenous daily or clindamycin plus primaquine may be considered. For individuals with documented or highly suspected disease, optimal duration of therapy has not been sufficiently studied outside the area of HIV but is recommended to continue for at least 14 days (Limper 1989). Transition to oral therapy may be considered in patients who have clinically improved and are able to tolerate drugs orally.

Viral Infections

Viral infections account for about 5% of infections in FN. Herpes simplex virus results from reactivation of a latent virus in patients who develop neutropenia and mucositis. Patients without prophylaxis who undergo induction or reinduction therapy for acute leukemia and who are seropositive for HSV based on pretreatment serology carry an 80% risk of reactivation and infection (Zaia 2009). Recipients of allogeneic HCT are at risk of HSV directly after receipt of their conditioning regimen; the HSV may occur later depending on level of immunosuppression. Although systemic disease is uncommon, disseminated HSV may be associated with mucosal damage and pain, which could limit nutrition and hydration, which in turn can increase the risk of bacterial and fungal superinfections. Similarly, varicella zoster virus (VZV) is associated with impaired cellular immunity. Patients at highest risk of reactivation of latent infection include those who require systemic immunosuppression beyond the prophylactic period. Acyclovir or valacyclovir is considered the treatment of choice for both HSV and VZV infections. Alternatively, famciclovir may be considered if acyclovir or valacyclovir cannot be used. Foscarnet should be reserved for individuals with acyclovir-resistant infection.

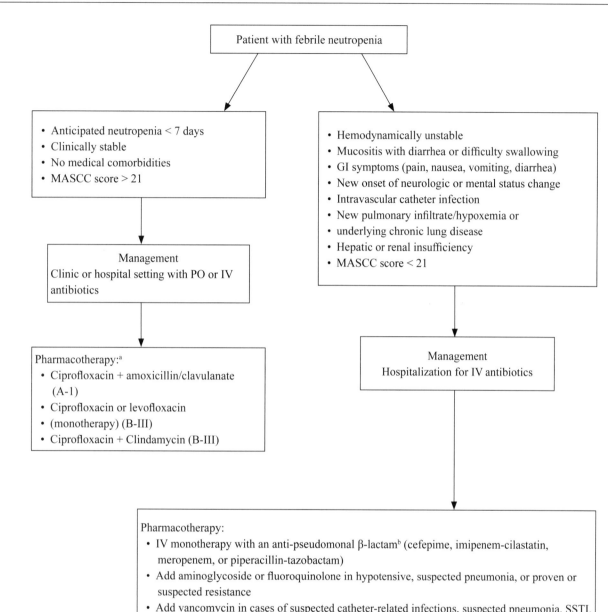

Figure 1-2. Empiric management of febrile neutropenia.

[a]Those on fluoroquinolone prophylaxis should not receive fluoroquinolone

[b]In those with a penicillin allergy, cephalosporins are typically tolerated but in cases requiring alternative therapy consider ciprofloxacin + clindamycin or aztreonam + vancomycin.

ESBL = extended-spectrum β-lactamase; KPC = *Klebsiella pneumoniae* carbapenemase; MRSA = methicillin-resistant *Staphylococcus aureus*; VRE = vancomycin-resistant *Enterococcus*.

Adapted with permission from Freifeld AG, Bow EJ, Sepkowitz KA, et al. Clinical practice guideline for the use of antimicrobial agents in neutropenic patients with cancer: 2010 update by the Infectious Diseases Society of America. Clin Infect Dis 2011;52:e56-e93.

Cytomegalovirus (CMV) is the most common opportunistic infection for those receiving allogeneic HCT or alemtuzumab therapy (Boeckh 2009; Keating 2002). Cytomegalovirus often occurs early postengraftment but can be seen late, especially in patients with graft-versus-host disease. Patients at highest risk of infection are HCT recipients who are CMV seropositive before transplantation or those who have seropositive donors. Cytomegalovirus activation can occur in up to 60% of patients regardless of surveillance and prophylaxis (George 2010). In addition, patients who are CMV seropositive and are receiving grafts from CMV-negative donors carry an increased risk of CMV disease and reactivation and have longer periods and more severe cases of reactivation (Pietersma 2011; Beck 2010). Allogeneic HCT recipients should have active surveillance for CMV for up to 6 months post-transplantation, whereas individuals receiving alemtuzumab should have active surveillance for at least 2 months after discontinuation.

Initiation of pre-emptive antiviral treatment should occur regardless of clinical presentation if the patient has a detectable antigen or viral DNA in the blood. Treatment should be initiated in cases of a single positive antigen in the blood or two consecutively positive polymerase-chain-reaction tests. Initiation with oral valganciclovir is commonly the antiviral of choice for CMV treatment in allogeneic HCT, including GI graft-versus-host disease. Valganciclovir is as effective as intravenous ganciclovir but is associated with fewer adverse effects; both agents may cause bone marrow suppression and prolong neutropenia. Foscarnet therapy is reserved for patients unable to tolerate either ganciclovir or valganciclovir or as alternative therapy given the above-mentioned toxicities of ganciclovir and valganciclovir. Cidofovir is commonly reserved for individuals whose disease failed to respond or relapsed on ganciclovir/valganciclovir, foscarnet, or combination therapy. The risk of nephrotoxicity with cidofovir and foscarnet limits their use in the management of viral infections. Treatment should be given for at least 14 days and until CMV is no longer detectable; treatment doses of antivirals are often followed by maintenance doses for 2 to 3 months.

Influenza

Patients with neutropenia who have exposure to or signs and symptoms of infection or in the event of an outbreak should begin antiviral treatment within 48 hours of exposure or onset of symptoms. Patients with lung infiltrates during high periods of influenza (October through March) should be considered for empiric antiviral therapy with a neuraminidase inhibitor. Oseltamivir 75 mg orally twice daily for 10 days should be initiated in patients who are highly immunocompromised and until the resolution of symptoms. Doses of up to 150 mg orally twice daily of oseltamivir have been used but have not demonstrated extensive benefit. Alternatively, zanamivir, two oral inhalations twice daily also for up to 10 days, may be considered. It is recommended to start either agent as close as possible to the onset of symptoms. Both agents have activity against influenza A and influenza B.

BK Virus

Infection with human polyomavirus type I, or BK virus (BKV), is usually asymptomatic; 50% to 90% of individuals may be infected with BKV by the age of 10 years (Knowles 2006). Although urinary shedding of BKV has been isolated in up to 80% of HCT recipients, only 5%–15% of HCT recipients will experience high-level replication leading to BKV-associated hemorrhagic cystitis (PVHC) 3 to 6 weeks post-transplant (Arthur 1988). Hematopoietic cell transplant recipients reporting dysuria, urinary urgency with hematuria, and high-level BKV replication are diagnosed with PVHC in the absence of other organisms. Although fluoroquinolones may inhibit BKV replication or decrease BKV levels in HCT patients, they have not been associated with a decrease in PVHC and may cause resistance among BKV isolates. In addition, cidofovir given in low-dose (up to

Table 1-2. Infection Risk and Prophylaxis in Neutropenia

	Risk Factors	Prophylaxis
Low (< 10%)	• Standard chemotherapy for solid tumors • Neutropenia expected to last < 7 days	• No bacterial, fungal, or viral prophylaxis indicated • Viral prophylaxis may be considered in prior HSV

Intermediate (10%–20%)	• Autologous HCT
	• CLL
	• Lymphoma
	• Multiple Myeloma
	• Purine analog therapy
	  ○ Clofarabine
	  ○ Cladribine
	  ○ Fludarabine
	  ○ Nelarabine
	• Neutropenia expected to last
	• 7–10 days
		Bacterial:
		• Consider fluoroquinolone
		
		Fungal:
		• Consider fluconazole or micafungin with Autologous HCT + mucositis (until neutropenia resolution)
		
		Viral[a]:
		• Initiate acyclovir, valacyclovir, or famciclovir during neutropenia and for 30 days after HCT (consider VZV prophylaxis for at least 1 year after HCT)

Table 1-2. Infection Risk and Prophylaxis in Neutropenia *(continued)*

	Risk Factors	Prophylaxis

High (>20%)	• Acute leukemia
	  ○ Induction
	  ○ Consolidation
	• Alemtuzumab
	• Allogeneic HCT
	• GVHD + High-dose steroids
	• Profound neutropenia
	• Proteasome Inhibitors
	  ○ Bortezomib
	  ○ Carfilzomib
	• MASCC score < 21
	• Neutropenia expected to last
	• > 10 days
		Bacterial: consider fluoroquinolone
		Fungal:
		• Consider fluconazole in ALL until neutropenia resolution
		• Consider fluconazole or micafungin in neutropenic allogeneic HCT (continue during neutropenia and for at least 75 days post-transplant)
		• Consider posaconazole in patients with MDS (until neutropenia resolution) or significant GVHD (until resolution of GVHD)
		Viral[a]:
		• Initiate acyclovir, valacyclovir, or famciclovir during neutropenia and for 30 days after HCT for HSV (Consider VZV prophylaxis for at least 1 year post HCT)
		• Proteasome inhibitors should receive VZV prophylaxis during therapy
		• Alemtuzumab recipients should receive HSV prophylaxis for at least 2 months after therapy and until CD4$^+$ > 200 cells/mm^3
		• CMV prophylaxis with valganciclovir, ganciclovir, foscarnet, or cidofovir in allogeneic HCT(1–6 months post-transplant or GVHD) OR alemtuzumab recipients (minimum of 2 months after therapy completion)[b]
		Pneumocystis: sulfamethoxazole/trimethoprim (preferred) or dapsone, atovaquone, pentamidine if intolerant to trimethoprim/sulfamethoxazole
		• Initiate prophylaxis:
		  ○ Alemtuzumab recipients
		  ○ ALL
		  ○ Allogeneic HCT
		• Consider prophylaxis:
		  ○ Autologous HCT
		  ○ Purine analog therapy Prolonged Corticosteroids
		  ○ Temozolomide + radiation
		Some institutions wait until engraftment occurs

[a]Viral prophylaxis for HSV and VZV include acyclovir, valacyclovir, or famciclovir

[b]Those receiving CMV prophylaxis with cidofovir, foscarnet, ganciclovir, or valganciclovir should have adequate coverage against HSV and VZV

ALL = acute lymphocytic leukemia; CLL = chronic lymphocytic leukemia; CMV = cytomegalovirus; GVHD = graft-versus-host disease; HCT = hematopoietic cell transplantation; HSV = herpes simplex virus; MASCC = Multinational Association of Supportive Care in Cancer; MDS = myelodysplastic syndrome; VZV = varicella zoster virus.

Information from Freifeld AG, Bow EJ, Sepkowitz KA, et al. Clinical practice guideline for the use of antimicrobial agents in neutropenic patients with cancer: 2010 update by the Infectious Diseases Society of America. Clin Infect Dis 2011;52:e56-e93; and Tomblyn M, Chiller Ta, Einsele H, et al. Guidelines for preventing infectious complications among hematopoietic cell transplantation recipients: a global perspective. Biol Blood Marrow Transplant 2009;15:1143-238.

1 mg/kg intravenous three times weekly without probenecid) or high-dose regimens (5 mg/kg intravenous weekly with probenecid) has been evaluated in HCT recipients with PVHC but has not been associated with improved efficacy. Currently, there are insufficient data to support initiation of prophylaxis or pre-emptive therapy for BKV. The cornerstone of management is to reduce the level of immunosuppression.

Prophylaxis
Antibacterial

Fluoroquinolone antibacterial therapy is commonly used in adults with chemotherapy-induced neutropenia. Although ciprofloxacin is recommended as preferred antibacterial prophylaxis, levofloxacin may be utilized because of its im-proved gram-positive coverage (Freifeld 2011). Antibacterial prophylaxis is not currently recommended in patients at low risk whose anticipated neutropenia is less than 7 days. Various studies found reduced incidences of documented infections, bloodstream infections, and febrile periods in patients who received antibacterial prophylaxis during the early afebrile stage of neutropenia. In addition, increasing concern for antibiotic resistance, fungal overgrowth, and antibacterial adverse effects has arisen. A meta-analysis evaluated 46 placebo-controlled or no-intervention studies compared with antibiotic prophylaxis and identified that antibiotic prophylaxis reduced all-cause mortality (RR 0.66; 95% CI, 0.55–0.79), infection-related death (RR 0.61; 95% CI, 0.48–0.77), occurrence of fever (RR 0.80; 95% CI, 0.74–0.87), and documented infections (clinically, RR 0.65; 95% CI, 0.56–0.76; microbiologically, RR 0.51; 95% CI, 0.42–0.62) (Gafter-Gvili 2012). Although no mortality difference between fluoroquinolone or trimethoprim/sulfamethoxazole prophylaxis was identified, fluoroquinolones were associated with fewer adverse effects and less resistance (Gafter-Gvili 2012). The majority of patients included in this analysis were deemed at high risk secondary to a hematologic malignancy or receipt of an HCT.

Although ciprofloxacin is recommended as preferred antibacterial prophylaxis, levofloxacin may be used because of its improved gram-positive coverage (Freifeld 2011). Studies have evaluated levofloxacin's similar spectrum of activity against gram-negative organisms and improved gram-positive activity against such organisms as streptococci. One study compared levofloxacin 500 mg orally daily with placebo in adults with ANCs of less than 1000 cells/mm^3 and neutropenia expected to last more than 7 days. Levofloxacin was found to result in fewer microbiologically documented infections and bacteremias compared with placebo in those with acute leukemia as well as those with solid tumors or lymphomas. Mortality was similar between the groups (Bucaneve 2005). An evaluation performed in Germany compared moxifloxacin 400 mg/day with levofloxacin 500 mg/day among patients with hematologic malignancies (excluding allogeneic HCT) and prolonged neutropenia (defined as neutropenia of more than 5 days). Although survival was similar between the two groups, an increased incidence of gram-negative bacteremia (p=0.04) and Clostridium difficile–associated diarrhea (p<0.001) was identified in the moxifloxacin group (von Baum 2006).

Fluoroquinolone prophylaxis may increase the risk for fluoroquinolone-resistant *E. coli*, MRSA, and *C. difficile*. It is not recommended to add gram-positive coverage with such

Table 1-3. Additions to Empiric Treatment for Febrile Neutropenia on the Basis of Clinical Signs and Symptoms

Abdominal Pain/Diarrhea	Oral metronidazole or oral vancomycin if suspected *Clostridium difficile* infection intravenous metronidazole should only be used in those unable to take oral therapy Ensure anaerobic coverage
Lung Infiltrates	Azithromycin or fluoroquinolone (unless receiving for prophylaxis or empiric treatment) Antifungal with mold activity (itraconazole, posaconazole, or voriconazole) for intermediate-high-risk patients Antivirals during influenza outbreaks Concern for *Pneumocystis jiroveci*, add trimethoprim/sulfamethoxazole Concern for MRSA, add vancomycin or linezolid
Cellulitis or skin and SSSI	Vancomycin Daptomycin, linezolid, or quinupristin/dalfopristin may be added as an alternative to vancomycin For papules or lesions, consider antifungal with mold activity in high-risk patients
Vascular Access Devices (ports)	Vancomycin May need to remove device
Vesicular Lesions	Acyclovir, famciclovir, or valacyclovir
CNS Infection	Concern for meningitis: antipseudomonal β-lactam with CSF penetration (may already be on board) (cefepime, meropenem) + vancomycin + ampicillin[a] Encephalitis suspected: high dose acyclovir

[a]If piperacillin/tazobactam or meropenem are used, ampicillin is unnecessary.

CNS = central nervous system; CSF = cerebrospinal fluid; MRSA = methicillin-resistant *Staphylococcus aureus*; SSSI = skin and soft tissue infection.

Information from Freifeld AG, Bow EJ, Sepkowitz KA, et al. Clinical practice guideline for the use of antimicrobial agents in neutropenic patients with cancer: 2010 update by the Infectious Diseases Society of America. Clin Infect Dis 2011;52:e56-e93.

agents as penicillins or macrolides because the addition does not improve infection-related mortality and is associated with GI upset. Those receiving antibacterial prophylaxis should be educated on the potential for rash or GI intolerance. Therefore, fluoroquinolone prophylaxis is recommended for patients at intermediate or high risk of infection during periods of prolonged neutropenia (see Table 1-2). Although timing as to when antibacterial prophylaxis should be discontinued is not well studied, it is recommended to discontinue prophylaxis at the end of neutropenia or on initiation of empiric antibiotic therapy in those who become febrile.

Fungal

Routine antifungal prophylaxis is recommended in patients at high risk with neutropenia. Fluconazole, itraconazole, posaconazole, voriconazole, caspofungin, and micafungin all are acceptable options as prophylaxis against *Candida* infections based on patient-specific factors such as previous antifungal prophylaxis, fungal infections, and tolerability. Antifungal prophylaxis is not recommended for patients at low risk with anticipated neutropenia lasting less than 7 days. Fluconazole prophylaxis in high-risk groups has decreased yeast colonization, lowered mucosal and invasive *Candida* infections, reduced mortality in allogeneic HCT recipients, and improved long-term survival (Marr 2000; Slavin 1995). Invasive *Aspergillus* prophylaxis is recommended in patients who are older than 13 years and receiving intensive chemotherapy for acute myeloid leukemia (AML) or myelodysplastic syndrome (Freifeld 2011; Cornely 2007). Mold prophylaxis may be considered in those with prior invasive aspergillosis, anticipated prolonged neutropenia (lasting longer than 14 days), or prolonged neutropenia immediately before HCT (Freifeld 2011).

Fluconazole prophylaxis was most beneficial in those receiving autologous HCT but not receiving colony-stimulating factors and patients with leukemia taking mucotoxic regimens such as cytarabine with an anthracycline. Patients receiving fluconazole and prophylaxis can predispose to colonization and bloodstream infection secondary to fluconazole-resistant *Candida* strains. Although low-dose amphotericin B and itraconazole have activity against invasive molds, no mortality benefit was observed when compared with fluconazole (Marr 2004; Koh 2002). In addition, aerosolized amphotericin B prevents invasive aspergillosis in those with prolonged neutropenia compared with placebo, but it lacks consistent device delivery and formulation as well as comparative data with mold-active azoles or echinocandins (Rijnders 2008). For those undergoing HCT, micafungin (50 mg intravenous once daily) was superior to fluconazole (400 mg intravenous once daily) based on the absence of suspected, proven, or probable invasive fungal infection during treatment and 4 weeks post-treatment and was associated with fewer invasive aspergillosis episodes in allogeneic HCT. Survival and adverse effects were similar in both groups (van Burik

2004). No difference was demonstrated in invasive-fungal-infection-free survival 180 days post allogeneic HCT between voriconazole (200 mg orally twice daily) and fluconazole (400 mg orally once daily), but a trend in favor of voriconazole was noted for reduced incidence of *Aspergillus* and invasive *Candida* infections (Wingard 2010). When posaconazole (200-mg oral suspension three times daily) was compared with fluconazole (400-mg oral suspension once daily) or itraconazole (200-mg oral solution twice daily) in neutropenic patients with AML or myelodysplastic syndrome receiving induction or reinduction chemotherapy, posaconazole significantly reduced invasive fungal and aspergillosis infections (Cornely 2007). In addition, posaconazole is recommended for patients at high risk, including allogeneic HCT recipients with graft-versus-host disease (grades II to IV or chronic extensive) or receiving intensive immunosuppression (high-dose corticosteroids, antithymocyte globulin, or a combination of at least two immunosuppressive agents).

Posaconazole oral suspension is limited by its ability to achieve detectable and therapeutic drug concentrations. Those with inadequate intake or diet, as well as patients who require concomitant proton pump inhibitor therapy, should avoid the oral suspension and receive treatment with either posaconazole delayed-release tablets or the intravenous formulation. Cimetidine also interacts with posaconazole suspension and should be avoided. Although the package insert states that no dosage adjustment is required for posaconazole suspension with concomitant use of antacids or other H_2-receptor antagonists, additional data suggests decreased absorption of posaconazole suspension when given with ranitidine or metoclopramide (Dolton 2012). Posaconazole suspension should be administered during a high-fat meal or immediately after (within 20 minutes) to enhance absorption and optimize levels. In addition, posaconazole suspension may be administered with a liquid nutritional supplement or an acidic carbonated beverage to improve absorption and optimize serum levels. Individuals unable to tolerate this drug should not receive it for prophylaxis. Although the duration of prophylaxis is unknown in patients at high risk, those with acute leukemia should discontinue antifungal prophylaxis with myeloid reconstitution. Allogeneic HCT should continue antifungal prophylaxis during the period of neutropenia and for at least 75 days post-transplantation or until completion of immunosuppressive treatment (Marr 2000). Secondary antifungal prophylaxis is recommended in chronic systemic *Candida* infection or for invasive filamentous (e.g., mucormycosis or aspergillosis) fungal infections.

Pneumocystis jiroveci Pneumonia

Prophylaxis with trimethoprim/sulfamethoxazole (1 double-strength 160-mg/800-mg tablet orally daily) should be initiated in patients with acute lymphocytic leukemia (throughout therapy), in allogeneic HCT recipients (at least 6

Table 1-4. Duration of Anti-Infective Therapy in Febrile Neutropenia

Undocumented Infection	
Regardless of Risk Factor	ANC > 500 cells /mm^3 and increasing
Documented Infection[a]	
Bacterial	
SSSI	10–14 days
BSI[b] Gram-negative Gram-positive[c]	10–14 days 7–14 days
Sinusitis	10–21 days
Pneumonia	10–21 days
Fungal (Mold or Yeast)	
Candida or yeast BSI	At least 14 days after first negative blood culture
Mold *(Aspergillus, Fusarium, Mucor)*	At least 12 weeks but can last months to years, duration based on clinical/radiographic response
Viral	
CMV	At least 14–21 days + until CMV is no longer detectable in the blood
HSV/VZV	7–10 days
Influenza	10 days and until symptom resolution

[a]If neutropenia still unresolved when adequate duration of therapy with anti-infective has occurred, anti-infective should be continued until ANC > 500 cells/mm^3 and increasing.
[b]Catheter removal should be considered with *Acinetobacter, Bacillus* spp., *Corynebacterium jeikeium, Candida,* atypical molds/mycobacterias/ yeast, *P. aeruginosa, S. aureus, Stenotrophomonas maltophilia,* VRE, septic arthritis, tunnel infection, or port infection.
[c]If *S. aureus* isolated, anti-infective therapy should continue for at least 2 weeks after the first negative blood cultures.
ANC = absolute neutrophil count; BSI = bloodstream infection; CMV = cytomegalovirus; HSV = herpes simplex virus; SSSI = skin and skin structure infection; VZV = varicella zoster virus.
Information from Freifeld AG, Bow EJ, Sepkowitz KA, et al. Clinical practice guideline for the use of antimicrobial agents in neutropenic patients with cancer: 2010 update by the Infectious Diseases Society of America. Clin Infect Dis 2011;52:e56-e93.

months and while receiving immunosuppression), in patients receiving alemtuzumab (at least 2 months after therapy and until CD4$^+$ > 200 cells/mm^3), and in patients receiving temozolomide plus radiotherapy (until recovery from lymphopenia). Prophylaxis may be considered in patients receiving purine analog (i.e., fludarabine) therapy (until CD4$^+$ >200 cells/mm^3), in those on rituximab therapy, autologous HCT recipients (3–6 months post-transplant), and in those receiving at least 20 mg or more of prednisone or its equivalent daily for at least 4 weeks for neoplastic disease (until recovery from lymphopenia). If trimethoprim/sulfamethoxazole is given, it also provides some coverage against *Nocardia*, toxoplasmosis, and *Listeria*. If trimethoprim/sulfamethoxazole cannot be used because of intolerance or allergy, then dapsone (assess for G6PD deficiency before initiation), inhaled pentamidine, or atovaquone may be used as an alternative.

Viral

Herpes simplex virus seropositive patients undergoing allogeneic or autologous HCT or receiving induction or reinduction therapy for acute leukemia should receive antiviral prophylaxis with acyclovir, valacyclovir, or famciclovir. Prophylaxis should continue throughout the neutropenic period, until resolution of mucositis, and for at least 30 days after HCT. Antiviral prophylaxis may be extended in those with recurrent HSV infections or in those with graft-versus-host disease or as VZV prophylaxis for up to 1 year. Those who do not receive appropriate antiviral prophylaxis may experience reactivation and infection in up to 80% of HCT (Meyers 1980). In those undergoing allogeneic HCT, the risk of HSV is most common within the first month post-transplantation but may also occur during periods of immunosuppression. Although acyclovir or valacyclovir is considered the prophylaxis of choice, foscarnet should be initiated in those with previous acyclovir-resistant infection. In those receiving antiviral prophylaxis with ganciclovir or foscarnet, CMV is also adequately covered by these agents, and additional HSV prophylaxis is not required. Patients with chronic lymphocytic leukemia receiving alemtuzumab should receive antiviral prophylaxis for at least 2 months after completion or until CD4$^+$

is more than 200 cells/mm^3 based on whichever happens later. Those considered at intermediate risk of HSV reactivation based on previous infection should receive HSV prophylaxis during future episodes of neutropenia caused by cytotoxic therapy.

Allogeneic HCT recipients with histories of VZV infection are at increased risk of reactivation of the infection if not receiving adequate antiviral prophylaxis. Those receiving proteasome inhibitors (e.g., bortezomib, carfilzomib) should receive antiviral prophylaxis during active treatment. Allogeneic HCT recipients who are seropositive for VZV before transplant should receive prophylaxis for at least 1 year post-transplantation, with the potential to extend beyond that time if the patient continues to receive immunosuppression. Antivirals used for HSV also have activity against VZV. Empiric use is not recommended in FN and should be reserved for active treatment of HSV or VZV.

Cytomegalovirus prophylaxis should be considered in allogeneic HCT or alemtuzumab therapy. Those at risk of reactivation, based on CMV serology before transplantation, should receive pre-emptive monitoring for infection and therapy if either the donor or the recipient is seropositive.

Individuals undergoing cancer treatment and members of their households should be vaccinated annually against influenza. Immunization for patients receiving treatment should be with the inactivated form of the virus; however, family members may receive the live attenuated formulation unless the patient received HCT. Although ideal timing for vaccination regarding therapy has not been established, responses may be best between chemotherapy cycles: either more than 7 days after a treatment cycle or more than 14 days before chemotherapy begins. Vaccination should not be administered in HCT recipients unless more than 6 months post-transplant, given the low likelihood of immune development early after HCT. Pending results of respiratory polymerase chain reaction testing and/or if a patient with neutropenia reports exposure to influenza, a 5-day course of oseltamivir or zanamivir should be initiated regardless of vaccination history. Some suggest a longer period of treatment in this population (CDC 2014).

Hematopoietic Growth Factors in FN

Individuals considered at intermediate to high risk of FN should be considered for prophylactic granulocyte-colony-stimulating factors (G-CSF) and receive filgrastim or pegfilgrastim unless treatment is symptomatic or palliative. The agent tbo-filgrastim received label approval in 2012 as a human leukocyte growth factor and can also be used for prophylaxis for patients at intermediate to high risk of developing FN. Similarly to other G-CSF, individuals receiving induction therapy for AML or HCT should be considered for granulocyte-macrophage-colony-stimulating factor.

Reduction of the incidence, duration, and severity of chemotherapy-induced neutropenia has been demonstrated in various cancers, but its high cost has limited its use for all patients receiving chemotherapy. Primary prophylaxis in high-risk FN with pegfilgrastim was evaluated in the setting of breast cancer and small-cell lung cancer. In the breast cancer study, a statistically significant reduction was seen in FN incidence, hospitalization, and requirement for intravenous antibiotics (Vogel 2007). In the small-cell lung cancer study, a reduction was seen in FN during the first cycle of chemotherapy with prophylactic antibiotics and G-CSF (p=0.01) but this was not observed with subsequent cycles of chemotherapy (Timmer-Bonte 2005). In addition, G-CSF improve the incidence of full-dose chemotherapy, although this has not been associated with improved response or survival. Meta-analyses have established G-CSF efficacy in decreasing infections, neutropenic risk, and infection-related mortality (Kuderer 2007; Sung 2007).

The patient's ANC should be evaluated before each cycle of chemotherapy. For patients who had FN or dose-limiting neutropenia in the presence of previous colony-stimulating factors, chemotherapy dose reduction or change in chemotherapy should be considered. Patients who experienced FN or dose-limiting neutropenia but had no previous exposure to colony-stimulating factors should be considered for the use of these agents. If FN occurs while a patient is receiving prophylactic filgrastim or sargramostim during a current chemotherapy cycle, the patient should continue receiving these agents; but if the patient was given prophylactic pegfilgrastim, no additional treatment is required with G-CSF. A patient who was not receiving G-CSF prophylaxis at time of FN but who presents with age older than 65 years (highest risk), sepsis, ANC of less than 100 cells/mm^3, neutropenia expected to last more than 10 days, pneumonia, invasive fungal infection, other documented infection, previous FN, or hospitalization at time of fever should be given filgrastim or sargramostim based on the type of treatment. Currently, only filgrastim and sargramostim are approved for therapy for FN, although fewer data are available supporting their use with adjunctive antibiotics. Sargramostim 250 mcg/m^2 intravenous daily should be given daily for the first 14 days, with 7 days off if engraftment does not occur, as manifested by increasing ANC. An additional cycle of sargramostim may be given with the same dose and duration. If after two cycles of sargramostim engraftment does not occur, the dose of sargramostim may be increased to 500 mcg/m^2 intravenous daily for 14 days. If engraftment does not occur after increasing the dose, it is unlikely to occur with subsequent administration.

The most common patient-reported adverse event is mild to moderate bone pain, which can typically be controlled with a nonnarcotic analgesic. Rare cases have been reported of splenic rupture, allergic reactions, acute respiratory distress syndrome, alveolar hemorrhage with hemoptysis, and sickle cell crisis in those with the disease.

Nonpharmacologic Management of FN

Various environmental precautions should occur in the management of FN. Hand hygiene is the most effective means of preventing health care–acquired infections during periods of neutropenia. All visitors and health care workers should wash their hands before and after entering the room of a patient with neutropenia. Protective gear or a single-patient room are not required in the setting of neutropenia unless the patient is a HCT recipient. In addition, in an attempt to prevent mold infections, allogeneic HCT recipients should be placed in private rooms with high-efficiency particulate air filtration.

Skin care during neutropenia should include daily bathing and inspection of sites likely to be entryways for infections. Oral and dental hygiene should be maintained during neutropenic periods. For patients with mucositis, oral rinsing with sterile water, normal saline, or sodium bicarbonate solutions should occur 4 to 6 times daily.

Dried flowers, fresh flowers, and other plants should not be allowed in the presence of patients with neutropenia because molds have been isolated from those sources. Finally, a patient with neutropenia should follow a neutropenic diet consisting of well-cooked foods and should avoid lunch meats. Fresh fruits and vegetables are permitted as long as they are thoroughly washed.

Conclusion

Neutropenia associated with treatment and malignancy puts cancer patients at risk of many infections. Our goals as pharmacists are to prevent morbidity, mortality, and infections; to identify and provide effective treatment and prophylaxis; to avoid unnecessary and excessive antimicrobial therapy; and to minimize toxicities while providing enhanced quality of life. Those undergoing chemotherapy, radiation, and transplantation should be evaluated with each treatment and assessed for the potential of those procedures to cause neutropenia.

References

American Cancer Society. Cancer Facts & Figures. 2014.

Arthur RR, Shah KV, Charache P, Saral R. BK and JC virus infections in recipients of bone marrow transplants. J Infect Dis 1988;158:563-569.

Auberger J, Lass-Flörl C, Ulmer H, et al. Significant alterations in the epidemiology and treatment outcome of invasive fungal infections in patients with hematological malignancies. Int J Hematol 2008;88:508-15.

Beck JC, Wagner JE, DeFor TE, et al. Impact of cytomegalovirus (CMV) reactivation after umbilical cord transplantation. Biol Blood Marrow Transplant 2010;16:215-22.

Boeckh M, Ljungman P. How we treat cytomegalovirus in hematopoietic cell transplant recipients. Blood 2009;113:5711-9.

Bollée G, Sarfati C, Thiéry G, et al. Clinical picture of Pneumocystis jiroveci pneumonia in cancer patients. Chest 2007;132:1305-10.

Bowers DR, Liew YX, Lye DC, et al. Outcomes of appropriate empiric combination versus monotherapy for Pseudomonas

---

Practice Points

In determining the optimal pharmacotherapy for the prevention and management of infections with patients with underlying malignancy, practitioners should consider the following: of malignancy, treatment of malignancy, anticipated duration of neutropenia, and Multinational Association of Supportive Care in Cancer index risk score, where a score of 21 or greater is associated with a low risk of complications in FN cancer patients.

- Risk stratification of bacterial, fungal, and viral infections in individuals with neutropenia is based on type of malignancy, treatment of malignancy, anticipated duration of neutropenia, and Multinational Association of Supportive Care in Cancer index risk score, where a score of 21 or greater is associated with a low risk of complications in FN cancer patients.
- Low-risk individuals requiring empiric management of FN may be managed in ambulatory care setting with orally/intravenous antibiotics such as ciprofloxacin plus amoxicillin/clavulanate, ciprofloxacin or levofloxacin monotherapy, or ciprofloxacin plus clindamycin.
- High-risk patients requiring empiric management should be hospitalized for intravenous antibiotics. Empiric management may include an anti-pseudomonal β-lactam antibiotic but caution should be used in those with frequent exposure to the health care setting and/or receiving prophylactic or empiric antibiotics. Therefore, it is important to consider

multi-drug resistant organisms in patients with immunocompromise, along with local susceptibility and epidemiologic patterns.
- Fungal origin of infection should be considered in individuals receiving empiric antibiotics for 4 days or longer who still experience FN or have recurrent fever while on antimicrobial therapy.
- The risk of viral infection is low with the use of appropriate viral prophylaxis in individuals with intermediate or high risk of infection. Allogeneic HCT seropositive for VZV before transplant should receive prophylaxis for at least 1 year and possibly longer if immunosuppression continues.
- Patients considered at intermediate or high risk of FN should be considered for prophylactic granulocyte-colony stimulating factors; however, many patients experience mild or moderate pain as an adverse event, which can be managed by a non-narcotic analgesic.

aeruginosa bacteremia. Antimicrob Agents Chemother 2013;57:1270-4.

Brusch JL, Weinstein L. Fever of unknown origin. Med Clin North Am 1988;72:1247-61.

Bucaneve G, Micozzi A, Menichetti F, et al. Levofloxacin to prevent bacterial infection in patients with cancer and neutropenia. N Engl J Med 2005;353:977-87.

Centers for Disease Control and Prevention. Preventing Infections in Cancer Patients. 2014.

Centers for Disease Control and Prevention. Seasonal Influenza. 2014.

Cornely OA, Maertens J, Winston DJ, et al. Posaconazole vs. fluconazole or itraconazole prophylaxis in patients with neutropenia. N Engl J Med 2007;356:348-359.

Dolton MJ, Ray JE, Chen SC, et al. Multicenter study of posaconazole therapeutic drug monitoring: exposure-response relationship and factors affecting concentration. Antimicrob Agents Chemother 2012;56:5503-10

Fausel CA. Neutropenia and agranulocytosis. In: Tisdale JE, Miller DA, eds. Drug-induced Diseases: Prevention, Detection, and Management. 2nd ed. Bethesda, MD: American Society of Health-System Pharmacists; 2010: 962-971.

Freifeld AG, Bow EJ, Sepkowitz KA, et al. Clinical practice guideline for the use of antimicrobial agents in neutropenic patients with cancer: 2010 update by the Infectious Diseases Society of America. Clin Infect Dis 2011;52:e56-e93.

Gafter-Gvili A, Fraser A, Paul M, et al. Antibiotic prophylaxis for bacterial infections in afebrile neutropenic patients following chemotherapy. Cochrane Database Syst Rev 2012 Jan 18;1:CD004386.

George B, Pati N, Gilroy N, et al. Pre-transplant cytomegalovirus (CMV) serostatus remains the most important determinant of CMV reactivation after allogeneic hematopoietic stem cell transplantation in the era of surveillance and preemptive therapy. Transpl Infect Dis 2010;12:322-9.

Hu Y, Li L, Li W, et al. Combination antibiotic therapy versus monotherapy for Pseudomonas aeruginosa bacteraemia: a meta-analysis of retrospective and prospective studies. Int J Antimicrob Agents 2013;42:492-6.

Keating MJ, Flinn I, Jain V, et al. Therapeutic role of alemtuzumab (Campath-1H) in patients who have failed fludarabine: results of a large international study. Blood 2002;99:3554-61.

Kern WV, Marchetti O, Drgona L, et al. Oral antibiotics for fever in low-risk neutropenic patients with cancer: a double-blind, randomized, multicenter trial comparing single daily moxifloxacin with twice daily ciprofloxacin plus amoxicillin/clavulanic acid combination therapy--EORTC infectious diseases group trial XV. J Clin Oncol 2013;31:1149-56.

Klastersky J, Paesmans M, Rubenstein EB, et al. The Multinational Association for Supportive Care in Cancer risk index: A multinational scoring system for identifying low-risk febrile neutropenic cancer patients. J Clin Oncol 2000;18:3038-51.

Klastersky J. Management of fever in neutropenic patients with different risks of complications. Clin Infect Dis 2004;39 Suppl 1:S32-7.

Klastersky J, Ameye L, Maertens J, et al. Bacteraemia in febrile neutropenic cancer patients. Int J Antimicrob Agents 2007;30 Suppl 1:S51-9.

Knowles W. Discovery and epidemiology of the human polyomaviruses BK virus (BKV) and JC virus (JCV). Adv Exp Med Biol 2006;577:19-45.

Koh LP, Kurup A, Goh YT, et al. Randomized trial of fluconazole versus low-dose amphotericin B in prophylaxis against fungal infections in patients undergoing hematopoietic stem cell transplantation. Am J Hematol 2002;71:260-7.

Kuderer NM, Dale DC, Crawford J, Cosler LE, et al. Mortality, morbidity, and cost associated with febrile neutropenia in adult cancer patients. Cancer 2006;106:2258-66.

Kuderer NM, Dale DC, Crawford J, et al. Impact of primary prophylaxis with granulocyte colony-stimulating factor on febrile neutropenia and mortality in adult cancer patients receiving chemotherapy: a systematic review. J Clin Oncol 2007;25:3158-67.

Limper AH, Offord KP, Smith TF, Martin WJ. Pneumocystis carinii pneumonia. Differences in lung parasite number and inflammation in patients with and without AIDS. Am Rev Respir Dis 1989;140:1204.

Marr KA, Carter RA, Boeckh M, et al. Invasive aspergillosis in allogeneic stem cell transplant recipients: changes in epidemiology and risk factors. Blood 2002;100:4358-66.
Marr KA, Crippa F, Leisenring W, et al. Itraconazole versus fluconazole for prevention of fungal infections in patients receiving allogeneic stem cell transplants. Blood 2004;103:1527-1533.

Marr KA, Seidel L, Slavin MA, et al. Prolonged fluconazole prophylaxis is associated with persistent protection against candidiasis-related death in allogeneic marrow transplant recipients: long-term follow-up of a randomized, placebo-controlled trial. Blood 2000;96:2055-2061.

Martin-Garrido I, Carmona EM, Specks U, et al. Pneumocystis pneumonia in patients treated with rituximab. Chest 2013;144:258-65.

Meyers JD, Flournoy N, Thomas ED. Infection with herpes simplex virus and cell-mediated immunity after marrow transplant. J Infect Dis 1980;142:338-346.

National Cancer Institute. Nutrition and cancer care (PDQ). 2011.

National Institutes of Health (NIH). Lymphocytopenia. 2013.

National Institutes of Health (NIH). Pets and the Immunocompromised Person. 2014.

Nguyen TD, Williams B, Trang E. Cefepime therapy all-cause mortality. Clin Infect Dis 2009;49:902-4.

Patel RA, Gallagher JC. Drug Fever. Pharmacotherapy 2010;30:57-69.

Paul M, Borok S, Fraser A, et al. Empirical antibiotics against gram-positive infections for febrile neutropenia: systematic review and meta-analysis of randomized controlled trials. J Antimicrob Chemother 2005;55:436-44.

Pietersma FL, van Dorp S, Minnema MC, et al. Influence of donor on cytomegalovirus (CMV) status on severity of viral reactivation after allogeneic stem cell transplantation in CMV-seropositive recipients. Clin Infect Dis 2011;52:e144-48.

Rijnders BJ, Cornelissen JJ, Slobbe L, et al. Aerosolized liposomal amphotericin B for the prevention of invasive pulmonary aspergillosis during prolonged neutropenia: a randomized, placebo-controlled trial. Clin Infect Dis 2008;46:1401-1408.

Schimpff SC. Empiric antibiotic therapy for granulocytopenic cancer patients. Am J Med 1986;80:13-20.

Slavin MA, Osborne B, Adams R, et al. Efficacy and safety of fluconazole prophylaxis for fungal infections after marrow transplantation-a prospective, randomized, double-blind study. J Infect Dis 1995;171:1545-52.

Sung L, Nathan PC, Alibhai SM, et al. Meta-analysis: effect of prophylactic hematopoietic colony-stimulating factors on mortality and outcomes of infection. Ann Intern Med 2007;147:400-11.

Timmer-Bonte JN, de Boo TM, Smit HJ, et al. Prevention of chemotherapy-induced febrile neutropenia by prophylactic antibiotics plus or minus granulocyte colony-stimulating factor in small-cell lung cancer: a Dutch Randomized Phase III Study. J Clin Oncol 2005;23:7974-84.

Trecarichi EM, Tumbarello M. Antimicrobial-resistant Gram-negative bacteria in febrile neutropenic patients with cancer: current epidemiology and clinical impact. Curr Opin Infect Dis 2014;27:200-10.

U.S. Food and Drug Administration (FDA). Information for Healthcare Professionals: Cefepime.2009.

U.S. Food and Drug Administration (FDA). Food Safety for People with Cancer. 2014.

van Burik J-AH, Ratanatharathorn V, Stepan DE, et al. Micafungin versus fluconazole for prophylaxis against invasive fungal infections during neutropenia in patients undergoing hematopoietic stem cell transplantation. Clin Infect Dis 2004;39:1407-1416.

Vogel CL, Wojtukiewicz MZ, Carroll RR, et al. First and subsequent cycle use of pegfilgrastim prevents febrile neutropenia in patients with breast cancer: a multicenter, double-blind, placebo-controlled phase III study. J Clin Oncol 2005;23:1178-84.

von Baum H, Sigge A, Bommer M, et al. Moxifloxacin prophylaxis in neutropenic patients. J Antimicrob Chemother 2006;58:891-4.

Vardakas KZ, Tansarli GS, Bliziotis IA, et al. β-Lactam plus aminoglycoside or fluoroquinolone combination versus β-lactam monotherapy for Pseudomonas aeruginosa infections: a meta-analysis. Int J Antimicrob Agents 2013;41:301-10.

Wald A, Leisenring W, van Burik JA, et al. Epidemiology of Aspergillus infections in a large cohort of patients undergoing bone marrow transplantation. J Infect Dis 1997;175:1459-66.

Walsh TJ, Pappas P, Winston DJ, et al. Voriconazole compared with liposomal amphotericin B for empirical antifungal therapy in patients with neutropenia and persistent fever. N Engl J Med 2002;346:225-34.

Walsh TJ, Teppler H, Donowitz GR, et al. Caspofungin versus liposomal amphotericin B for empirical antifungal therapy in patients with persistent fever and neutropenia. N Engl J Med 2004;351:1391-402.

Wingard JR, Carter SL, Walsh TJ, et al. Randomized, double-blind trial of fluconazole versus voriconazole for prevention of invasive fungal infection after allogeneic hematopoietic cell transplantation. Blood 2010;116:5111-8.

Yahav D, Paul M, Fraser A, et al. Efficacy and safety of cefepime: a systematic review and meta-analysis. Lancet Infect Dis 2007;7:338-48.

Zaia J, Baden L, Boeckh MJ, et al. Viral disease prevention after hematopoietic cell transplantation. Bone Marrow Transplant 2009;44:471-82.

SELF-ASSESSMENT QUESTIONS

1. A 37-year-old man (height 72 inches, weight 80 kg) who has stage III colorectal cancer comes to your clinic for follow-up. He reports that he is feeling well and is tolerating his first cycle of chemotherapy with good oral intake of food and fluids. He does not report any symptoms. His medical history is significant for ulcerative colitis and seasonal allergies. He is allergic to penicillin (rash/hives) and shellfish. His drug regimen includes FOLFOX (fluorouracil, leucovorin, oxaliplatin), last cycle 7 days ago; infliximab 5 mg/kg intravenous every 8 weeks; and a multivitamin one tablet orally daily. His vital signs include temperature 101.9°F, blood pressure 128/78 mm Hg, respiratory rate 14 breaths/minute, and heart rate 83 beats/minute. His laboratory values are as follows:

Sodium	134 mEq/L
Potassium	3.8 mEq/L
Chloride	101 mmol/L
Carbon dioxide	23 mmol/L
Blood urea nitrogen	16 mg/dL
Creatinine	0.9 mg/dL
Glucose	106 mg/dL
Hemoglobin	12.3 g/dL
Hematocrit	34.8%
Platelets	99/mm^3
White blood cells (WBC)	9 x 10^3 cells/mm^3
WBC differential	Lymphocytes: 60%
	Neutrophils: 44%

Which one of the following is the best antibiotic regimen to initiate in this patient?
- A. Ciprofloxacin 500 mg orally twice daily plus clindamycin 300 mg orally every 8 hours.
- B. Ciprofloxacin 500 mg orally twice daily plus amoxicillin/clavulanate 500 mg orally every 8 hours.
- C. Piperacillin/tazobactam 4.5 g intravenously every 6 hours.
- D. Cefepime 2 g intravenously every 8 hours.

2. A 50-year-old patient with chronic myeloid leukemia (CML) recently started dasatinib as well as a 10-day course of sulfamethoxazole/trimethoprim, one double-strength tablet orally twice daily, for cellulitis. In addition, the patient takes prednisone 5 mg orally daily (rheumatoid arthritis) and reports an episode of oral candidiasis 12 months ago. Which one of the following factors places this patient at the highest risk of developing neutropenia?
- A. Age.
- B. Corticosteroid use.

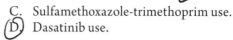

- C. Sulfamethoxazole-trimethoprim use.
- D. Dasatinib use.

Questions 3–5 pertain to the following case.

D.B. is a 48-year-old woman on your transplant service. She was diagnosed with AML and received an allogeneic hematopoietic cell transplantation (HCT) 10 days ago. Her ANC is 80 cells/mm^3 and she is currently afebrile.

3. Which one of the following is the most appropriate anti-infective prophylaxis for D.B.?
- A. Levofloxacin 500 mg orally daily plus fluconazole 400 mg orally daily plus acyclovir 800 mg orally twice daily plus sulfamethoxazole/trimethoprim 400/80 mg orally daily.
- B. Levofloxacin 500 mg orally daily plus fluconazole 400 mg orally daily.
- C. Levofloxacin 500 mg orally daily.
- D. Moxifloxacin 400 mg orally daily plus posaconazole 200 mg orally twice daily plus sulfamethoxazole/trimethoprim 400/80 mg orally daily.

4. Which one of the following is best to recommend to the medical team regarding D.B.'s sargramostim therapy?
- A. Discontinue sargramostim.
- B. Continue sargramostim 250 mcg/m^2 intravenously daily for a total of 14 days; followed by 7 days off sargramostim; may repeat.
- C. Increase sargramostim to 500 mcg/m^2 intravenously daily.
- D. Discontinue sargramostim, initiate pegfilgrastim 6 mg subcutaneously every 7 days.

5. D.B. reports a dull, aching pain in her bones. Which one of the following is best to recommend managing D.B.'s pain?
- A. Change to pegfilgrastim.
- B. Reduce the dose of sargramostim.
- C. Start a fentanyl patch.
- D. Start acetaminophen.

Questions 6 and 7 pertain to the following case.

E.B. is a 32-year-old woman (height 65 inches, weight 60 kg). Her medical history includes non-Hodgkin lymphoma and AIDS. She is taking tenofovir/emtricitabine/atazanavir/ritonavir. E.B. recently received a diagnosis of maxillary *Aspergillus*. She was started on intravenous amphotericin B 60 mg daily but her kidney function worsened from baseline on day 7 of therapy (baseline SCr: 0.9 mg/dL; current SCr: 2.8 mg/dL).

6. Which one of the following is the optimal agent and dose for E.B.?

A. Intravenous amphotericin B 30 mg daily once SCr decreases to baseline.
B. Posaconazole oral suspension 200 mg orally four times daily.
C. Fluconazole 400 mg intravenous/orally daily.
D. Voriconazole 400 mg orally daily

7. E.B. has improved since starting appropriate treatment and is getting ready to be discharged. She has received a total of 14 days of treatment. The medical team asks for discharge recommendations. Which one of the following is best to recommend for E.B.?

A. Discontinue antifungal therapy.
B. Continue posaconazole 200 mg orally QID for at least an additional 10 weeks.
C. Continue fluconazole 400 mg orally daily for at least an additional 12 weeks.
D. Continue voriconazole 400 mg orally daily for at least an additional 6 weeks.

Questions 8–9 pertain to the following case.

T.T. is a 60-year-old man (height 74 inches, weight 86 kg) who has stage IV non-small cell lung cancer with metastasis to the brain. He has received three cycles of cisplatin/docetaxel (last dose was 10 days ago) and pegfilgrastim (last dose was 9 days ago). He is brought to the emergency department because he has a fever (102.1°F) and is lethargic. His current ANC is 319 cells/mm³. He has not had any hospitalizations in the last 6 months. T.T.'s medical history is significant for a previous *C. glabrata* (fluconazole resistance) infection, hypertension, bipolar depression, and seizures. He has no known drug allergies. His drug regimen includes cisplatin/docetaxel, pegfilgrastim, levetiracetam 1500 mg orally twice daily, lorazepam 0.5 mg orally twice daily, metoprolol tartrate 25 mg orally twice daily, mirtazapine 30 mg orally at bedtime, quetiapine 50 mg orally at bedtime, and omeprazole 20 mg orally daily. His vital signs are temperature 102.1°F, blood pressure 108/78 mm Hg, respiratory rate 12 breaths/minute, and heart rate 62 beats/minute. T.T.'s laboratory values are as follows:

Sodium	138 mEq/L
Potassium	4.2 mEq/L
Chloride	108 mmol/L
Carbon dioxide	20 mmol/L
Blood urea nitrogen	20 mg/dL
Creatinine	0.7 mg/dL
Glucose	99 mg/dL
Hemoglobin	10.4 g/dL
Hematocrit	31.9%
Platelets	100/mm³
White blood cells (WBC)	8 x 10³ cells/mm³

8. Which one of the following is best to recommend for T.T.?

A. Ceftazidime intravenous 2 g every 8 hours
B. Piperacillin/tazobactam intravenous 4.5 g every 6 hours
C. Moxifloxacin intravenous 400 mg daily plus vancomycin intravenous 1000 mg every 8 hours
D. Piperacillin/tazobactam intravenous 4.5 g every 6 hours plus vancomycin intravenous 1000 mg every 8 hours

9. Four days later, T.T. has persistent neutropenic fever. Which one of the following is the best empiric agent to recommend for T.T.?

A. Voriconazole 400 mg orally twice daily.
B. Fluconazole intravenous 400 mg daily.
C. Micafungin intravenous 100 mg daily.
D. Posaconazole oral suspension 400 mg orally twice daily.

10. A 32-year-old woman with Hodgkin lymphoma has received intravenous cefepime and vancomycin for the past 4 days for febrile neutropenia. Blood cultures drawn from a peripherally inserted central catheter (PICC) line reveal MRSA. She continues to be febrile but the rest of her vital signs are stable. You call down to the lab and request the MIC the patient's isolate for vancomycin. You are told that vancomycin has an MIC of 2 mcg/mL. Which one of the following is best to recommend for this patient?

A. Remove the PICC line.
B. Remove the PICC line and continue vancomycin for 10 more days.
C. Continue vancomycin for 10 more days.
D. Start daptomycin.

11. A woman with esophageal cancer will be starting chemotherapy in 3 weeks. She asks if influenza vaccination will be administered before starting chemotherapy. The patient's last influenza vaccination was around 12 months ago. Which one of the following is best to recommend regarding influenza vaccine for this patient?

A. Administer today.
B. Administer 1 week before chemotherapy.
C. Administer on the day of chemotherapy.
D. Administer 6 months after the completion of chemotherapy.

12. A patient is started on levofloxacin prophylaxis because of anticipated neutropenia lasting more than 10 days. After completing all cycles of chemotherapy, the patient's ANC is 1319 cells/mm³ (2 days ago it was 800 cells/mm³). Which one of the following is best to recommend for this patient's levofloxacin prophylaxis?

A. Discontinue today.
B. Continue until the ANC is greater than 10,000 cells/mm^3.
C. Discontinue and initiate pegfilgrastim once weekly.
D. Continue indefinitely.

13. A study is comparing Drug A with placebo for its ability to decrease the risk of neutropenia in chemotherapy patients by 75%. Hepatotoxic effects were more common in the Drug A group than in the placebo group, as follows:

Treatment	Subjects	Death/liver failure
Drug A	512	32
Placebo	500	12

What is the number needed to harm for Drug A in this study?
A. 3
B. 26
C. 32
D. 54

$$\left(\frac{32}{512}\right) - \left(\frac{12}{500}\right)$$

$0.0625 - 0.024 = 0.0385$

$1/0.0385 = 26 = NNH$

14. In a cohort study to determine an association between the consumption of fresh fruits and vegetables and the development of infection in FN patients, the relative risk of infection in the group consuming fresh fruits and vegetables compared with the group not consuming fresh fruits and vegetables was 0.90 (95% confidence interval [CI], 0.53–1.09). Which one of the following p-values best reflects these results?

A. < 0.01
B. < 0.05
C. > 0.01
D. > 0.05

15. A 28-year-old woman who recently underwent an allogeneic HCT had routine blood work and was found to have another cytomegalovirus (CMV)-positive polymerase chain reaction (PCR) test of 23,361 copies/mL. Two weeks ago her CMV PCR was also found to be positive (18,765 copies/mL). She does not report any active signs or symptoms of CMV. She has no known drug allergies and has an estimated CrCL of 96 mL/minute. Which one of the following is best to recommend for this patient?

A. Cidofovir.
B. Ganciclovir.
C. Valganciclovir.
D. Foscarnet.

Questions 16 and 17 pertain to the following case.

T.Z.'s physician contacts you about initiating voriconazole for suspected aspergillosis. He asks you to go over T.Z.'s drug list to make sure there are no interacting agents. A complete drug list from the patient's medical records includes the following: allopurinol 100 mg orally daily, hydrochlorothiazide 25 mg orally daily, metformin 1000 mg orally twice daily, pantoprazole 40 mg orally daily, and simvastatin 40 mg orally at bedtime.

16. Which one of the following is best to recommend for T.Z.?

A. Voriconazole is contraindicated with the use of pantoprazole and should be switched to posaconazole.
B. Simvastatin is contraindicated with the use of voriconazole and should be switched to lovastatin.
C. Simvastatin is contraindicated with the use of voriconazole and should be switched to atorvastatin.
D. Allopurinol, hydrochlorothiazide, and voriconazole should not be used together.

17. After 7 days of voriconazole therapy (200 mg orally twice daily), T.Z.'s trough concentration is 0.8 mcg/mL. Which one of the following is best to recommend for T.Z.?

A. Voriconazole 300 mg orally twice daily.
B. Voriconazole 350 mg orally twice daily.
C. Voriconazole 400 mg orally twice daily.
D. Change to posaconazole oral suspension 200 mg orally twice daily.

Questions 18 and 19 pertain to the following case.

M.R. is a 29-year-old woman who recently received a diagnosis of metastatic breast cancer. She comes to the emergency department and after having blood cultures is started on empiric imipenem/cilastatin. M.R.'s vital signs are: temperature 102.7°F; heart rate 121 beats/minute; blood pressure 78/42 mm Hg, and respiratory rate 30 breaths/minute. Chest radiography reveals pulmonary infiltrates.

18. Which one of the following is best to recommend for M.R.?

A. Change imipenem/cilastatin to linezolid.
B. Change imipenem/cilastatin to cefepime.
C. Add vancomycin.
D. Add daptomycin.

19. On day 3 of M.R.'s therapy, the Gram stain performed on the blood cultures shows growth of gram-negative rods. M.R's temperature is 98.8°F. Which one of the following is best to recommend for M.R.?

A. Discontinue vancomycin.
B. Discontinue daptomycin.
C. Change to ertapenem.
D. Change to levofloxacin.

20. A patient comes to clinic today and laboratory tests reveal a WBC of 0.5 x 10^3 cells/mm^3 and neutrophils 15%. Which one of the following chemotherapy agents would be best to avoid in this patient?

A. Capecitabine.
B. Erlotinib.
C. Paclitaxel.
D. Sorafenib.

LEARNER CHAPTER EVALUATION: INFECTIONS IN PATIENTS WITH MALIGNANCIES.

As you take the posttest for this chapter, also evaluate the material's quality and usefulness, as well as the achievement of learning objectives. Rate each item using this 5-point scale:

- Strongly agree
- Agree
- Neutral
- Disagree
- Strongly disagree

1. The content of the chapter met my educational needs.
2. The content of the chapter satisfied my expectations.
3. The author presented the chapter content effectively.
4. The content of the chapter was relevant to my practice and presented at the appropriate depth and scope.
5. The content of the chapter was objective and balanced.
6. The content of the chapter is free of bias, promotion, or advertisement of commercial products.
7. The content of the chapter was useful to me.
8. The teaching and learning methods used in the chapter were effective.
9. The active learning methods used in the chapter were effective.
10. The learning assessment activities used in the chapter were effective.
11. The chapter was effective overall.

Use the 5-point scale to indicate whether this chapter prepared you to accomplish the following learning objectives:

12. Demonstrate an understanding of the risk factors and causes of bacterial, viral, and fungal infections in those with hematologic or solid-tumor malignancies.
13. Distinguish between patients at high risk, moderate risk, and low risk for febrile neutropenia.
14. Develop an infectious diseases pharmacotherapeutic plan for treatment and prophylaxis of antibacterial, antifungal, and antiviral infections in a patient with malignancy (solid and hematologic).
15. Assess the safety profiles of anti-infective drugs used to manage and prevent antibacterial, antifungal, and antiviral infections.
16. Evaluate drug therapy for the presence of drug-drug interactions in those receiving treatment or prophylaxis for febrile neutropenia.
17. Evaluate the role of hematopoietic growth factors in the prevention of febrile neutropenia.
18. Please provide any specific comments relating to any perceptions of bias, promotion, or advertisement of commercial products.
19. Please expand on any of your above responses, and/or provide any additional comments regarding this chapter:

Advances in Hepatitis C Therapy

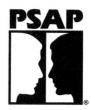

By Michelle T. Martin, Pharm.D., BCPS, BCACP;
and Ian R. McNicholl, Pharm.D., FCCP, BCPS (AQ–ID), AAHIVP

Reviewed by Paulina Deming, Pharm.D.; Carolyn Orendorff, Pharm.D., BCPS; and Quynh-Chi Duong, Pharm.D., BCPS

Learning Objectives

1. Analyze recent trends in hepatitis C virus (HCV) transmission, diagnosis, and management.
2. Evaluate patient characteristics for appropriate timing of HCV treatment.
3. Devise a genotype-based treatment plan for treatment-naive HCV patients.
4. Construct a management strategy for treatment-experienced patients with HCV.
5. Design a plan to optimize HCV treatment outcomes in patients who are cirrhotic, post-transplant, or HIV coinfected.
6. Develop a monitoring plan for drug interactions and adverse events associated with HCV treatment.
7. Assess patients for clinical outcomes and HCV treatment response.

Introduction

Hepatitis C virus (HCV) is the most common blood-borne infection in the United States (Armstrong 2006). More Americans are infected with and die from HCV than from human immunodeficiency virus (HIV) (Ly 2012). Chronic HCV infection is (1) the primary reason for liver transplant and (2) the leading cause of end-stage liver disease, liver-related death, and hepatocellular carcinoma (HCC) in the United States (Alter 2007; Kim 2002). Groundbreaking changes in HCV treatment have occurred in the past 4 years with the approval of several novel direct-acting antiviral (DAA) agents with improved sustained virologic response (SVR) rates and shorter treatment durations compared with treatment with pegylated interferon and ribavirin.

Unlike other viral diseases, HCV is curable. Currently available HCV treatments have success rates in the 90% range—depending on the patient's HCV genotype (GT), progression of disease, and previous treatment experience (AASLD 2014). Patients whose therapy previously failed or who are ineligible for treatment with pegylated interferon now have an improved chance to achieve SVR. However, continued obstacles accompany these new agents.

Before initiating HCV treatment, providers must consider drug-drug interactions (DDIs), adverse effect profiles, concomitant diagnoses, the patient's ability to adhere to treatment regimens, necessary lab monitoring, and lifestyle changes. Adherence is imperative for successful response to HCV treatment. Medication access is vital, but the extremely high cost of the new DAAs could have a crippling effect on the health care system. Several more

---

Baseline Knowledge Statements

Readers of this chapter are presumed to be familiar with the following:

- Basic virology and replication of HCV
- Currently available direct-acting antivirals and other agents used for HCV treatment, including dosing, adverse events, drug reactions, monitoring parameters, and regimens
- Futility rules of response-guided therapy for the treatment of genotype 1
- Complications of cirrhosis

Additional Readings

The following free resource is available for readers wishing additional background information on this topic.

- American Association for the Study of Liver Diseases, Infectious Diseases Society of America, and International Antiviral Society–USA. Recommendations for testing, managing, and treating hepatitis C.

antiviral agents are in various stages of clinical trials, and HCV treatment will continue to evolve rapidly in the next few years.

Epidemiology

The World Health Organization estimates that 150 million people are infected with HCV worldwide and that 350,000 people die from HCV-related causes annually (WHO 2014). The Centers for Disease Control and Prevention (CDC) estimates that HCV affects about 4 million Americans, or 1.3%–1.9% of the population (Armstrong 2006; CDC 2014). These epidemiological data are based on the National Health and Nutrition Examination Survey (NHANES), which does not include homeless, incarcerated, active military, or institutionalized patients. At 3.2 million, the NHANES estimate is conservative; an expanded prevalence model estimates HCV prevalence at 5.2 million. Unfortunately, only 50% of patients are diagnosed and aware of their HCV infection, and only 17% have been prescribed HCV treatment (Yehia 2014). Hepatitis C infection is estimated to cause about 17,000 deaths annually in the United States (CDC 2014). The number of new cases of HCV reported annually decreased from 291,000 in 1989 to 16,500 in 2011 (CDC 2011a).

Although the incidence of HCV declined in the 2000s, there has been a recent increase in cases among young patients in nonurban settings, which is thought to be a result of increased heroin use among that population (CDC 2011b). Injection drug use is the most common mode of HCV transmission in the United States (Armstrong 2006). Worldwide, the use of unsafe injection practices accounts for up to 40% of cases of HCV in other countries (WHO 2014). Box 2-1 lists risk factors and modes of HCV transmission.

Patients infected with HCV who were born from 1945 to 1965 were most likely exposed to HCV from injection drug use and tainted blood transfusions; recent screening initiatives have been directed at that population (Armstrong 2006). The American Association for the Study of Liver Diseases (AASLD), the CDC, the Centers for Medicare & Medicaid Services, and the U.S. Preventive Services Task Force endorse a one-time screening of patients born from 1945 to 1965 regardless of risk factors, as well as screening of all patients with risk factors (Moyer 2013; CDC 2012).

Hepatitis C virus is a single-stranded, enveloped RNA virus from the Flaviviridae family of the *Hepacivirus* genus. Before the discovery of HCV in 1989, it had been identified as non-A, non-B hepatitis (Houghton 2009). The virus lacks a proofreading polymerase, which allows mutations to occur during viral replication, and evasion of the immune system. No vaccine is currently available for HCV, but researchers are investigating several approaches (Swadling 2013). No pre- or postexposure prophylaxis is available for HCV.

Although the six major GTs of HCV have treatment recommendations, researchers have isolated additional GTs and at least 67 different subtypes (e.g., GT 1a, 1b, 2a, 2b, 2c, 3a) (Smith 2014). Genotype prevalence differs by geographic location. Genotype 1 is the most common form in the United States, accounting for about 75% of infections nationally, with GT 1a more prevalent than GT 1b. Genotypes 2 and 3 constitute about 20% of HCV infections in the United States (CDC 2011a). Genotypes 1–3 are the most common found in Europe. Genotype 4 is found predominantly in the Middle East, GT 5 in South Africa, and GT 6 in Asia (Nakano 2012).

Pathophysiology
Acute HCV Infection

After acute HCV infection, the virus is transferred by way of the blood to the liver, where it binds to host receptors on hepatocytes and enters the cell by means of receptor-mediated endocytosis. The fusion of the viral

---

Box 2-1. Risk Factors for Hepatitis C Virus Transmission

- Intravenous drug use
- Illicit intranasal drug use
- Human immunodeficiency virus or hepatitis B virus
- Blood transfusions or solid organ transplants (before July 1992)
- Clotting factors (before 1987)
- Hemodialysis
- Occupational exposure
- Receiving injections with used/contaminated needles
- Tattoos, acupuncture, or body piercing with unsterilized instruments
- Perinatal transmission (children born to mother with hepatitis C virus)
- Sexual transmission (multiple sex partners, men who have sex with men, or history of sexually transmitted disease)
- Patients born between 1945 – 1965

Information from: Ghany MG, Strader DB, Thomas DL, et al. American Association for the Study of Liver Diseases. Diagnosis, management, and treatment of hepatitis C: an update. Hepatology 2009;49:1335-74.

envelope and the cell membrane allows the uncoating and release of viral RNA into the cell. Next, the RNA gets translated into a large polyprotein, which in turn is cleaved into smaller, functional proteins by the HCV protease complex NS3/4A. The RNA is replicated, and the new virus is assembled. Upon release from the cell, the virus spreads to other hepatocytes for further replication (Cisek 2011; Schlutter 2011; Hoofnagle 2002). In an infected liver, up to 1 trillion virions are produced every day. Although HCV can be found in nonliver cells, it replicates in hepatocytes. The virus activates an immune response, and inflammatory mediators lead to varying degrees of hepatic fibrosis over time.

Acute HCV may present with mild to severe—albeit vague—symptoms such as fatigue, nausea, vomiting, and diarrhea (Box 2-2). If symptoms occur, they usually present within the average incubation period of 6–7 weeks after HCV exposure, but they can appear any time from 2–26 weeks after exposure. Up to 80% of patients have no symptoms after contracting the virus (WHO 2002).

About 15%–25% of patients who are exposed to HCV spontaneously clear the virus and eliminate the infection. The remaining 75%–85% of patients develop chronic HCV, defined as HCV viral RNA detectable for more than 6 months (Ghany 2009; WHO 2002).

Chronic HCV Infection

Often, patients transition from acute to chronic HCV infection, unaware of their infection (WHO 2002). The HCV causes inflammation with progression of hepatic fibrosis, and the hepatocytes lose their ability to function. Chronic HCV infection can take decades to transform a healthy liver to a cirrhotic liver. Roughly 20% of patients with chronic HCV develop cirrhosis; subsequently, portal hypertension can develop and result in esophageal varices. Other sequelae of advanced liver disease include ascites and encephalopathy. On physical examination, patients may have jaundice, palmar erythema, and spider angioma (WHO 2002). Patients with chronic HCV and cirrhosis are at risk of the development of hepatocellular carcinoma, which occurs at a rate of about 1%–4% per year in this population (McHutchison 2005). Figure 2-1 illustrates the progression of HCV. In addition, steatosis has been linked with progression to cirrhosis among patients infected with GT 3 (Rubbia-Brandt 2004).

CLINICAL EVALUATION AND DIAGNOSIS

The HCV antibody blood test is the initial screening test for HCV. If the patient has a positive HCV antibody, a blood test for HCV RNA quantitative viral load should be drawn to determine whether the patient has replicating virus or current chronic infection. Patients with chronic infections have detectable virus levels. All patients who have been exposed to HCV have positive HCV antibodies (detectable 4–10 weeks after exposure) regardless of whether they have a chronic infection. Patients who were exposed to HCV but only had an acute infection and cleared the virus have positive HCV antibodies and undetectable HCV RNA quantitative levels. Patients who were treated successfully for HCV and cleared the virus also have undetectable HCV RNA quantitative virus levels. Table 2-1 describes the interpretation of these tests.

Unlike antibodies for hepatitis A and B, the HCV antibody does not protect against future HCV infection. Because no protective IgG antibodies develop in patients who have cleared HCV either spontaneously or by means of treatment, patients are at continued risk of HCV reinfection if reexposure occurs (Ghany 2009). Patients with chronic infection should undergo an additional blood test to determine their HCV GT, which is used for selecting proper treatment. The viral load should be measured at 12 weeks after completion of therapy to determine SVR. A patient with an undetectable HCV viral load at 12 weeks after treatment completion is considered cured. Treatment with pegylated interferon and ribavirin historically used SVR24 to assess cure. Concordance between SVR12 and SVR24 in regimens including DAAs has increased; SVR12 has become the trend for assessment of cure with new DAAs (Chen 2013).

Genetic Testing

Historically, testing for the IL28B genotype was occasionally used to help predict responsiveness to HCV treatment with pegylated interferon and ribavirin: patients with the CC genotype responded most favorably; those with the CT and TT genotypes responded less favorably. The use of DAA agents in addition to or in lieu of pegylated interferon and ribavirin greatly improves the SVR rates for patients with HCV GT 1 regardless of IL28B genotype. Hence, there is no clinical need for IL28B testing, and it is no longer routinely done in practice (Ghany 2011).

Before initiation of the HCV treatment regimen with simeprevir, pegylated interferon, and ribavirin for GT 1a infections, a Q80K mutation lab panel (costing more than $700) is recommended. If the patient has the Q80K polymorphism, treatment with an alternative HCV regimen is recommended because the simeprevir-based regimen

---

Box 2-2. Symptoms of Acute Hepatitis C Virus

- Fatigue
- Abdominal Pain
- Loss of Appetite / Nausea / Vomiting
- Diarrhea
- Fever
- Myalgia / Arthralgia
- Jaundice
- Dark urine / Clay-colored stool

Information from: World Health Organization. Hepatitis C Global Alert and Response, 2002.

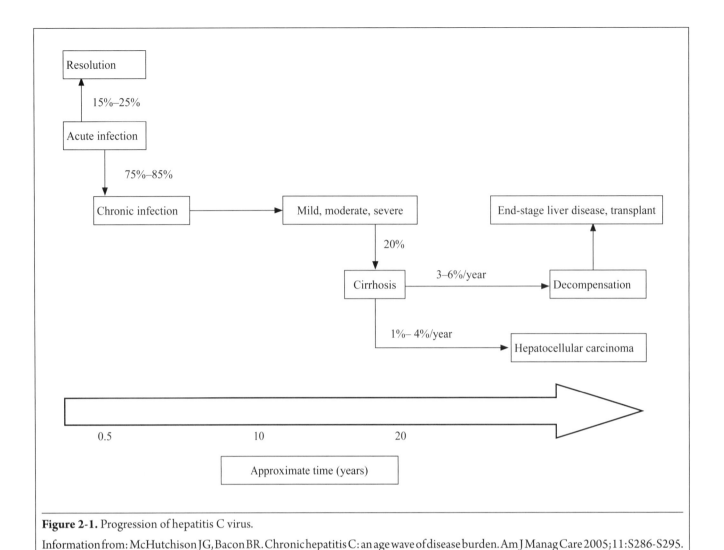

Figure 2-1. Progression of hepatitis C virus.

Information from: McHutchison JG, Bacon BR. Chronic hepatitis C: an age wave of disease burden. Am J Manag Care 2005;11:S286-S295.

did not improve SVR rates significantly over treatment with pegylated interferon and ribavirin in the QUEST and PROMISE clinical trials (Jacobson 2013a; Lawitz 2013a; Manns 2013). Because the simeprevir, pegylated interferon, and ribavirin regimen is not first line for GT 1a patients, most providers initiate more effective HCV treatment with sofosbuvir-based regimens, which eliminates the need for a costly lab test. The Q80K polymorphism does not affect treatment outcomes with sofosbuvir and simeprevir treatment and does not need to be ordered before initiating this combination.

Procedures and Noninvasive Measures of Disease Progression
Liver Biopsy

Liver biopsy has been considered the gold standard for evaluating both degree of inflammation (grade) and extent of scarring or fibrosis (stage) to evaluate the severity of a patient's liver disease (Ghany 2009). Severity of liver disease is often categorized according to a METAVIR fibrosis score of F0 (no scarring) to F4 (cirrhosis), and an activity,

or inflammation, score of A0 (no activity) to A3 (severe activity). With an increasing rate of SVR with HCV treatment with DAAs for GT 1, consensus on the utility of liver biopsy is in flux—and provider specific. Because of the invasive nature of a biopsy and the associated risks with the procedure, some patients or providers may opt for noninvasive tests.

Transient Elastography and Serum Biomarkers

Transient elastography is an ultrasound-based technology that estimates the degree of liver stiffness, which is used as a marker of fibrosis. This painless procedure takes about 5 minutes and can be performed easily either at bedside or in a clinic setting. However, narrow intercostal space, obesity, and ascites pose challenges or can inhibit accurate results. A liver stiffness measurement of more than 12.5 kPa indicates cirrhosis, whereas scores of 2.5–7 kPa indicate mild or absent fibrosis (Castera 2008).

The degree of fibrosis and inflammation can also be estimated by liver biomarker blood tests that measure components of the extracellular hepatic matrix (Poynard

2012). Such tests use the METAVIR score to indicate the degree of scarring and inflammation in the liver. Other surrogate measures that can indicate the presence of cirrhosis include platelet levels below 150,000/mcL, INR greater than 1 in the absence of anticoagulation, and albumin less than 3.5 mg/dL.

The FIB-4 index uses the equation [(age x AST) ÷ (platelets x ALT)] to assess likelihood of fibrosis level. The AST-to-platelet ratio index (APRI) can estimate presence of cirrhosis: APRI values of 0.4 or less do not indicate significant fibrosis and cirrhosis, whereas a value of 1.5 or more indicates significant fibrosis (Snyder 2006). Providers may opt to use noninvasive markers of cirrhosis such as these in both complicated and uncomplicated patients in the era of highly successful HCV treatment.

Imaging

Patients with cirrhosis must undergo imaging of the liver every 6 months to screen for HCC (AASLD 2014). Abdominal ultrasonography is used to screen for lesions; it can also identify splenomegaly, ascites, and other abnormalities. If lesions are detected on ultrasonography, computed tomography scans or magnetic resonance imaging is used for more precise evaluation. Early detection and treatment of HCC yield better response rates (Ghany 2009; WHO 2002). Ultrasonography and alpha fetoprotein testing every 6 months has resulted in a 90.2% sensitivity of HCC detection and a 63.4% sensitivity of early stage HCC compared with 43.9% and 31.7%, respectively, with ultrasonography alone (Singal 2012). Therefore, some providers use this combination for HCC surveillance.

Endoscopy

Endoscopy is used for screening for esophageal varices, a clinical sequela of portal hypertension. Variceal banding can decrease the risk of rupture, as can pharmacologic therapy with nonselective β-blockers that are used for decreasing portal pressure and lowering the risk of bleeding (Garcia-Tsao 2007).

TREATMENT

The ultimate goal of HCV treatment is eradication of the HCV infection to prevent complications and death from liver disease. Successful treatment with SVR can halt the progression of liver fibrosis and prevent cirrhosis, end-stage liver disease, HCC, and the need for liver transplantation (AASLD 2014). Treatment for HCV infection has also been shown to reverse fibrosis (LaBarca 2014). Even patients with late-stage fibrosis had decreased all-cause mortality rates after SVR (van der Meer 2012). The right timing for HCV treatment depends on a thorough assessment of social and medical factors, including patient readiness, comorbidities, concomitant medications, and insurance coverage in order to individualize treatment, ensure patient safety, and increase favorable outcomes.

Two DAA agents were approved by the U.S. Food and Drug Administration (FDA) in 2013, and a combination agent was approved in October 2014 for HCV treatment; all offer superior SVR rates compared with previous regimens. Other, potentially all-oral treatment options for GT 1 currently in phase 3 trials include combinations of sofosbuvir and daclatasvir; daclatasvir, asunaprevir, and beclabuvir (BMS-791325); and paritaprevir/ritonavir, ombitasvir, and dasabuvir; with or without ribavirin. Shorter treatment length for GT 3 is also probable during the next year.

In January 2014 the AASLD, the International Antiviral Society, and the Infectious Diseases Society of America published their joint guidelines for HCV management; these guidelines are updated periodically with new developments in HCV management. Pharmacologic treatment regimens and treatment duration differ based on HCV GT. Figure 2-2 presents a treatment algorithm based on GT as recommended by the joint guidelines; updates are expected in December 2014—after the printing of this chapter.

Both simeprevir and sofosbuvir are effective in GT 1 and 4, but only sofosbuvir is effective in treating GT 2, 3, 5, and 6. The fixed-dose combination of ledipasvir and sofosbuvir is FDA approved for GT 1 but was also approved by the European Union for use in GT 3 and 4. Current guidelines

Table 2-1. Interpretation of HCV Blood Tests

		HCV RNA Quantitative	
		Detectable	**Not Detected**
HCV Antibody	Positive	Acute or chronic HCV infection	Resolved HCV infection (spontaneous resolution or successful treatment)
	Negative	Early acute infection or chronic HCV infection in an immunocompromised patient	No HCV infection

HCV = hepatitis C virus.

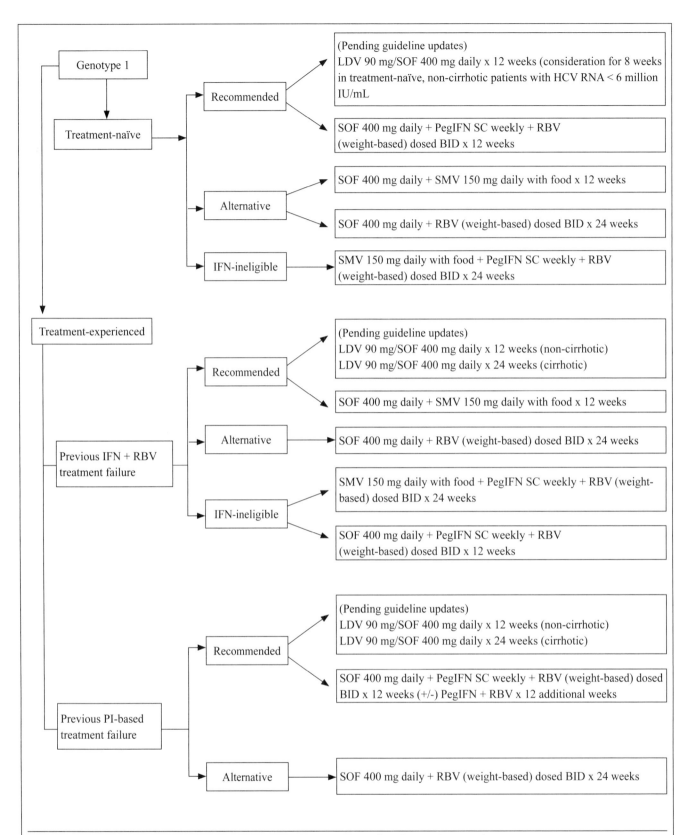

Figure 2-2a. Treatment algorithm based on hepatitis C virus genotype 1 (as of December 2014).

BID = twice daily; IU = international units; LDV = ledipasvir; PegIFN = pegylated interferon; RBV = ribavirin; SC = subcutaneously; SMV = simeprevir; SOF = sofosbuvir.

Information from: American Association for the Study of Liver Diseases, Infectious Diseases Society of America, and International Antiviral Society-USA. Recommendations for testing, managing, and treating hepatitis C, 2014 [homepage on the Internet].

recommend use of sofosbuvir or simeprevir over the older protease inhibitors (PIs), boceprevir, and telaprevir (AASLD 2014). Table 2-2 describes the agents used for HCV treatment. Regimen components, pill burden, and duration of therapy vary based on patient comorbidities, level of fibrosis, and HCV treatment history.

Hepatitis C virus treatment is usually not an urgent recommendation, except in peritransplantation patients. Deferring HCV treatment may be an option in patients with minimal or no fibrosis and no evidence of significant extrahepatic disease. However, it is difficult to predict which patients will progress in their liver disease and at what rate. As of press time, the guidelines recommend the immediate treatment of patients with advanced fibrosis (METAVIR F3) or compensated cirrhosis (METAVIR F4), liver transplant recipients, and patients with severe extrahepatic manifestations of HCV such as cryoglobulinemia and glomerulonephritis. High priority is recommended for patients with HIV coinfection; hepatitis B virus; other liver disease, including nonalcoholic steatohepatitis; and other conditions.

Previously, treatment duration and medication toxicities were considerations in the timing of HCV treatment. But because new treatment has shorter duration and less toxicity, increasing numbers of patients may elect to undergo treatment. Other patients may elect to wait for future treatment options that have near 100% SVR rates, short durations, minimal adverse drug reactions, and possibly lower costs. Waiting until an all-oral treatment is the standard of care will prevent unnecessary exposure to the known adverse effects associated with pegylated interferon.

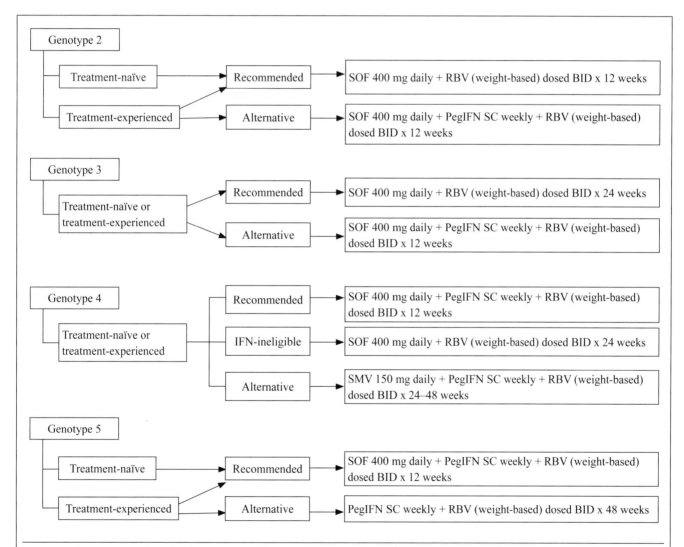

Figure 2-2b. Treatment algorithm based on hepatitis C virus genotypes 2–6 (as of December 2014).

BID = twice daily; PegIFN = pegylated interferon; RBV = ribavirin;
SC = subcutaneously; SMV = simeprevir; SOF = sofosbuvir.
Information from: American Association for the Study of Liver Diseases, Infectious Diseases Society of America, and International Antiviral Society-USA. Recommendations for testing, managing, and treating hepatitis C, 2014 [homepage on the Internet].

Table 2-2. Currently Approved HCV Medications

Medication	PegIFN alfa-2a	PegIFN alfa-2b	Ribavirin	Sofosbuvir	Ledipasvir / Sofosbuvir	Simeprevir
Mechanism of Action	Immunomodulation Inhibition of viral replication and cell proliferation		Antiviral Synthetic nucleoside analog; exact mechanism unknown Causes improvement in ETR; decrease in relapse rate when used with PegIFN	Direct-acting antiviral; NS5B polymerase inhibitor	Direct-acting antiviral fixed dose combination; NS5A replication complex inhibitor + NS5B polymerase inhibitor	Direct-acting antiviral; NS3/4A protease inhibitor
Dose and Dosage Forms	180 mcg SC weekly (adjusted for renal impairment) Available in prefilled 180 mcg/0.5 mL syringe, or 180 mcg/1 mL vial	1.5 mcg/kg weekly SC (adjusted for renal impairment). Available in prefilled pen: 50, 80, 120, or 150 mcg	Doses split twice daily (adjusted by weight and for renal impairment) Based on genotype and PegIFN used: ≤75 kg: 1000 mg/day; >75 kg: 1200 mg/day Available in 200-mg tablets or capsules	400 mg by mouth daily	90 mg/400 mg by mouth daily	150 mg by mouth daily with food
Coadministration	Historically used as monotherapy in patients who could not tolerate RBV Current use with RBV is limited to GT 5, 6. Used with SOF + RBV in GT 1 – 6, or used with SMV + RBV in GT 1, 4.		Must be taken with PegIFN or SOF, or SOF + SMV. Not effective as monotherapy.	To be taken with PegIFN and RBV for use in GT 1, 4, 5, 6 May be taken with RBV for use in GT 1, 4 Must be taken with RBV for use in GT 2 – 3 Can be taken with SMV +/- RBV in GT 1 Also used in fixed dose combination with LDV for GT 1	None (or with RBV off label as of 12/ 10/2014)	Only approved for use in GT 1 Must be taken with PegIFN and RBV, or with SOF +/- RBV
Common Adverse Drug Reactions	Flu-like symptoms: headaches, myalgias, arthralgia, fevers, chills, fatigue Psychiatric (depression, irritability, emotional lability) Injection site reactions Neutropenia Alopecia Thrombocytopenia Insomnia Endocrine/metabolic: diabetes, hyperlipidemia, thyroid abnormalities Nausea/anorexia		Hemolytic anemia: fatigue, dyspnea, chest pain Nausea/vomiting/diarrhea/ constipation Anorexia Rash/dry skin Cough	Headache	Headache Fatigue	Rash Photosensitivity

Table 2-2. Currently Approved HCV Medications (*continued*)

Medication	PegIFN alfa-2a	PegIFN alfa-2b	Ribavirin	Sofosbuvir	Ledipasvir / Sofosbuvir	Simeprevir
Cautions	Psychiatric conditions, thyroid conditions, endocrine disorders must be well-controlled and monitored during the course of treatment		Pregnancy category X (teratogenic). Patients must use 2 forms of contraception during treatment and for 6 months after discontinuation	No recommendations for use in patients with CrCl <30mL/min (trial in progress at the time of editing)	No recommendations for use in patients with CrCl <30 mL/min as of 12/10/2014	Do not miss doses; resistance may occur No recommendations for use in patients with CrCl <30 mL/min as of 12/10/2014 Not labeled for use in Child Pugh Class B or C
24-hour- Phone Patient Assistance	Genentech: pegylated interferon alfa-2a Pegassist 1-888-941-3331	Merck: pegylated interferon alfa-2b 1-866-939-HEPC (4372)	Contact Genentech or Merck	1-855-7-MYPATH (69-7284)	1-855-7-MYPATH (69-7284)	1-855-5-OLYSIO (65-9746)
Financial Assistance	Genentech: pegylated interferon alfa-2a Access Solutions	Merck: pegylated interferon alfa-2b ACT Program	Genentech: will provide ribavirin with pegylated interferon alfa-2a Access Solutions	Gilead Sciences	Gilead Sciences	Jannsen
FDA approval date	10/17/2002	1/2001	12/3/2002	12/6/2013	10/10/2014	11/22/2013

DCV = daclatasvir; ETR = end-of-treatment response; FDA = food and drug administration; GT = genotype; HCV = hepatitis c virus; PegIFN = pegylated interferon; RBV = ribavirin; SC = subcutaneously; SMV = simeprevir; SOF = sofosbuvir; VL = viral load

Pegylated Interferon and Ribavirin

Pegylated interferon alfa-2a or alfa-2b and ribavirin are FDA approved to treat HCV GTs 1–6. Before 2011, the combination of those two agents was the standard of care for HCV treatment. With the advent of DAA agents, the use of pegylated interferon has declined sharply, and several regimens have eliminated the need for ribavirin as well. Pegylated interferon is self-administered by the patient by way of a once-weekly subcutaneous injection and must be dose adjusted for renal function. Pegylated interferon is associated with significant laboratory abnormalities and a substantial adverse-effect profile, which limit its use. Patients with uncontrolled depression, decompensated liver disease, autoimmune disease, cardiac disease, absolute neutrophil counts less than 1500/mm^3, platelets less than 90,000/mm^3, or hemoglobins less than 10 g/dL are considered interferon ineligible. Flu-like symptoms, mood changes (and the potential for suicidal or homicidal ideation), and cytopenias are among the many adverse drug reactions that patients may experience while on pegylated interferon; patients typically feel sicker during HCV treatment with pegylated interferon than when they were not treating the disease.

Ribavirin is an antiviral that works in conjunction with pegylated interferon or other DAAs and must not be used as monotherapy for HCV treatment. It is dosed orally twice daily based on a patient's weight and renal function. Ribavirin causes anemia and can cause a rash. It is also teratogenic; pregnancy should be avoided, and effective contraception must be practiced during treatment and for 6 months after the last ribavirin dose regardless of the patient's sex.

NS3/4A Protease Inhibitors

The PIs prevent the virus from cleaving the replicated polyprotein into smaller proteins and thus, by inhibiting the NS3/4A complex, interfere with the virus's ability to replicate (Schlutter 2011). Protease inhibitors induce rapid resistance if used alone; thus, they are used in combination with pegylated interferon and ribavirin or with other DAA agents. To avoid the development of resistance to PIs, patients must be counseled on the importance of adherence.

Telaprevir and Boceprevir

In 2011, the PIs boceprevir and telaprevir were the first two DAA agents approved for HCV treatment in combination with pegylated interferon and ribavirin as triple therapy for GT 1. If a patient failed to meet the futility rules for boceprevir or telaprevir treatment, or if the patient experienced viral breakthrough while on treatment, the HCV treatment was to be discontinued. Because of complicated futility rules, dosing every 8 hours, pill burden, less-than-optimal efficacy, drug-drug interactions, and a high incidence of adverse drug events, current guidelines do not recommend use of the first-wave PIs (AASLD

2014). In addition, the manufacturer discontinued telaprevir in August 2014. Therefore, this chapter focuses on simeprevir and other recently approved or pipeline PIs.

Simeprevir

The second-wave NS3/4A PI, simeprevir, was approved in November 2013; its advantages over first-wave PIs include once-daily dosing, decreased pill burden, less-specific food coadministration requirements, and fewer DDIs. Simeprevir is used in combination with pegylated interferon and ribavirin for GT 1 and 4 patients and with sofosbuvir for GT 1 patients. Incremental adverse effects incurred by the addition of simeprevir to treatment with pegylated interferon and ribavirin include rash, photosensitivity, pruritus, and nausea. Although simeprevir contains a sulfa moiety, there is insufficient evidence to indicate higher incidence of rash in sulfa-allergic patients; providers have used simeprevir without problems in sulfa-allergic patients.

Protease inhibitors also have the potential for significant DDIs because of their inhibition of cytochrome P450 (CYP450) 3A4. Table 2-3 lists the pharmacokinetics of select HCV agents. Although simeprevir causes far fewer DDIs than the first-wave PIs do, concerns about clinically significant DDIs remain. The package insert lists contraindicated drug classes. To avoid potentially dangerous interactions, patients must be counseled on the importance of disclosing of all of their medications and supplements to their health care providers.

Paritaprevir

Paritaprevir, a PI that is ritonavir boosted and coformulated with ombitasvir, was studied in combination with dasabuvir as part of AbbVie's HCV regimen, as discussed later in the chapter. As of press time, the manufacturer was awaiting FDA approval.

NS5B Polymerase Inhibitors
Sofosbuvir

Sofosbuvir, a first-in-class NS5B nucleotide polymerase inhibitor, was FDA approved in December 2013. It was the first HCV agent to allow for the all-oral treatment of HCV GT 2 and 3. Sofosbuvir is also recommended in combination with simeprevir in GT 1 patients who are interferon ineligible or post-transplant. A few thousand patients were treated in six phase 3 trials with the combinations of sofosbuvir and ribavirin with or without pegylated interferon, and in the phase 2 COSMOS trial with the combination of sofosbuvir and simeprevir. Because sofosbuvir is not dependent on CYP450, DDIs are generally limited and involve agents that induce p-glycoprotein, because it is a p-glycoprotein substrate. These agents include carbamazepine, phenytoin, phenobarbital, oxcarbazine, rifamycins, and St. John's wort; all can potentially decrease sofosbuvir concentrations. The package insert gives more details and a listing of contraindicated drugs and drug classes.

Patients with GT 2 and 3 who were intolerant of, ineligible for, or unwilling to take pegylated interferon were evaluated in the randomized, double-blind, placebo-controlled 12-week POSITRON trial. This study found that the SVR12 rate for GT 2 cirrhotic patients was considerably higher (94%) than for GT 3 cirrhotic patients (21%) (Jacobson 2013b). In the FUSION trial, which enrolled patients treated previously with pegylated interferon and ribavirin (nearly 30% of patients with cirrhosis), the SVR12 rate for GT 3 was 30% after 12 weeks of treatment versus 62% after 16 weeks of treatment (Jacobson 2013b). In FISSION, SVR12 rates for GT 2 patients were improved with sofosbuvir and ribavirin after 12 weeks: 97% compared with 78% with pegylated interferon and ribavirin after 24 weeks. Genotype 3 patients had similar SVR12 rates (56% for sofosbuvir and ribavirin, 63% for pegylated interferon and ribavirin) (Lawitz 2013b). Those three GT 2 and 3 trials demonstrated that GT 3 patients did not respond as well as GT 2 patients to 12-week treatment with sofosbuvir and ribavirin. That result prompted modifications in the VALENCE trial to extend treatment length to 24 weeks for GT 3 patients in order to achieve GT 3 SVR rates that would be closer to GT 2 rates. The sofosbuvir study findings that GT 3 patients did not respond as well as GT 2 patients did were unexpected because those two GTs had previously been viewed as similar in their responses to pegylated interferon and ribavirin. Moving forward, it is expected that those two GTs will be assessed differently in clinical trials.

Treatment-naive patients with GT 1, 4, 5, and 6 experienced a 90% SVR rate when sofosbuvir was combined with pegylated interferon and ribavirin for 12 weeks, compared with a historical control of 60% (p<0.001) in NEUTRINO (Lawitz 2013b). The study comprised 292 GT 1 patients and 35 non–GT 1 patients (28 with GT 4, 1 with GT 5, and 6 with GT 6). Although this regimen still included pegylated interferon and ribavirin, patients with all four GTs had significantly higher SVRs compared with pegylated interferon and ribavirin treatment without a DAA, as well as shorter treatment durations.

Discontinuation rates caused by adverse events were low in GT 2 and 3 sofosbuvir- and ribavirin-based treatment regimens; some of the placebo arms had higher discontinuation rates than did treatment arms (2% in the sofosbuvir and ribavirin arm, 4% in the placebo arm) (Jacobson 2013b). Discontinuation rates caused by adverse events were 1% in the sofosbuvir and ribavirin 12-week arm; 2% in the sofosbuvir, pegylated interferon, and ribavirin 12-week arm; and 11% in the pegylated interferon and ribavirin 24-week arm in GT 1 patients (Lawitz 2013b). Common adverse events in patients treated with sofosbuvir, pegylated interferon, and ribavirin included fatigue, headache, nausea, insomnia, and anemia. Notably, no resistance-associated mutations were found in any of the phase 3 sofosbuvir trials.

Dasabuvir

Dasabuvir is the NS5B nonnucleoside polymerase inhibitor that was studied in combination with paritaprevir/ritonavir and ombitasvir as part of AbbVie's HCV regimen, discussed later in the chapter. The manufacturer expects FDA approval in late December 2014.

NS5A Replication Complex Inhibitors

The NS5A inhibitors work by preventing new replication complexes, which are sites of RNA synthesis for HCV. These agents constitute a new DAA class for HCV

Table 2-3. Pharmacology of Select HCV Direct Acting Antivirals

Drug	Class	t1/2	Metabolism	Elimination
Simeprevir	NS3/4A protease inhibitor	10–13 hours (healthy volunteers); 41 hours (HCV-infected patients)	Substrate of CYP3A4; Mild inhibitor of CYP3A4; Substrate of P-gp; Inhibitor of P-gp; Substrate of OATP1B1/3; Inhibitor of OATP1B1/3	Biliary excretion
Sofosbuvir	NS5B polymerase inhibitor	0.4 hours for sofosbuvir; 27 hours for active metabolite	Non-CYP450, non-UGT mediated metabolism	Urine (80%)
Ledipasvir	NS5A replication complex inhibitor	47 hours	Slow oxidative metabolism by an unknown mechanism	Biliary excretion

CYP = cytochrome P450; HCV = hepatitis C virus; NS3/4A = nonstructural protein 3/4A; NS5B = nonstructural protein 5B; P-gp = P-glycoprotein; OATP1B1/3 = organic anion transporting polypeptide 1B1; UGT = uridine diphosphate glucuronyltransferase.

Information from manufacturer's package inserts.

treatment and were approved in late 2014. Overall class benefits include fewer adverse events and DDIs when compared with PIs. Resistance is a concern with this class of drugs; the agents must be coadministered with other DAAs. Some studies have indicated improved SVR rates when these inhibitors are used in combination with a PI and an NS5B polymerase inhibitor rather than just one additional DAA. Pipeline second-generation NS5A inhibitors have demonstrated improved resistance panels compared with first-generation NS5As.

Ledipasvir

Ledipasvir is a first-in-class NS5A inhibitor with once-daily dosing that has potent antiviral activity against GT 1a and 1b. Three phase 3 ION trials evaluated a fixed-dose combination of ledipasvir 90 mg/sofosbuvir 400 mg with or without ribavirin for 8, 12, or 24 weeks in 1952 GT 1 treatment-naive and prior nonresponders, including 224 cirrhotic patients. Those trials were modeled after the phase 2 study LONESTAR, which demonstrated 95%–100% SVR4 rates in a smaller cohort of treatment-naive and some treatment-experienced, non-cirrhotic patients treated with the same treatment arms (Lawitz 2014a). Key findings of the ION studies included comparable SVR12 rates regardless of race, concomitant ribavirin, non-CC IL28b genotype status, high baseline HCV viral load, or the presence of cirrhosis. Results of the ION studies yielded SVR rates ranging from 93.1% to 99.1% (Afdhal 2014b, Afdhal 2014c, Kowdley 2014). Ledipasvir is generally well tolerated when combined with sofosbuvir. Adverse drug events included nausea and headache. The fixed-dose combination of ledipasvir/sofosbuvir without ribavirin won FDA approval in October 2014 for the treatment of GT 1 patients.

Package labeling for ledipasvir/sofosbuvir states that non-cirrhotic treatment-naive patients with HCV RNA levels less than 6 million IU/mL may be considered for 8 weeks of treatment, because 97% of those 123 patients achieved SVR12 in ION-3. After 12 weeks of treatment, 99% of the 213 cirrhotic and non-cirrhotic treatment-naive patients achieved SVR12 in ION-1; 95% of the 87 non-cirrhotic treatment-experienced patients achieved SVR12 in ION-2. Therefore, the package labeling states that both (1) cirrhotic and non-cirrhotic treatment-naive and (2) non-cirrhotic treatment-experienced GT 1 patients should receive 12 weeks of treatment. After 24 weeks of treatment, 100% of the 22 treatment-experienced cirrhotic patients achieved SVR12 in ION-2; the FDA label reflects the extended length of therapy for that difficult-to-treat patient population.

This drug combination has simplified the HCV regimen to one tablet once daily for patients who can obtain medication insurance coverage. Several insurers have not yet added it to their formularies because the cost is $94,500 for a 12-week supply. But it is roughly the same cost of the combination of sofosbuvir, pegylated interferon, and ribavirin for 12 weeks, which was first line for GT 1 treatment-naive patients in early 2014.

Daclatasvir

Daclatasvir is an NS5A inhibitor with activity against GT 1–6. Bristol-Myers Squibb is investigating (1) a combination of daclatasvir, asunaprevir, and beclabuvir in GT 1 and (2) daclatasvir in combination with other DAAs for multiple GTs. A randomized, open-label phase 2 study assessed an interferon-free combination of daclatasvir and sofosbuvir in treatment-naive GT 1–3 patients and in GT 1 patients for whom previous therapy with first-generation PIs had failed (Sulkowski 2014). The SVR rates were 88%–100% for GT 2 and 3 patients and 95%–100% for GT 1 patients. However, the small number of patients included in each arm makes it difficult to know whether any differences among treatment arms would be significant in larger trials.

Only 2 out of 211 study patients (<1%) discontinued therapy because of adverse events (fibromyalgia, stroke), and those events were deemed not related to HCV treatment. The incidence of serious adverse events and grade 3 or 4 laboratory abnormalities did not differ substantially between treatment groups and ranged from 0 to 14% (0–4 patients per arm, with each arm containing a different number of patients). The most common grade 3 or 4 adverse event was anemia (occurring only in ribavirin-containing treatment arms), and 5 of the 90 patients in ribavirin-containing arms had subsequent reductions in ribavirin doses. No grade 3 or 4 AST, ALT, or bilirubin elevations were seen. The most common adverse events were fatigue, nausea, and headache (Sulkowski 2014). Efficacy and safety results from daclatasvir and sofosbuvir trials have been favorable. The results of several more daclatasvir trials are expected soon.

Ombitasvir

Ombitasvir is the NS5A inhibitor that is coformulated with paritaprevir and ritonavir that was studied in combination with dasabuvir as part of AbbVie's HCV regimen, as discussed later in the chapter. The manufacturer expects FDA approval in late December 2014.

Direct-Acting Antiviral Combinations
Sofosbuvir and Simeprevir

The phase 2 COSMOS trial evaluated the use of sofosbuvir 400 mg daily and simeprevir 150 mg daily with or without ribavirin for 12 or 24 weeks in 167 GT 1 patients who were treatment naive or previous null responders (Lawitz 2014b). The study evaluated patients with METAVIR scores of F0–F2 (cohort 1, n=80) and patients with METAVIR scores of F3–F4 (cohort 2, n=87). The overall SVR12 rate was 92% (90% in cohort 1, 94% in cohort 2). The most common adverse events were fatigue, headache, and nausea; anemia occurred only in patients who received ribavirin. Four patients (2%) discontinued all study drugs because of adverse events (Lawitz 2014b). Overall, the combination of sofosbuvir and simeprevir had high SVR rates and was well tolerated. Although the combination did not receive FDA approval until November 2014, AASLD guidelines had recommended its use since January 2014.

Support for the use of sofosbuvir and simeprevir stems from a small phase 2 trial, so the response rates in real-world populations have disappointed some providers. The TRIO Network evaluated the real-world data from 955 patients who were started on 12 weeks of a sofosbuvir-based regimen for GT 1, 2, 4, 5, and 6. The intent-to-treat SVR rates for treatment-naive and treatment-experienced GT 1 were 81% and 72% for patients treated with sofosbuvir, pegylated interferon, and ribavirin, and 83% and 81% for patients treated with sofosbuvir and simeprevir with or without ribavirin, respectively (Dieterich 2014).

Asunaprevir, Daclatasvir, and Beclabuvir

With the paradigm shift toward an all-oral regimen, manufacturers evaluated asunaprevir 100 mg twice daily and daclatasvir 60 mg daily for 24 weeks as a dual regimen for GT 1b patients in Japan. Historically, GT 1b patients have had higher SVR rates with DAAs and have been an easier-to-treat subpopulation. The SVR24 rates were 87.4% in the 135 interferon-ineligible or -intolerant group and 80.5% in the 87 previous nonresponders group (Kumada 2014). In February 2014, the FDA granted breakthrough designation for the dual regimen of asunaprevir and daclatasvir for the treatment of GT 1b patients, but the manufacturer withdrew the New Drug Application in October 2014 because the regimen would have little utility or desirability in the era of more-effective, shorter-duration treatment options. Bristol-Myers Squibb is investigating asunaprevir 200 mg, daclatasvir 30 mg, and beclabuvir (an NS5B polymerase inhibitor) 75 mg as a single-tablet regimen dosed twice daily (the "daclatasvir trio") in phase 3 trials. The UNITY 1 trial (daclatasvir + asunaprevir + beclabuvir x 12 weeks) has enrolled treatment-naive and treatment-experienced non-cirrhotic patients with GT 1; the UNITY 2 trial (daclatasvir + asunaprevir + beclabuvir + ribavirin x 12 weeks) has enrolled treatment-naive cirrhotic GT 1 patients. The results of those and other daclatasvir trials are expected soon.

Paritaprevir/Ritonavir, Ombitasvir, and Dasabuvir

This three-drug DAA combination consists of a coformulation of the ritonavir-boosted paritaprevir (a HCV NS3/4A PI) and ombitasvir (an NS5A inhibitor), and dasabuvir (a nonnucleoside NS5B polymerase inhibitor). In February 2014, data were presented on the final four studies in the pivotal phase 3 program: PEARL-II, PEARL-III, PEARL-IV, and TURQUOISE-II. Although the SVR rates were impressive with the regimens of paritaprevir/ritonavir/ombitasvir (150 mg/100 mg/25 mg) and dasabuvir 250 mg, study results indicated that the combination with ribavirin is still a required component of HCV GT 1a treatment. PEARL-IV yielded a higher SVR rate in GT 1a patients who received ribavirin compared with those that did not (97% vs. 90%). PEARL-III, presented in early 2014, was a monoinfection study of treatment-naive, GT 1b patients who received paritaprevir/ritonavir,

ombitasvir, and dasabuvir with or without ribavirin for 12 weeks. The SVR12 rate was 99% for both GT 1b arms regardless of the inclusion of ribavirin.

A dual regimen of paritaprevir/ritonavir/ombitasvir (150 mg/100 mg/25 mg) for 12 weeks in the phase 3 PEARL-I study resulted in cure rates of 95% in GT 1b patients. A lower SVR rate (90%) was observed with previous null responders compared with treatment-naive patients, suggesting that a third DAA is required in this more-difficult-to-treat subpopulation. AbbVie has filed for FDA approval of a fixed-dose combination of paritaprevir/ritonavir with ombitasvir for once-daily dosing. In some patients, that combination will need to be further combined with dasabuvir 250 mg dosed twice daily. Adverse drug reactions to this drug combination included headache, fatigue, and nausea.

SPECIAL POPULATIONS

Currently available HCV treatment is neither FDA approved nor appropriate in all patient populations. Some providers are postponing patient treatment until more data are available and until agents have been shown to be safe and efficacious for patients' specific conditions or until agents become FDA approved.

Cirrhosis

Patients who undergo treatment before developing cirrhosis usually tolerate treatment better than those with cirrhosis. Decompensation was more likely to occur, and SVR was less likely to occur with boceprevir- and telaprevir-based treatment for GT 1 cirrhotic patients than for patients with less-advanced disease (Hézode 2014). Cirrhotic patients treated with sofosbuvir experience high SVR rates in clinical trials, and the current HCV guidelines recommendations are the same for treatment-naive patients with or without compensated cirrhosis (AASLD 2014). It is important to note that SVR rates have increased for patients with cirrhosis who receive DAAs compared with SVR rates after previous treatment with a pegylated interferon and ribavirin backbone. In general, SVR rates in cirrhotic patients are still lower when compared with the rates of patients without cirrhosis. Labeled use of simeprevir is limited to patients with compensated liver disease, given the theoretical accumulation of simeprevir in patients with cirrhosis and the lack of data in this population; package inserts state simeprevir should not be used in cirrhotic patients with Child–Pugh Class B or C. Some providers choose to use simeprevir in cirrhotic patients who can obtain insurance coverage, and they monitor patients closely. The treatment of cirrhotic patients is further discussed in the following.

Renal Impairment

Current DAA treatments are not FDA approved for patients on dialysis or patients with CrCl less than 30 mL/minute. A clinical trial is under way to evaluate the currently approved sofosbuvir 400-mg daily dose and a 200-mg daily dose in combination with ribavirin for 24 weeks in renally impaired patients and patients on dialysis with GT 1 and 3 (NIH 2014). More safety data are needed before recommending the use of sofosbuvir in patients with renal impairment. AbbVie is studying an HCV regimen for GT patients who are on dialysis or have CrCl less than 30 mL/minute; Bristol-Myers Squibb is investigating asunaprevir, daclatasvir, and beclabuvir in the setting of renal impairment; and several other pipeline DAA agents are under investigation in patients with renal impairment.

Previous Treatment Nonresponse or Relapse

Treatment with sofosbuvir and/or simeprevir was not studied in patients for whom PI-based treatment with boceprevir or telaprevir failed. The ION-2 trial resulted in 94% SVR12 rates in the 66 patients treated with ledipasvir/sofosbuvir for 12 weeks of treatment after PI-based treatment had failed (Afdhal 2014b). The combination of sofosbuvir and daclatasvir has also been studied in patients whose first-wave PIs failed. Current HCV guidelines do not recommend using simeprevir for patients whose PI-based treatment has failed; that population would likely benefit from an alternative combination of DAAs.

Liver Transplantation

Ideally, to protect a new liver from infection, HCV should be eliminated before orthotopic liver transplantation or living related donor liver transplantation. If the patient either cannot receive HCV treatment or is unable to achieve SVR before transplantation, HCV treatment should be initiated post-transplantation because a post-transplant liver experiences accelerated rates of fibrosis with HCV infection. Successful HCV treatment in the post-transplant setting can protect the graft function and extend the time between transplant and liver decompensation.

Now that all-oral regimens are available and successful, the use of pegylated interferon in post-transplant patients should be avoided; many post-transplant patients are interferon ineligible, and interferon use can increase the risk of rejection. In sofosbuvir and ribavirin studies in the post-transplant population, the ribavirin dose was initiated at and titrated up from 200 mg twice daily based on patient tolerance and provider preference. In early 2014, sofosbuvir and ribavirin began to be used in the post-transplant population.

In January 2014, AASLD guidelines recommended the use of sofosbuvir and simeprevir for the treatment of post-transplant patients despite the lack of supporting clinical trial data. The TARGET longitudinal observational study evaluated data from 245 post-transplant patients who were started on sofosbuvir-based regimens for GT 1–3. The SVR4 rate was 90% for 68 GT 1 patients who had reached 4 weeks post-treatment and were treated with sofosbuvir

and simeprevir with or without ribavirin (86% for cirrhotic patients, 94% for non-cirrhotic patients) (Jensen 2014). The SVR12 data have not yet been presented, but the SVR4 data are similar to the COSMOS data that did not include transplant patients.

HIV/HCV Coinfection

Patients with HIV/HCV coinfection should be treated for HCV because SVR will prevent accelerated hepatic fibrosis (Labarga 2014). The use of simeprevir with pegylated interferon and ribavirin has resulted in an overall 74% SVR rate in GT 1 coinfected patients (Dieterich 2013). The PHOTON trial evaluated use of sofosbuvir-based regimens in HIV-coinfected patients, and SVR rates were 67%–88% based on GT. The ERADICATE trial enrolled GT 1 treatment-naive, stable, HIV-coinfected patients who were treated with ledipasvir/sofosbuvir for 12 weeks. An interim analysis of the trial yielded a 98% SVR rate in 40 of the 50 patients who had reached 12 weeks post-treatment. Current information suggests that HIV/HCV coinfected patients can be enrolled in the same trial as monoinfected HCV patients because SVR rates no longer appear to be significantly different if these patients are receiving modern DAAs.

Drug-drug interactions are common between HCV DAAs and antiretroviral agents, particularly with non-nucleoside reverse transcriptase inhibitors and PIs. When making decisions about the management of DDIs between HCV and HIV drugs, providers must carefully assess patient-specific factors such as stage of liver disease, previous HCV treatment, comorbid conditions, HIV viral load, immunodeficiency status, HIV genotype or phenotype, and medication access. One strategy is to substitute the patient's HIV treatment with an alternative regimen that does not interact with HCV DAAs. Another approach is to select alternative HCV agents that do not interact with the patient's HIV treatment. In the second scenario, simeprevir should be avoided because it is a CYP450 3A4 inhibitor and, consequently, has many DDIs with antiretrovirals.

Patients with HIV and their health care providers also may defer HCV treatment until HCV DAA combinations with fewer DDIs become available. Delay in HCV treatment should be considered only if the severity of a patient's liver disease does not warrant immediate treatment. Patients with concomitantly diagnosed HIV and HCV may delay treatment of HIV until after completion of HCV treatment if DDIs would be prohibitive on concurrent therapy—depending on careful consideration of CD4[+] count and other clinical factors.

PATIENT AND PROVIDER EDUCATION

Pharmacoeconomics

Because of the high prices of the newer DAA agents (more than $84,000 for 12 weeks of sofosbuvir alone and $94,500 for 12 weeks of ledipasvir/sofosbuvir), some providers find it challenging to obtain insurance approval of their preferred regimens for HCV treatment. To minimize the financial burden, some insurers have implemented HCV therapy formulary restrictions, high co-pays, or cost sharing for specialty pharmacy medications. Most insurance plans (1) require completion of multiple-page prior authorization forms, (2) limit the duration of approval time, and (3) request additional clinical documentation or justification from prescribers. Some plans limit lifetime HCV treatment coverage to one course of treatment; others deny coverage for off-label DAA combinations. Several state insurance plans and Medicaid managed care plans limit HCV medication approval to patients with cirrhosis or F3–F4 staging and deny coverage for patients with less severe disease. In some situations, patients cannot afford the out-of-pocket co-pay. Other patients lack insurance coverage. Historically, expensive treatment was unobtainable in those circumstances, but several manufacturers now offer patient assistance programs, co-pay cards, and discount coupons. Some nonprofit organizations also offer assistance (see Table 2-2). Pharmacists can facilitate the use of these programs in community and clinical settings. They can also decrease the cost burden on payers by reducing and correcting improper prescribing.

Medication Selection

Pharmacists are in a position to help guide providers in selecting HCV drugs that allow for optimal patient access to medication. To further aid in proper prescribing, pharmacists can provide new referral evaluation for appropriateness of therapy. The pharmacist should be aware of current treatment recommendations and make sure that patients are prescribed regimens appropriate for their GTs, treatment status, comorbidities, medications, and other patient concerns. Box 2-3 lists additional resources for HCV education for both patients and providers.

Adherence

For HCV treatment success, adherence is required; nonadherence negatively affects SVR rates (Weiss 2009) and potentially leads to the development of resistance. If delay in treatment would not be harmful, providers should recommend waiting until the patient is fully committed to begin HCV treatment. The importance of medication adherence should be emphasized at treatment initiation, at all follow-up visits, and at the time of medication refills. Pharmacists can counsel patients on the importance of adherence to minimize risk of treatment failure. Patients should be encouraged to use adherence aids such as pillboxes, alarms, and medication charts, and be given specific instructions on what to do if they miss a dose of HCV treatment. The pharmacist's expertise and provision of education for providers and patients increase the likelihood of selecting appropriate treatment candidates and of patient adherence to the HCV regimen.

Patient Counseling

The initial conversation with the patient about HCV treatment should include a discussion about its risks and benefits. It is important that patients understand the mode of HCV transmission and be counseled on avoiding behaviors that can lead to spread of the virus. Patients should be informed about currently available classes of agents for treatment of their specific HCV GT and treatment history status. Pharmacists can provide group patient education classes, extensive one-on-one patient education at the initiation of HCV treatment, and ongoing follow-up assessment to assist in patient comprehension and safety. The patient should be informed about the meaning of HCV laboratory tests, SVR, the next step if the current course of treatment fails, and how the disease could progress. The pharmacist is the ideal provider to inform patients about the proper storage of their HCV drugs, the potential adverse effects of the treatment, steps that can be taken to alleviate or minimize adverse reactions, and the procedure to follow if an adverse effect occurs. Successfully treated patients should be counseled that no immunity is conferred and that reinfection is possible with re-exposure.

Box 2-3. HCV Resources for Patients and Providers

HCV Guidelines
- American Association for the Study of Liver Diseases, Infectious Disease Society of America, and International Antiviral Society

Drug-Drug Interaction Sources
- Lexicomp, Inc
- Micromedex Solutions
- University of Buffalo – AIDS Clinical Trial Group
- University of California at San Francisco
- University of Liverpool
  - http://www.hep-druginteractions.org
  - http://www.hiv-druginteractions.org

Government-Sponsored HCV Information
- Centers for Disease Control and Prevention
- U.S. Department of Veterans Affairs

HIV and Hepatitis Information
- HIVandHepatitis.com
- National AIDS Treatment Advocacy Project

Online HCV Courses and Certificate Programs
- National Association of Specialty Pharmacy
- University of Washington

Free Online HCV Textbook
- inPractice Hepatology

HCV Clinical Information
- Clinical Care Options
- ViralEd

Patient Support Groups
- American Liver Foundation
- HCV Advocate
- HCV Support

Education about the importance of lifestyle changes can also be provided by pharmacists. Obese and overweight patients should be encouraged to make healthy diet choices and engage in regular exercise to achieve a healthy body mass index. All patients should be urged to begin a low-fat diet that includes plenty of fruits, vegetables, and whole grains and to maintain adequate hydration during HCV treatment. Obese patients are more likely to have nonalcoholic fatty liver disease, which is a risk factor in HCV fibrosis progression (Ortiz 2002). Alcohol consumption accelerates scarring of the liver, and all HCV patients should be counseled to begin abstention upon HCV diagnosis (AASLD 2014). Patients should abstain from illicit drug use during the course of HCV treatment because concomitant and frequent drug use can have a negative impact on SVR and adherence in some settings (Robaeys 2013; Grebely 2011; Alvarez-Uria 2009; Sylvestre 2007). However, illicit drug use is not a contraindication for treatment. From a public health concern, some clinics are attempting to treat active illicit drug users as a way of decreasing the transmission of HCV. Smoking is associated with a risk of developing HCC, and patients who use tobacco products should be offered smoking-cessation services based on stage of readiness to quit (Koh 2011). Similarly, daily marijuana smoking is associated with progression of fibrosis and should be discouraged (Hézode 2005). Patients should be counseled to avoid herbal supplements because such substances lack FDA approval, can be hepatotoxic, and may interact with HCV regimens. See Box 2-3 for additional resources for HCV education for patients and providers.

Monitoring

During previous HCV treatment with PI-based regimens that included pegylated interferon and ribavirin, providers used response-guided therapy to make decisions on length of treatment based on HCV RNA quantitative level. With the advent of DAAs in 2011, updated liver guidelines recommend that the lower limit of detection for the HCV level should be from less than 10 to 15 IU/mL. Several commercial HCV RNA assays are available, and it was important to know the lower limit of detection to select the most sensitive assay available that would ensure proper response-guided therapy with use of PIs. However, in the era of combination DAA agents, response-guided therapy is no longer necessary.

Historically, baseline thyroid-stimulating hormone and fasting lipid profile were recommended both before starting pegylated interferon treatment and during the course of therapy. The need for and the frequency of laboratory monitoring are less clear with a 12-week treatment duration and are not addressed in the updated guidelines. Table 2-4 provides recommendations for laboratory monitoring during HCV treatment combinations. The regimen

of ledipasvir/sofosbuvir does not require specific monitoring, although providers (and insurers) may request HCV RNA levels at week 4. Renal function should be monitored in patients with decreased CrCl (more than 30 mL/minute is recommended) and in patients taking tenofovir. To facilitate communication among providers, providers should document follow-up visits, education provided, laboratory assessments, drug-drug interactions, medication changes, adverse drug reactions, and management plans in patients' medical records.

Drug Interactions

To enable providers to monitor for and prevent DDIs, patients should be counseled on the need to inform the pharmacist and other health care providers about their current HCV drugs. Several resources assist providers in the detection and explanation of DDIs with HCV medications (see Box 2-3). Access to drug information resources such as Lexicomp and Micromedex is provided by many employers, and several databases offer convenient applications for handheld devices. The University of Liverpool has an extensive and free online interactive DDI information system. Users may select the proposed hepatitis or HIV regimens and add additional medications to review for DDIs. The Web site also includes fact sheets on select phase III HCV pipeline agents. The AIDS Clinical Trials Group Network DDI database, developed with the University at Buffalo, offers users free access to a searchable database with supporting evidence for HIV/HCV DDIs with the selected agent. However, an alternative source must be consulted for non-HIV/HCV DDIs. Providers who work with HIV/HCV coinfected patients may prefer to use the University of California, San Francisco, database, which lets users select a patient's HIV regimen and then search for interactions by agent, drug class, or all interactions. Prescribers may also use a variety of other available sources; the above are examples of sources with information specific to HCV and HIV.

Adverse Drug Events

Rash and pruritus can occur with simeprevir and ribavirin use. Hematologic changes can occur with pegylated interferon and ribavirin, and complete blood count should be monitored at baseline and at least every 4 weeks during treatment. Studies have indicated that managing ribavirin-induced anemia with ribavirin dose reduction does not affect SVR compared with managing ribavirin-induced anemia with the addition of epoetin-stimulating agents. Therefore, ribavirin dose reduction is the preferred anemia management technique.

Treatment with pegylated interferon can cause thrombocytopenia, and patients with thrombocytopenia should be monitored for bleeding during the course of treatment. Prescribers may reduce the dose of pegylated interferon when the platelet count falls below 50,000/mm³;

Table 2-4. Laboratory Monitoring for PegIFN HCV Regimens with or without Ribavirin

Treatment Combination	Lab	Frequency
SOF + RBV	CBC with differential	Baseline Every 4 weeks during treatment
	Comprehensive Metabolic Profile	Baseline Every 4 weeks during treatment
	HCV PCR Quantitative	Baseline Some insurance plans request at week 4 End of treatment 12 weeks after treatment
	Pregnancy test (women of childbearing capacity)	Baseline Every 4 weeks during treatment
SOF + RBV + PegIFN or SMV + RBV + PegIFN	CBC with differential	Baseline Every 4 weeks during treatment
	Comprehensive Metabolic Profile	Baseline Every 4 weeks during treatment
	HCV PCR Quantitative	Baseline Some insurance plans request at week 4 End of treatment 12 weeks after treatment
	TSH	Baseline Every 12 weeks during treatment
	Lipids	Baseline Every 12 weeks during treatment
	Pregnancy test (women of childbearing capacity)	Baseline Every 4 weeks during treatment

CBC = complete blood count; HCV PCR = hepatitis C virus polymerase chain reaction; PegIFN = pegylated interferon; RBV = ribavirin; SMV = simeprevir; SOF = sofosbuvir; TSH = thyroid stimulating hormone.

Information from: American Association for the Study of Liver Diseases, Infectious Diseases Society of America, and International Antiviral Society-USA. Recommendations for Testing, Managing, and Treating Hepatitis C; and Ghany MG, Strader DB, Thomas DL, et al; for the American Association for the Study of Liver Diseases. Diagnosis, management, and treatment of hepatitis C: an update. Hepatology 2009;49:1335-74.

pegylated interferon alfa-2b is reduced to 1 mcg/kg/week, and pegylated interferon alfa-2a is reduced to 90 mcg per week. Eltrombopag was FDA approved in 2012 to preserve platelet counts for patients with HCV and thrombocytopenia; although its use successfully increased platelets, allowing for initiation or continuation of HCV treatment with pegylated interferon, it has not been universally adopted by providers. Eltrombopag is not currently recommended for use with the new DAAs, and it is not recommended in the AASLD guidelines (Afdhal 2014a). Dose reduction of pegylated interferon is more cost-effective than use of eltrombopag. Use of eltrombopag in HCV is expected to diminish as pegylated interferon is phased out of treatment practice.

INVESTIGATIONAL TREATMENT AGENTS

The field of treatment of HCV is changing rapidly, and newer treatments hold the promise of greater success in clearing HCV in more diverse patient populations. Several all-oral treatment options for GT 1 are currently in phase 3 trials, and several phase 2 trials are evaluating shortened-duration HCV treatment for multiple GTs. Bristol-Myers Squibb has announced plans to file in early 2015 for FDA approval of the triple DAA combination of asunaprevir, daclatasvir, and beclabuvir; that combination was studied as a fixed-dose combination. Merck is evaluating the use of grazoprevir (an NS3/4A PI) and elbasvir (an NS5A inhibitor) in GT 1–6 and in HIV/HCV coinfection.

Gilead is investigating the use of a fixed-dose combination of sofosbuvir and GS-5816 (an NS5A inhibitor) for GT 1–6. Several other pharmaceutical companies, including Roche and Achillion, have DAAs in varying phases of clinical trials. It is hoped that new DAA combinations will offer greater tolerability and ease of administration than do regimens with pegylated interferon and ribavirin, as well as shorter durations of treatment than the combinations now available. Table 2-5 lists selected recently-approved or pipeline medications and classes under investigation for treatment of HCV.

Conclusion

Hepatitis C virus affects about 5 million Americans. Recent advancements in pharmacologic treatment and the FDA approval of DAAs have greatly increased SVR rates in patients with all HCV GTs but with the drawback of increased treatment costs. Several pipeline agents are in various phases of drug development. Future developments in antiviral therapy are expected to yield HCV treatments with decreased pill burdens, improved adverse effect profiles, and shorter durations of therapy. Pharmacists can play an integral role in improving the safety and outcomes of HCV treatment by providing patient counseling and by advising on proper timing and medication selection.

References

fdhal NH, Dusheiko GM, Giannini EG, et al. Eltrombopag increases platelet numbers in thrombocytopenic patients with HCV infection and cirrhosis, allowing for effective antiviral therapy. Gastroenterology 2014;146:442-52.

Afdhal N, Rajender Reddy K, Nelson DR, et al for the ION-2 Investigators. Ledipasvir and sofosbuvir for previously treated HCV genotype 1 infection. New Engl J Med 2014;370:1483-93.

Afdhal N, Zeuzem S, Kwo P, et al for the ION-1 Investigators. Ledipasvir and sofosbuvir for untreated HCV genotype 1 infection. N Engl J Med 2014;370:1889-98.

Patient Care Scenario

A 59-year-old non-cirrhotic woman with HCV GT 1a presents to the liver clinic to inquire about HCV treatment options. She was treated once with PegIFN and RBV in 2004, but she had to stop treatment at week 15 because of psychiatric adverse events that led to a suicide attempt, and her HCV relapsed after treatment discontinuation. Her medical history includes HIV infection, bipolar disorder, hypertension, and asthma. Her home drugs include efavirenz/emtricitabine/tenofovir disoproxil fumarate 600 mg/200 mg/300 mg daily, lithium 300 mg twice daily, amlodipine 10 mg daily, fluticasone/salmeterol 250/50 mcg inhalation twice daily, and albuterol 90 mcg inhalation every 6 hours as needed. Which HCV treatment regimen is most appropriate for this patient?

   A. Sofosbuvir plus simeprevir
   B. Ledipasvir/sofosbuvir
   C. Daclatasvir plus asunaprevir plus beclabuvir
   D. Paritaprevir/r plus ombitasvir plus dasabuvir

Answer

Option B is preferred. NS5B and NS5A inhibitors have fewer DDIs than PIs, so this regimen would be appropriate for use in a patient with the listed antiretroviral agents. The provider should monitor for tenofovir-associated adverse reactions in patients receiving ledipasvir/sofosbuvir with the combination of efavirenz, emtricitabine and tenofovir DF. Refer to VIREAD, TRUVADA, or ATRIPLA prescribing information for recommendations on renal monitoring. Option A would include a DDI with simeprevir and efavirenz that could lead to a decreased exposure to and therapeutic effect of simeprevir. Option C would include a DDI with asunaprevir and efavirenz that could lead to a decreased exposure to and therapeutic effect of asunaprevir. Option D would include a DDI with paritaprevir/r and both efavirenz (that could lead to a decreased exposure to and therapeutic effect of paritaprevir) and fluticasone (that could lead to an increased exposed to fluticasone).

1. Lexicomp, Inc: http://www.lexi.com
2. Micromedex Solutions: http://www.micromedex.com
3. University of Buffalo – AIDS Clinical Trial Group: http://tprc.pharm.buffalo.edu/home/di_search
4. University of California at San Francisco: http://hivinsite.ucsf.edu/insite?page=ar-00-02
5. University of Liverpool: http://www.hep-druginteractions.org and http://www.hiv-druginteractions.org

---

Practice Points

- Several new HCV agents will likely be FDA-approved around the time of publication and later in 2015. Review the current treatment guidelines for the most up-to-date information for clinical practice.
- Current guidelines recommend use of SOF-based regimens over use of SMV + PegIFN + RBV.
  - SVR rates with SMV are less than SVR rates with SOF (though not compared in a head-to-head trial).
  - SOF-based regimens were well-tolerated, do not induce resistance, and do not require response-guided therapy (no futility rules), making treatment easier for both patients and providers
- Current treatment with SOF- or SMV-based regimens may not be appropriate for all patients at this time, including:
  - Patients with renal impairment
  - Patients without insurance coverage who do not qualify for financial assistance programs
  - Patients without interest in or dedication to treatment

Alter MJ. Epidemiology of hepatitis C virus infection. World J Gastroenterol 2007;13:2436-41.

Alvarez-Uria G, Day JN, Nasir AJ, Russell SK, Vilar FJ. Factors associated with treatment failure of patients with psychiatric diseases and injecting drug users in the treatment of genotype 2 or 3 hepatitis C chronic infection. Liver Int 2009;29:1051-5. American Association for the Study of Liver Diseases, Infectious Diseases Society of America, and International Antiviral Society-USA. Recommendations for Testing, Managing, and Treating Hepatitis C.

Armstrong GL, Wasley A, Simard EP, McQuillan GM, Kuhnert WL, Alter MJ. The prevalence of hepatitis C virus infection in the United States, 1999 through 2002. Ann Intern Med 2006;144:705-14.

Castera L, Forns X, Alberti A. Non-invasive evaluation of liver fibrosis using transient elastography. J Hepatol 2008;48:835-47.

Centers for Disease Control and Prevention (CDC). Disease Burden from Viral Hepatitis A, B, and C in the United States, 2014.

Centers for Disease Control and Prevention (CDC). Division of Viral Hepatitis - Statistics and Surveillance 2011a.

Centers for Disease Control and Prevention (CDC). Notes from the field: risk factors for hepatitis C virus infections among young adults—Massachusetts, 2010. MMWR 2011b;60:1457–8.

Centers for Disease Control and Prevention (CDC). Hepatitis C virus infections among adolescents and young adults—Rural Wisconsin 2010, 2002–2009. MMWR 2011b;60:537–41.

Centers for Disease Control and Prevention. Recommendations for the Identification of Chronic Hepatitis C Virus Infection Among Persons Born During 1945–1965. MMRW 2012;61;1-18.

Ciesek, S, Manns MP. Hepatitis in 2010: the dawn of a new era in HCV therapy. Nat Rev Gastroenterol Hepatol 2011;8:69-71.

Chen J, Florian J, Carter W, et al. Earlier sustained virologic response end points for regulatory approval and dose selection of hepatitis C therapies. Gastroenterology 2013;144:1450-55.

Dieterich D, Bacon BR, Flamm SL, et al. Evaluation of sofosbuvir and simeprevir-based regimens in the TRIO network: academic and community treatment of a real-world, heterogeneous population. American Association for the Study of Liver Diseases (AASLD) Liver Meeting. Boston, November 7-12, 2014. Abstract 46.

Dieterich D, Rockstroh J, Orkin C, et al. Simeprevir (TMC435) plus peginterferon/ribavirin in patients co-infected with HCV genotype-1 and HIV-1: primary analysis of the C212 study. 14th European AIDs Conference (EACS 2013). Brussels. October 16-19, 2013. Abstract PS9/5.

Table 2-5. Classes of Select Recently-Approved and Investigational Agents for HCV Treatment

Class	Target / Mechanism	Examples
Direct-acting antivirals	NS3 and NS3/4A protease inhibitors	Paritaprevir/ritonavir (AbbVie)
		Asunaprevir (Bristol-Myers Squibb)
		Grazoprevir (MK-5172) (Merck)
		Danoprevir (Roche)
	NS5A replication complex inhibitors	Daclatasvir (Bristol-Myers Squibb)
		Ledipasvir (Gilead)
		Ombitasvir (AbbVie)
		ACH-3102 (Achillion)
		GS-5816 (Gilead)
		Elbasvir (MK-8742) (Merck)
	NS5B polymerase inhibitors: non-nucleoside inhibitors and nucleoside analogues	Beclabuvir (BMS-791325) (Bristol-Myers Squibb)
		Dasabuvir (AbbVie)
		Mericitabine (Roche)
Host-targeting agents	Cyclophilin A (anti-viral)	Alisporivir (Novartis)
	microRNAs	Miravirsen (Santaris)
	Interferons (immunomodulatory)	PegIFN lambda (Bristol-Myers Squibb)
	HCV infectivity inhibitor 1 (HCV II-1)	GS-563253 (Gilead)

HCV= hepatitis C virus.

Information from: Schlutter J. Therapeutics: new drugs hit the target. Nature 2011;474:S5-S7. Clinicaltrials.gov.

Garcia-Tsao G, Sanyal AJ, Grace ND et al. Prevention and management of gastroesophageal varices and variceal hemorrhage in cirrhosis. Hepatology 2007;46:922-38.

Ghany MG, Nelson DR, Strader DB, Thomas DL, Seeff LB. American Association for the Study of Liver Diseases. An update on treatment of Genotype 1 Chronic Hepatitis C Virus Infection: 2011 practice guideline by the American Association for the Study of Liver Diseases. Hepatology 2011;54:1433-44.

Ghany MG, Strader DB, Thomas DL, Seeff LB. American Association for the Study of Liver Diseases. Diagnosis, management, and treatment of hepatitis C: an update. Hepatology 2009;49:1335-74.

Grebely J, Matthews GV, Hellard M, et al. Adherence to treatment for recently acquired hepatitis C virus (HCV) infection among injecting drug users. J Hepatol 2011;55:76-85

Hézode C, Fontaine H, Dorival C, et al for the CUPIC Study Group. Effectiveness of telaprevir or boceprevir in treatment-experienced patients with HCV genotype 1 infection and cirrhosis. Gastroenterology 2014;147:132-42.

Hézode C, Roudot-Thoraval F, Nguyen S, et al. Daily cannabis smoking as a risk factor for progression of fibrosis in chronic hepatitis C. Hepatology 2005;42:63-71.

Hoofnagle JH. Course and outcome of hepatitis C. Hepatology 2002;36:S21-S29.

Houghton M. The long and winding road leading to the identification of the hepatitis C virus. Journal of Hepatology 2009;51:939-48.

Jacobson I, Dore GJ, Foster GR, et al. Simeprevir (TMC435) with peginterferon/ribavirin for chronic HCV genotype 1 infection in treatment-naïve patients: results from QUEST-1, a phase III trial. The International Liver Congress 2013, 48th Annual Meeting of the European Association for the Study of the Liver; April 24–28, 2013; Amsterdam, The Netherlands. J Hepatol Suppl 2013a;58:S574.

Jacobson IM, Gordon SC, Kowdley KV, et al. Sofosbuvir for hepatitis C genotype 2 or 3 in patients without treatment options. N Engl J Med 2013b;368:1867–77.

Jensen DM, O'Leary JG, Pockros PJ, et al. Safety and Efficacy of Sofosbuvir-Containing Regimens for Hepatitis C: Real-World Experience in a Diverse, Longitudinal Observational Cohort. American Association for the Study of Liver Diseases (AASLD) Liver Meeting. Boston, November 7-12, 2014. Abstract 45.

Kim WR. The burden of hepatitis C in the United States. Hepatology 2002;36:S30-S34.

Koh WP, Robien K, Wang R, et al. Smoking as an independent risk factor for hepatocellular carcinoma: the Singapore Chinese Health Study. Br J Cancer 2011;105:1430-35.

Kowdley KV, Gordon SC, Reddy KR, et al. Ledipasvir and sofosbuvir for 8 or 12 weeks for chronic HCV without cirrhosis. N Engl J Med 2014;370:1879-88.

Kumada H1, Suzuki Y, Ikeda K, et al. Daclatasvir plus asunaprevir for chronic HCV genotype 1b infection. Hepatology 2014;59:2083-91.

Labarga P, Fernandez-Montero JV, Barreiro P, et al. Changes in liver fibrosis in HIV/HCV-coinfected patients following different outcomes with peginterferon plus ribavirin therapy. J Viral Hepat 2014;21:475-9.

Lawitz E, Forns X, Zeuzem S, et al. Simeprevir (TMC435) with peg-interferon/ribavirin for treatment of chronic HCV genotype 1 infection in patients who relapsed after previous interferon-based therapy: results from PROMISE, a phase III trial. Digestive Disease Week 2013; May 18–21, 2013; Orlando, FL. Gastroenterology 2013;144:S–151.

Lawitz E, Mangia A, Wyles D, et al. Sofosbuvir for previously untreated chronic hepatitis C infection. N Engl J Med 2013;368:1878-87.

Lawitz E, Poordad FF, Pang PS, et al. Sofosbuvir and ledipasvir fixed-dose combination with and without ribavirin in treatment-naïve and previously treated patients with genotype 1 hepatitis C virus infection (LONESTAR): an open-label, randomized, phase 2 trial. Lancet 2014;383:515-23.

Lawitz E, Sulkowski MS, Ghalib R, et al. Simeprevir plus sofosbuvir, with or without ribavirin, to treat chronic infection with hepatitis C virus genotype 1 in non-responders to pegylated interferon and ribavirin and treatment-naive patients: the COSMOS randomised study. Lancet 2014;384:1756-65.

Ly KN, Xing J, Klevens RM, Jiles RB, Ward JW, Holmberg SD. The increasing burden of mortality from viral hepatitis in the United States between 1999 and 2007. Ann Intern Med 2012;156:271-8.

Manns M, Marcellin P, Poordad FP, et al. Simeprevir (TMC435) with peginterferon/ribavirin for treatment of chronic HCV genotype-1 infection in treatment-naive patients: results from QUEST-2, a phase III trial. The International Liver Congress 2013, 48th Annual Meeting of the European Association for the Study of the Liver; April 24–28, 2013; Amsterdam, The Netherlands. J Hepatol Suppl 2013;58:S568.

McHutchison JG, Bacon BR. Chronic hepatitis C: an age wave of disease burden. Am J Manag Care 2005;11:S286-S295.

Moyer VA; U.S. Preventive Services Task Force. Screening for hepatitis C virus infection in adults: u.s. Preventive services task force recommendation statement. Ann Intern Med 2013;159:349-57.

Nakano T, Lau GM, Sugiyama M. An updated analysis of hepatitis C virus genotypes and subtypes based on the complete coding region. Liver Int 2012;32:339-45.

NIH. Sofosbuvir Plus Ribavirin in Subjects With HCV Infection and Renal Insufficiency. In: ClinicalTrials.gov [Internet]. Bethesda (MD): National Library of Medicine (US). 2014. NLM Identifier: NCT01958281.

Ortiz V, Berenguer M, Rayon JM, Carrasco D, Berenguer J. Contribution of obesity to hepatitis C-related fibrosis progression. Am J Gastroenterol 2002;97:2408-14.

Poynard T, de Ledinghen V, Zarski JP, et al for the Fibrosis-TAGS group. Relative performances of FibroTest, Fibroscan, and biopsy for the assessment of the stage of liver fibrosis in patients with chronic hepatitis C: a step toward the truth in the absence of a gold standard. J Hepatol 2012;56:541-8.

Robaeys G, Grebely J, Mauss S, et al. Recommendations for the management of hepatitis C virus infection among people who inject drugs. Clin Infect Dis 2013;57:S129-S137.

Rubbia-Brandt L, Fabris P, Paganin S et al. Steatosis affects chronic hepatitis C progression in a genotype specific way. Gut 2004;53:406-12.

Schlutter J. Therapeutics: new drugs hit the target. Nature 2011;474:S5-S7.

Singal AG, Conjeevaram HS, Volk ML, et al. Effectiveness of hepatocellular carcinoma surveillance in patients with cirrhosis. Cancer Epidemiol Biomarkers Prev 2012;21:793-9.

Smith DB, Bukh J, Kuiken C, et al. Expanded classification of hepatitis C virus into 7 genotypes and 67 subtypes: updated criteria and genotype assignment Web resource. Hepatology 2014;59:318-27.

Snyder N, Gajula L, Xiao SY, et al. APRI: an easy and validated predictor of hepatic fibrosis in chronic hepatitis C. J Clin Gastroenterol 2006;40:535-42.

Sulkowski MS, David F. Gardiner DF, Maribel Rodriguez-Torres M, et al for the AI444040 Study Group. Daclatasvir plus Sofosbuvir for Previously Treated or Untreated Chronic HCV Infection. N Engl J Med 2014;370:211-21.

Swadling L, Klenerman P, Barnes E. Ever closer to a prophylactic vaccine for HCV. Expert Opin Biol Ther 2013;13:1109-24.

Sylvestre DL, Clements BJ. Adherence to hepatitis C treatment in recovering heroin users maintained on methadone. Eur J Gastroenterol Hepatol 2007;19:741-7.

van der Meer AJ, Veldt BJ, Feld JJ, et al., Hofmann WP, de Knegt RJ, Hansen BE, Janssen HL. Association between sustained virological response and all-cause mortality among patients with chronic hepatitis C and advanced hepatic fibrosis. JAMA 2012;308:2584-93.

Weiss JJ, Bräu N, Stivala A, Swan T, Fishbein D. Review article: adherence to medication for chronic hepatitis C - building on the model of human immunodeficiency virus antiretroviral adherence research. Aliment Pharmacol Ther 2009;30:14-27.

World Health Organization (WHO). Hepatitis Factsheet, 2014.

World Health Organization. Hepatitis C Global Alert and Response, 2002.

Yehia BR, Schranz A, Umscheild C, Lo Re V. The treatment cascade for people with chronic hepatitis C virus infection in the United States [abstract 669]. Top Antivir Med 2014;22:332-3.

SELF-ASSESSMENT QUESTIONS

21. Which one of the following U.S. patients is most at risk for the transmission of hepatitis C virus (HCV)?

    A. A 51-year-old man with chronic kidney disease.
    B. A 35-year-old woman who uses intravenous heroin.
    C. An infant born at 32 weeks gestation to a 28-year-old mother with HCV.
    D. A 42-year-old man who has sex with men (MSM).

22. A 21-year-old treatment-naïve cirrhotic man with HCV genotype (GT) 1a presents for initial evaluation of HCV. The patient is a heroin user, but he has halved his heroin usage in the last 3 months. The patient has demonstrated appointment adherence and medication adherence in the past. The patient is on the state's Medicaid insurance plan, which does not cover any combination of two or more direct acting antivirals. According to the current guidelines, which one of the following is best to recommend for this patient?

    A. Treat with pegylated interferon plus ribavirin plus sofosbuvir for 12 weeks.
    B. Treat with simeprevir plus sofosbuvir for 24 weeks.
    C. Do not treat because the patient is likely to be reinfected through continued injection drug use (IDU).
    D. Do not treat because the patient is likely to be nonadherent.

23. A 42-year-old treatment-naïve cirrhotic woman with HCV GT 1b sickle cell presents for initial evaluation of HCV. The patient requests HCV treatment. Which one of the following treatment regimens is best to recommend for this patient?

    A. Sofosbuvir plus pegylated interferon plus ribavirin for 12 weeks.
    B. Sofosbuvir plus ribavirin for 24 weeks.
    C. Simeprevir plus sofosbuvir for 12 weeks.
    D. Ledipasvir/sofosbuvir plus ribavirin for 12 weeks.

24. A non-cirrhotic patient with HCV GT 1a was a null-responder to treatment with pegylated interferon and ribavirin in 2007–2008. Which one of the following is best to recommend for this patient per the current AASLD guidelines?

    A. Sofosbuvir plus pegylated interferon plus ribavirin for 12 weeks.
    B. Simeprevir plus pegylated interferon plus ribavirin for 24 weeks.
    C. Sofosbuvir plus simeprevir for 12 weeks.
    D. Ledipasvir/sofosbuvir for 24 weeks.

25. A 42-year-old treatment-naïve, non-cirrhotic HIV/HCV coinfected man presents to liver clinic for HCV treatment evaluation. The patient's HIV regimen consists of atazanavir 300 mg at bedtime, ritonavir 100 mg daily, and emtricitabine/tenofovir 200 mg/300 mg tablet daily. He is also well controlled on sertraline 25 mg daily, levetiracetam 500 mg twice daily, and sildenafil 25 mg as needed. Which one of the following is best to recommend for this patient's HCV GT 1a treatment?

    A. Sofosbuvir plus pegylated interferon plus ribavirin for 12 weeks.
    B. Sofosbuvir plus simeprevir for 12 weeks.
    C. Paritaprevir/ritonavir/ombitasvir plus dasabuvir plus ribavirin for 12 weeks.
    D. Daclatasvir plus asunaprevir for 24 weeks.

26. Which one of the following patients would most likely be considered interferon-ineligible?

    A. A 62-year-old woman with a history of depression 10 years ago; not on antidepressants for the last 4 years.
    B. A 43-year-old woman with hypothyroidism; TSH within normal limits on levothyroxine.
    C. A 25-year-old man with bipolar disorder who refuses psychiatric treatment; history of suicide attempt 2 years ago.
    D. A 57-year-old man with compensated cirrhosis.

27. A woman with HCV GT 1 (weight 85 kg) is on treatment (sofosbuvir 400 mg daily, pegylated interferon alpha-2a 180 mcg weekly, ribavirin 600 mg twice daily); she develops anemia with a hemoglobin of 10.5 g/dL at week 2 of treatment. Baseline hemoglobin was 13.4 g/dL. Which one of the following is best to recommend for this patient?

    A. Stop ribavirin.
    B. Stop sofosbuvir.
    C. Add an erythrocyte-stimulating agent.
    D. Reduce ribavirin to 200 mg every morning and 400 mg every evening.

28. Which one of the following patients most requires immediate treatment for HCV?

A. A 56-year-old woman with GT 2b; no biopsy available; with platelet count of 138,000/mcL, INR 1.1.

B. A 54-year-old man with GT 1, cirrhosis, and HCC status post transcatheter arterial chemoembolization; awaiting liver transplant with a model for end-stage liver disease score of 23.

C. A 63-year-old treatment-naïve man with HCV GT 3a; biopsy reveals stage 2 with steatosis.

D. A 21-year-old woman with GT 1a; newly diagnosed after HCV screening because of a history of intravenous drug use (5 years).

29. A 56-year-old woman has just moved and is establishing care with her new provider. Her medical records are not available but after the initial visit, the patient admits to a remote history of intravenous drug use and now has worsening fatigue. Which one of the following would best assess this patient for the presence of chronic HCV?

A. Liver biopsy.

B. Positive HCV antibody.

C. Positive HCV antibody and detectable HCV RNA viral load.

D. Positive HCV antibody, detectable HCV RNA viral level, and liver biopsy.

30. A 54-year-old non-cirrhotic man (weight 78 kg) with HCV genotype 3a presents to liver clinic. He states that he has never been treated for HCV. Which one of the following is best to recommend for this patient's HCV treatment?

A. Sofosbuvir 400 mg daily plus pegylated interferon alfa-2a 180 mcg subcutaneously every week plus ribavirin 600 mg twice daily for 12 weeks.

B. Sofosbuvir 400 mg daily plus ribavirin 600 mg twice daily for 24 weeks.

C. Pegylated interferon alfa-2a 180 mcg subcutaneously every week plus ribavirin 600 mg twice daily for 12 weeks.

D. Sofosbuvir 400 mg daily plus ribavirin 600 mg twice daily for 12 weeks.

31. Of the following recent advancements in HCV treatment, which one is most important?

A. GT 2 patients with cirrhosis may now be treated with all-oral treatment.

B. SVR12 is used as a measure of cure instead of SVR24.

C. GT 1 sustained viral response (SVR) rates are in the 90% range.

D. HIV/HCV coinfected patients have SVR rates similar to HCV monoinfected patients.

32. A 62-year-old man is referred for HCV treatment initiation with simeprevir and sofosbuvir for GT 1a. The patient's home drugs include amlodipine 10 mg daily, hydrochlorothiazide 25 mg daily, tadalafil 10 mg as needed for erectile dysfunction, carbamazepine 500 mg twice daily, and atorvastatin 10 mg daily. Which one of the following is best to recommend for this patient?

A. Discontinue atorvastatin during HCV treatment.

B. Refer to the patient to neurology clinic for potential change in his treatment regimen.

C. Advise patient to discontinue tadalafil during HCV treatment.

D. Switch amlodipine to an alternate antihypertensive agent.

33. A 47-year-old cirrhotic man with HCV GT 1a presents to clinic after transferring care from out of state. His medical records indicate that he was treated with boceprevir, pegylated interferon plus ribavirin in 2013, but the treatment was discontinued at week 12 because the patient did not pass the futility rules. The patient requests retreatment of his HCV with new agents. Which one of the following treatment regimens would be most appropriate for this patient?

A. Sofosbuvir plus pegylated interferon plus ribavirin for 12 weeks.

B. Sofosbuvir plus simeprevir for 12 weeks.

C. Daclatasvir plus ASV for 24 weeks.

D. Ledipasvir/sofosbuvir for 24 weeks.

34. For which patient would treatment with ledipasvir/sofosbuvir for 24 weeks be most appropriate?

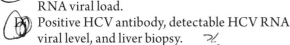

A. A 55-year-old patient with METAVIR score of F4 disease on lab tests who failed treatment with telaprevir, pegylated interferon, and ribavirin in 2012.

B. A 58-year-old patient with METAVIR score of F3 disease on lab tests who experienced treatment failure with pegylated interferon and ribavirin in 2003.

C. A 63-year-old patient with cirrhosis documented by liver biopsy in 2012 who is treatment-naïve.

D. A 68-year-old patient without documented cirrhosis who experienced treatment failure with sofosbuvir and ribavirin in 2014.

35. A 52-year-old treatment-experienced woman (weight 56 kg) with HCV GT 1a on dialysis presents to clinic requesting HCV treatment. She was a partial responder to HCV treatment with pegylated interferon and ribavirin in 2009. She is now awaiting a kidney transplant. Her laboratory values include CrCl 6 mL/minute and hemoglobin 10.1 mg/dL. Which one of the following would best manage this patient's HCV?

A. Start HCV treatment now with sofosbuvir 200 mg daily and simeprevir 75 mg daily for 12 weeks.

B. Start HCV treatment now with reduced-dose pegylated interferon and ribavirin 200 mg daily.

C. Treat the HCV as soon as patient is discharged after receiving her kidney transplant.

D. Wait until her CrCl is greater than 30 mL/minute after the kidney transplant before starting HCV treatment.

36. A 49-year-old patient with HCV GT 1a presents at week 4 of treatment with sofosbuvir plus pegylated interferon plus ribavirin. The patient's HCV RNA level was detected but less than 43 IU/mL. Which one of the following is best to recommend for this patient?

A. Check the HCV RNA level at treatment completion at week 12.

B. Check the viral level at week 8; if positive, discontinue all treatment at that time.

C. Discontinue treatment because the positive viral load indicates that the patient will not achieve SVR12.

D. Discontinue treatment because the detectable viral load indicates nonadherence.

37. A 57-year-old cirrhotic MSM has a medical history of HIV/HCV coinfection. He also has a continued history of methamphetamine use and unprotected sexual encounters. The patient was treated for HCV GT 1a, and had an undetectable HCV RNA upon completion of HCV treatment with sofosbuvir plus simeprevir for 12 weeks. He returns at 24 weeks after treatment and has a viral load of 3,275,000 IU/mL, and GT 3a. Which one of the following best explains this patient's viral load?

A. The patient's virus relapsed after HCV treatment.

B. The patient was re-infected after treatment completion.

C. The patient had a super-infection with GT 1a and GT 3 at baseline

D. The wrong GT was reported because of a laboratory error.

38. A 58-year-old man (weight 87 kg) has coinfection with HCV GT 1a and HIV. He also has a history of orthotopic liver transplantation (OLT) in May of 2009. His laboratory results include hemoglobin 11.9 mg/dL and platelets 75,000/mm³. His home drugs include abacavir 600 mg/lamivudine 300 mg daily, darunavir 800 mg daily, ritonavir 100 mg daily, amlodipine 10-mg oral tablet daily, docusate sodium 100-mg oral capsule twice a day, multivitamin daily, omeprazole 40-mg oral delayed release capsule daily, dapsone 100-mg inhalation once monthly, tacrolimus 3-mg oral capsule every 12 hours, and ursodiol 300-mg oral capsule three times daily. Which one of the following is best to recommend for this patient's HCV?

A. Sofosbuvir 400 mg daily plus pegylated interferon alfa-2a 180 mcg subcutaneously every week plus ribavirin 600 mg twice daily for 12 weeks.

B. Paritaprevir/ritonavir/ombitasvir (150 mg/100 mg/25 mg) daily plus dasabuvir 250 mg twice daily for 12 weeks.

C. Sofosbuvir 400 mg daily plus ribavirin 200 mg twice daily for 24 weeks.

D. Sofosbuvir 400 mg daily plus simeprevir 150 mg daily for 12 weeks.

39. Which one of the following patients would most require counseling on the importance of using two forms of contraception during the course of HCV treatment and for 6 months after completion of treatment?

A. A 29-year-old woman on sofosbuvir plus ribavirin.

B. A 47-year-old woman on sofosbuvir plus simeprevir.

C. A 53-year-old woman on sofosbuvir plus daclatasvir.

D. A 36-year-old woman on ledipasvir/sofosbuvir.

40. A 47-year-old woman with HCV GT 2 on treatment with sofosbuvir 400 mg daily and ribavirin 400 mg twice daily presents to the clinic after her week 4 blood draw. The HCV RNA virus level is 107 IU/mL. What one of the following is best to recommend for this patient?

A. Stop all HCV treatment because the HCV level is detectable.

B. Add simeprevir to the patient's regimen as rescue therapy.

C. Check HCV RNA level at week 8; discontinue all treatment if the patient still has a detectable viral level.

D. Continue HCV treatment for the full 12-week course.

Learner Chapter Evaluation: Hepatitis C.

As you take the posttest for this chapter, also evaluate the material's quality and usefulness, as well as the achievement of learning objectives. Rate each item using this 5-point scale:

- Strongly agree
- Agree
- Neutral
- Disagree
- Strongly disagree

20. The content of the chapter met my educational needs.
21. The content of the chapter satisfied my expectations.
22. The author presented the chapter content effectively.
23. The content of the chapter was relevant to my practice and presented at the appropriate depth and scope.
24. The content of the chapter was objective and balanced.
25. The content of the chapter is free of bias, promotion, or advertisement of commercial products.
26. The content of the chapter was useful to me.
27. The teaching and learning methods used in the chapter were effective.
28. The active learning methods used in the chapter were effective.
29. The learning assessment activities used in the chapter were effective.
30. The chapter was effective overall.

Use the 5-point scale to indicate whether this chapter prepared you to accomplish the following learning objectives:

31. Analyze recent trends in hepatitis C virus (HCV) transmission, diagnosis, and management.
32. Evaluate patient characteristics for appropriate timing of HCV treatment.
33. Devise a genotype-based treatment plan for treatment-naive HCV patients.
34. Construct a management strategy for the treatment of partial responders, nonresponders, and relapsers with HCV.
35. Design a plan to optimize HCV treatment outcomes in patients who are cirrhotic, posttransplant, or HIV coinfected.
36. Develop a monitoring plan for drug interactions and adverse events associated with HCV treatment.
37. Assess patients for clinical outcomes and HCV treatment response.
38. Please provide any specific comments relating to any perceptions of bias, promotion, or advertisement of commercial products.
39. Please expand on any of your above responses, and/or provide any additional comments regarding this chapter:

HIV Infection

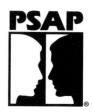

By Craig R. Ballard, Pharm.D., AAHIVP;
and Lucas Hill, Pharm.D., AAHIVP

Reviewed by Taylor K. Gill, Pharm.D., BCPS, AAHIVP; and Thomas J. Kleyn, Pharm.D., BCPS, AAHIVP

Learning Objectives

1. Evaluate patient characteristics to determine the optimal regimen for treatment-naive patients with HIV infection.
2. Apply available data in determining the use of new antiretrovirals in both treatment-experienced and treatment-naive patients with HIV infection.
3. Assess the appropriateness of HIV pre-exposure prophylaxis on an individual-patient basis
4. Assess the appropriateness of and design a regimen for HIV postexposure prophylaxis.
5. Design an appropriate treatment regimen for a patient presenting with transmitted HIV resistance or an antiretroviral-therapy-treatment-experienced patient.

6. Develop a monitoring plan for drug interactions and adverse events associated with HIV treatment.

Introduction

Epidemiology

As the AIDS epidemic continues to evolve, encouraging epidemiologic trends have emerged. Globally, 2012 saw 2.3 million new human immunodeficiency virus (HIV) infections, a 33% decline since 2001. Following a similar trend, the number of deaths from AIDS decreased from 2.3 (2.1–2.6) million in 2005 to 1.6 (1.4–1.9) million in 2012. That decrease in the number of deaths from AIDS has resulted in an increase in the number of people living with HIV infection, estimated at 35.3 (32.2–38.8) million (UNAIDS 2013).

Baseline Knowledge Statements

Readers of this chapter are presumed to be familiar with the following:
- Antiretroviral (ARV) medications, doses, common or significant adverse drug reactions, drug interactions and recommended monitoring parameters for U.S. Department of Health and Human Services recommended regimens for treatment-naive patients
- Identification of ARVs requiring dose adjustment for renal or hepatic insufficiency
- Criteria (CD4+ based) for initiation and discontinuation of both primary and secondary opportunistic infection prophylaxis (e.g., Pneumocystis jiroveci pneumonia, *Mycobacterium avium-intracellulare* complex, Cryptococcus meningitis, tuberculosis)

Additional Readings

The following free resources are available for readers wishing additional background information on this topic.
- CDC, NIH, HIVMA-IDSA. Guidelines for Prevention and Treatment of Opportunistic Infections in HIV-Infected Adults and Adolescents.
- Department of Health and Human Services. Panel on Antiretroviral Guidelines for Adults and Adolescents. Guidelines for the Use of Antiretroviral Agents in HIV-1-Infected Adults and Adolescents.
- U.S. Public Health Service. Preexposure prophylaxis for the prevention of HIV infection in the United States–2014. A clinical practice guideline.
- U.S. Public Health Service. Preexposure prophylaxis for the prevention of HIV infection in the United States–2014. Clinical Providers' Supplement.

The Centers for Disease Control and Prevention (CDC) estimates that 1.1 million people are living with HIV in the United States, with the incidence remaining stable at about 50,000 new infections annually (CDC 2013). The most recent CDC surveillance data indicates that men who have sex with men, African-Americans, Hispanics, and women of color continue to be at higher risk of the acquisition of HIV. Trends indicate that the number of people living with HIV will continue to increase with patients living longer, resulting in greater numbers of patients taking antiretrovirals (ARVs) for extended periods and highlighting the importance of management of adverse effects related to antiretroviral therapy (ART) as well as skilled treatment of experienced patients.

Transmission and Testing

The incidence of new HIV infections in the United States has remained relatively stable despite treatment and prevention efforts. The CDC's sexually-transmitted-infection (STI)-treatment guidelines recommend high-intensity behavioral counseling for all sexually active adolescents and adults at risk of STI/HIV infection. The counseling should focus on personal behavioral modifications that can reduce the risk of infection and should include evaluation and counseling regarding injection-drug, noninjection-drug, and alcohol abuse. It is recommended that all patients aged 13–64 years in health care settings be tested for HIV regardless of the presence of high-risk behavior, because early detection is essential for linkage to care that reduces the risk of HIV transmission (Workowski 2010).

Advancements in HIV Testing

In July 2012, the U.S. Food and Drug Administration (FDA) approved the first home HIV test (OraQuick In-Home HIV Test) for individuals 17 years or older. The cost is around $40 per kit. The kit provides results in 20 minutes and does not require sending a specimen to a laboratory. The manufacturer offers full online instructions on how to use the test. The user should not eat, drink, or use oral care products such as mouthwash, toothpaste, or whitening strips 30 minutes before the test. The test stick is swiped along the upper and lower gums, then inserted into the developer tube. If a line appears next to the C and no line appears next to the T, then the result is negative. If there are lines next to both the C and the T, then the result is positive. The home HIV test has been shown to be 99.98% specific. If the result is positive, it is recommended that follow-up laboratory testing be conducted (e.g., for the HIV RNA viral load). The in-home test may report a false-negative result if the person was infected within the previous 3 months.

Another advancement in HIV testing is the development of a fourth-generation immunoassay, approved by the FDA in 2010. In addition to antibody detection, this assay detects the p24 antigen, which becomes detectable before an antibody response and thereby allows for earlier detection of acute HIV infection (MMWR 2013).

Treatment as Prevention

Initiation of antiretroviral treatment of the infected person in a serodiscordant couple reduces the risk of transmission to the uninfected person. That prevention strategy, known as *treatment as prevention*, was evaluated in heterosexual contact in the HPTN 052 study; this multicontinent, randomized, controlled trial compared early versus delayed ART in patients with CD4$^+$ counts of 350–550 cells/mm^3 in a stable sexual relationship with a person who was not infected. Serodiscordant couples were assigned in a 1:1 ratio to either early or delayed receipt of ART; the early-therapy group received ART regardless of CD4$^+$ count, and the delayed-therapy group initiated therapy after either two consecutive CD4$^+$ measurements of 250 cells/mm^3 or less or after development of an illness related to AIDS. The primary prevention end point consisted of linked HIV transmission in the HIV-negative partner; the primary clinical end point was the earliest occurrence of pulmonary tuberculosis, severe bacterial infection, a WHO (World Health Organization) stage 4 event, or death. By the end of the study, 39 transmissions had been observed, with 28 of them virologically linked to the infected partner. Only one linked transmission occurred in the early-therapy group (hazard ratio [HR] 0.04; 95% confidence interval [CI], 0.01–0.27). The early-therapy group also had fewer clinical end points (HR 0.59; 95% CI, 0.4–0.88). This demonstrates that early initiation of ART reduces the rate of sexual transmission of HIV (Cohen 2011). The study was carried out in heterosexual couples, and the same benefit has yet to be demonstrated in men who have sex with men and in intravenous-drug users.

Other Considerations
Early Infection

Although 50,000 new HIV infections occur in the United States each year, very few people seek care or are diagnosed after being acutely infected (CDC 2012). The term *early HIV infection* describes both acute infection (defined as immediately after HIV infection and before seroconversion) and recent HIV infection (defined as within 6 months of initial infection). Early HIV infection is characterized by extremely high HIV replication rates resulting in high HIV serum viral loads (more than 1 million copies/mL) in the newly infected individual. The very high HIV serum load during the acute phase of HIV infection reflects HIV replication in reservoirs such as the genital tract, which makes the transmission of HIV more likely during this time.

The complete eradication of HIV by ART is not possible because of the viral reservoirs established during early infection. It has been shown that resting CD4 T cells carry integrated viral DNA in the genome of these host cells and that these cells are capable of producing replication-competent virus. These T cells tend to be memory cells and therefore are long lived; and they do not express viral antigens on their surface, which enables them to avoid recognition by the immune system. Studies have also demonstrated that ongoing HIV replication may continue in treated aviremic patients—typically, in lymphoid tissue. An important area of focus has been gut-associated lymphoid tissue (GALT) as a significant viral reservoir, with an overall higher HIV burden in GALT than in the blood of patients receiving treatment (Chun 2012). This understanding has led to research into various strategies for targeting those viral reservoirs.

Pharmacists working in the areas of HIV, infectious diseases, STI clinics, or primary care or in emergency departments need to be aware of the clinical presentation of acute retroviral infection. Acute HIV symptoms can be general or nonspecific and may be explained by other causes such as a viral syndrome or other sexually transmitted disease. Acute HIV infection is generally defined as a transient symptomatic illness that will begin days to weeks after HIV infection and that can last from a few days to several months. Acute HIV infection can also occur asymptomatically, although 75% of patients have mononucleosis-like syndromes that often include rash, fever, pharyngitis, and headache within 2–6 weeks of infection (Table 3-1).

To add to the difficulty of acute HIV diagnosis, HIV may mimic symptoms considered in the differential diagnosis (e.g., Epstein-Barr virus, cytomegalovirus, influenza, viral hepatitis, streptococcal infection, syphilis). If a patient presents with symptoms of an STI such as gonorrhea, chlamydia, or syphilis and is diagnosed and treated for that event, it is possible that what had been an acute HIV transmission event could be missed. If rapid testing for HIV gets completed at this time, it may result in a false negative because most HIV screening tests for the presence of antibodies, which may not be detectable for several weeks or longer after initial HIV exposure.

Detection of P24 antigen by the fourth-generation immunoassay can occur 14–20 days after infection; however, p24 detection can be transient based on immune

Table 3-1. Symptoms of Acute HIV Infection

Signs and symptoms	Incidence (%)
Fever	96
Adenopathy	74
Pharyngitis	70
Rash	70
Myalgia/arthralgia	54
Diarrhea	32
Headache	32
Nausea / vomiting	27

complex formation's interference with the assay (CDC 2014). An HIV RNA test could help in the diagnosis at this time, but it is unlikely that a general health care practitioner would check serum HIV RNA unless the patient discloses a high-risk encounter for acquisition of HIV. The serum HIV RNA test also adds cost to the visit, and the result may take several days to be obtained, which creates additional barriers to the early diagnosis of HIV. It is for those reasons that a complete sexual history should be obtained to be able to assess for risk of HIV exposure. It is critical to provide education for the patient together with instructions on monitoring for acute retroviral syndrome.

Sanctuary Sites

The HIV infection is a chronic infection because of its ability to remain in anatomic sanctuary sites or cellular reservoirs of virus in the body. Those latent reservoirs—thought to remain present in the brain, lymphoid tissue, bone marrow, and genital tract—allow HIV persistence and latency. Sanctuary sites create challenges for current ART because the available antiretroviral drugs do not distribute evenly throughout the body. It is highly probably that suboptimal concentrations in in the central nervous system (CNS), genital tract, or colorectal tissue (Table 3-2) allow active HIV replication and selection of resistant viral variants (Cory 2013; Cohen 2012).

One study examined paired semen/blood samples from 145 HIV-infected men on ART and showed that 6% of patients had detectable HIV RNA in semen but not in serum (Lambert-Niclot 2012). This is a concerning finding because it suggests that residual HIV RNA shedding can occur in the semen of patients with undetectable serum viral loads and increase the risk of HIV transmission. Discordant HIV replication and drug resistance have been observed between cerebral spinal fluid (CSF) and serum compartments, suggesting that HIV can replicate independently from virus in the blood compartment (Letendre 2011; Tashima 2002).

Table 3-2. Antiretroviral Drugs with Genital Tract Fluid and Tissue to Blood Plasma Ratio of 1 or Greater

	CVF	SP	Colorectal tissue
NRTI	Emtricitabine Lamivudine Tenofovir Zidovudine	Abacavir Emtricitabine Lamivudine Tenofovir Zidovudine	Emtricitabine Tenofovir
NNRTI	Etravirine	none	Etravirine
PI	Indinavir/r	Indinavir/r	Darunavir/r Ritonavir
CCR5 inhibitor	Maraviroc	none	Maraviroc
INSTI	Raltegravir	Raltegravir	Raltegravir

ᵃComparisons are tissue/blood (BP) paired samples. Genital tract exposure within 2 and 1 hour of dosing for women and men, respectively. Dolutegravir, elvitegravir/cobicistat, rilpivirine not included.
AUC = blood serum area under the curve; CVF = cervicovaginal fluid; SP = seminal plasma.
Information from Cohen MS, Muessig KE, Smith MK, et al. Antiviral agents and HIV prevention: controversies, conflicts, and consensus. AIDS 2012;26:1585-98.

Uncontrolled HIV replication and immune activation in CSF have been associated with neurobehavioral disturbances resulting from HIV-mediated neural damage (Letendre 2011). Those CNS disturbances can manifest as anxiety, depression, insomnia, mania, and psychosis. They can also manifest as HIV-associated neurocognitive disorder (HAND), three subgroups of CNS disturbances that are classified as asymptomatic neurocognitive impairment, mild neurocognitive disorder, and HIV-associated dementia. The HIV can persist in the CSF despite a suppressive systemic HIV serum viral load.

The ability of ART to suppress HIV RNA levels in the CSF may be limited by the ability of those drugs to cross the blood-brain barrier. If adequate antiretroviral drug levels are achieved in the CNS, leading to improved CNS HIV suppression, then it would be clinically relevant to monitor for improvement in neurocognitive performance. Studies that estimate the ability of antiretroviral drugs to penetrate into the CNS (Figure 3-1) and be used as CNS compartment-targeted ART, or CNS-T ART, have been attempted. One study assessed the association of the proportion of patients with detectable CSF HIV viral load and CNS penetration effectiveness (CPE) of the antiretroviral regimen. The study showed a significant benefit of achieving undetectable CSF HIV viral load associated with higher CPE (>7) of the ART regimen (Letendre 2011). A recent randomized controlled trial randomized study subjects 1:1 to CNS-T ART or non–CNS-T ART with a primary outcome of change in neurocognitive performance as measured by change in global deficit score from baseline to week 16. Unfortunately, the study was terminated early because of slow accrual and the low likelihood of detecting a difference in the primary outcome. No evidence of neurocognitive benefit for a CNS-T strategy in HIV-associated neurocognitive disorders was found, but the authors noted that a benefit for a subgroup or small overall benefits could not be excluded (Ellis 2014).

The pharmacist must be aware of HIV sanctuary sites and the limitations of current ART such as the variability in penetrating important target sites in the body. Although no study has definitively demonstrated improvements in neurocognitive function with higher-CPE drugs, many practitioners optimize the CPE of ART when a patient is identified with HAND. Further studies are needed to test strategies that would improve antiretroviral penetration into sanctuaries; these may involve (1) modification of drugs to enhance absorption and distribution characteristics, (2) blockade of drug metabolism or influx/efflux transporters, or (3) targeting specific sites such as the CNS (Cory 2013).

Resistance

Resistance to HIV drugs remains an important threat to long-term ART goals. The careful selection and monitoring of combination ART is crucial to prevent or delay of resistance and maintain the durability of the regimen. Combination ART delays the onset of drug resistance, but many patient and health system variables can cause suboptimal drug exposure (Osterberg 2012) and the selection of drug resistance, thereby leading to reduced drug efficacy and treatment failure. Resistance to one or more drugs in a regimen can lead to cross-resistance that can limit the activity of unused antiretroviral drugs and exhaust effective combination ART in a short time if issues of health literacy, adherence, individualized treatment selection, and monitoring of ART are not thoughtfully considered.

Transmitted drug resistance continues to be a clinical concern in the initial selection of ART. Genotypic resistance testing should be part of the initial workup once a patient tests positive for HIV. Transmission of drug-resistant HIV to any class of ART has been estimated at 18% in the United States, with mutations in the non-nucleoside reverse transcriptase inhibitor (NNRTI) class being the most common. A retrospective analysis was performed of serum samples taken before treatment initiation in four phase 3 studies from 2000 to 2013. That study showed a stable presence of transmitted nucleoside reverse transcriptase inhibitor (NRTI) resistance mutations; however, there were increases in transmitted NNRTI and PI resistance mutations across the study period. The study found little evidence of transmitted integrase strand transfer inhibitor (INSTI) resistance (Margot 2014).

Currently, HIV-drug-resistance testing is recommended at entry into care whether ART will be immediate or deferred; if deferred, repeat testing should be considered at the time of ART initiation. The HIV drug-resistance test most commonly used in baseline testing is a genotypic assay that detects mutations known to confer drug resistance in the reverse transcriptase and protease HIV genes. It is not standard practice to screen for mutations in the integrase gene; although this assay is commercially available, it adds to the cost of screening. Surveillance of future transmitted INSTI resistance is important because the use of INSTI-based initial ART will likely increase with the addition of four INSTI-based regimens to the U.S. Department of Health and Human Services (DHHS)-recommended list of regimens for ARV therapy-naive patients.

Although the overall U.S. rate of transmitted drug resistance is stable, there is concern about higher rates in some U.S. cities. HPTN 061 is a longitudinal cohort study of African-American men who have sex with men in Atlanta, Boston, Los Angeles, New York, San Francisco, and Washington. That cohort study found 23.1% of newly infected men in this population had drug-resistant HIV and 11.2% showed multiclass resistance. In three cities, the incidence of drug resistance exceeded 40%, and that did not include genotype testing for integrase mutations (Chen 2014).

As the use of INSTI-based therapy in both treatment-naive regimens and treatment-experienced regimens—including simplification strategies—increases, it will be important to maintain awareness of the potential for transmitted INSTI resistance to trend upward. Pharmacists involved in optimizing ART will see increased use of genotypic resistance assays that include the integrase gene.

TREATMENT

Treatment Initiation
Early Infection

Treatment of early infection has been controversial. Early treatment has been associated with the risks of toxicity from ART over a lifetime, and most patients have normal CD4+ cell counts after recovery from early HIV infection and remain asymptomatic for many years. Conversely, there are recognized benefits to treating early infection (Box 3-1, Box 3-2). The recent availability of

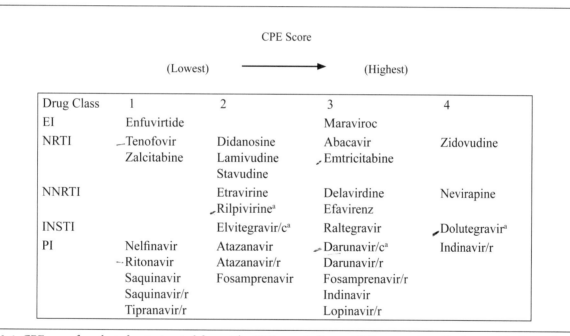

CPE Score

(Lowest) ⟶ (Highest)

Drug Class	1	2	3	4
EI	Enfuvirtide		Maraviroc	
NRTI	Tenofovir Zalcitabine	Didanosine Lamivudine Stavudine	Abacavir Emtricitabine	Zidovudine
NNRTI		Etravirine Rilpivirine[a]	Delavirdine Efavirenz	Nevirapine
INSTI		Elvitegravir/c[a]	Raltegravir	Dolutegravir[a]
PI	Nelfinavir Ritonavir Saquinavir Saquinavir/r Tipranavir/r	Atazanavir Atazanavir/r Fosamprenavir	Darunavir/c[a] Darunavir/r Fosamprenavir/r Indinavir Lopinavir/r	Indinavir/r

Figure 3-1. CPE score for selected antiretroviral drugs. The CPE score indicates CNS penetration effectiveness. The larger CPE score reflect estimates of better penetration or effectiveness in the CNS. ART regimens with combination CPE scores greater than 7 have been associated with lower CNS HIV viral loads compared with ART regimens with CPE Scores of 7 or less.

[a]Personal communication.

EI = Entry/fusion inhibitors; NRTI = nucleoside reverse transcriptase inhibitors; NNRTI = nonnucleoside reverse transcriptase inhibitors; INSTI = integrase strand transfer inhibitors; PI = protease inhibitors; /r = ritonavir boosted; /c = cobicistat boosted.

Information from Letendre S. Central nervous system complications in HIV disease: HIV associated neurocognitive disorder. Top Antivir Med 2011;19:137-42.

better-tolerated and easier-to-administer antiretroviral drugs leaves fewer reasons to argue against the treatment of early infection, and pharmacists should be aware of the evidence that supports early HIV treatment.

The identification of early HIV infection warrants genotypic drug-resistance testing before the initiation of ART, with the results guiding selection of the ART regimen. Use of the genotypic drug-resistance test in early HIV infection provides the optimal time to test for transmitted drug resistance. Initiation of ART with early HIV infection has been changed from "should be considered optional" (CIII) to "should be offered" (BII), although definitive data are lacking as to whether that approach will result in long-term virologic, immunologic, or clinical benefits for the individual patient. Some data suggest several potential benefits of ART during early HIV infection—including the public health benefit of decreased transmission rates—but there are risks associated with the initiation of chronic ART.

Multiple studies have supported the benefit of early HIV treatment. ACTG A5217 was an open-label trial that randomized patients within 6 months of HIV seroconversion to either 36 weeks of ART (immediate treatment) or no treatment (deferred treatment). The treatment arm used emtricitabine/tenofovir 200 mg/300 mg plus lopinavir/ritonavir 800 mg/200 mg. The primary end point was a composite of requiring treatment or retreatment and the $\log_{10}$ HIV-1 RNA level at week 72 (both groups) and week 36 (delayed-treatment group). The immediate-treatment group had a better outcome than the delayed-treatment group at week 72 (50% vs. 10%; p=0.005) and at week 36 (0% vs. 27.5%; p=0.002) (Hogan 2012). The Data and Safety Monitoring Board recommended stopping the study because further follow-up was unlikely to change those findings.

Another prospective observational study involved 468 patients (95% men) with early HIV infection. A total of 213 subjects initiated ART early, and a subset of 97 subjects initiated within 4 months of the estimated date of infection. The ART regimens were not specified, but 64% of patients treated early achieved the primary end point (CD4$^+$ greater than 900 cells/mm^3 during 48 months of observation) versus 34% of those treated later (p<0.001). The study concluded that initiating ART in the 4-month window after HIV-1 infection enhanced the likelihood of recovery of CD4$^+$ counts to 900 or more cells/mm^3 (Le 2013).

The open-label SPARTAC trial looked at short-course ART in adults with primary HIV infection. Patients were randomized to ART for 48 weeks, 12 weeks, or no ART (standard of care). Treatment was initiated within 6 months after seroconversion, and the primary end point was a CD4$^+$ less than 350 cells/mm^3 or long-term ART initiation. During a median follow-up of 4.2 years, only the 48-week treatment group demonstrated a delay to a CD4$^+$ less than 350 cells/mm^3, with 29% falling to that level versus 40% of the 12-week group and 39% of the no-ART group. Among study participants in the 48-week group, treatment starting closer to the estimated time of infection appeared to confer greater benefit (Fidler 2013).

Chronic HIV Infection

The rationale for ART is that viral suppression preserves and improves immune function in most patients regardless of baseline CD4$^+$ count. Recent data suggest that during chronic HIV infection, earlier initiation of ART results in better immunologic responses and clinical outcomes, including reductions in both AIDS- and non-AIDS-associated morbidity and mortality. There also is increasing evidence that earlier ART reduces HIV-associated inflammation and associated complications (McComsey 2014).

Studies such as NA-ACCORD and HPTN 052 provide supporting evidence to initiate ART earlier in chronic infection, and ART is now recommended for all HIV-infected individuals to reduce the risk of disease progression. The strength of evidence for that recommendation varies by pretreatment CD4$^+$ count, with the strongest evidence supporting treatment in asymptomatic persons with CD4$^+$ counts less than 500 cells/mm^3 and with expert opinion supporting treatment in asymptomatic persons with CD4$^+$ counts more than 500 cells/mm^3. Although the exact CD4$^+$

Box 3-1. Potential Benefits of Treating Early HIV Infection

- Improves laboratory markers of disease progression
  - Decrease viral replication
  - Increase CD4$^+$ cell counts
- Decrease severity of disease
- Lower viral set point
- Reduce size of viral reservoir
- Decrease rate of viral mutation by suppressing viral replication
  and preserving HIV-specific immune function
- Reduce profound loss of gastrointestinal lymphoid tissue (GALT)
  that occurs during first weeks of infection
- Reduce the risk of HIV transmission

Box 3-2. Potential Risks of Treating Early HIV Infection

- Drug toxicities (increased total time on medication)
- Development of ART resistance
- Poor adherence with chronic therapy
- Adverse effect on well-being and quality of life
- Premature use of ART before better/safer future options available
- Transmission of drug-resistant virus if virologic suppression not maintained
- Cost

---

count for initiation of therapy is not known, evidence points to starting at higher counts; and the current general recommendation is to treat everyone with chronic HIV infection unless a patient is unable to commit to treatment and fails to understand the benefits and risks of therapy, including the consequences of suboptimal adherence and selection of viral resistance. Patients may choose to postpone therapy and, in consultation with providers on a case-by-case basis, may defer therapy on the basis of clinical or psychosocial factors.

Earlier initiation of ART also is recommended for the prevention of transmission of HIV. That recommendation pertains to all HIV-infected pregnant women for the prevention of perinatal transmission and for all HIV-infected people at risk of transmitting HIV to sex partners. Earlier initiation of ART is also recommended for patients with AIDS-defining conditions, acute opportunistic infections, lower CD4[+] counts, HIV-associated nephropathy, early infection, hepatitis B virus, or hepatitis C virus coinfection, rapidly declining CD4[+] counts, or higher viral loads.

Determining the Optimal Treatment Regimen

As of May 2014, there are seven recommended DHHS initial regimens for ART-naive patients that have shown potent virological efficacy as measured by the proportion

of subjects achieving and maintaining viral suppression in comparative clinical trials. Each regimen has the strongest (AI) DHHS guidelines rating (Table 3-3). An additional three initial regimens are recommended but only for patients with pre-ART serum HIV RNA less than 100,000 copies/mL. Regimen selection for ART-naive patients should be individualized based on multiple variables such as a patient's comorbid conditions, potential adverse drug effects, known or potential drug interactions with other medications or supplements, pregnancy or pregnancy potential, results of genotypic drug-resistance testing, pretreatment viral load, sex, pretreatment CD4[+] count if considering nevirapine or rilpivirine, HLA-B*5701 testing (if considering abacavir), coreceptor tropism testing (if considering maraviroc), patient preferences and adherence potential, convenience, and insurance coverage.

The most significant change in the May 2014 DHHS guidelines was the inclusion of three additional INSTI-based regimens for a total of four INSTI-based regimens as recommended for initial treatment (see Table 3-3). The coformulated regimen of elvitegravir/cobicistat/ tenofovir/emtricitabine was changed from alternative INSTI status to the recommended category based on additional data through 144 weeks from two phase 3 studies. Two dolutegravir-based regimens were added to the

Table 3-3. DHHS Initial Recommended Regimens for the Antiretroviral-Naïve Patient[a,b]

Regardless of Pre-ART Plasma HIV RNA	
NNRTI based	• Efavirenz/tenofovir/emtricitabine[c,d,e] (AI)
PI based	• Atazanavir/ritonavir[i] + tenofovir/emtricitabine[d,e] (AI)
	• Darunavir/ritonavir (daily) + tenofovir/emtricitabine[d,e] (AI)
INSTI based	• Raltegravir + tenofovir/emtricitabine[d,e] (AI)
	• Elvitegravir/cobicistat/tenofovir/emtricitabine[e,f] (AI)
	• Dolutegravir (daily) + abacavir/lamivudine[d,g] (AI)
	• Dolutegravir (daily) + tenofovir/emtricitabine[d,e] (AI)

Only for Patients with Pre-ART serum HIV RNA less than 100,000 copies/mL	
NNRTI based	• Efavirenz[c] + abacavir/lamivudine[d,g]
	• Rilpivirine/tenofovir/emtricitabine[d,e,h]
PI based	• Atazanavir/ritonavir[i] + abacavir/lamivudine[d,g]

[a]Selection of a regimen should be individualized on the basis of virologic efficacy, toxicity, pill burden, dosing frequency, drug-drug interaction potential, resistance testing results, and comorbid conditions.

[b]Based on individual patient characteristics and needs, in some instances, an alternative or other regimen may be an optimal regimen for a specific patient.

[c]Consider alternative to efavirenz in women who plan to become pregnant or are not using effective contraception.

[d]Lamivudine can be used in place of emtricitabine and vice versa.

[e]Tenofovir: caution if renal insufficiency.

[f]Elvitegravir/cobicistat/tenofovir/emtricitabine should not be started if CrCl < 70 mL/minute.

[g]Abacavir should not be used in patients who test positive for HLA-B*5701.

[h]Only for patients with CD4[+] count >200 cells/mm[3] and HIV RNA viral load < 100,000 copies/mL

[i]Atazanavir/ritonavir should not be used in patients who take >20 mg omeprazole or equivalent proton pump inhibitor per day.

AI = highest DHHS guideline rating; ART = antiretroviral therapy.

list of recommended regimens in the DHHS guidelines only 2 months after FDA approval. In three phase 3 randomized, controlled trials, dolutegravir 50 mg once daily plus 2 NRTIs was compared with three DHHS guideline–designated recommended regimens.

NEW ANTIRETROVIRALS

Since 2011, three new antiretrovirals and one new boosting agent have been approved for the treatment of HIV. The antiretrovirals are two INSTIs (elvitegravir in August 2012, dolutegravir in August 2013) and one NNRTI (rilpivirine in May 2011). Cobicistat was approved in August 2012 as a boosting agent in the coformulated tablet of elvitegravir/cobicistat/emtricitabine/tenofovir and is now also available as a single agent. Those new agents introduce new options for once-daily single-tablet regimens as well as some unique resistance profiles compared with other agents in the same class.

Integrase Strand Transfer Inhibitors

Since approval of the first INSTI, raltegravir, in 2007, this class of antiretrovirals has received significant attention. The INSTIs are potent antiretrovirals with excellent efficacy and are very well tolerated. First-generation INSTIs raltegravir and elvitegravir are considered to have relatively low barriers to resistance, whereas the second-generation INSTI dolutegravir may have a higher barrier to resistance (Table 3-4).

Elvitegravir

Elvitegravir is available as a stand-alone agent and in a fixed-dose combination tablet containing elvitegravir/cobicistat/emtricitabine/tenofovir. Elvitegravir is currently the only integrase inhibitor that requires cytochrome P450 (CYP) 3A4 inhibition with a boosting agent to allow for once-daily dosing. The approval of elvitegravir in the fixed-dose combination was based on 48-week data from two studies in treatment-naive patients: studies 102 and 103. In study 102, patients were randomly assigned to receive elvitegravir/cobicistat/emtricitabine/tenofovir or efavirenz/emtricitabine/tenofovir once daily plus matching placebo, with a primary end point of HIV RNA less than 50 copies/mL at week 48. Patients had to have estimated glomerular filtration rates (GFRs) of at least 70 mL/minute. The results demonstrated noninferiority with 87.6% versus 84.1% of patients having HIV RNA less than 50 copies/mL in the elvitegravir/cobicistat/emtricitabine/

Table 3-4. Comparison of Integrase Inhibitors

Drug	Dosing	Advantages	Disadvantages
Dolutegravir	• Treatment naïve or experienced but integrase naïve: 50 mg daily • Integrase experienced: 50 mg twice daily • Treatment naïve with 3A4 inducers: 50 mg twice daily	• One pill once a day option • Once daily dosing in treatment naïve patients • Multiple clinical trials in treatment naïve and experienced patients • Well tolerated • Few drug interactions • High barrier to resistance	• Need for twice-daily dosing in integrase experienced patients • Need for twice-daily dosing when administered with CYP3A4 inducers such as efavirenz, rifampin, tipranavir/ritonavir • Limited clinical experience
Elvitegravir	150 mg daily	• One pill once a day option • Well tolerated	• Must be taken with food • Low barrier to resistance • Many drug interactions due to administration with boosting agent • Limited data in treatment experienced patients • Restrictions in renal impairment
Raltegravir	400 mg twice daily	• 5 years of clinical trial data available • Effective in treatment experienced and naïve patients • Few drug interactions • Well tolerated	• Twice-daily dosing • Low barrier to resistance

tenofovir arm versus the efavirenz/emtricitabine/tenofovir arm, respectively (difference 3.6%; 95% CI, -1.6% to 8.8%). Nausea was more common in the elvitegravir/cobicistat/emtricitabine/tenofovir arm, and dizziness, abnormal dreams, insomnia, and rash were more common in the efavirenz/emtricitabine/tenofovir arm. Serum creatinine increased more in the elvitegravir arm, with a median increase of 0.15 mg/dL and median decrease in GFR of 14.3 mL/minute, with most change occurring by week 2 (Sax 2012). More recently, 144-week data were reported, with 80.2% versus 75.3% in the elvitegravir arm versus the efavirenz arm maintaining viral suppression, respectively (difference 4.9%; 95% CI,-1.3% to 11.1%) (Wohl 2014). Resistance mutations were detected in 10 of 21 patients in the elvitegravir arm who were eligible for resistance testing, with 9 patients demonstrating integrase resistance and all 10 indicating NRTI resistance. Fourteen of 28 patients in the efavirenz arm demonstrated reverse transcriptase mutations. The median change in SCr at week 144 was 0.14 mg/dL in the elvitegravir arm versus 0.01 mg/dL in the efavirenz arm and was similar to week 48 results.

Study 103 was also a phase 3 noninferiority study that randomly assigned patients to receive elvitegravir/cobicistat/emtricitabine/tenofovir or atazanavir/ritonavir plus emtricitabine/tenofovir plus matching placebos. The primary end point was HIV RNA 50 copies or less per mL at 48 weeks with 12% noninferiority margin. A total of 708 patients were treated, with 89.5% in the elvitegravir arm and 86.8% in the atazanavir arm achieving the primary outcome (adjusted difference 3%; 95% CI, -1.9% to 7.8%). There were fewer increases in AST and ALT in the elvitegravir arm. Median change in estimated GFR (mL/minute) was -14.1 in the elvitegravir arm and -9.6 in the atazanavir/ritonavir arm (DeJesus 2012). Viral suppression was maintained at week 144 in 77.6% in the elvitegravir arm and in 74.6% in the atazanavir arm (difference 3.1%; 95% CI, -3.2% to 9.4%) (Clumeck 2014). Development of resistance failed in 8 patients in the elvitegravir arm versus 2 in the atazanavir/ritonavir arm, with only M184V/I present in the atazanavir/ritonavir arm. The safety findings were similar at weeks 48, 96, and 144, with effects on GFR seen around 2 to 4 weeks, plateauing around 18 to 24 weeks, and remaining stable through week 144.

Elvitegravir has also been approved as an individual agent in treatment-experienced patients when given with a ritonavir-boosted protease inhibitor and another antiretroviral agent. Once-daily elvitegravir was compared with twice-daily raltegravir when given with a ritonavir-boosted protease inhibitor and optimized background regimen in a prospective, randomized, double-dummy, noninferiority phase 3 study. Almost two-thirds of patients in the study had baseline mutations to two or more classes of agents. Through week 96, 52% and 53% maintained HIV RNAs less than 50 copies/mL in the elvitegravir and raltegravir arms, respectively. Through week 96, integrase resistance was detected in

6.6% of patients in the elvitegravir arm and in 7.4% in the raltegravir arm. Adherence to 90% or more of study drug was 78.3% for elvitegravir and 65.3% for raltegravir through week 96. Incidences of adverse events attributed to study drug were similar between the two arms, as was change in GFR because cobicistat was not administered in this study (Elion 2013). Elvitegravir has been approved for treatment-experienced patients at a dose of 85 mg once daily when given with atazanavir 300 mg/ritonavir 100 mg once daily or lopinavir 400 mg/ritonavir 100 mg twice daily. Elvitegravir should be dosed at 150 mg once daily when given in combination with darunavir 600 mg/ritonavir 100 mg twice daily, fosamprenavir 700 mg/ritonavir 100 mg twice daily, or tipranavir 500 mg/ritonavir 200 mg twice daily. It is not recommended to give elvitegravir with cobicistat-boosted protease inhibitors.

As the phase 3 studies demonstrated, the fixed-dose combination containing elvitegravir/cobicistat causes increases in SCr and decreases estimated CrCl because of inhibition of active tubular secretion of creatinine by cobicistat. It is recommended that if patients experience increases in SCr of more than 0.4 mg/dL from baseline, they should be evaluated for evidence of tubulopathy. The fixed-dose combination of elvitegravir/cobicistat/emtricitabine/tenofovir is recommended only for patients with baseline CrCl of more than 70 mL/minute, and therapy should be discontinued if CrCl falls below 50 mL/minute.

Elvitegravir/cobicistat/tenofovir/emtricitabine offers a one-pill, once-a-day option in treatment-naive patients; however, it must be taken with food. The once-daily dosing may provide advantage over the use of raltegravir, but the renal effects of the fixed-dose combination with cobicistat may limit its use in some patients. This medication has been demonstrated to be effective in treatment-experienced patients as well when given with a ritonavir-boosted protease inhibitor. It provides a once-daily integrase inhibitor option versus twice daily with raltegravir, but elvitegravir often will be required to be given with a twice-daily protease inhibitor in this patient population. Given the short half-life of elvitegravir (2.3 hours), boosting with cobicistat or ritonavir is required for once-daily dosing (Ramanathan 2011). Because cobicistat is a potent CYP3A4 and CYP2D6 inhibitor, the fixed-dose combination tablet can result in significant drug interactions with CYP3A4 and CYP2D6 substrates. However, cobicistat in the fixed-dose combination should not be considered an equivalent alternative to ritonavir for boosting of protease inhibitors or other CYP3A4 substrates. Last, elvitegravir does not provide any benefit over raltegravir in terms of resistance profile because both agents have relatively low barriers to resistance.

Dolutegravir
Approved in August 2013, dolutegravir is the newest INSTI and is considered second-generation based on its improved resistance profile. Dolutegravir is available as an individual agent as well as a fixed-dose combination including dolutegravir/abacavir/lamivudine. Dolutegravir

is approved for use in both treatment-naive and treatment-experienced patients. Approval in treatment-naive patients was based on 48-week results from three studies. SPRING-2 was a phase 3, randomized, double-blind, active-controlled noninferiority study in which treatment-naive adults were randomly assigned dolutegravir 50 mg daily or raltegravir 400 mg twice daily in combination with emtricitabine/tenofovir or abacavir/lamivudine. The primary end point was the proportion of patients with HIV RNA less than 50 copies/mL at 48 weeks with a 10% noninferiority margin. At 48 weeks, 88% of patients in the dolutegravir arm and 85% in the raltegravir arm had achieved HIV RNA of less than 50 copies/mL (adjusted difference 2.5%; 95% CI, -2.2 to 7.1). Patient $CD4^+$ counts increased by a median of 230 cells/mm^3 in each group. The most common adverse events were nausea, headache, nasopharyngitis, and diarrhea and were similar in frequency in both treatment arms. There were no treatment failures in the dolutegravir arm caused by treatment emergent integrase resistance, whereas in the raltegravir arm, 1 patient who experienced virologic failure (6%) developed integrase resistance and 4 patients (21%) developed NRTI resistance (Raffi 2013). More recently, 96-week data have been presented, with 81% and 76% in the dolutegravir and raltegravir arms, respectively, maintaining HIV RNA less than 50 copies/mL (adjusted difference 4.5%; 95% CI, -1.1 to 10) with median increases in $CD4^+$ count similar between the two groups (Raffi 2013). In the FDA snapshot analysis of patients with baseline viral load of more than 100,000 copies/mL, 78% in the dolutegravir arm and 63% in the raltegravir arm achieved HIV RNA less than 50 copies/mL (difference 15%; 95% CI, 3.5–26.8). There were no additional patients with treatment-emergent mutations after 48 weeks in either arm. Mean change in estimated CrCl in the dolutegravir arm was -19.6 mL/minute and -9.3 mL/minute in the raltegravir arm.

SINGLE was a randomized, double-blind, phase 3 study in which patients were randomized to receive dolutegravir 50 mg daily with abacavir/lamivudine or the fixed-dose combination of efavirenz/emtricitabine/tenofovir. The primary end point was the proportion of patients with HIV RNA less than 50 copies/mL at 48 weeks. Eighty-eight percent and 81% of patients in the dolutegravir and efavirenz arms, respectively, achieved HIV RNA less than 50 copies/mL (adjusted difference 7%; 95% CI, 2–12), demonstrating superiority of dolutegravir. The dolutegravir arm also demonstrated a greater increase in $CD4^+$ count (267 vs. 208 cells/mm^3, p<0.001). Ten percent of patients in the efavirenz arm and 2% in the dolutegravir arm discontinued treatment because of adverse events, with rash and psychiatric events more common in the efavirenz arm and insomnia more often reported in the dolutegravir arm. No patients in the dolutegravir arm demonstrated treatment-emergent mutations, whereas 4 patients in the efavirenz arm developed efavirenz-associated mutations and 1 patient a tenofovir-associated mutation.

FLAMINGO was an open-label, noninferiority study in which HIV-1 treatment-naive patients were randomized to receive dolutegravir 50 mg daily or darunavir 800 mg daily plus ritonavir 100 mg daily, given with investigator-selected emtricitabine/tenofovir or abacavir/lamivudine. The primary end point was the proportion of patients with HIV-1 RNA less than 50 copies/mL at week 48. This was a noninferiority study with a 12% noninferiority margin. At week 48, 90% of patients receiving dolutegravir and 83% of patients receiving darunavir had HIV RNA less than 50 copies/mL (adjusted difference 7.1%; 95% CI, 0.9–13.2), demonstrating superiority of dolutegravir (p=0.25). No treatment-emergent resistance mutations were detected in either group. Discontinuation because of adverse events contributed to differences in response rates, with 2% in the dolutegravir group and 4% in the darunavir group. Patients in the dolutegravir group also had significantly fewer low-density-lipoprotein values of grade 2 or higher (p=0.0001) (Clotet 2014).

Dolutegravir has also been studied in treatment-experienced patients. The SAILING study was a 48-week, phase 3, randomized, double-blind, active-controlled noninferiority study. Patients were eligible with two consecutive HIV RNA values of 400 copies/mL or more, resistance to two or more classes of antiretrovirals, and one or two fully active drugs for background therapy. Patients received either dolutegravir 50 mg daily or raltegravir 400 mg twice daily added to investigator-selected background therapy. The primary end point was proportion of patients with HIV RNA less than 50 copies/mL at 48 weeks, with noninferiority of 12%. The proportion of patients with treatment-emergent integrase inhibitor resistance was a secondary end point. Some 71% in the dolutegravir arm and 64% in the raltegravir arm had HIV RNAs less than 50 copies/mL at 48 weeks (adjusted difference 7.4%; 95% CI, 0.7–14.2) demonstrating superiority of dolutegravir, with protocol-defined failure occurring earlier and more often in the raltegravir arm (6% vs. 12%). Four patients in the dolutegravir arm and 17 patients in the raltegravir arm demonstrated treatment-emergent integrase inhibitor resistance (adjusted difference -3.7%; 95% CI, -6.1 to -1.2; p=0.003); however, none of the integrase resistant mutations in the dolutegravir arm conferred phenotypic resistance to dolutegravir or raltegravir. Significantly more patients in the raltegravir arm developed resistance to their background regimens (3% vs. 1%). Adverse events were similar between the two treatment arms (Cahn 2013).

The VIKING-3 study was a single-arm, open-label phase 3 study in which treatment-experienced patients with integrase inhibitor resistance received dolutegravir 50 mg twice daily for 7 days while continuing the failing regimen without raltegravir or elvitegravir. Patient regimens were then optimized to one or more fully active drugs plus dolutegravir. The primary end points were the mean change from baseline in HIV RNA at day 8 and the proportion of patients with HIV RNAs less than 50 copies/

mL at week 24. At day 8, the mean change in HIV RNA was $-1.43 \log_{10}$ copies/mL, and 69% of patients had HIV RNAs less than 50 copies/mL at week 24. The presence of a Q148 mutation with at least two other integrase-resistance-associated mutations resulted in the most-reduced response (11% of patients at baseline) and decreased by 96% the likelihood of achieving HIV RNA less than 50 copies/mL at 24 weeks. Some 24% of patients with Q148 mutations and at least two other integrase-associated mutations achieved HIV RNAs less than 50 copies/mL at 24 weeks versus 58% for patients with Q148 and one additional integrase mutation and 79% for patients with no Q148 mutation (Castagna 2014).

In summary, dolutegravir is well tolerated and has an improved resistance profile compared with first-generation INSTIs. The SAILING study, although a noninferiority study, demonstrated superiority of dolutegravir over raltegravir in treatment-experienced patients; and for many treatment-experienced but integrase-naive patients, dolutegravir is a once-daily, potent antiretroviral. Table 3-4 compares available integrase inhibitors.

Non-nucleoside Reverse Transcriptase Inhibitors
Etravirine

Second-generation NNRTIs were developed to overcome resistance that often developed from first-generation NNRTIs. That resistance included the selection of K103N mutation, conferring complete loss of activity. Second-generation NNRTIs retain activity against first-generation NNRTI resistance. Etravirine is a second-generation NNRTI that is approved for use in treatment-experienced patients at a dose of 200 mg twice daily with food. Etravirine can be used as part of a potent salvage regimen in combination with darunavir/ritonavir and an integrase inhibitor in patients with NRTI and NNRTI resistance mutations. Although the agent is not new, recent studies have demonstrated that etravirine pharmacokinetics support the use of a dose of 400 mg once daily.

The Monetra study was an open-label pilot study that switched treatment-experienced patients who were stable on twice-daily etravirine to once-daily etravirine. A total of 24 patients were enrolled, and the on-treatment analysis showed rates of viral suppression of 95% at week 24 and

---

Pivotal Study that May Change Practice

Walmsley SL, Antela A, Glumeck N, et al. Dolutegravir plus abacavir-lamivudine for the treatment of HIV-1 infection. N Engl J Med 2013;369(19):1807-18.

Setting: SINGLE examined the effectiveness of dolutegravir, the first second-generation integrase inhibitor, in comparison with efavirenz in treatment-naïve patients. Efavirenz has been the standard comparator in many treatment-naïve studies as its coformulation as a one-pill once-daily regimen provides

Design: Patients were eligible if they were 18 years of age or older, had not previously received ART, had a plasma HIV RNA greater than 1000 copies/mL and negative for HLA-B*5701 allele. Patients were randomly assigned to receive dolutegravir 50 mg with abacavir/lamivudine or

Outcomes: 414 patients were randomized to the dolutegravir arm and 419 patients to the efavirenz arm. At week 48, 88% of patients in the dolutegravir arm and 81% in the efavirenz arm had plasma HIV RNA less than 50 copies/mL with an adjusted treatment difference of 7% (95% CI 2 to 12) demonstrating superiority of dolutegravir (p=0.003). Overall difference in response was due primarily to discontinuations because of adverse events (2% in the dolutegravir group and 10% in the efavirenz group) in the intention to treat analysis. Treatment difference was maintained despite stratification of baseline viral load, race, sex, and age. The median time to viral suppression was 28 days in the dolutegravir group

IMPACT: This study demonstrates superiority of dolutegravir compared to efavirenz when combined with two NRTIs in treatment-naïve patients, and is the first time superiority has been demonstrated over efavirenz. The difference in response rate was primarily due to improved

an excellent option in treatment-naïve patients. However treatment with efavirenz can be limited by the presence of baseline resistance, a low barrier to resistance, and neuropsychological adverse effects.

efavirenz/emtricitabine/tenofovir with matching placebos. The primary efficacy endpoint was the proportion of patients with plasma HIV RNA less than 50 copies/ml at week 48. Secondary outcomes included the time to viral suppression and the change from baseline CD4+ T-cell count.

and 84 days in the efavirenz group (p<0.001). The adjusted mean change from baseline in CD4+ T-cell count was 267 in the dolutegravir group versus 208 in the efavirenz group (p<0.001). Grade 3 or 4 adverse events were reported in 10% of patient in the dolutegravir group and 16% in the efavirenz group with rash and neuropsychiatric events significantly more common with efavirenz and insomnia more common with dolutegravir. 4% of patients in each group met the definition of virologic failure. No major NRTI or integrase inhibitor mutations were found in the dolutegravir group, and in the efavirenz group there was 1 patient with tenofovir resistance and 4 with NNRTI resistance.

tolerability of dolutegravir. Dolutegravir in combination with abacavir/lamivudine provides an excellent regimen that is very well tolerated with a high barrier to resistance for treatment-naïve patients.

Cahn P, Pozniak AL, Mingrone H, et al. **Dolutegravir versus raltegravir in antiretroviral-experienced, integrase-inhibitor-naïve adults with HIV: week 48 results from the randomised, double-blind, non-inferiority SAILING study.** Lancet 2013;382(9893):700-8.

Setting: SAILING examined the effectiveness of dolutegravir, the first second-generation integrase inhibitor, in comparison with raltegravir. Raltegravir has been an excellent option in salvage regimens and treatment-experienced patients. However, raltegravir does have limitations in twice daily dosing and a low barrier to resistance.

Design: Patients were eligible if they had two consecutive HIV RNA values of 400 copies per mL or higher (unless greater than 1000 copies per mL at screening), resistance to two or more classes of antiretroviral drugs, and had one to two fully active drugs for background therapy. 354 patients were randomized to receive dolutegravir 50 mg daily and 361 received raltegravir twice daily with matching placebo plus investigator-selected background regimen. The primary end point was the proportion of patients with HIV RNA less than 50 copies per mL at week 48, with a non-inferiority margin of 12%. A secondary end point was the proportion of patients with treatment-emergent integrase-inhibitor resistance.

Outcomes: At week 48, 251 (71%) of patients on dolutegravir and 230 (64%) or patients on raltegravir had HIV RNA less than 50 copies per mL (adjusted difference 7.4%; 95% CI 0.7 to 14.2). This demonstrated superiority of dolutegravir versus raltegravir (p=0.03). CD4 counts increased in both groups with a mean change of 162 cells per microliter in the dolutegravir arm and 153 cells per microliter in the raltegravir arm. Four patients (1%) in the dolutegravir arm and 17 patients (5%) in the raltegravir arm developed treatment emergent integrase-inhibitor resistance (adjusted difference -3.7%; 95% CI -6.1 to -1.2; p=0.003), with protocol defined virologic failure occurring earlier and more frequently in the raltegravir arm (12% versus 6% by week 48). However these four mutations in the dolutegravir arm did not confer phenotypic resistance to dolutegravir or raltegravir. 12 patients in the raltegravir arm (3%) and 4 patients in the dolutegravir arm (1%) had treatment-emergent resistance to their background regimen at week 48. Adverse event frequency was similar among both groups.

IMPACT: This study demonstrates the superiority of dolutegravir compared to raltegravir in treatment-experienced patients. This drug has a high barrier to resistance with no patients in this study taking dolutegravir developing phenotypic resistance to dolutegravir or raltegravir. Very few patients with virologic failure develop resistance to their background regimen when taking dolutegravir as well. Dolutegravir is an excellent option for treatment-experienced patients on a salvage regimen as it is well tolerated with once-daily dosing in integrase-naïve patients.

85% at week 48, with two of the three virological failures having baseline resistance to etravirine. The median C_{24} trough was 100 times higher than the EC50, or concentration of drug that gives half-maximal response, for wild-type HIV (Schneider 2012). This small trial demonstrated the efficacy of once-daily etravirine in treatment-experienced patients who are susceptible to etravirine.

The data are supported by the SENSE trial, in which once-daily etravirine was shown to be noninferior to efavirenz in treatment-naive patients, with significantly fewer neuropsychiatric adverse events (Gazzard 2011). With a favorable metabolic profile compared with profiles of protease inhibitors, etravirine provides an excellent option in the management of treatment-experienced patients.

Rilpivirine

Rilpivirine is a new second-generation NNRTI. It was approved in May 2011 as a single agent and as coformulated emtricitabine/rilpivirine/tenofovir, a once-daily ART regimen; it must be taken with food. Rilpivirine was approved for treatment-naive patients based on the results of two phase 3 trials (ECHO and THRIVE) for which there are now 96-week data (Cohen 2013). Patients were randomized to receive either rilpivirine 25 mg daily or efavirenz 600 mg daily along with an NRTI backbone with a noninferiority margin of 12% at week 48. The response rate at week 96 was 78% in both groups, but there were more virologic failures in the rilpivirine arm in patients with less than 95% adherence or baseline viral loads greater than 100,000/mL. Data were similar at week 48, and therefore rilpivirine should be used with caution in patients with baseline viral loads more than 100,000 copies/mL or CD4+ counts less than 200 cell/mm³. When compared with efavirenz, rilpivirine had fewer discontinuations because of adverse events (4% vs. 9%), grades 2–4 adverse events (17% vs. 33%), rash (4% vs. 15%), dizziness (8% vs. 27%), abnormal dreams/nightmares (8% vs. 13%), and grades 2–4 lipid abnormalities.

Emtricitabine/rilpivirine/tenofovir provides a very well-tolerated fixed-dose-combination option for patients who are treatment naive, because it is generally better tolerated than the fixed-dose combination containing efavirenz. Rilpivirine also plays a role in patients who are treatment experienced because it maintains activity in patients who have developed single resistance mutations to first-generation NNRTIs that typically confer cross-resistance on all first-generation NNRTIs. Patients who are stable and virologically suppressed on the single-tablet regimen of efavirenz/emtricitabine/tenofovir can safely be switched to the rilpivirine-containing single-tablet regimen and maintain virologic suppression (Mills 2013). Rilpivirine also is not a potent inhibitor or inducer of CYP enzymes and therefore is a useful option to avoid drug interactions.

The benefits of rilpivirine must be weighed against certain barriers to use, including a food requirement (it should be administered with at least 400 calories of solid food). Rilpivirine must be avoided with proton pump inhibitors and administered at least 4 hours before or 12 hours after H_2-receptor antagonists. Rilpivirine is associated with decreased efficacy at high HIV viral loads and low CD4$^+$ counts.

Boosting Agents
Cobicistat

Cobicistat is considered a pharmacokinetic enhancer that has no antiretroviral activity. In the fixed-dose combination tablet elvitegravir/cobicistat/emtricitabine/tenofovir the presence of cobicistat and its CYP3A4 inhibition allows for once-daily dosing of elvitegravir. As an individual agent, cobicistat is used to boost atazanavir 300 mg once daily or darunavir 800 mg once daily. A potential benefit of cobicistat is that it can be used as a pharmacokinetic enhancer in place of ritonavir because it is more selective for CYP3A4 inhibition and has fewer induction effects; this could lead to more-predictable drug interactions. Cobicistat does inhibit renal tubular secretion of creatinine and therefore causes increases in SCr but does not affect actual renal glomerular function (German 2012). It is not recommended to coadminister cobicistat with tenofovir disoproxil fumarate in patients who have estimated CrCl less than 70 mL/minute.

Cobicistat has been studied in combination with darunavir and atazanavir in place of ritonavir. In a 48-week randomized, double-blind, double-dummy, active-controlled trial, treatment-naive patients were randomized to receive either cobicistat or ritonavir in combination with atazanavir and emtricitabine/tenofovir. At week 48, 85.2% of patients in the cobicistat group and 87.4% of patients in the ritonavir group had HIV viral loads less than 50 copies/mL, demonstrating noninferiority of cobicistat (Gallant 2013). Those results were confirmed in patients with high baseline viral loads. The rates of serious adverse events and discontinuations because of adverse events were similar between the two arms, and the median SCr increase in the cobicistat group was 0.13 mg/dL versus 0.09 mg/dL in the ritonavir arm. As mentioned earlier, cobicistat has been approved as an individual boosting agent and will soon be available as a coformulated tablet with atazanavir and darunavir, thereby helping reduce pill burden. Cobicistat is not recommended for use as a boosting agent with twice-daily darunavir.

COINFECTION MANAGEMENT
Hepatitis C

A primary consideration in the treatment of hepatitis C in patients coinfected with HIV is drug interaction between antiretrovirals and direct-acting antivirals used in treating hepatitis C. Sofosbuvir, the first nucleoside NS5B inhibitor, has very few drug interactions and is compatible with all antiretrovirals except tipranavir/ritonavir because of P-glycoprotein (P-gp) induction. Sofosbuvir is neither a significant inhibitor nor significant inducer of hepatic or intestinal enzymes. Simeprevir, a second-generation NS3/4A protease inhibitor, is a CYP3A substrate and intestinal CYP3A4 inhibitor, an organic anion transport protein (OATP), and a P-gp inhibitor. Simeprevir, therefore, should not be administered with any ART regimen containing cobicistat, efavirenz, delavirdine, nevirapine, etravirine, or protease inhibitors. That leaves regimens composed of NRTIs, raltegravir, dolutegravir, rilpivirine, maraviroc, and enfuvirtide.

Asunaprevir is another protease inhibitor that will likely be approved in 2015. It is metabolized by CYP3A4 and is a substrate of P-gp and OATP1B1. Asunaprevir is a weak inducer of CYP3A4 and P-gp and a moderate inhibitor of CYP2D6 (Eley 2013). Although data regarding drug interactions with antiretrovirals are limited, drug interactions will likely exist with protease-inhibitor-based antiretroviral regimens because it is a CYP3A4 substrate.

Ledipasvir, the first NS5A inhibitor, was recently approved (in fixed-dose combination with sofosbuvir); and daclatasvir will likely become available soon. Daclatasvir likely will be compatible with various ARV regimens using dose adjustments for daclatasvir. Ledipasvir has been studied with ARV regimens containing emtricitabine/tenofovir with efavirenz, rilpivirine, and raltegravir (Osinusi 2014). Ledipasvir is not a CYP inhibitor or inducer and is a weak inhibitor of P-gp, breast cancer resistance protein, OATP1B1, and OATP1B3 (Kiser 2013). Ledipasvir is minimally metabolized and eliminated primarily in the feces and has minimal drug interactions (Kirby 2013). It is recommended to monitor for increases in tenofovir-related adverse effects when ledipasvir is given with efavirenz/emtricitabine/tenofovir. Similarly, increases in tenofovir exposure are expected when ledipasvir is given in combination with regimens containing tenofovir and ritonavir-boosted protease inhibitors; considering an alternative ARV regimen or careful monitoring is recommended. Ledipasvir has not been studied with elvitegravir/cobicistat/emtricitabine/tenofovir, and coadministration is not recommended. Despite those considerations, ledipasvir is compatible with a variety of ARV regimens and generally has more-manageable drug interactions with ARVs than the hepatitis C virus protease inhibitor class does.

Lastly, it is expected that a three-drug hepatitis C regimen will become available by the end of 2014 that contains a protease inhibitor (ABT450) boosted with 100 mg of ritonavir daily; an NS5A inhibitor (ombitasvir); and a non-nucleoside NS5B polymerase inhibitor (dasabuvir) given with or without ribavirin. Although drug interaction data for this regimen are limited, the regimen does contain ritonavir 100 mg daily, and therefore it can be expected that the known drug interactions between ritonavir and other antiretrovirals will apply.

Pre-exposure Prophylaxis

In July 2012, a combination tablet of emtricitabine/tenofovir received label approval by the FDA as pre-exposure prophylaxis (PrEP) for sexually active adults at risk of HIV infection, which represents the first time ARVs received approval for use in patients without HIV infection. The approval for that indication was based on the results of several studies, the largest of which was the iPrEx study, which included 2499 HIV-seronegative men or transgender women who have sex with men. The patients were randomized to receive emtricitabine/tenofovir or placebo daily. All patients received HIV testing, risk reduction counseling, condoms, and management of STIs. During a median of 1.2-year and maximum of 2.8-year follow-up, 100 patients became infected with HIV—36 in the emtricitabine/tenofovir group and 64 in the placebo group—indicating a 44% relative risk reduction in the incidence of HIV (95% CI, 15–63; p=0.005). Study drug was detected in 51% of patients who were seronegative and 9% of patients who were HIV infected (p<0.001). Similar rates of adverse events were seen in both groups. No emtricitabine or tenofovir resistance was detected in patients who were newly infected (Grant 2010).

Two studies have also been conducted in heterosexual patients. The TDF2 study was conducted in Botswana, where 1219 HIV-seronegative men and women (45.7% women) were randomized to receive emtricitabine/tenofovir or placebo once daily. Patients were visited monthly and given prevention services, including HIV testing, counseling on adherence, management of STIs, monitoring for adverse events, and counseling on risk reduction. Serious adverse events were similar, but the treatment group did have higher rates of nausea, vomiting, and dizziness. In the modified intent-to-treat analysis, 33 patients became infected during the study—9 in the treatment group and 24 in the placebo group—with a prevention efficacy of 62.2% (95% CI, 21.5%–83%; p=0.03). The only detected resistance to study drug was in a patient who had had an unrecognized acute infection at baseline. Two of 4 patients tested in the treatment group had detectable drug levels, whereas 80% of the 69 patients tested who did not undergo seroconversion had detectable drug levels (Thigpen 2012). Of note, a sample of patients were followed for bone mineral density, and patients in the treatment arm had significantly greater decline in T-scores and Z-scores.

The Partners PrEP study enrolled HIV-1 serodiscordant couples from Kenya and Uganda; seronegative partners were randomized to either tenofovir, emtricitabine/

tenofovir, or placebo (Baeten 2012). Eighty-two infections occurred during the study (7 in the tenofovir group, 13 in the emtricitabine/tenofovir group, 52 in the placebo group), indicating a relative reduction in the incidence of HIV of 67% with tenofovir and 75% with emtricitabine/tenofovir. Eight patients receiving treatment were found to have had HIV infection at baseline, and 2 developed resistance. No patients who were infected during the study had detected resistance. Of the 29 patients in the treatment groups that were infected, 31% had detectable tenofovir levels versus 82% in the control group who did not acquire HIV.

Two studies in women found no significant reduction in HIV incidence with the use of PrEP. The FEM-PrEP randomized, double-blind, placebo-controlled trial enrolled 2120 HIV-negative women in Kenya, South Africa, and Tanzania; the women were randomized to receive emtricitabine/tenofovir or placebo once daily. HIV infections occurred in 33 of the patients in the treatment group and 35 in the placebo group. A significantly higher proportion of patients in the treatment group experienced nausea, vomiting, or elevated aminotransferase levels. However, less than 40% of HIV-uninfected women in the treatment group had evidence of recent pill use at the visits that matched with HIV infection for the patients who seroconverted (Damme 2012).

The VOICE trail was a double-blind, placebo-controlled trial in which HIV-negative women were randomized to receive tenofovir, emtricitabine/tenofovir, tenofovir gel, or placebo daily. Incidence rates per 100 person-years were 6.3 for tenofovir versus 4.2 for placebo, 4.7 for emtricitabine/tenofovir versus 4.6 for placebo, and 5.9 for tenofovir gel versus 6.8 for placebo, thus showing no benefit. Tenofovir was detected in serum in 30% of patients receiving tenofovir, 29% of patients receiving emtricitabine/tenofovir, and 25% of patients receiving tenofovir gel (Marazzo 2013). These results contradict evidence found in other patient populations and are thought to be attributed to poor adherence.

Pre-exposure prophylaxis with emtricitabine/tenofovir appears to be effective in reducing the incidence of HIV in both homosexual and heterosexual patients at risk of acquiring HIV. However, the literature indicates that the success of PrEP is closely tied to adherence. Although serious adverse events were similar between treatment groups and placebo, studies demonstrated increased adverse effects of nausea and vomiting, which may affect adherence. Decreases in bone mineral density must be considered as potential adverse effects of PrEP containing tenofovir. The development of resistance does not seem to be a concern in patients who acquire HIV infection while taking PrEP. However, care must be taken to ensure patients have negative HIV tests within 1 week of starting PrEP before exposing them to emtricitabine/tenofovir, because of the potential for resistance to develop in patients already HIV infected. It is also recommended that patients be tested for HIV every 3 months while taking PrEP.

Postexposure Prophylaxis

Occupational

Use of ART as occupational postexposure prophylaxis (PEP) was introduced in the 1990 CDC guidelines. In 2013, the U.S. Public Health Service updated PEP guidelines, replacing the 2005 guidelines. The updated guidelines reflect the many ARVs approved since 2005 and recommend HIV PEP regimens that are better tolerated and that facilitate improved adherence. Specifically, the new guidelines (1) eliminate the recommendation to assess the level of risk associated with individual exposures to determine the number of drugs recommended for PEP, (2) modify and expand the list of ARV drugs that can be considered for use as PEP, and (3) offer an option for concluding HIV follow-up testing of exposed personnel sooner than 6 months after exposure (Kuhar 2013).

The preferred HIV PEP regimen is now the use of emtricitabine/tenofovir and raltegravir. Alternative regimens are recommended (Table 3-5), as are alternative antiretroviral drugs that should be used only with expert consultation and that include abacavir, efavirenz, enfuvirtide, fosamprenavir, maraviroc, saquinavir, and stavudine. Antiretroviral agents that are not recommended or are considered contraindicated include didanosine, nelfinavir, tipranavir, and nevirapine.

The duration of treatment with PEP is 28 days and should be discontinued early only if (1) the source individual is shown to be HIV negative; (2) the exposed individual is found to be HIV positive; (3) the adverse effects of PEP therapy are intolerable, resulting in suboptimal adherence and no other alternative treatment is available; and (4) the exposed individual has reevaluated the benefits and risks of PEP therapy and decides to discontinue therapy. Those reasons also apply to nonoccupational postexposure prophylaxis (nPEP) cases.

Nonoccupational Postexposure Prophylaxis

The use of nPEP is one of many strategies for preventing new HIV infections; it involves the use of ART immediately (within 72 hours) after exposure to HIV to prevent infection. Nonoccupational postexposure prophylaxis is considered when an individual is potentially exposed to HIV outside the workplace (e.g., sexual assault, episodes of unprotected sex, needle-sharing injection-drug use). No randomized clinical trials have assessed the efficacy of nPEP. Recommendations have been based on animal studies, human work on occupational PEP, mother-to-child-transmission studies, ongoing treatment of chronic established HIV infection, and, more recently, prospective human trials in serodiscordant couples. However, similar guidelines in the management of occupational exposures to HIV can be applied to guide treatment choices for nPEP cases (Figure 3-2, Figure 3-3).

Nonoccupational postexposure prophylaxis should be used only for infrequent, unanticipated exposures and is not a substitute for risk reduction behaviors. Use of nPEP does not completely eliminate the risk of HIV infection,

Table 3-5. HIV Postexposure prophylaxis (PEP) regimens

Preferred Regimen	
Tenofovir/emtricitabine 1 tab PO daily plus raltegravir 400 mg PO BID	
Alternative Regimens	
Column A[a]	Column B[b]
Raltegravir 400 mg PO BID	(Tenofovir + lamivudine) or (zidovudine + lamivudine or emtricitabine)
Darunavir 800 mg PO daily + Ritonavir 100mg PO daily	Tenofovir/emtricitabine or (tenofovir + lamivudine) or (zidovudine + lamivudine or emtricitabine)
Atazanavir 300 mg PO daily + Ritonavir 100 mg PO daily	Tenofovir/emtricitabine or (Tenofovir + lamivudine) or (zidovudine + lamivudine or emtricitabine)
Lopinavir/ritonavir 2 tabs PO BID	Tenofovir/emtricitabine or (Tenofovir + lamivudine) or (zidovudine + lamivudine or emtricitabine)
Etravirine 200 mg PO BID	Tenofovir/emtricitabine or (Tenofovir + lamivudine) or (zidovudine + lamivudine or emtricitabine)
Rilpivirine 25 mg PO daily	Tenofovir/emtricitabine or (Tenofovir + lamivudine) or (zidovudine + lamivudine or emtricitabine)

[a]May combine 1 drug or drug pair from Column A and 1 pair of nucleoside/nucleotide reverse transcriptase inhibitors from Column B.
[b]Another alternative for PEP is a fixed-dose combination regimen elvitegravir/cobicistat/emtricitabine/tenofovir1 tab daily

Adapted from U.S. Public Health Service. PHS Guideline for Reducing Human Immunodeficiency Virus, Hepatitis B Virus, and Hepatitis C Virus Transmission Through Organ Transplantation Guidelines for Occupational Exposures to HIV. Public Health Reports 2013;128;247-353.

and extensive harm- or risk-reduction counseling should be attempted for individuals whose behaviors result in frequent, recurrent exposures to HIV (e.g., people who have HIV-infected sex partners and rarely use condoms, injection drug users who share equipment) (Box 3-3). These individuals could also be considered for PrEP if they are willing to take medication that reduces the chance of HIV infection.

The use of nPEP can be expensive, with many 28-day treatment courses costing more than $2000. Many of the patients who present to emergency departments for nPEP do not have medical insurance or are underinsured. Pharmacists may become involved in developing a mechanism to assist patients in occupational PEP and nPEP programs. At the University of California, San Diego, Medical Center, pharmacists in the Medication Error Reduction Program, emergency department, and HIV clinic collaborated on a multidisciplinary project with the emergency department, the occupational medicine department, and the HIV clinic to update and improve access to ART for health care workers and patients with potential HIV exposure (see Figure 3-2, Figure 3-3). The use of patient assistance programs has helped provide ART for nPEP patients with no medication coverage (Box 3-4).

Conclusion

Advances in the treatment of HIV infection have dramatically changed the course of HIV disease. Current HIV treatment regimens are simpler so as to better assist with adherence while improving efficacy and safety. Multiclass combination single-tablet regimens are available for non-nucleoside and integrase-strand-transfer-inhibitor-based regimens. Future treatment will include single-tablet regimens for protease-inhibitor-based regimens. Progress continues in the discovery of strategies for preventing transmission of HIV to uninfected individuals through the use of preprophylaxis, postexposure prophylaxis, and

---

Box 3-3. Factors that Increase the Risk of HIV Transmission

- High serum viral load (a high HIV viral load when seroconverting or with advanced untreated disease)
- Sexually transmissible infection(s) in the source or exposed individual, especially genital ulcer disease and symptomatic gonococcal infections
- Breach in genital mucosal integrity (e.g., trauma, genital piercing or genital tract infection)
- Breach in oral mucosal integrity when performing oral sex
- Penetrating, percutaneous injuries with a hollow bore needle, direct intravenous or intra-arterial injection with a needle or syringe containing HIV infected blood
- Uncircumcised status of the insertive HIV negative partner practicing insertive anal intercourse or insertive vaginal intercourse

---

Box 3-4. Resources for Nonoccupational HIV Postexposure

HIV prophylaxis programs or pharmaceutical manufacturer patient assistance programs to access drugs for nonoccupational postexposure:
- Lopinavir/ritonavir (Abbvie): 1-800-222-6885
- Raltegravir (Merck): 1-800-850-3430
- Tenofovir/emtricitabine (Gilead Sciences): 1-800-226-2056

Practice Points

In determining whether the patient should consider PEP therapy, the clinician has several considerations to piece together in reviewing the benefits and risks of treatment:
- There have been no randomized prospective trials undertaken in humans to assess the efficacy of PEP or nPEP.
- Guidelines have been developed based on data from animal studies and human studies on MTCT prophylaxis, HPTN 052 and on-going treatment for established HIV infection.
- Early initiation of PEP within 72 hours is recommended. PEP should not be offered more than 72 hours after exposure unless expert consultation is provided because benefits after 72 hours are undefined.
- A 28-day treatment course of PEP has been accepted as the standard treatment duration
- HIV antibody testing is conducted at baseline, 6 weeks, 3 and 6 months after potential exposure of HIV. If there is a possibility of co-infection, expert advice should be obtained.
- If a fourth-generation combination HIV p24 antigen-HIV antibody test is utilized, then HIV testing can be changed to baseline, 6 weeks and 4 months after exposure.
- HIV transmission risk should be discussed. If a condom fails it is assumed that a similar risk is incurred as for unprotected sex.
- Transmission risk through receptive anal intercourse is estimated at 1.4%–1.7% (with ejaculation) and 0.65% (with withdrawal before ejaculation). Anal intercourse is associated with high transmission rates of HIV and nPEP should strongly be recommended.
- Transmission risk through receptive vaginal intercourse is estimated at 0.08%. Use of ART has been found to greatly reduce heterosexual transmission of HIV (PARTNER Study).
- Transmission through re-use of injection equipment is estimated at 0.8% per act.

other prevention methodologies. Despite those improvements with the current use of ART, however, the presence of pharmacologic sanctuaries is an impediment to achieving a functional cure of HIV. Future HIV therapeutics will require creative strategies to improve drug concentrations in those sanctuaries by increasing serum concentrations, increasing drug penetration, or improving drug delivery.

Unfortunately, only 30% of people with HIV currently living the United States have achieved viral suppression. Efforts to successfully control HIV in the future will require the health care system to substantially improve upon HIV testing and diagnosis, linking people with HIV to medical care and retaining them in care, prescribing HIV treatment regimens, and achieving durable viral suppression.

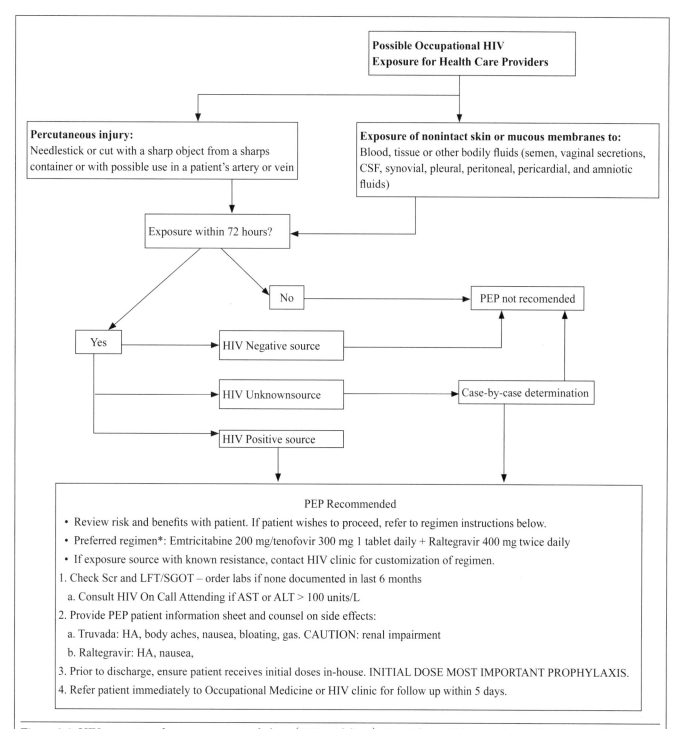

Figure 3-2. HIV occupational postexposure prophylaxis (PEP guidelines). Note: This guideline is to be used to assist in clinical efficiency, but is not a substitute for sound clinical judgement.

Information from University of California, San Diego Medical Center PEP Guidelines

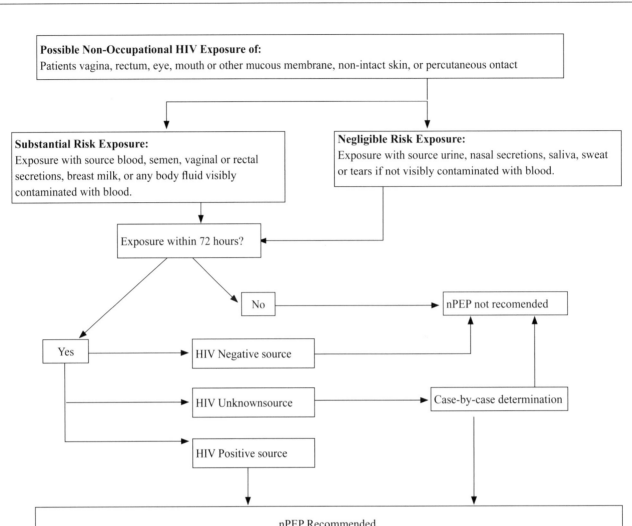

Possible Non-Occupational HIV Exposure of:
Patients vagina, rectum, eye, mouth or other mucous membrane, non-intact skin, or percutaneous ontact

Substantial Risk Exposure:
Exposure with source blood, semen, vaginal or rectal secretions, breast milk, or any body fluid visibly contaminated with blood.

Negligible Risk Exposure:
Exposure with source urine, nasal secretions, saliva, sweat or tears if not visibly contaminated with blood.

Exposure within 72 hours?

No

nPEP not recomended

Yes

HIV Negative source

HIV Unknownsource

Case-by-case determination

HIV Positive source

nPEP Recommended
- Review risk and benefits with patient. If patient wishes to proceed, refer to regimen instructions below.
- Preferred regimen*: Emtricitabine 200 mg/tenofovir 300 mg 1 tablet po daily + Raltegravir 400 mg twice daily for 28 days total.

* If funding issues, consider the following regimen which can be provided free of charge by the HIV Clinic (equally effective, but more GI adverse effects): Emtricitabine/tenofovir 1 tablet daily + Lopinavir 200 mg/Ritonavir 50 mg 2 tablets twice daily for 28 days total.

- If exposure source with known resistance, contact HIV clinic for customization of regimen.
1. Check Scr and LFT/SGOT – order labs if none documented in last 6 months
   a. Consult HIV On Call Attending if AST or ALT > 100 units/L
2. Provide PEP patient information sheet and counsel on side effects:
   a. Emtricitabine/tenofovir: HA, body aches, nausea, bloating, gas. CAUTION: renal impairment
   b. Raltegravir: HA, nausea
   c. Lopinavir/ritonavir: diarrhea, nausea, HA, fatigue; CAUTION: CA++ channel blockers, p450 metabolized drugs
3. Prior to discharge, ensure patient receives initial doses in-house. INITIAL DOSE MOST IMPORTANT PROPHYLAXIS.
4. Refer patient to HIV Clinic for follow up within 5 days unless patient has a primary care provider that can see the patient in the next 5 days.

Figure 3-3. HIV non-occupational postexposure prophylaxis (nPEP guidelines). Note: This guideline is to be used to assist in clinical efficiency but is not a substitute for sound clinical judgement.

Information from University of California, San Diego Medical Center nPEP Guidelines.

REFERENCES

Baeten JM, Donnell D, Ndase P, et al. Antiretroviral prophylaxis for HIV prevention in heterosexual men and women. N Engl J Med 2012;367:399-410.

Bennett NJ, Gilroy SA, Glatt A, et al; for Medscape. HIV disease [homepage on the Internet].

Cahn P, Pozniak AL, Mingrone H, et al. Dolutegravir versus raltegravir in antiretroviral-experienced, integrase-inhibitor-naïve adults with HIV: week 48 results from the randomised, double-blind, non-inferiority SAILING study. Lancet 2013;382:700-8.

Castagna A, Maggiolo F, Penco G et al. Dolutegravir in antiretroviral-experienced patients with raltegravir- and/or elvitegravir-resistant HIV-1: 24-week results of the phase III VIKING-3 study. J Infect Dis 2014 Epub ahead of print.

Centers for Disease Control and Prevention (CDC). Antiretroviral postexposure prophylaxis after sexual, injection-drug use, or other nonoccupational exposure to HIV in the United States: recommendations from the U.S. Department of Health and Human Services. MMWR 2005;54:1-20.

Centers for Disease Control and Prevention (CDC). Detection of Acute HIV Infection in Two Evaluations of a New Diagnostic Testing Algorithm – United States, 2011-2013. Morbidity and Mortality Weekly Report June 21, 2013.

Centers for Disease Control and Prevention (CDC). Estimated HIV incidence in the United States, 2007-2010. HIV surveillance supplemental report 2012;17.

Centers for Disease Control and Prevention (CDC). HIV in the United States: At a glance. November 2013.

Centers for Disease Control and Prevention (CDC). Laboratory Testing for the Diagnosis of HIV Infection: Updated Recommendations. Published June 27 2014.

Chun TW, Fauci A. HIV reservoirs: pathogenesis and obstacles to viral eradication and cure. AIDS 2012;26:1261-8.

Chan CN, Dietrich I, Hosie, MJ, et al. Recent developments in human immunodeficiency virus-1 latency research. J Virol 2013;94:917-32.

Chen I, Cummings V, Wang L, et al. Antiretroviral drug resistance among HIV-infected black men who have sex with men in the US. Program and abstracts of the 21st Conference on Retroviruses and Opportunistic Infections; March 3-6, 2014; Boston, MA. Abstract 581.

Clotet B, Feinberg J, Lunzen JV, et al. Once-daily dolutegravir versus darunavir plus ritonavir in antiretroviral-naïve adults with HIV-1 infection (FLAMINGO): 48 week results form the randomized open-label phase 3b study. The Lancet.

Published online April 1 2014. http://dx.doi.org/10.1016/S0140-6736(14)60084-2.

Clumeck N, Molina JM, Henry K, et al. A randomized, double-blind comparison of single-tablet regimen elvitegravir/cobicistat/emtricitabine/tenofovir DF vs ritonavir-boosted atazanavir plus emtricitabine/tenofovir DF for initial treatment of HIV-1 infection: analysis of week 144 results. J Acquir Immune Defic Syndr 2014;65:121-4.

Cohen CJ, Molina JM, Cassetti I, et al. Week 96 efficacy and safety of rilpivirine in treatment-naïve, HIV-1 patients in two Phase III randomized trials. AIDS 2013;27:939-50.

Cohen MS, Chen YQ, McCauley M, et al. Prevention of HIV-1 infection with early antiretroviral therapy. N Engl J Med 2011;365:493-505.

Cohen MS, Muessig KE, Smith MK, et al. Antiviral agents and hiv prevention: controversies, conflicts, and consensus. AIDS 2012; 26:1585-98.

Van Damme L, Corneli A, Ahmed K, et al. Pre-exposure prophylaxis for HIV infection among African women. N Engl J Med 2012;367;411-22.

DeJesus E, Rockstroh JK, Henry K, et al. Co-formulated elvitegravir, cobicistat, emtricitabine, and tenofovir disoproxil fumarate versus ritonavir-boosted atazanavir plus co-formulated emtricitabine and tenofovir disoproxil fumarate for the initial treatment of HIV-1 infection: a randomised, double-blind, phase 3, non-inferiority trial. Lancet 2012;379:2429-38.

Dieterich D, Tural C, Nelson M, et al. Faldaprevir Plus Pegylated Interferon Alfa-2a/ Ribavirin in HIV/HCV Coinfection: STARTVerso4. Conference on Retroviruses and Opportunistic Infections (CROI 2014). Boston, March 3-6. Abstract 23.

Eley T, Li W, Huang S-P, et al. Evaluation of pharmacokinetic drug-drug interactions between BMS-791325, an NS5b nonnucleoside polymerase inhibitor, daclatasvir, and asunaprevir in triple combination in hepatitis C virus genotype-1 infected patients. EASL 48th Annual Meeting. Amsterdam, April 25-28,2013.

Elion R, Molina JM, Ramon Arribas Lopez J, et al. A randomized phase 3 study comparing once daily elvitegravir with twice-daily raltegravir in treatment-experienced subjects with HIV-1 infection: 96-week results. J Acquir Immune Defic Syndr 2013;63:484-7.

Ellis RJ, Letendre S, Vaida F, et al. Randomized trial of central nervous system-targeted antiretrovirals for hiv-associated neurocognitive disorder. Clin Inf Dis 2014; 58:1015-22.

Else LJ, Taylor S, Back Dj, et al. Pharmacokinetics of antiretroviral drugs in anatomical sites : the male and female genital tract. Antivir Ther 2011;16:1149-67.

Eron JJ, Cooper DA, Steigbigel RT, et al. Efficacy and safety of raltegravir for treatment of HIV for 5 years in the

BENCHMRK studies: final results of two randomised, placebo-controlled trials. Lancet Infect Dis 2013;13:587-96.

Fidler S., Porter K, Ewings F, et al; SPARTAC Trial Investigators. Short-course antiretroviral therapy in primary HIV infection. N Engl J Med 2013;368:207-17.

Gazzard B, Duvivier C, Zagler C, et al. Phase 2 double-blind, randomized trial of etravirine versus efavirenz in treatment-naive patients: 48-week results. AIDS 2011;25:2249-58.

Gallant JE, Koenig E, Andrade-Villanueva J, et al. Cobicistat versus ritonavir as a pharmacoenhancer of atazanavir plus emtricitabine/tenofovir disoproxil fumarate in treatment-naïve HIV type 1-infected patients: week 48 results. J Infect Dis 2013;208:32-9.

Grant R, Lama J, Anderson P, et al. Preexposure chemoprophylaxis for HIV prevention in men who have sex with men. N Engl J Med 2010;363:2587-99.

German P, Liu H, Szwarcberg J et al. Effect of cobicistat on glomerular filtration rate in subjects with normal and impaired renal function. J Acquir Immune Defic Syndr 2012;61:32-40.

Hogan CM, DeGruttola V, Sun X, et al. The setpoint study (ACTG A5217) : effect of immediate versus deferred antiretroviral therapy on virologic set in recently HIV-1-infected individuals. J Infect Dis 2012;205:87-96.

Joint United Nations Programme on HIV/AIDS (UNAIDS). Global report: UNAIDS report on the global AIDS epidemic 2013. Geneva: UNAIDS.

Kirby B, Mathias A, Yang C, et al. Metabolism and excretion of ledipasvir in humans. Eighth International Workshop on Clinical Pharmacology of Hepatitis Therapy. June 2013, Cambridge, MA. Poster #O22.

Kiser, JJ, Burton JR, Everson GT. Drug-drug interactions during antiviral therapy for chronic hepatitis C. Nat Rev Gastroenterol Hepatol 2013;10:596-606.

Kuhar DT, Henderson DK, Struble KA, et al. Updated US Public Health Service guidelines for the management of occupational exposures to human immunodeficiency virus and recommendations for post exposure prophylaxis. Infect Control Hosp Epidemiol 2013;34:875-92.

Lambert-Niclot S, Tubiana R, Beaudoux C, et al. Detection of HIV-1 RNA in seminal plasma samples from treated patients with undetectable HIV-1 RNA in blood plasma on a 2002-2011 survey. AIDS 2012;26:971-5.

Le T, Wright E, Smith D, et al. Enhanced CD4+ T-Cell Recovery with Earlier HIV-1 Antiretroviral Therapy. N Engl J Med 2013;368:218-30.

Lennox JL, DeJesus E, Lazzarin A, et al. Safety and efficacy of raltegravir-based versus efavirenz-based combination therapy in treatment-naïve patients with HIV-1 infection: a

multicentre, double-blind randomized controlled trial. Lancet 2009;374:796-806.

Margot NA, Martin R, Miller MD, et al. Drug resistance mutations in treatment-naive HIV-infected patients 2000-2013. Program and abstracts of the 21st Conference on Retroviruses and Opportunistic Infections. March 3-6, 2014; Boston, MA. Abstract 578.

Marrazzo J, Ramjee G, Nair G, et al. Preexposure prophylaxis for HIV in women: daily oral tenofovir, oral tenofovir/emtricitabine, or vaginal tenofovir gel in the VOICE study. 20th Conference on Retroviruses and Opportunistic Infections. March 3-6, 2013. Atlanta. Abstract 26LB.

McComsey GA, Kitch D, Sax PE, et al. Associations of inflammatory markers with AIDS and non-AIDS clinical events after initiation of antiretroviral therapy : AIDS Clinical Trials Group A5224s, a substudy of ACTG A5202. J Acquir Immune Defic Syndr 2014;65:167-74.

Mills AM, Cohen C, Dejesus E, et al. Efficacy and safety 48 weeks after switching from efavirenz to rilpivirine using emtricitabine/tenofovir disoproxil fumerate-based single-tablet regimens. HIV Clin Trials 2013;14:216-23.

Osinusi A, Townsend K, Nelson A, et al. 49th European Association for the Study of the Liver International Liver Congress (EASL 2014). London, April 9-13, 2014. Abstract O14.

Osterberg L, Blaschke T. Adherence to medication. N Engl J Med 2005;353:487-97.

Raffi F, Jaeger H, Quiros-Roldan E, et al. Once-daily dolutegravir versus twice-daily raltegravir in antiretroviral-naïve adults with HIV-1 infection (SPRING-2 study): 96 week results from a randomised, double-blind, non-inferiority trial. Lancet Infect Dis 2013;13:927-35.

Raffi F, Rachlis A, Stellbrink HJ, et al. Once-daily dolutegravir versus raltegravir in antiretroviral-naïve adults with HIV-1 infection: 48 week results from the randomised, double-blind, non-inferiority SPRING-2 study. Lancet 2013;381:735-43.

Ramanathan S, Mathis A, German P, et al. Clinical Pharmacokinetic and Pharmacodynamic Profile of the HIV Integrase Inhibitor Elvitegravir. Clin Pharmacokinet 2011;50.

Rockstroh JK, DeJesus E, Lennox J, et al. Durable efficacy and safety of raltegravir versus efavirenz when combined with tenofovir/emtricitabine in treatment naïve HIV-1 infected patients: final 5-year results from STARTMRK. J Acquir Immune Defic Syndr 2013;63:77-85.

Rosen RC, Catania JA, Ehrhardt AA, et al. The Bolger conference on pde-5 inhibition and HIV risk: implications for health policy and prevention. J Sex Med 2006;3:960-75.

Sax PE, DeJesus E, Mills A, et al. Co-formulated elvitegravir, cobicistat, emtricitabine, and tenofovir versus co-formulated efavirenz, emtricitabine, and tenofovir for initial treatment of HIV-1 infection: a randomised, double-blind, phase 3 trial, analysis of results after week 48. Lancet 2012;379(9835):2439-48.

Schneider L, Ktorza N, Fourati S, et al. Switch from etravirine twice daily to once daily in non-nucleoside reverse transcriptase inhibitor resistant HIV-infected patients with suppressed viremia: The monetra study. HIV Clin Trials 2012;13:284-8.

Tashima KT, Flanigan TP, Kurpewski J, et al. Discordant human immunodeficiency virus type 1 drug resistance mutations, including K103N, observed in cerebrospinal fluid and plasma. Clin Infect Dis 2002;35:82-3.

Thigpen M, Kebaabetswe P, Paxton L. Antiretroviral pre-exposure prophylaxis for heterosexual HIV transmission in Botswana. N Engl J Med 2012;367:423-34.

Walmsley SL, Antela A, Glumeck N, et al. Dolutegravir plus abacavir-lamivudine for the treatment of HIV-1 infection. N Engl J Med 2013;369:1807-18.

Wohl DA, Cohen C, Mills A, et al. A randomized, double-blind comparison of single-tablet regimen elvitegravir/cobicistat/emtricitabine/tenofovir DF versus single-tablet regimen efavirenz/emtricitabine/tenofovir DF for initial treatment of HIV-1 infection: analysis of week 144 results. J Acquir Immune Defic Syndr 2014;65:118-20.

Workowski KA, Berman S. Sexually transmitted diseases treatment guidelines, 2010. MMWR Recomm Rep Dec 17 2010;59:1-110.

SELF-ASSESSMENT QUESTIONS

Questions 41 and 42 pertain to the following case.

J.B., a 20-year old man, comes to the emergency department (ED) complaining of dysuria and discharge. He identifies as a man who has sex with men (MSM) and reports unprotected receptive and insertive anal sex 2 days ago with an anonymous male partner who disclosed after the encounter that he is HIV positive. J.B.'s rapid HIV test is negative; the gonococcal test is positive; a rapid plasma reagin test is nonreactive for syphilis. The HSV-2 IgG is negative and the Hep B surface antigen is negative. J.B. is treated for gonorrhea. He is counseled that he may be at risk of HIV infection and is offered nonoccupational post-exposure prophylaxis (nPEP), but he is concerned that he doesn't have insurance and may be unable to pay for medication. He does not take any medications currently. He is given 5 days of nPEP medication and advised to go to the HIV clinic for help with continued supply of medication.

41. Which one of the following regimens would be best to recommend for nPEP for J.B.?

    A. Abacavir/lamivudine plus dolutegravir.
    B. Tenofovir/emtricitabine plus raltegravir.
    C. Zidovudine/lamivudine plus raltegravir.
    D. Elvitegravir/cobicistat/emtricitabine/tenofovir.

42. J.B. takes 5 days of nPEP medication but does not go to the clinic for the remainder of the 28-day supply. He returns to the ED 2 weeks later with complaints of fever, sweats, rash, myalgias, diarrhea, and headache. He asks for more nPEP medication. He is diagnosed with an acute retroviral syndrome and is referred to the HIV clinic. He comes into clinic 3 weeks later feeling better. Tests drawn at the ED visit return with these results: HIV-1 RNA 1.5 million copies/mL, CD4$^+$ count is 575 cells/mm^3; resistance test reveals a K103N mutation. The HLA-B*5701 test result was reported as present. The physician wants to treat J.B. today because she has read an update about treatment of HIV primary infection; however, J.B. is only willing to take one pill a day. The physician asks you to recommend a single tablet regimen (STR). Which one of the following is best to recommend for J.B.?

    A. Efavirenz/tenofovir/emtricitabine.
    B. Rilpivirine/emtricitabine/tenofovir.
    C. Elvitegravir/cobicistat/emtricitabine/tenofovir.
    D. Abacavir/lamivudine/dolutegravir.

43. A community physician calls the HIV pharmacist for advice on a heavily treatment-experienced patient. The patient is taking tenofovir/emtricitabine/rilpivirine plus dolutegravir plus darunavir and ritonavir once daily and is having some subtle CNS cognitive decline. The serum viral load is undetectable, but the physician did a lumbar puncture and the patient has 20 copies/mL detectable in the CSF. The physician wants to look at what the CNS penetration effectiveness (CPE) score would be but cannot find rilpivirine or dolutegravir in the CPE chart published by Letendre. Which one of the following is best to recommend for this patient?

    A. Maintain the regimen because there are no CNS data for dolutegravir or rilpivirine.
    B. Intensify the regimen by adding zidovudine to increase the CPE regimen score.
    C. Maintain the regimen because the CPE regimen score is > 7 which means it has a better chance of decreasing the CNS viral load than regimens ≤ 7.
    D. Change the regimen because the CPE regimen is < 7 and is causing some cognitive deficit.

44. The Center for Occupational and Environmental Medicine nurse practitioner calls the HIV on-call physician about a 33-year old male employee who had a needle exposure. The needle caused deep tissue injury and was from a patient with known HIV infection and a detectable HIV RNA of 187,000 copies/mL in the past 24 hours. The source patient had not been taking antiretroviral therapy (ART) but was an established patient at the HIV clinic. The source patient previously had been taking maraviroc 150 mg twice daily plus tenofovir/emtricitabine 1 tablet daily plus raltegravir 400 mg twice daily plus darunavir 600 mg twice daily with ritonavir 100 mg twice daily. Which one of the following is the best plan for initiating occupational postexposure prophylaxis (PEP) for this employee?

    A. Do not use PEP because the risk is small.
    B. Start tenofovir/emtricitabine plus darunavir/ritonavir.
    C. Start tenofovir/emtricitabine plus raltegravir.
    D. Start maraviroc plus tenofovir/emtricitabine plus raltegravir plus darunavir plus ritonavir.

45. A 55-year-old man with HIV and hepatitis C co-infection is referred to the clinic for pharmacist-assisted management of ART. His HIV is currently well controlled on tenofovir/emtricitabine plus atazanavir plus ritonavir with HIV RNA < 20 copies/mL and CD4$^+$ count 630 cells/mm^3. His hepatitis C is genotype 1A, HCV RNA 15 million copies/mL but has never been treated. The patient has a history of methamphetamine use, and although he quit 5 months ago, he admits to a relapse 1 week ago. His liver biopsy from 2 years ago shows F3 fibrosis. The liver clinic attending physician wants to treat the patient's

hepatitis C with the combination of sofosbuvir 400 mg daily plus simeprevir 150 mg daily for 12 weeks because of his cirrhosis. A review of his ART history includes the use of zidovudine/lamivudine, stavudine, indinavir, ritonavir, darunavir, and his current regimen. Past HIV genotype resistance testing shows mutations M184V, K103N in reverse transcriptase conferring resistance to emtricitabine, lamivudine, efavirenz, and nevirapine and D30N in protease conferring resistance to nelfinavir. Which one of the following is the best ART regimen for this patient's HIV while his hepatitis C is treated with sofosbuvir and simeprevir?

A. Continue tenofovir/emtricitabine plus atazanavir and ritonavir.

B. Change to elvitegravir/cobicistat/emtricitabine/tenofovir.

C. Change to emtricitabine/tenofovir/rilpivirine plus dolutegravir.

D. Change to emtricitabine/tenofovir plus etravirine plus dolutegravir.

46. A 65-year-old man is referred to the HIV clinic for initiation of ART. He was admitted to a community hospital 2 months ago where he was diagnosed with extrapulmonary tuberculosis and HIV. He has been taking rifampin, pyrazinamide, and ethambutol for 6 weeks because he developed hepatotoxicity from isoniazid. He is also taking azithromycin 1200 mg PO once weekly for *Mycobacterium avium-intracellulare* complex (MAC) prophylaxis and co-trimoxazole DS 1 tablet PO daily for *Pneumocystis jiroveci* pneumonia (PCP) prophylaxis. The patient reports that his urine is bright orange. He denies nausea, but his appetite is poor and he eats only one small meal daily. He participates in a direct observed therapy (DOT) referral program. His HIV-1 RNA is 408,000 copies/mL and CD4$^+$ count is 45 cells/mm^3. An HIV resistance test shows no treatment limiting mutations. HLA-B*5701 is not present. The patient's SCr is 1.5 mg/dL and GFR is 48 mL/minute; ALT and AST are within normal limits. The patient is very eager to start treatment today. Which one of the following is the best ART regimen to initiate in this patient?

A. Elvitegravir/cobicistat/emtricitabine/tenofovir 1 tablet daily.

B. Rilpivirine/emtricitabine/tenofovir 1 tablet daily.

C. Dolutegravir 50 mg daily with abacavir plus lamivudine.

D. Dolutegravir 50 mg twice daily with abacavir plus lamivudine.

Questions 47 and 48 pertain to the following case.

C.C. is a 42-year-old African American woman with treatment experience referred for management of HIV drug resistance.

In 2006 she presented to the HIV clinic after moving to San Diego from Washington DC. At that time her HIV-1 RNA was 23,000 copies/mL and her CD4$^+$ count was 28 cells/mL and she reported being treatment-naïve. Her baseline (before treatment) genotype resistance tests showed the following mutations: K219E (NRTI), G190A, V108I and Y181C. C.C. was started on tenofovir/emtricitabine with atazanavir and ritonavir and her HIV-1 RNA became undetectable. In 2011 she fell out of care and interrupted her treatment. She returned to the clinic in December 2012 with HIV-1 RNA of 111,000 copies/mL and CD4$^+$ count of 230 cells/mL. She requested a simple regimen because she found it difficult to adhere to her treatment. She was started on elvitegravir/cobicistat/emtricitabine/tenofovir with atazanavir. She took this regimen for 3 months and then dropped the atazanavir. She returned to clinic 6 months later with detectable viral load while taking only elvitegravir/cobicistat/emtricitabine/tenofovir. Another resistance test showed the following mutations: K65R, M184V, K219E (nucleoside reverse transcriptase inhibitors [NRTIs]); K106I, V108I, Y181C, G190A (non-nucleoside reverse transcriptase inhibitors [NNRTIs]); T66A, S147G, Q148R, E138K (integrase strand transfer inhibitor [INSTI]); M36I/T (protease inhibitor [PI]). Tropism R5. As the pharmacist on call, you check the Stanford University HIV Drug Resistance Database to better understand C.C.'s resistance profile.

47. Which one of the following would have the best chance of antiretroviral activity given C.C.'s integrase mutations?

A. Elvitegravir 150 mg boosted with cobicistat 150 mg.

B. Dolutegravir 100 mg daily.

C. Dolutegravir 50 mg twice daily.

D. Raltegravir 800 mg twice daily.

48. Which one of the following is the best regimen to treat C.C.'s resistant HIV?

A. Elvitegravir/cobicistat/tenofovir/emtricitabine 1 tablet daily plus atazanavir 300 mg daily.

B. Maraviroc 150 mg daily plus tenofovir/emtricitabine daily plus dolutegravir 50 mg daily plus darunavir 800 mg daily plus ritonavir 100 mg daily.

C. Maraviroc 150 mg twice daily plus zidovudine/lamivudine 1 tablet twice daily plus dolutegravir 50 mg twice daily plus darunavir 600 mg twice daily plus ritonavir 100 mg twice daily.

D. Emtricitabine/tenofovir 1 tablet daily plus etravirine 200 mg twice daily plus raltegravir 800 mg twice daily plus darunavir 600 mg twice daily plus ritonavir 100 mg twice daily.

49. A 56-year old man with HIV infection comes to the clinic to be evaluated for restarting ART; he was recently discharged from the hospital for right

lower extremity cellulitis. He had been on efavirenz/emtricitabine/tenofovir combination regimen for several years but stopped 3 months ago because of an insurance lapse. He does not want to restart it because it makes him "float." He states he stopped his efavirenz/emtricitabine/tenofovir combination altogether rather than taking it sporadically. The ID fellow asks if resistance testing should be done because the patient is new to the clinic and doesn't remember if he ever had one done. Which one of the following is best to recommend for this patient?

A. Genotype sequencing reverse transcriptase and protease.
B. Genotype sequencing reverse transcriptase, integrase and protease.
C. Genotype and phenotype combination tests.
D. There is no need for resistance testing since he was off ART for > 4 weeks.

50. A 37-year-old man who has had HIV infection for 6 years comes into the clinic to restart ART. He had previously been only on tenofovir/emtricitabine/efavirenz but took it inconsistently. A resistance test was completed last month and showed a K103N mutation. The HIV attending provider has read substantial resistance literature describing the M184V mutation can be often linked with a K103N mutation, but that the standard genotype resistance test would often not identify both mutations unless there was drug selection pressure from lamivudine or emtricitabine. She recommends that the next regimen should be designed as if the report included a M184V mutation. The patient's most recent HIV-1 RNA is 210,000 copies/mL and his CD4$^+$ count is 190 cells/mL. The patient wants to know what he should use next, because he was told he is resistant to tenofovir/emtricitabine/efavirenz. Which one of the following regimens is best to recommend for this patient?

A. Elvitegravir/cobicistat/emtricitabine/tenofovir.
B. Rilpivirine/emtricitabine/tenofovir.
C. Abacavir/lamivudine/dolutegravir.
D. Darunavir plus ritonavir plus emtricitabine/tenofovir.

51. A treatment-naïve patient with HIV infection presents to clinic to discuss initiating ART. He states he is motivated and ready to start treatment, and is adherent with his other daily medications. The patient's current HIV viral load is 117,000 copies/mL and his CD4+ count is 452 cells/mm^3. His baseline CrCl is 93 mL/minute, and ALT and AST are within normal limits. The patient has a history of depression that is somewhat controlled but he still complains of depressed mood. His only medication is citalopram 20 mg daily. He reports he has an erratic sleeping schedule because he works nights as an

event organizer. He also states he has heard about one pill once-daily regimens and would strongly prefer such a regimen if available. HLAB*5701 testing has not been performed. Which one of the following is the best initial antiretroviral treatment for this patient?

A. Efavirenz/emtricitabine/tenofovir.
B. Rilpivirine/emtricitabine/tenofovir.
C. Elvitegravir/cobicistat/emtricitabine/tenofovir.
D. Dolutegravir/abacavir/lamivudine.

52. A 34-year-old man asks about "a pill you can take to prevent HIV." The patient is a man who has sex with men and reports he is not in a relationship. He says he understands the importance of using protection during intercourse but does have multiple sexual partners. He last had an HIV test 3 months ago; the test was negative. He does not currently take any other medications. The patient asks if he can receive pre-exposure prophylaxis (PrEP). Which one of the following is the best answer to give this patient?

A. No, PrEP is only indicated for heterosexual serodiscordant couples.
B. Yes, he is an excellent candidate for PrEP and he can start right away.
C. Yes, but he must get a more recent HIV test before starting PrEP.
D. Yes, he should take PrEP only before he has a sexual encounter.

53. A physician in your clinic would like to start a patient who is treatment naïve on elvitegravir/cobicistat/emtricitabine/tenofovir. She asks you for the appropriate plan for monitoring this patient's renal function while taking this ARV combination. Which one of the following is best to recommend for this patient?

A. Monitor SCr, urine glucose, and urine protein at baseline and during treatment; start treatment as long as CrCl is greater than 70 mL/minute and discontinue if CrCl decreases to less than 50 mL/minute.
B. Monitor SCr, urine glucose, and urine protein at baseline and during treatment; start treatment as long as CrCl is greater than 70 mL/minute and discontinue if CrCl decreases to less than 70 mL/minute.
C. Check SCr at baseline and as long as CrCl is greater than 70 mL/minute start treatment with monitoring for the development of adverse events.
D. Monitor CrCl, urine glucose, and urine protein at baseline and during treatment; start treatment as long as CrCl is greater than 50 mL/minute, and discontinue if CrCl decreases to less than 50 mL/minute.

54. A physician in your clinic would like to initiate ART in a treatment-naïve patient and would like your opinion. He is considering using either efavirenz/emtricitabine/tenofovir or dolutegravir/abacavir/lamivudine because the patient states he heard about adverse effects of protease inhibitors and does not want to take them. The physician would like you to explain if there is a benefit to taking dolutegravir/abacavir/lamivudine because efavirenz/emtricitabine/tenofovir is also a first-line recommended regimen for treatment-naïve patients. Which one of the following is the best response to give the physician?

   A. Efavirenz/emtricitabine/tenofovir is a first-line regimen; however, in clinical trials dolutegravir was superior to efavirenz because of better tolerability, but it has a lower barrier to resistance.
   B. Efavirenz/emtricitabine/tenofovir is a first-line regimen; however, in clinical trials dolutegravir was superior to efavirenz because of better tolerability, and it has a higher barrier to resistance.
   C. Efavirenz/emtricitabine/tenofovir is a first-line regimen; however, in clinical trials dolutegravir was superior but is not recommended in patients with a baseline viral load of greater than 100,000 copies/mL.
   D. Efavirenz/emtricitabine/tenofovir is a first-line regimen; however, in clinical trials dolutegravir was superior to efavirenz in efficacy, but it has more adverse effects.

55. A physician is seeing a treatment-naïve patient in clinic who he would like to start on a new ARV regimen. The patient is taking rivaroxaban, a CYP3A substrate, for atrial fibrillation. Which one of the following is best to recommend for this patient?

   A. Darunavir plus ritonavir plus emtricitabine/tenofovir.
   B. Elvitegravir/cobicistat/emtricitabine/tenofovir.
   C. Etravirine plus emtricitabine/tenofovir.
   D. Rilpivirine/emtricitabine/tenofovir.

56. A treatment-experienced patient presents to clinic for modification of his current ARV regimen because his current regimen of efavirenz/emtricitabine/tenofovir is failing. A test demonstrates resistance to all NRTIs and first-generation NNRTIs (efavirenz and nevirapine). The resistance test demonstrates susceptibility to second-generation NNRTIs and protease inhibitors. Before his current regimen he was long ago exposed to several NRTIs but has never been exposed to PIs or INSTIs. He states he feels he would struggle with a regimen that was more than one pill once daily.

Which one of the following is best to recommend for this patient?

   A. Etravirine plus darunavir plus ritonavir plus raltegravir.
   B. Etravirine plus darunavir plus ritonavir plus dolutegravir.
   C. Elvitegravir/cobicistat/emtricitabine/tenofovir.
   D. Emtricitabine/tenofovir plus dolutegravir.

57. A 35-year-old woman with HIV infection who is treatment-naïve presents to clinic to discuss initiation of ART. Her baseline viral load is 84,000 copies/mL and her CD4$^+$ count is 325 cells/mm^3. Her physician would like to avoid a PI–based regimen because of a history of hyperlipidemia and hyperglycemia; the physician also would like to avoid efavirenz because the patient is of childbearing potential. He is somewhat concerned about adherence because the patient has had trouble adhering to her diabetes medications. He would like to start her on an INSTI-based regimen. Her current medications include fluticasone/salmeterol inhaler, albuterol inhaler, metformin, and glipizide. Testing has been performed and HLAB*5701 is present. Which one of the following is best to recommend for this patient?

   A. Emtricitabine/tenofovir plus dolutegravir 50 mg daily.
   B. Emtricitabine/tenofovir plus raltegravir 400 mg twice daily.
   C. Dolutegravir/abacavir/lamivudine daily.
   D. Elvitegravir/cobicistat/emtricitabine/tenofovir daily.

58. A 58-year-old man presents to your clinic for follow up. He is currently taking elvitegravir/cobicistat/emtricitabine/tenofovir with his last HIV viral load less than 50 copies/mL and CD4$^+$ count of 487 cells/mm^3. The patient has a history of diabetes and hypercholesterolemia. He wants to discuss treatment of his high cholesterol, for which he is not taking any medications. His physician would like to treat the patient with simvastatin and seeks your opinion on starting this new medication. Which one of the following is best to recommend for this patient?

   A. Any statin should be appropriate for the patient; simvastatin is an appropriate choice.
   B. No statin should be used with the patient's current ART regimen, another class of medications must be considered.
   C. It is important to control the patient's cholesterol but his current ARV regimen is not compatible with simvastatin; change the ARV regimen to rilpivirine/emtricitabine/tenofovir.

D. To prevent drug interactions with his ARV regimen, rosuvastatin would be a better alternative than simvastatin.

59. A 47-year-old man presents to your clinic for follow up on his current ARV regimen of rilpivirine/emtricitabine/tenofovir that was started 6 months ago. His HIV viral load is less than 50 copies/mL and his CD4+ count is 562 cell/mm³. This is his first ARV regimen, and although he is tolerating it well he reports a recent burning sensation in his chest almost every day. He thinks it is caused by heartburn. The patient talked to a pharmacist about it at his local pharmacy who made several nonpharmacologic recommendations that have not helped. He has also tried using over-the-counter antacids; these have helped a little bit but have not provided enough relief. He is requesting a medication for relief. Which one of the following is best to recommend for this patient?

A. Order omeprazole 20 mg daily and instruct the patient to separate his ARVs by taking rilpivirine/emtricitabine/tenofovir 4 hours before or 12 hours after omeprazole.

B. Order famotidine 20 mg daily and instruct the patient to separate his ARVs by taking rilpivirine/emtricitabine/tenofovir 4 hours before or 12 hours after famotidine.

C. Prescribe an alternative ARV regimen and order famotidine 20 mg daily.

D. Prescribe famotidine 20 mg daily because this is compatible with his ARV regimen.

60. A 32-year-old man returns to clinic for follow up on his ARV regimen of efavirenz/emtricitabine/tenofovir which he has been taking for 1 year. His last HIV viral load (1 month ago) was less than 50 copies/mL and his CD4+ count was 465 cells/mm³. The patient also has active hepatitis B infection. He reports he really likes the one pill once-daily option that his current regimen provides, but he is having abnormal dreams that are bothersome and sometimes cause difficulty sleeping. He has not missed any doses since starting his ARV regimen. He wants to know if there are any other options for switching his ARV regimen. The patient has a history of depression that is well controlled on fluoxetine 40 mg daily and anxiety well controlled on alprazolam 0.5 mg twice daily as needed. Which one of the following ARV regimens is best to recommend for this patient?

A. Elvitegravir/cobicistat/emtricitabine/tenofovir.

B. Dolutegravir/abacavir/lamivudine.

C. Rilpivirine/emtricitabine/tenofovir.

D. Continue on his current ARV regimen.

Learner Chapter Evaluation: HIV Infection.

As you take the posttest for this chapter, also evaluate the material's quality and usefulness, as well as the achievement of learning objectives. Rate each item using this 5-point scale:

- Strongly agree
- Agree
- Neutral
- Disagree
- Strongly disagree

40. The content of the chapter met my educational needs.
41. The content of the chapter satisfied my expectations.
42. The author presented the chapter content effectively.
43. The content of the chapter was relevant to my practice and presented at the appropriate depth and scope.
44. The content of the chapter was objective and balanced.
45. The content of the chapter is free of bias, promotion, or advertisement of commercial products.
46. The content of the chapter was useful to me.
47. The teaching and learning methods used in the chapter were effective.
48. The active learning methods used in the chapter were effective.
49. The learning assessment activities used in the chapter were effective.
50. The chapter was effective overall.

Use the 5-point scale to indicate whether this chapter prepared you to accomplish the following learning objectives:

51. Evaluate patient characteristics to determine the optimal regimen for treatment-naive patients with HIV infection.
52. Apply available data in determining the use of new antiretrovirals in both treatment-experienced and treatment-naive patients with HIV infection.
53. Assess the appropriateness of HIV preexposure prophylaxis on an individual-patient basis
54. Assess the appropriateness of and design a regimen for HIV postexposure prophylaxis.
55. Design an appropriate treatment regimen for a patient presenting with transmitted HIV resistance or an antiretroviral-therapy-treatment-experienced patient.
56. Develop a monitoring plan for drug interactions and adverse events associated with HIV treatment.
57. Please provide any specific comments relating to any perceptions of bias, promotion, or advertisement of commercial products.
58. Please expand on any of your above responses, and/or provide any additional comments regarding this chapter:

Questions 59–61 apply to the entire learning module.

59. How long did it take you to read the instructional materials in this module?
60. How long did it take you to read and answer the assessment questions in this module?
61. Please provide any additional comments you may have regarding this module:

INFECTIOUS DISEASES IV PANEL

Series Editors:

John E. Murphy, Pharm.D., FCCP, FASHP
Professor of Pharmacy Practice and Science
Associate Dean for Academic and Professional Affairs
University of Arizona College of Pharmacy
Tucson, Arizona

Mary Wun-Len Lee, Pharm.D., FCCP, BCPS
Vice President and Chief Academic Officer
Pharmacy and Health Sciences Education
Midwestern University
Professor of Pharmacy Practice
Midwestern University
Chicago College of Pharmacy
Downers Grove, Illinois

Faculty Panel Chair

Ian R. McNicholl, Pharm.D., FCCP,
BCPS (AQ-ID), AAHIVP
Associate Director, Medical Affairs
Gilead Sciences
Foster City, California

CNS INFECTION IN IMMUNOCOMPETENT HOSTS

Author

P. Brandon Bookstaver, Pharm.D.,
FCCP, BCPS (AQ-ID), AAHIVP
Associate Professor and Vice Chair
Department of Clinical Pharmacy
and Outcomes Sciences
South Carolina College of Pharmacy,
University of South Carolina
Columbia, South Carolina

April Miller Quidley, Pharm.D., FCCM, BCPS
Critical Care Pharmacist
PGY2 Critical Care Pharmacy Residency Director
Department of Pharmacy
Vidant Medical Center
Adjunct Associate Professor
Department of Pharmacy Practice
Campbell University College of
Pharmacy and Health Sciences
Greenville, North Carolina

Reviewers

Vanthida Huang, Pharm.D., BSPharm, FCCP
Associate Professor
Department of Pharmacy Practice
Midwestern University College of Pharmacy-Glendale
Glendale, Arizona

Sandra C. Bartlett, Ph.D., Pharm.D., BCPS
Associate Professor
Department of Pharmacy Practice
Husson University School of Pharmacy
Bangor, Maine

Abby R. Marrero, Pharm.D., BCPS
Clinical Pharmacy Supervisor/Coordinator
PGY1 Pharmacy Residency Director
Department of Pharmacy
West Kendall Baptist Hospital
Miami, Florida

FOOD- AND WATERBORNE ILLNESSES

Authors

Allana J. Sucher, Pharm.D., BCPS
Associate Professor of Pharmacy Practice
Department of Pharmacy Practice
Regis University
Rueckert-Hartman College for Health Professions
Denver, Colorado

Elias B. Chahine, Pharm.D., BCPS (AQ-ID)
Associate Professor of Pharmacy Practice
Department of Pharmacy Practice
Palm Beach Atlantic University
Lloyd L. Gregory School of Pharmacy
West Palm Beach, Florida
Clinical Pharmacist
Department of Pharmacy
JFK Medical Center
Atlantis, Florida

Reviewers

Katie J. Suda, Pharm.D., M.S.
Research Health Scientist
Center of Innovation for Complex Chronic Healthcare
Department of Veterans Affairs
Research Associate Professor
Department of Pharmacy Systems,
Outcomes, and Policy
University of Illinois at Chicago
Chicago, Illinois

Kari A. McCracken, Pharm.D. , BCPS
Clinical Pharmacy Manager/Infectious
Diseases Clinical Specialist
PGY-1 Pharmacy Residency Director
Department of Pharmacy
St. John Medical Center
Tulsa, Oklahoma

Jennifer Phillips, Pharm.D., BCPS
Assistant Professor
Department of Pharmacy Practice
Midwestern University
Downers Grove, Illinois

QUALITY AND SAFETY IN ANTIMICROBIAL PRACTICE

Authors

Monica V. Mahoney, Pharm.D., BCPS (AQ-ID)
Clinical Pharmacy Coordinator, Infectious Diseases
Department of Pharmacy
Beth Israel Deaconess Medical Center
Boston, Massachusetts

Christopher McCoy, Pharm.D., BCPS
Clinical Coordinator, Antimicrobial Stewardship
PGY2 Infectious Diseases/Antimicrobial
Stewardship Residency Director
Department of Pharmacy
Beth Israel Deaconess Medical Center
Boston, Massachusetts

Reviewers

Kimberly Luk, Pharm.D.
Ambulatory Care Pharmacist/Case Manager
Department of Infectious Diseases
Kaiser Permanente
Martinez, California

Carol Heunisch, Pharm.D., BCPS
Director, Pharmacy Services
NorthShore University HealthSystem
Evanston, Illinois

Michael C. Ott, Pharm.D., BCPS
Clinical Coordinator Pharmacy Services
Department of Pharmacy Services
Erie County Medical Center Corporation
Buffalo, New York

The American College of Clinical Pharmacy and the authors thank the following individuals for their careful review of the Infectious Diseases IV chapters:

Ralph H. Raasch, Pharm.D., BCPS
Associate Professor of Pharmacy (retired)
Division of Practice Advancement
and Clinical Education
Eshelman School of Pharmacy
The University of North Carolina at Chapel Hill
Chapel Hill, North Carolina

Emilie L. Karpiuk, Pharm.D., BCPS, BCOP
Oncology Pharmacist
Department of Pharmacy
Froedtert Hospital
Milwaukee, Wisconsin

Marianne McCollum, Ph.D., BSPharm, BCPS
Assistant Dean for Assessment
School of Pharmacy
Rueckert-Hartman College for Health Professions
Regis University
Denver, Colorado

CNS Infections in Immunocompetent Hosts

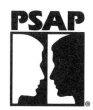

By P. Brandon Bookstaver, Pharm.D., FCCP, BCPS (AQ-ID), AAHIVP; and April Miller Quidley, Pharm.D., FCCM, BCPS

Reviewed by Vanthida Huang, Pharm.D., FCCP; Sandy C. Bartlett, Ph.D., Pharm.D., BCPS; and Abby R. Marrero, Pharm.D., BCPS

Learning Objectives

1. Use patient demographics, risk factors, and results of a lumbar puncture to distinguish the common pathogens associated with meningitis.
2. Assess a patient for medications associated with drug-induced aseptic meningitis.
3. Using the impact of immunization practices on national epidemiologic trends in meningitis and encephalitis, justify antimicrobial prophylaxis of meningitis.
4. Design a treatment regimen and monitoring plan for a patient with community- or hospital-acquired bacterial meningitis, bacterial brain abscess, or viral meningoencephalitis.
5. Using an understanding of medication penetration into central nervous system compartments, justify the use of intraventricular or intrathecal administration of antimicrobials.

Introduction

Central nervous system (CNS) infections have a low overall incidence but remain significant causes of morbidity and mortality in the United States and worldwide. Vaccinations, antimicrobial resistance, and increased numbers of invasive procedures have changed the epidemiology and management of these infections. However, the involvement of bacteria, viruses, and parasites may complicate the diagnosis and treatment of CNS infections.

Prompt initiation of antimicrobial therapy is the cornerstone of treatment for CNS infections. Based on the patient history and risk factors, optimally dosed therapy with adequate CNS penetration aimed at the likely pathogens is essential. In general, patients who are not at extremes of age and who have community-acquired bacterial disease should receive empirical therapy with a third-generation cephalosporin and vancomycin targeting *Streptococcus pneumoniae*, *Neisseria meningitidis*, and

Baseline Knowledge Statements

Readers of this chapter are presumed to be familiar with the following:
- Pharmacokinetics/pharmacodynamics of antibiotics used in central nervous system (CNS) infections
- Common spectrum of activity of antibiotics used in CNS infections
- Infectious Diseases Society of America guidelines on bacterial meningitis
- Centers for Disease Control and Prevention Advisory Committee on Immunization Practices updated guidelines for adults and children

Additional Readings

The following free resources are available for readers wishing additional background information on this topic.
- Advisory Committee on Immunization Practices (ACIP). 2014 Updated Recommendations.
- Centers for Disease Control and Prevention (CDC). Immunizations and Vaccines.
- Tunkel AR, Hartman BJ, Kaplan SL, et al. IDSA practice guidelines for the management of bacterial meningitis. Clin Infect Dis 2004;39:1267-84.
- Tunkel AR, Glaser CA, Bloch KC, et al. The management of encephalitis: clinical practice guidelines by the Infectious Diseases Society of America. Clin Infect Dis 2008;47:303-27.

Haemophilus influenzae. Infants as well as adults older than 50 years should receive additional therapy targeting *Listeria monocytogenes*. For nosocomial infections related to trauma or neurosurgery, broad-spectrum antibiotic therapy against methicillin-resistant *Staphylococcus aureus* (MRSA) and gram-negative organisms is required. Additional therapies may be used when viral or parasitic infections are suspected (Tunkel 2004).

Epidemiology of CNS Infections
Risk Factors

In immunocompetent hosts, bacterial CNS infections are usually community acquired and occur spontaneously. Meningitis can affect all age groups, but infants are at the greatest risk (as many as 88 cases per 100,000) (Thigpen 2011). The disease also tends to occur where individuals gather in large confined groups (e.g., prisons, dormitories, military settings), enabling infection to spread rapidly (CDC 2012). Globally, the meningitis belt of the sub-Saharan regions of Africa places individuals at highest risk of meningococcal disease (WHO 2014).

By contrast, health care–associated CNS infections usually involve invasive procedures or neurotrauma. Neurosurgical procedures, including placement of indwelling devices and treatment of traumatic brain injuries, put patients at risk of nosocomial CNS infections (CDC/NHSN 2014).

Incidence and Microbiology

Bacteria are a common cause of CNS infections, with 1.38 to 2 cases per 100,000 people from 2004 to 2007 (Thigpen 2011). Common pathogens of CNS infections are *S. pneumoniae*, *N. meningitidis*, *H. influenzae*, *L. monocytogenes*, and Group B *Streptococcus* with age-related differences in likely pathogens (Box 1-1) (MacNeil 2011; Tunkel 2004).

Although the incidence of *S. pneumoniae* has declined, it is still the most common pathogen, with a rate of 0.81 cases per 100,000 people in 2006–07. An almost 35% decline in incidence is attributed to routine use of pneumococcal vaccination, including both the 7-valent pneumococcal vaccine (PCV7) and the more recently introduced 13-valent pneumococcal vaccine (PCV13).

The incidence of health care–associated intracranial infections varies with the procedure types and patient-specific risk factors. Ventriculostomy-related infections occur at a rate of 2%–27%, whereas the rate of infection with extraventricular drains is about 8% (Beer 2011; Kitchen 2011). Risk factors for ventriculostomy-related infections include intraventricular or subarachnoid hemorrhage; cerebrospinal fluid (CSF) leak associated with intracranial fracture; systemic infection; and extended duration of catheterization (Stenehjem 2012). The incidence of infection after traumatic brain injury is also variable, being less than 2% among patients with CSF leakage only and as high as 25% among patients with basilar skull fractures (Derber 2012; Beer 2011). In this population, *S. aureus* and *S. epidermidis* account for 80% of infections. Gram-negative pathogens account for most of the remaining cases, with anaerobes and fungal pathogens being infrequent causes of health care–associated intracranial infections.

Worldwide, in areas with poor vaccine access, mumps and measles remain significant causes of viral meningitis

---

Box 1-1. Common Bacterial Pathogens in CNS Infections

Community-Acquired CNS Infections

  Less than 1 month of age
    Group B *Streptococcus*
    Escherichia coli
    Klebsiella pneumoniae
    Listeria monocytogenes
    Gram-negative bacilli

  1 month to less than 18 years
    Streptococcus pneumoniae
    Neisseria meningitidis
    Haemophilus influenzae

  18 years to less than 50 years
    Streptococcus pneumoniae
    Neisseria meningitidis
    Gram-negative bacilli (in immunocompromised individuals)

  Greater than 50 years
    Streptococcus pneumoniae
    Listeria monocytogenes
    Gram-negative bacilli

Health Care-Associated CNS Infections
    Staphylococcus aureus
    Staphylococcus epidermidis
    Gram-negative bacilli (including *Pseudomonas aeruginosa*)

(also known as aseptic meningitis). Japanese B encephalitis virus is an important pathogen in worldwide epidemic meningitis. However, these viruses are less common causes of CNS infections in the United States. Instead, enteroviruses, arboviruses, and varicella zoster viruses (VZVs) are common in the United States, with 11 cases per 100,000 individuals annually (Takhar 2011; Desmond 2006). The incidence of viral infections decreases with increasing patient age. Herpes simplex virus (HSV) is the most common cause of encephalitis, with an increasing incidence caused by the rising rates of HIV infection and associated immunodeficiency.

PATHOPHYSIOLOGY

Central nervous system infections manifest primarily as meningitis and may also be related to encephalitis. Such infections occur when pathogens enter the CNS through either contiguous spread or hematogenous routes. Contiguous spread occurs through the dispersion of adjacent infections, including the sinus cavities and the middle ear. These infections may be acquired after local trauma or neurosurgery.

The specialized blood flow of the blood-brain barrier (BBB) protects the CNS from infection. Bacteria trigger the release of cytokines that stimulate vasodilation and increase vascular permeability. This disrupts the normal blood flow at the BBB and allows pathogens to enter. Once pathogens enter the CNS, cerebral edema occurs, and patients develop the signs and symptoms of meningitis.

Cerebral edema can decrease cerebral flood flow, causing local or globalized ischemia, cortical destruction, cranial nerve damage, and vasculitis. Ischemia, cortical destruction, and ischemia can result in temporary or permanent neurologic deficits. Cranial nerve damage commonly occurs at the eighth cranial nerve, causing hearing loss. Meningitis, especially *N. meningitidis*, can also cause severe sepsis and shock.

Anatomy of CNS Infections

Central nervous system infections present significant treatment challenges for clinicians. An important aspect in management is an understanding of the anatomy of the CNS and of the location of infections within the CNS. A lipid membrane cell layer with tight junctions in the BBB and blood-CSF surrounds the CNS compartments. This barrier limits antimicrobial penetration, especially in the absence of inflammation. The CSF is often devoid of a rapid immune response to bacterial infections, with its slow migration of cells and naturally low levels of immunoglobulins that account for less than 0.5% of serum. The compartments in the CNS can be divided into the CSF space, the extracellular space of the brain tissue, and the intracellular space that includes neurons, glial cells, and other circulating cells. Furthermore, the compartments within the CNS and in the CSF space specifically do not equilibrate, leading

to significant differences in drug concentrations. Of note, meningitis occurs in the arachnoid space, and encephalitis is an infection of the brain tissue itself.

CLINICAL PRESENTATION AND DIAGNOSIS OF CNS INFECTIONS

The acuity of most CNS infections requires a high index of suspicion in patients at risk of the disease. Prompt recognition and diagnosis are essential as part of early management. A medical history (including risk factors for infection and recent exposures) and physical examination yield important information to help guide the diagnosis and treatment. About 95% of patients with meningitis present with two of the following signs and symptoms: fever, headache, nuchal rigidity, or photophobia (Tenkel 2004). A diffuse petechial rash may be present in up to 50% of patients with meningococcemia. In encephalitis and more-extensive CNS disease, patients may also present with altered mental status, stupor, and seizures. Box 1-2 outlines the signs and symptoms that contribute to clinical suspicion of CNS infections. Common meningeal signs are atypical in infants, and nonspecific signs and symptoms such as excessive irritability or crying, vomiting or diarrhea, tachypnea, altered sleep pattern, and poor eating should be noted. In critically ill patients (who are often intubated and sedated), fever combined with a potential CNS source such as recent neurosurgery, CNS trauma, or presence of implantable material should prompt suspicion of a CNS infection (Beer 2010; Baumeister 2008; Boviatis 2004).

Diagnosis of CNS infections starts with clinical suspicion and, unless contraindicated, should include a lumbar puncture (LP). A computed tomography (CT) scan is often performed before LP to rule out a central mass or other risk of herniation. Radiologic evidence also distinguishes meningeal or ventricular involvement and, depending on the type of infection, may include magnetic resonance imaging. An opening pressure at the time of LP should be obtained and, if elevated, may suggest infection. The CSF is evaluated for the following variables: appearance, glucose, protein, WBC with differential, and RBC. Common diagnostic and normal values in the CSF are listed in Table 1-1.

Box 1-2. Clinical Signs and Symptoms of CNS Infections

- Altered mental status (more common in encephalitis)
- Focal neurologic deficits (positive Brudzinski and Kernig sign)
- Seizures (less common in meningitis)
- Malaise
- Skin lesions: specifically in Meningococcal meningitis presents as diffuse petechial rash meningitis

---

Compared with older children and adults, newborns generally have higher CSF-to-serum ratios and greater variability in CSF glucose. Protein values in the CSF of newborns are generally higher than those reached by 6 or 12 months of age, which are similar to those of adults. Other laboratory findings should include CSF lactate and C-reactive protein. A concurrent serum glucose at the time of LP aids in the interpretation of CSF glucose. Although variable under normal conditions, CSF glucose is about two-thirds of serum values. In bacterial meningitis, patients usually have turbid-appearing CSF with neutrophilic-predominant pleocytosis, marked decrease in glucose (e.g., <40% of serum), elevated protein, and elevated opening pressure.

Nearly 90% of bacterial meningitis cases have elevated CSF WBCs of more than 1000 cells/mm[3.] Although decreased CSF glucose is consistent with bacterial meningitis, some reports demonstrate 50% of cases have normal glucose profiles. Comparatively, the CSF profile in viral meningitis often demonstrates normal glucose and protein, with a lymphocytic-predominant pleocytosis, although the CSF WBCs may also be normal. Red blood cells in the CSF may indicate severe acute bleeding such as subarachnoid hemorrhage or evidence of a traumatic LP, often referred to as a *traumatic tap*. Measuring RBCs in three consecutive tubes distinguishes a traumatic tap from other origins. The RBC values that continue to fall in consecutive tubes are often indicative of a traumatic tap. With a traumatic tap, WBC count and protein levels are falsely elevated and require correction: protein (subtract 1 mg/dL for every 1000 RBCs); WBCs (subtract 1 cell/mm[3] for every 500–1000 RBCs).

A CSF Gram stain and culture should always be performed. A positive Gram stain is sufficient for diagnosis in up to 70% of cases of bacterial meningitis. Blood cultures should also be obtained as part of the initial workup.

Ideally, the LP and all cultures should be obtained immediately before initiating antibiotic therapy.

For clinicians, one of the more challenging diagnoses is that of partially treated meningitis. This is the case when a patient may have received an oral antibiotic such as a fluoroquinolone or amoxicillin/clavulanate as an outpatient for a suspected bacterial infection (e.g., sinusitis). Despite the suboptimal therapy for bacterial meningitis, the oral antibiotic may interfere with CSF findings, including the Gram stain and culture results. Additional rapid diagnostics, including bacterial antigen testing (BAT), may be considered; BAT is available for the most common bacterial pathogens (e.g., *S. pneumoniae*, *N. meningitidis*, *H. influenzae* type B). The data are inconsistent on the actual value of BAT; however, some clinicians may opt to obtain BAT, especially in patients with negative Gram stains or recent histories of antibiotic exposure (Karre 2010).

Polymerase chain reaction (PCR) is a useful modality for the detection of viral meningitis. It is especially useful in the diagnosis of enterovirus, which helps rule out bacterial etiologies and avoid the overuse of antimicrobials. PCR is also a sensitive means of diagnosis of cytomegalovirus (CMV) and HSV infections (Seehusen 2003). In-house PCR testing can significantly reduce turnaround time for a potentially negative test—allowing for antimicrobial de-escalation—and possibly expedite earlier hospital discharge (Rand 2005).

Drug-Induced Aseptic Meningitis

The overall incidence of drug-induced aseptic meningitis (DIAM) is unknown, but DIAM is thought to be relatively rare. Nonsteroidal anti-inflammatory drugs (e.g., ibuprofen) are the most commonly implicated drug class. Sulfonamide antibiotics (e.g., sulfamethoxazole) represent the most common antimicrobials associated with DIAM (Jolles 2000). Other agents associated with

Table 1-1. Comparative Cerebrospinal Fluid Profile in Meningitis by Pathogen

Variable	Normal Conditions	Bacterial Meningitis	Viral Meningitis/ Encephalitis	Fungal Meningitis/ Meningo-encephalitis
Opening Pressure	60–200 mm H$_2$0[a]	Increased (>250 mm H$_2$O)	Rarely increased	Frequently increased
WBC count (cells/mm^3)	Up to 5 (20 in newborns)	1,000–5,000	100–500	100–500
Dominant Cell Type	Lymphocytes (70%)	Neutrophil (>80%)	Lymphocytes	Lymphocytes
Protein	20–60 mg/dL[b]	Usually increased (100–500 mg/dL)	Normal/Slightly increased	Moderately increased
Glucose	Two-thirds of serum	Low (<40 mg/dL or 40% of concurrent serum)	Rarely low	Often low

[a]In children < 8 years of age 10–100 mm H$_2$O.
[b]Up to 150 mg/dL in newborns.

DIAM are listed in Box 1-3. Intraventricular drug administration has also been associated with DIAM, likely caused by a direct chemical irritant effect. Risk factors for DIAM appear to be the presence of a connective tissue disorder (e.g., systemic lupus erythematosus) and repeat exposure to an offending agent(s). The mechanism by which systemic drug administration causes DIAM is not fully understood; however, it is hypothesized to be a type 4 or 5 hypersensitivity reaction. Intravenous immunoglobulin-associated DIAM is thought to be secondary to activation of tumor necrosis factor-α–primed neutrophils by antineutrophil cytoplasmic antibodies.

Clinical symptomatology is similar to other etiologies of meningitis, making differentiation a challenge. Symptoms may appear within hours to days from initiation of the offending agent. Repeat exposure is associated with decreased time to onset. An LP may be abnormal, with slightly elevated opening pressure and WBC count, but results may be quite variable. Drug-induced aseptic meningitis is considered a diagnosis of exclusion that is made by ruling out other common bacterial, fungal, or viral causes of infection. Establishing a temporal relationship to drug exposure and symptoms is important. Because of the ubiquitous availability of over-the-counter agents associated with DIAM, taking a careful medication history is important. Empirical treatment for bacterial meningitis and, potentially, viral encephalitis is warranted until infectious causes can be ruled out.

MANAGEMENT OF CNS INFECTIONS

Principles of Treatment

Systemic antimicrobial therapy and supportive care during the acute disease are essential in the management of CNS infections. Reducing mortality and associated neurologic sequelae are the primary goals of therapy. In bacterial meningitis, early administration of antibiotic therapy is associated with improved clinical outcomes and fewer long-term deficits. Antibiotic therapy should be administered immediately after a diagnostic LP.

Clinicians are often hesitant to obtain an LP without a CT scan in order to rule out intracranial mass lesions or severe brain edema. Risk factors for cerebral edema that could lead to herniation secondary to LP include age 60 years or older, immunocompromise, CNS disease history, seizures during the week before presentation, and neurologic abnormalities (Tunkel 2004). Significant time spent in obtaining diagnostic tests should not delay early antibiotic therapy. If clinicians are unable to obtain an LP in a timely manner, antimicrobial therapy should be initiated as soon as blood cultures are taken. Antibiotic therapy administered more than 1 to 2 hours before LP can reduce the yield of CSF cultures (Shin 2012; Tunkel 2004,). Supportive care includes fluid management; control of seizures; maintenance of intracranial pressure; and preservation of other organ functions, which could

Box 1-3. Medications Associated with Drug-Induced Aseptic Meningitis

Nonsteroidal anti-inflammatory drugs (e.g., ibuprofen)
Aminopenicillins (e.g., amoxicillin, ampicillin)
Carbamazepine
Intravenous immunoglobulin
Sulfonamides
Lamotrigine
Ranitidine
Muromonab
Medications administered intrathecally or intraventricularly

include maintaining hemodynamic and mechanical ventilation as needed. Many of these principles apply for most of the invasive CNS infections. Infections that involve a protected focus such as a brain abscess will include surgical intervention for treatment and diagnosis.

Antibiotic Penetration into CNS

Knowledge of antimicrobial penetration to the site of infection is essential for delivering therapy in this deep-seated compartment. In the majority of CNS infections, crossing the BBB is required. In general, most antimicrobials do not actively cross those tight junctions, especially in the absence of inflamed meninges. Inflammation disrupts the junctions between the endothelial cells, increasing permeability.

Antibiotics do not undergo active metabolism within the CSF; therefore, concentrations are based on drug properties (Nau 2010; Lutsar 1998). Drug characteristics associated with enhanced CSF concentrations include lipophilicity, small molecular weight, low degree of ionization, and low degree of protein binding. Highly lipophilic agents (e.g., fluoroquinolones and rifampin) penetrate rapidly into the CSF and maintain adequate concentrations. Many β-lactams are hydrophilic and highly ionized at a physiological pH and do not penetrate the BBB well, especially in the absence of meningeal inflammation. Ceftriaxone is highly protein bound (90%–95%), leading to delayed entry into the CSF; however, the half-life in the CSF is prolonged (Gaillard 1994; Nau 1993). Active transport mechanisms may also be present, further lowering the CSF concentrations of some agents. Meningeal inflammation occurs secondary to infection and generally increases the permeability—and thus the penetration—of antimicrobials, especially hydrophilic agents. Although controversial, the administration of dexamethasone is often recommended in many CNS infections, especially bacterial meningitis. Dexamethasone's anti-inflammatory effects may decrease the permeability of some agents, including β-lactams, aminoglycosides, and vancomycin (Nau 2010; Ricard 2007; Gaillard 1994).

Despite the potential decrease in CSF concentrations, aggressive dosing for CNS infections provides adequate concentrations against the majority of pathogens. Because

Table 1-2. CSF Penetration of Select Antimicrobials

Drug Class/Agent	CSF Penetration (presented as % of serum) or Ratio of AUC_{CSF}/AUC_{serum}[a] (presented as decimal)
Carbapenems	
Meropenem	0.39 (inflamed); 0.21–0.25 (non-inflamed)
Doripenem	14% (inflamed); 7% (non-inflamed)
Ertapenem	4%–7.1% (inflamed); 2.4% (non-inflamed)
Cephalosporins	
Cefazolin	11.3%–14.8% (inflamed); 2.7% (non-inflamed)
Cefuroxime	11.6%–13.7% (inflamed)
Cefotaxime	0.17 (inflamed); 0.12 (non-inflamed)
Ceftriaxone	1.5%–16% (inflamed); 0.007 (non-inflamed)
Cefepime	0.103 (inflamed); 0.078 (non-inflamed);
Ceftazidime	18%–45% (inflamed); 0.057 (non-inflamed)
Ceftaroline	14% (inflamed)
Cephamycins	
Cefoxitin	2.5%–35% (inflamed); 1–3% (non-inflamed)
Penicillins	
Penicillin G	5%–10% (inflamed)
Ampicillin	13%–35% (inflamed)
Piperacillin	0.32 (inflamed); 0.034 (non-inflamed)
Monobactam	
Aztreonam	16%–22% (inflamed)
β-lactamase inhibitors	
Clavulanate	0.084 (inflamed); 0.037 (non-inflamed)
Sulbactam	25% (inflamed)
Tazobactam	32%–36% (inflamed); 0.106 (non-inflamed);
Fluoroquinolones	
Ciprofloxacin	0.92 (inflamed); 0.24–0.45 (non-inflamed)
Levofloxacin	0.71 (non-inflamed)
Moxifloxacin	0.71–0.94 (inflamed); 0.46 (non-inflamed)
Aminoglycosides	
Gentamicin	0.27 (inflamed)
Tobramycin	8%–23% (inflamed)
Amikacin	8%–25% (inflamed); <3% (uninflamed)

Drug Class/Agent	CSF Penetration (presented as % of serum) or Ratio of AUC_{CSF}/AUC_{serum}[a] (presented as decimal)
Oxazolidinones[b]	
Linezolid	0.90 (non-inflamed)
Glycopeptides	
Vancomycin	0.30 (inflamed); 0.14–0.18 (non-inflamed)
Lipoglycopeptides[c]	
Telavancin	2% (inflamed); 1% (non-inflamed)
Oritavancin	1%–5% (inflamed)
Lipopeptide	
Daptomycin	5%–6% (inflamed); 2% (non-inflamed)
Tetracyclines[d]	
Doxycycline	0.20 (inflamed); 0.2 (non-inflamed)
Other Anti-infectives	
Metronidazole	0.87 (inflamed)
Sulfamethoxazole	0.24–0.30 (inflamed); 0.12 (non-inflamed)
Trimethoprim	0.42–0.51 (inflamed); 0.18 (non-inflamed)
Rifampin	0.22 (non-inflamed)

[a]AUC ratio of CSF to serum was included where available as a more accurate marker of true CSF penetration. However, these should be interpreted with caution, as the timing of calculation (first dose versus steady-state) is unclear.
[b]Data are not available for tedizolid
[c]Data are not available for dalbavancin. CSF penetration in 2 patients in early clinical studies was undetectable (FDA 2014).
[d]Data are not available for the glycylcycline, tigecycline.

of the delay in antibiotic penetration and elimination, the percentage of CSF penetration at a single point may not be the most appropriate measure to correlate true antimicrobial concentrations. The CSF to serum area under the concentration curve (AUC) ratio is likely the more appropriate measure. The CSF penetration of selected antimicrobials is summarized in Table 1-2. Data from studies with human subjects were preferentially included; however, animal data were used if relevant human data were unavailable. In addition, CSF measurements varied by presence of inflammation, antimicrobial dosages, and dosing schedule (e.g., single dose vs. multidose) and should be interpreted accordingly.

Antimicrobial Therapy
Bacterial Meningitis

The diagnosis of acute bacterial meningitis should be considered a neurologic emergency, and timely administration of antibiotics is critical. The exact timing of

Table 1-3. Bacterial Meningitis: Empirical Treatment by Population

Patient Population	Recommended Empirical Therapy & Dosing
Neonate (< 28 days)	Ampicillin 200-400 mg/kg/day divided IV q 8-12 hours *plus* Cefotaxime 50 mg/kg/dose IV q 8-12 hours or gentamicin (or tobramycin) 5 mg/kg/day IV q 24 hours
> 1 month to 50 years	**Peds:** Vancomycin 60 mg/kg/day IV divided q 6-8 hours[a] *plus* cefotaxime 50 mg/kg/dose IV q 6–8 hours (max: 12 g/day) *or* ceftriaxone 50 mg/kg/dose IV q 12 hours (Max 4 g/day) **Adults:** Vancomycin 15 mg/kg/dose IV q 8–12 hours *plus* ceftriaxone 2 g IV q 12 hours or cefotaxime 2 g IV q 4 hours[b]
>50 years	Vancomycin 15 mg/kg/dose IV q 8-12 hours plus ceftriaxone 2 g IV q 12 hours plus ampicillin 2 g IV q 4 hours
Penetrating Head Trauma or Postneurosurgery[c]	Vancomycin 15 mg/kg/dose IV q 8-12 hours *plus* cefepime 2 g IV q 8 hours or meropenem 2 g IV q 8 hours
CSF shunt in place[c,d]	Vancomycin 15 mg/kg/dose IV q 8-12 hours *plus* cefepime 2 g IV q 8 hours or meropenem 2 g IV q 8 hours

[a]Vancomycin dosing should be modified to target troughs of 15–20 mcg/mL.
[b]Cefotaxime doses up to 24 g/day have been studied in adults.
[c]Ceftazidime 2 g IV q 8 hours may also be an option in place of cefepime or meropenem.
[d]Vancomycin monotherapy may be reasonable in pediatrics without risk or a positive Gram stain for gram-negative organisms.
Adapted from The Infectious Diseases Society of America Practice Guidelines for the Management of Bacterial Meningitis, 2004.

onset of symptoms is typically unknown; hence there is no specific target administration time, but delay in therapy is associated with increased morbidity and mortality (Miranda 2009). Recommendations for the management of bacterial meningitis have not been updated since the Infectious Diseases Society of America's (IDSA's) 2004 guidelines (Tunkel 2004). The recommended empirical therapies, together with dosing information, are summarized in Table 1-3. Children younger than 1 month are at increased risk of *S. agalactiae* (Group B *Streptococcus*) and gram-negative Enterobacteriaceae (e.g., *Escherichia coli*). The recommended treatment regimen includes ampicillin plus cefotaxime or an aminoglycoside (e.g., gentamicin). Ceftriaxone is generally avoided in neonates younger than 28 days because of the potential for kernicterus and for ceftriaxone-calcium precipitation leading to clinically significant adverse events. Specifically, ceftriaxone-calcium precipitation has resulted in fatalities secondary to precipitate formation in the lungs and kidneys of neonates (Steadman 2010). In children older than 1 month and in adults younger than 50 years, vancomycin plus a third-generation cephalosporin (e.g., ceftriaxone) is recommended. Ceftriaxone-nonsusceptible strains of *S. pneumoniae* occur at rates of 10% or higher in many areas of the United States (Mendes 2014); this has prompted the need for the addition of vancomycin until culture and susceptibility reports are available. Adults older than 50 years should also be treated empirically with ampicillin to cover for *L. monocytogenes* as a possible pathogen. Duration of therapy is based on the isolated pathogen and ranges from 1 to 3 weeks. In the case of a

parameningeal focus or other concurrent primary infection (e.g., pulmonary source), duration may need to be adjusted. Box 1-4 contains recommend treatment durations.

Patients with penetrating trauma or those who have undergone neurosurgical procedures require broader empirical coverage because of the risk of gram-negative aerobic bacilli (e.g., *E. coli*), *Pseudomonas aeruginosa*, and methicillin-resistant *Staphylococcus* spp. (Shin 2012; Beer 2010). Empirical regimens should include vancomycin plus an antipseudomonal β-lactam with adequate CSF concentrations such as cefepime or meropenem. Vancomycin CSF concentrations approximate 30% of serum concentrations, and therefore dosing to minimum trough concentrations of 15–20 mg/L is required to achieve pharmacodynamic targets in the CSF (Ricard 2007). Staphylococcal isolates, specifically *S. aureus*, with minimum inhibitory concentrations (MICs) of 2 mg/L or more will prevent the achievement of adequate AUC/MIC targets (i.e., > 400), especially within the CSF. Other anti-MRSA agents include daptomycin and linezolid.

Box 1-4. Duration of Antibiotic Therapy for Bacterial Meningitis by Pathogen

Neisseria meningitidis: 7 days
Streptococcus pneumoniae: 10–14 days
Staphylococcus aureus: 10–14 days
Streptococcus agalactiae: 14–21 days
Gram negative bacilli: 21 days
Listeria monocytogenes: ≥ 21 days

Meropenem is recommended as the carbapenem of choice, according to the IDSA guidelines (Tunkel 2004). In a rabbit model of meningitis, doripenem demonstrated efficacy comparable to that of cefepime (Stucki 2012). Doripenem's penetration into the CSF is about 14% of serum penetration, but a lack of clinical data limits the recommendation for doripenem use (Margetis 2011). Ertapenem lacks activity against *P. aeruginosa* but has proved effective in animal models of pneumococcal meningitis despite limited CSF penetration (Cottagnoud 2003). However, routine use of ertapenem cannot be recommended. Among β-lactams, carbapenems are thought to have the highest epileptogenic potential, although this potential risk does not preclude their use in CNS infections (Miller 2011). Available data indicate a comparatively lower risk with meropenem, whereas imipenem/cilastatin has the highest risk of drug-induced seizures and typically is avoided in CNS infections.

Adjuvant Corticosteroids

The use of adjunctive corticosteroids is recommended in many cases of bacterial meningitis to reduce inflammatory-related sequelae secondary to disease and bacterial lysis. The American Academy of Pediatrics recommends dexamethasone in children at least 6 weeks old with known *H. influenzae* meningitis; the agent has been shown to reduce the incidence of residual hearing loss. However, data in neonates are limited and do not demonstrate a benefit in using adjunctive dexamethasone (Daoud 1999). A large multicenter study failed to demonstrate mortality benefit using dexamethasone in children with meningococcal or pneumococcal meningitis, but it may provide benefit in preventing long-term hearing deficits.

Clinical benefit with adjunctive steroids, including reduced mortality, has been demonstrated in randomized controlled trials for adults with suspected or proven pneumococcal meningitis (de Gans 2002). Although these findings are not as convincing for other pathogens, a reasonable approach is to consider adding dexamethasone empirically until definitive data, such as CSF or blood culture findings, are available. Dexamethasone should be dosed at 0.15 mg/kg intravenously every 6 hours for 2–4 days and given concomitantly or within 10–20 minutes of the first antibiotic dose. The benefit is unclear if dexamethasone is given after antibiotics have been initiated, and thus is not recommended at that time.

Table 1-4. Empirical Antibiotic Treatment of Brain or Epidural Abscess

Infection Source	Common Pathogens	Antibiotic Therapy
Dental abscess or orthodontic procedure	*Streptococcus* spp. Gram-positive anaerobes	Penicillin G 12–24 million units IV per day (given as continuous infusion or divided doses q 4 hours) plus metronidazole 500 mg IV q6 hours (may consider 1 g IV q6 hours); *or* third-generation cephalosporin (ceftriaxone or cefotaxime) *plus* metronidazole Addition of vancomycin may be considered if *S. aureus* is suspected (e.g., recent surgical procedure)
Sinusitis, Otitis media, Mastoiditis	*Streptococcus* spp., including *S. pneumoniae* Gram-positive anaerobes *S. aureus* (less common)	Third-generation cephalosporin (ceftriaxone 2 g IV q12 hours *or* cefotaxime 2 g IV q4 hours) *plus* metronidazole Addition of vancomycin may be considered if *S. aureus* is suspected (e.g., recent surgical procedure)
Pulmonary abscess or bronchiectasis	*Streptococcus* spp., including *S. pneumoniae* Gram-positive anaerobes	Third-generation cephalosporin (ceftriaxone or cefotaxime) *plus* metronidazole
Penetrating trauma or recent neurosurgery	Gram-negative bacilli including *P. aeruginosa* *S. aureus*, including MRSA	Vancomycin 15 mg/kg IV q8-12 hours *plus* cefepime 2 g IV q8 hours *or* meropenem 2 g IV q8 hours; *or* ceftazidime 2 g IV q8 hours
Congenital heart disease	*Streptococcus* spp. *Haemophilus* spp. *Enterococcus* spp. (less common)	Third-generation cephalosporin (ceftriaxone or cefotaxime) ± ampicillin 2 g IV q4 hours (if *Enterococcus* is suspected)
Endocarditis	*Streptococcus* spp. *Staphylococcus* spp. *Enterococcus* spp. (less common)	Treatment directed by underlying endocarditis management (refer to infective endocarditis guidelines)

Limited data in patients with resistant pneumococcal meningitis have demonstrated some increased treatment failures with the administration of adjunctive dexamethasone. Dexamethasone's anti-inflammatory effects can decrease permeability of the BBB and therefore reduce the penetration of vancomycin, although the clinical significance is unclear (Ricard 2007). That decreased permeability prompted study of rifampin as a component of the treatment regimen. In animal models, the addition of rifampin to the treatment regimen demonstrated some improved outcomes. However, routine use of rifampin in patients with adjunctive steroids is not routinely recommended.

Infections of the Parenchyma–Epidural/Brain Abscess

The management of brain and epidural abscesses requires complex, multimodal approaches to therapy by using an interdisciplinary team. Brain abscesses occur secondary to a contiguous, hematogenous, or direct inoculation from trauma and require a combination of surgical and antimicrobial therapy. Surgical intervention (e.g., craniotomy, CT-guided aspiration) will provide source control and avoid potential abscess rupture into the ventricles, which could increase mortality by more than 50% (Derber 2012; Beer 2010; De Louvois 2000). Empirical antimicrobial therapy should be broad so as to cover the most common aerobic (e.g., *Streptococcus, Staphylococcus, Enterobacteriaceae*) and anaerobic organisms (e.g., *Prevotella* and *Bacteroides* spp.) (Derber 2012; De Louvois 2000).

The etiology varies greatly depending on the source (Table 1-4). Antimicrobial strategies should include (1) agents that penetrate the BBB and (2) dosing that delivers adequate concentrations at the site of the infection. Agents that have demonstrated good penetration into intracranial pus include ampicillin, cefuroxime, ceftazidime, and metronidazole (Nau 2010; Fong 1984). Although other agents (e.g., penicillin, vancomycin, ceftriaxone, cefepime, and meropenem) lack concentration data specific to intracranial abscess, each achieves adequate penetration across the BBB and has demonstrated clinical success in the management of brain abscesses (Derber 2012; De Louvois 2000).

Empirical treatment for anaerobes is recommended for most of the contiguous sources of brain abscesses (e.g., oral cavity) and those resulting from direct trauma or pulmonary abscess. Metronidazole is considered the agent of choice for treatment of anaerobes because it has good penetration into the CSF and abscess. Although penicillins with β-lactamase inhibitors (e.g., piperacillin/tazobactam) typically provide adequate anaerobic coverage, they do not penetrate optimally into the CNS. Ampicillin/sulbactam at 8 g of ampicillin daily has been used successfully in infections secondary to multidrug-resistant organisms (e.g., *Acinetobacter* spp.). If meropenem is used in the primary treatment regimen, a second agent with anaerobic activity is not needed in most cases (see Table 1-4).

Antimicrobial stewardship efforts to de-escalate therapy to targeted pathogens are essential once cultures and susceptibility data are available. The duration of treatment for brain abscess is 4–6 weeks of intravenous therapy when surgical drainage has occurred. In the absence of surgical intervention, antibiotic therapy should extend to 6–12 weeks. Brain abscesses with less-common pathogens (e.g., *Nocardia* spp.) may require extended courses of treatment up to 1 year in duration in addition to surgical intervention (Mamelak 1994).

Spinal epidural abscesses (SEAs) or cerebral and spinal subdural abscesses should be evaluated as surgical emergencies (Derber 2012; Wong 2011; Tompkins 2010). Up to 71% of patients with SEAs have neurologic deficits on examination that may require acute intervention because of the unpredictable and sometimes rapid changes in symptomatology (Tompkins 2010).

Empirical antimicrobial therapy is indicated in all patients and should target the primary organisms *Staphylococcus* spp. (e.g., MRSA) and gram-negative bacilli (e.g., *E. coli, P. aeruginosa*). Less commonly, SEAs may involve mixed anaerobic pathogens. The empirical treatment for SEAs is vancomycin plus an antipseudomonal β-lactam (e.g., cefepime). The addition of metronidazole should be considered, especially if a carbapenem is not used as the antipseudomonal agent. Antibiotics should not be delayed in patients with neurologic deficits; however, antibiotic therapy may be delayed in stable, immunocompetent patients in order to obtain an unadulterated culture by CT-guided aspiration. Regardless of the timing of antibiotics, culture and susceptibilities are important to guide definitive therapy. Recommended treatment duration is 6–8 weeks of intravenous therapy; however, it may be extended because of risk of recurrence or in immunocompromised hosts. There are no data to support the use of oral antibiotic therapy for long-term infection suppression (Tompkins 2010).

Viral Encephalitis

Pharmacotherapeutic management of viral encephalitis is limited primarily to herpesvirus, including HSV, CMV, VZV, and human herpesvirus-6 (HHV-6) (Nath 2013; Studahl 2013). Because of the complex management and the relatively low prevalence of many of these invasive viral infections, an interdisciplinary team approach that includes infectious diseases specialists should be considered.

Herpes simplex virus (e.g., HSV-1) is the most common type of viral encephalitis in the United States, and empirical therapy with intravenous acyclovir should be initiated as soon as possible until HSV can be ruled out. The use of intravenous acyclovir therapy is highly effective, reducing mortality to less than 10% in proven cases of HSV encephalitis when initiated within 4 days of symptoms (Tunkel 2008). Acyclovir is typically dosed at 10 mg/kg/dose intravenously every 8 hours in patients with normal renal function. Ideal body weight (IBW) has been proposed as the most appropriate dosing weight, although that recommendation is based on limited data (Davis 1991). Acyclovir therapy can be associated with acute kidney injury (AKI) because of obstruction caused by crystallization. When the maximal solubility is exceeded, acyclovir can precipitate in the tubular lumens. Hydration with oral or intravenous fluids is effective in reducing the likelihood of AKI. Rapid administration of intravenous doses may also contribute to early acyclovir-induced AKI (Hernandez 2009). Less-common adverse events include headache, altered mental status, and bone marrow suppression. Some institutions designate a maximal single dose of IV acyclovir to be 800 mg because of dose-dependent adverse effects (e.g., IBW of 80 kg and 10 mg/kg dose).

Valacyclovir, an oral prodrug of acyclovir, provides higher bioavailability than oral acyclovir and is often used in non-CNS infections secondary to HSV. Cerebrospinal fluid penetration of valacyclovir 1000 mg orally every 8 hours has been shown to exceed the target inhibitory concentrations for HSV-1 over a sustained period of 20 days of therapy (Pouplin 2011; Smith 2010). Safety and tolerability have also been demonstrated in doses up to 8000 mg daily (Pouplin 2011). The clinical data are very limited; however, valacyclovir may be considered if intravenous acyclovir is unavailable. It is rare that HSV-1 may be associated with acyclovir resistance because of alterations in thymidine kinase. In this case, foscarnet may be an alternative therapy.

Cytomegalovirus encephalitis is associated with significant morbidity and mortality. Although ganciclovir and foscarnet have antiviral activity against CMV and are effective in the management of CMV disease outside the CNS, treatment outcomes have not been improved with either drug as monotherapy (Tunkel 2008). The CSF penetration is limited with both agents. The current recommendation is combination therapy with ganciclovir 5 mg/kg intravenously every 12 hours plus foscarnet 60 mg/kg intravenously every 8 hours or 90 mg/kg intravenously every 12 hours (Tunkel 2008). The suggested dosing weight is the IBW, although data are limited for extremely obese patients. Ganciclovir is commonly associated with significant adverse drug events (ADEs) including hematologic disorders (primarily, neutropenia and thrombocytopenia). Foscarnet toxicity is common with severe ADEs, including AKI, anemia, and gastrointestinal effects. The use of these agents requires careful dosing assessment and strict management of potential end organ damage. Maintaining adequate hydration, limiting concurrent nephrotoxic agents, and adjusting the necessary dose reductions with changes in renal function are important strategies for minimizing toxic effects. A majority of patients with CMV encephalitis are immunocompromised as a result of either a disease process or drug therapy; therefore, management of the immunocompromised state should be a priority.

Varicella zoster virus encephalitis is relatively uncommon, and clinical outcomes data are limited to case series and anecdotal reports of success with acyclovir 10–15 mg/kg/dose given intravenously every 8 hours (Studahl 2013; Tunkel 2008). Based on limited clinical use, ganciclovir also has in vitro activity against VZV and may be considered as an alternative to acyclovir. The management of encephalitis caused by additional viruses (e.g., Epstein-Barr virus) is limited mostly to supportive care. The use of antiviral therapy has not been shown to improve outcomes. In the case of Epstein-Barr virus encephalitis, corticosteroids for patients with increased intracranial pressure are modestly effective in reducing disease-associated morbidity. Other causes of encephalitis, including rickettsial diseases and rare zoonotic-related viruses (e.g., West Nile, rabies), are not discussed in this chapter.

Multidrug-Resistant Pathogens: Vancomycin-Resistant Enterococcus, Extended-Spectrum β-lactamase, and Carbapenem-Resistant Enterobacteriaceae

Alternative agents may be needed for patients with severe allergies to primary treatment or those who have multidrug-resistant pathogens, such as vancomycin-resistant Enterococcus (VRE) or gram-negative Enterobacteriaceae. Although VRE is rarely encountered, its management poses a significant challenge to clinicians given the paucity of bactericidal agents with favorable CNS pharmacokinetic profiles. Administration of combination agents or use of alternative methods of administration such as intrathecal (IT) or intraventricular (IVT) therapy may be considered for those patients. Consultation with infectious diseases specialists is recommended. Primary therapeutic options may include daptomycin, linezolid, or quinupristin/dalfopristin either alone or in combination. Chloramphenicol possesses activity against VRE and has been used clinically, although availability and concern about serious adverse effects (e.g., bone marrow suppression, aplastic anemia, peripheral neuropathy, gray baby syndrome) make this a less desirable option.

Daptomycin is a bactericidal agent, highly protein bound, and possesses about 5%–6% penetration into the CSF. Daptomycin in combination with linezolid and/or gentamicin has resulted in clinical or microbiological cure in several published cases (Le 2010). Daptomycin at 8–12 mg/kg intravenously daily for multidrug-resistant pathogens is higher than the approved dose of 6 mg/kg every 24 hours. The higher dose maximizes dose-dependent bactericidal activity and enhances CSF penetration. Creatine phosphokinase elevation is the most commonly encountered ADE; it is typically benign, although some patients may experience myalgias and, rarely, rhabdomyolysis. The risks may increase with exposure to higher doses and in patients with concomitant kidney dysfunction and those receiving concurrent statins. Eosinophilic pneumonitis has also been documented with daptomycin (Bookstaver 2013; Bland 2014).

In vitro data support evidence of synergy when daptomycin is combined with rifampin or ampicillin. Limited clinical evidence supports the potential of gentamicin synergy. Most of the recent clinical data, not specifically in CNS infections, suggest the potential benefits of the ampicillin-plus-daptomycin regimen for invasive, deep-seated VRE infections, including those with an endovascular source (Sierra-Hoffman 2012).

Linezolid has been used successfully as monotherapy in the management of CNS infections caused by VRE, as well as in combination with daptomycin (Le 2010). Linezolid is bacteriostatic; however, an AUC_{CSF}/AUC_{serum} ratio of 0.9 has been documented, which suggests good CNS concentrations with a favorable pharmacokinetic profile for deep-seated infections. Published reports have described conventional linezolid dosing of 600 mg twice daily (Knoll 2013; Le 2010). Linezolid is associated with serious ADEs including thrombocytopenia, anemia, and, less commonly, leukopenia. Blood dyscrasias typically manifest in 7–10 days of therapy. Peripheral neuropathy, optic neuritis, and arthralgia have also been reported and are typically associated with protracted courses of therapy (e.g., > 2–3 weeks). Coadministration of serotonergic agents (e.g., selective serotonin-reuptake inhibitors) with linezolid increases the risk of serotonin syndrome because of the monoamine oxidase inhibition properties of linezolid. The only proven method of reducing that risk is avoidance of coadministration.

Quinupristin/dalfopristin has intrinsic activity against *E. faecium*—including vancomycin-resistant strains—but *E. faecalis* strains are inherently resistant. Quinupristin/dalfopristin has limited CSF penetration but in scarce reports has been shown to be effective in combination with daptomycin (Le 2010). Intraventricular quinupristin/dalfopristin has been used as effective adjunct therapy in VRE meningitis (Williamson 2002). With the availability of other agents and because of its significant drug-related adverse events (e.g., arthralgias and myalgias), quinupristin/dalfopristin is rarely used as a first-line agent.

Multidrug-resistant gram-negative organisms—including *Acinetobacter* spp., extended-spectrum β-lactamase (ESBL)–producing, and carbapenem-resistant Enterobacteriaceae (CRE)—are emerging pathogens in CNS infections. The majority of these infections are nosocomial in nature, although at least three cases of community-acquired meningitis by ESBL-producing *E. coli* have been reported (Elaldi 2013). Neonates are at high risk of gram-negative meningitis, including ESBLs. Mortality associated with those pathogens is high, and survivors may have neurologic sequelae including hearing loss, memory deficits, and seizures (Yaita 2012; López-Álvarez 2008).

A large review of meningitis secondary to *Acinetobacter* spp. suggests that combination therapy with direct IT or IVT plus systemic therapy is recommended (Karaiskos 2013). Although controlled trials are not available, one study suggested a reduction in mortality (from 74% to 20%) when combination therapy became standard practice (Cascio 2010). In many cases, the use of polymyxins is required because of the extensive class resistance among *Acinetobacter* spp. Aminoglycosides also remain susceptible in many cases. Ampicillin/sulbactam, which possesses good activity against *Acinetobacter*, has been evaluated at doses up to 8 g of sulbactam daily.

Carbapenems, specifically meropenem, are agents of choice for meningitis caused by ESBL-producing organisms. When susceptible, fluoroquinolones or aminoglycosides may be alternative treatment options, especially in combination with β-lactam. Another consideration is IVT aminoglycosides therapy. Reported cases of combination therapy have demonstrated varying degrees of success (Elaldi 2013). The combination of intravenous antibiotics plus IVT gentamicin compared with systemic antibiotics alone resulted in decreased mortality in gram-negative meningitis. Combination antibiotic therapy, including IVT administration, may be considered for MDRO gram-negative CNS infections because of the high mortality.

The management of meningitis or ventriculitis caused by CRE is similar to that of multidrug-resistant *Acinetobacter* spp. Combination therapy—often with polymyxins and aminoglycosides administered by IT or IVT routes—will be required. One case of carbapenemase-producing *Klebsiella pneumoniae* ventriculitis was treated successfully with a combination of tigecycline, amikacin, IVT gentamicin, and colistin (Nevrekar 2014). The penetration of tigecycline across the BBB is unknown; however, a case report of pediatric VRE meningitis supported the use of tigecycline in combination (Jaspan 2010).

Alternative Routes of Administration: Intrathecal and Intraventricular

As mentioned previously, direct CNS administration of antimicrobials by way of IT or IVT routes may be required as an adjunct to systemic therapy in patients with CNS infections caused by MDROs or severe ventriculitis unresponsive to conventional therapy. Agents such as vancomycin, colistin, and aminoglycosides are the most commonly used and studied; these agents are difficult to titrate because of significant systemic adverse effects. Direct CNS administration of β-lactams should be avoided because of reports of significant seizures in animals receiving cefazolin, aztreonam, and carbapenems (Nau 2010). The pharmacokinetics of the cerebrospinal fluid in directly administered agents have significant inter-patient variability caused by the critically ill state, variability in EVDs, and the presence of other agents that may enhance CSF clearance of the drug. The use of IT or IVT antimicrobials as adjuncts to systemic therapy is supported by IDSA guidelines (Tunkel 2004).

Although much of the data with IT or IVT administration are from single case reports and series, combination therapy of IT or IVT agents plus systemic therapy has been shown to improve outcomes in CNS infections caused by MDROs (Cascio 2010). A recent review of colistin IT and IVT administration in adults and children reported overall positive clinical outcomes, with reversible chemical meningitis being the most common severe adverse event. The data consistently showed that most IT or IVT antimicrobials are initiated more than 72 hours after initial suspicion of CNS infection and initiation of concurrent systemic antimicrobial therapy. The reason is likely based on delay in MDRO diagnosis and on hesitancy to use an invasive administration technique. It is not unreasonable to delay in therapy until necessary. Routine use of IVT aminoglycosides in combination with systemic therapy in infants was associated with a 3-fold increase in mortality compared with systemic therapy alone. Further study is required to determine whether a causal relationship exists between IVT therapy and an increase in mortality. The adverse effects of other agents (e.g., aminoglycosides and vancomycin) include reversible hearing loss and aseptic meningitis. The potential for seizures should be considered at the currently recommended antimicrobial doses, although seizures are rarely reported. Dosing recommendations for the most commonly used antibiotics in direct CNS administration are listed in Table 1-5.

Intraventricular administration is more commonly used clinically and is preferred over the IT route. The presence of an EVD allows for ease of both administration and therapeutic drug monitoring of the CNS. Despite limited data, the monitoring of drug concentrations may be beneficial if there is concern about adequate penetration of systemic antimicrobials. Intraventricular administration provides higher drug concentrations into the ventricles compared with IT administration. This is likely because of the natural circulation of the CSF from the ventricles down the spinal cord. In addition, IVT administration, specifically with colistin, may be associated with decreased adverse events such as chemical meningitis; however, data are limited. Either IVT or IT administration requires an interdisciplinary management team, including neurosurgical specialists, an infectious diseases specialist, and a pharmacist.

Vaccinations

Routine vaccination has had a major impact on the microbiological epidemiology and incidence of bacterial meningitis in the United States. Pediatric vaccinations against *S. pneumoniae, H. influenzae,* and *N. meningitidis* have decreased the incidence of those pathogens as causes of infection. Table 1-6 gives a brief overview of the primary recommendations and vaccine options targeting those pathogens. Further details are discussed in the following and can also be accessed at the CDC Advisory Committee on Immunization Practices (ACIP) Web site.

Routine vaccination of infants and children by using heptavalent polysaccharide *S. pneumoniae* vaccine (PCV7) decreased the incidence of invasive pneumococcal disease in children and in adults 65 years or older. Protection against serotypes 4, 6B, 9V, 14, 18C, 19F, and 23F had a significant impact on the incidence and types of invasive disease. Notably, in seven states, the total incidence of invasive pneumococcal disease decreased by 77% in children younger than 5 years, with a 98% reduction in disease among vaccine-protected serotypes. The incidence of disease caused by bacterial strains not included in the vaccine increased by 29%.

In 2010, PCV13 became approved by the U.S. Food and Drug Administration (FDA) for the prevention of six additional pneumococcal serotypes: 1, 3, 5, 6A, 7F, and 19A. Promptly thereafter, the ACIP added it to the recommended vaccine schedule. Specific data on the impact of PCV13 vaccine on invasive pneumococcal disease including meningitis are unavailable. However, incidence data from 2008 indicate that 12.7 cases of invasive pneumococcal disease per 100,000 people were caused by PCV13 serotypes compared with 8.2 cases per 100,000 people caused by non-PCV13 serotypes. A single dose of PCV13 is now recommended in previously unvaccinated adults older than 65 years, followed by a dose of 23-valent

Table 1-5. Intraventricular administration: Antimicrobial Dosing and Adverse Events of Selected Agents

Antimicrobial Agent	Dosing (Adult)	Adverse Events
Vancomycin	5–20 mg q 24 hours	Temporary hearing loss
Gentamicin & Tobramycin	5 mg q 24 hours	Temporary hearing loss; seizures; aseptic meningitis
Amikacin	30 mg q 24 hours	Temporary hearing loss; seizures; aseptic meningitis
Streptomycin	Maximum of 1 mg/kg q 24 to 48 hours	Temporary hearing loss; seizures; radiculitis; transverse myelitis; arachnoiditis
Daptomycin	5–10 mg q 72 hours	Fever
Colistin	10 mg q 24 hours	Dose-dependent meningeal inflammation/chemical meningitis; seizures; agitation; pain; edema

Information from Nau, R, Sorgel F, Eiffert H. Penetration of drugs through the blood-cerebrospinal fluid/blood-brain barrier for treatment of central nervous system infections. Clin Micro Rev 2010;23:858-83.

pneumococcal polysaccharide vaccine (PPSV23) 6–12 months later. Adults older than 65 years who previously received PPSV23 should receive a single dose of PCV13 at least 12 months after the PPSV23 vaccine (Nuorti 2010).

The PPSV23 vaccine is recommended for use in immunocompromised children older than 2 years and adults older than 50 years and for routine use in adults older than 65 years. It confers protection against 11 additional serotypes—2, 8, 9N, 11A, 12F, 15B, 17F, 19F, 20, 22F, and 33F—as well as one serotype (6A) fewer than PCV13. As a result, the incidence of invasive disease caused by *S. pneumoniae* declined from 1.09 to 0.81 cases per 100,000 people from 1998 to 2007.

Routine vaccination of infants and children with *H. influenzae* B (Hib) conjugate vaccine (PRP-T; ActHIB and Hiberix) has reduced both the incidence and the mortality rate of *H. influenzae* meningitis. Introduction of the Hib vaccine in 1991 reduced the incidence of meningitis by 99%. Because of the effectiveness of vaccination, unimmunized or partially immunized children are at the greatest risk of disease.

Routine vaccination against *N. meningitidis* began in 2005, and because of limited supply of the vaccine, early efforts focused on the immunization of adolescents (Cohn 2013). Since then, multiple vaccine formulations have been produced. Two formulations of quadrivalent meningococcal conjugate vaccines (MCV4) provide protection against serogroups A, C, Y, and W-135, which can be used in individuals from ages 2 to 55 years of age. An additional meningococcal polysaccharide vaccine (MPSV4) for individuals older than 55 years provides protection against serogroups A, C, Y, and W-135. The bivalent vaccine is formulated in combination with *H. influenzae* conjugate vaccine (PRP-OMP) to provide protection in infants and young children (aged 6 weeks to 18 months) against serogroups C and Y. The ACIP recommends routine vaccination with quadrivalent vaccines for children older than 2 months and in adolescents aged 11–18 years. The initial primary dose is recommended at age 11–12 years, with a booster following the

Table 1-6. Advisory Committee on Immunization Practices Recommendations for Bacterial Meningitis Associated Pathogens

Targeted Pathogen	Vaccine Product	Serotypes	Recommendation
N. meningitidis	Menactra	A, C, W, and Y	**Primary (1 dose):**
	Menveo	A, C, W, and Y	Age 11–12 years
			Age 13–18 years: Recommended if not previously vaccinated
			Age 19–21 years: May be given as catch-up if not received a dose after 16th birthday
			Booster (1 dose):
			Recommended if first dose received before 16th birthday
H. influenzae	PedvaxHIB; Comvax (combination vaccine)	B	**Primary (2 doses):** Age 2, 4 months **Booster (1 dose):** 12–15 months
	ActHIB; Pentacel (combination vaccine); MenHibRix (combination vaccine)	B	**Primary (3 doses):** Age 2, 4, 6 months **Booster (1 dose):** 12–15 months
S. pneumoniae	Prevnar 13 (PCV13)	1, 3, 4, 5, 6A, 6B, 7F, 9V, 14, 18C, 19A and 23F	**Primary (4 doses):** Age 2, 4, 6 and 12–15 months **Additional (1 dose):** Age > 65 years
	Pneumovax 23 (PPSV23)	1, 2, 3, 4, 5, 6B, 7F, 8, 9N, 9V, 10A, 11A, 12F, 14, 15B, 17F, 18C, 19F, 19A, 20, 22F, 23F, and 33F	**Additional (1 dose):** Age > 65 years

Adapted from information available from Vaccine Recommendations of the Advisory Committee for Immunization Practices (ACIP)..

age of 16 years. The incidence of invasive meningococcal disease declined from a peak in the late 1990s to an all-time low incidence of 0.2 case per 100,000 people in the early 2000s (Cohn 2010). Data in specific age-groups are unavailable at this time. No available vaccine provides protection against serotype B (Cohn 2013). Further details on <u>childhood and adult immunization schedules</u> are available online.

Anatomic or functional asplenia is a unique condition that warrants additional vaccination to protect individuals against a variety of bacterial (specifically, encapsulated organisms) and viral illnesses that are commonly associated with meningitis (Box 1-5). Hematologic, oncologic, and immunologic indications are the primary reasons for splenectomy, with 15% of operations performed secondary to traumatic injury (Di Sabatino 2011). To prevent overwhelming postsplenectomy infection, vaccination or revaccination with pneumococcal, Hib, and meningococcal vaccine is recommended. In previously unvaccinated adults older than 18 years, a single dose of PCV13 followed by a dose of PPSV23 at least 8 weeks later is recommended. Previously vaccinated adults should receive a single dose of PCV13 at least 1 year after the last dose of PPSV23. If previous vaccination with Hib vaccine is confirmed, a booster is not necessary, although it may still be administered. Two doses of MCV4 given at least 2 months apart are recommended. A yearly influenza vaccine is also recommended in all asplenic patients. The ideal timing of splenectomy vaccines is not known, but it has been suggested that vaccines be administered 2 weeks before planned splenectomy or 14 days after a spontaneous splenectomy.

Antimicrobial Prophylaxis of Meningitis

In *N. meningitidis* meningitis outbreaks, especially in the setting of residential facilities (e.g., dormitories, barracks, skilled nursing facilities, prisons), antimicrobial prophylaxis of close contacts is a key modality in disease prevention. Close contact is defined as members of the same household, individuals who share sleeping quarters, day care contacts, and anyone who shares oral secretions. Prophylaxis helps reduce nasopharyngeal carriage of meningitis-causing organisms and should be initiated as soon as possible after exposure. Prophylaxis can be effective up to 14 days following disease exposure. However, antimicrobial prophylaxis is not useful in the management of outbreaks of disease caused by *S. pneumoniae* or *L. monocytogenes*.

Rifampin, ciprofloxacin, and intramuscular ceftriaxone are effective prophylaxis in adults involved in outbreaks of *N. meningitidis*, but despite the recommendation, it is unknown whether individuals previously vaccinated against *N. meningitidis* receive additional benefit from antimicrobial prophylaxis. Ciprofloxacin may be used in children, considering the low risk of ADEs with a single dose; however, some clinicians may avoid it for children

---

Box 1-5. Vaccine Administration Recommendations in Splenectomy or Functional Asplenia

S. pneumoniae vaccine

Previously unvaccinated ≥ 18 years: PCV13 x 1 dose, followed by PPSV23 x 1 dose after a minimum of 8 weeks elapsed

Previously vaccinated: PCV13 x 1 dose at least 1 year following last PPSV23 dose

N. meningitidis vaccine

MCV4 x 2 doses, minimum of 2 months apart

H. influenzae vaccine

Previously unvaccinated: Hib x 1 dose

Previously vaccinated: Hib booster (1 dose) may be considered but not required

Influenza virus vaccine

Annual vaccine recommended

---

younger than 5 years, especially if alternative agents are readily available. Ceftriaxone is the preferred agent for pregnant women. Rifampin prophylaxis is also recommended for unvaccinated individuals exposed to *H. influenzae* meningitis. Rifampin prophylaxis is not recommended in pregnant women.

In clinical practice, it is important to verify the vaccination status of all individuals exposed to *H. influenzae*, because vaccination might not occur based on parental vaccine fears or vaccine shortages. Table 1-7 details antimicrobial prophylaxis doses by population. Prophylaxis is not recommended for individuals exposed during outbreaks of Group B *Streptococcus*, and pregnant women should receive penicillin or ampicillin prophylaxis during delivery if they are group B *Streptococcus* carriers, have a history of group B *Streptococcus* bacteriuria during pregnancy, or previously delivered an infant with the disease.

CONCLUSION

The complexities of CNS infections dictate the benefit of an interdisciplinary-team approach to management, which should include infectious diseases specialists, neurosurgeons, and pharmacists. Knowledge of pharmacokinetic/pharmacodynamic principles is essential for antimicrobial selection and dose optimization that will increase the likelihood of obtaining optimal concentrations in the CNS compartment. Based on the initial multidrug approach taken in suspected CNS infections, pharmacists can help ensure appropriate de-escalation of therapy, as confirmatory results become available. Furthermore, pharmacists can play a vital role in prevention and should promote routine vaccination among all age groups.

Table 1-7. Antibiotic Chemoprophylaxis in Close Contacts of Confirmed Bacterial Meningitis Cases

Pathogen	Prophylactic Antibiotic	Dosing Scheme
S. pneumoniae	None recommended	
L. monocytogenes	None recommended	
H. influenzae	Rifampin	Neonates: 10 mg/kg PO once daily x 4 days Children > 1 month/adults: 20 mg/kg (max 600 mg) PO once daily x 4 days *(→ pregnant)(unvaccinated)*
N. meningitidis	Ciprofloxacin	Children > 1 month: 20 mg/kg (max 500 mg) PO x 1 dose Children > 12 years/adults: 500 mg PO x 1 dose
	Rifampin	Neonates: 5 mg/kg PO q12 hours x 2 days Children > 1 month/adults: 10 mg/kg (max 600 mg) PO q12 hours x 2 days
	Ceftriaxone	Children < 12 years: 125 mg IM x 1 dose Children ≥ 12 years/adults: 250 mg IM x 1 dose *(pregnant.)*

Adapted from: Tunkel AR, Glaser CA, Bloch KC, et al. The management of encephalitis: clinical practice guidelines by the Infectious Diseases Society of America. Clin Infect Dis 2008;47:303-27.

REFERENCES

Baumeister S, Peek A, Friedman A, et al. Management of postneurosurgical bone flap loss caused by infection. Plast Reconstr Surg 2008;122:195e-208e.

Beer R, Pfausler B, Schmutzhard E. Infectious intracranial complications in the neuro-ICU patient population. Curr Opin Crit Care 2010;16:117-22.

Bland CM, Bookstaver PB, Lu ZK, et al. Musculoskeletal safety outcomes of patients receiving high doses of daptomycin with HMG-CoA reductase inhibitors. Antimicrob Agents Chemother 2014;58:5726-31.

Bookstaver PB, Bland CM, Qureshi ZP, et al. Safety and effectiveness of daptomycin across a hospitalized obese population: results of a multicenter investigation in the Southeastern United States. Pharmacotherapy 2013;33:1322-30.

Boviatsis EJ, Kouyialis AT, Boutsikakis I, et al. Infected CNS infusion pumps. Is there a chance for treatment without removal? Acta neurochirurgica 2004;146:463-7.

Burgess DS, Frei CR, Lewis Ii JS, et al. The contribution of pharmacokinetic-pharmacodynamic modelling with Monte Carlo simulation to the development of susceptibility breakpoints for Neisseria meningitidis. Clin Microbiol Infect 2007;13:33-9.

Cascio A, Conti A, Sinardi L, et al. Post-neurosurgical multidrug-resistant *Acinetobacter* baumannii meningitis successfully treated with intrathecal colistin. A new case

and a systematic review of the literature. Int J Infect Dis 2010;14:e572-9.

Centers for Disease Control and Prevention (CDC) National Healthcare Safety Network. Surveillance Definitions for Specific Types of Infections, 2014 [home page on the internet]. Centers for Disease Control and Prevention (CDC). Progress in introduction of pneumococcal conjugate vaccine--worldwide, 2000-2008. MMWR Morbidity and mortality weekly report 2008;57:1148-51.

Centers for Disease Control and Prevention (CDC). Bacterial meningitis [homepage on the Internet]. 2012.

Cohn AC, MacNeil JR, Clark TA, et al. Prevention and control of meningococcal disease: recommendations of the Advisory Committee on Immunization Practices (ACIP). MMWR Recomm Rep 2013;62:1-28.

Cohn AC, MacNeil JR, Harrison LH, et al. Changes in *Neisseria meningitidis* disease epidemiology in the United States, 1998-2007: implications for prevention of meningococcal disease. Clin Infect Dis 2010;50:184-91.

Cottagnoud P, Pfister M, Cottagnoud M, et al. Activities of ertapenem, a new long-acting carbapenem, against penicillin-sensitive or -resistant pneumococci in experimental meningitis. Antimicrob Agents Chemother 2003;47:1943-7.

De Louvois and Infection in Neurosurgery Working Party of the British Society of Antimicrobial Chemotherapy. The rational use of antibiotics in the treatment of brain abscess. Br J Neurosurg 2000;14:525-30.

Daoud AS, Baticha A, Al-Sheyyab M, et al. Lack of effectiveness of dexamethasone in neonatal bacterial meningitis. Eur J Pediatr 1999;158:230-3.

de Gans J, van de Beek D. Dexamethasone in adults with bacterial meningitis. N Engl J Med 2002;347:1549-56.

Derber CJ, Troy SB. Head and neck emergencies: bacterial meningitis, encephalitis, brain abscess, upper airway obstruction, and jugular septic thrombophlebitis. Med Clin North Am 2012;96:1107-26.

Di Sabatino A, Carsetti R, Corazza GR. Post-splenectomy and hyposplenic states. Lancet 2011;378:86-97.

Elaldi N, Gozel MG, Kolayli F, et al. Community-acquired CTX-M-15-type ESBL-producing Escherichia coli meningitis: a case report and literature review. J Infect Dev Ctries 2013;7:424-31.

Fong IW, Tomkins KB. Penetration of ceftazidime into the cerebrospinal fluid of patients with and without evidence of meningeal inflammation. Antimicrob Agents Chemother 1984;26:115-6.

Gaillard JL, Abadie V, Cheron G, et al. Concentrations of ceftriaxone in cerebrospinal fluid of children with meningitis receiving dexamethasone therapy. Antimicrob Agents Chemother 1994;38:1209-10.

Hasbun R, Abrahams J, Jekel J, et al. Computed tomography of the head before lumbar puncture in adults with suspected meningitis. N Engl J Med 2001;345:1727-33.

Jaspan HB, Brothers AW, Campbell AJ, et al. Multidrug-resistant Enterococcus faecium meningitis in a toddler: characterization of the organism and successful treatment with intraventricular daptomycin and intravenous tigecycline. Pediatr Infect Dis J 2010;29:379-81.

Jolles S, Sewell WA, Leighton C. Drug-induced aseptic meningitis: diagnosis and management. Drug Saf 2000;22:215-6.

Karaiskos I, Galani L, Baziaka F, et al. Intraventricular and intrathecal colistin as the last therapeutic resort for the treatment of multidrug-resistant extensively drug-resistant Acinetobacter baumannii ventriculitis and meningitis: a literature review. Int J Antimicrob Agents 2013;41:499-508.

Karre T, Vetter EA, Mandrekar JN, et al. Comparison of bacterial antigen test and gram stain for detecting classic meningitis bacteria in cerebrospinal fluid. J Clin Microbiol 2010;48:1504-5.

Kitchen WJ, Singh N, Hulme S, et al. External ventricular drain infection: improved technique can reduce infection rates. Br J Neurosurg 2011;25:632-5.

Knoll BM, Hellmann M, Kotton CN. Vancomycin-resistant Enterococcus faecium meningitis in adults: case series and review of the literature. Scan J Infect Dis 2013;45:131-9.

Le J, Bookstaver PB, Rudisill CN, et al. Treatment of meningitis caused by vancomycin-resistant Enterococcus faecium: high-dose and combination daptomycin therapy. Ann Pharmacother 2010;44:2001-6.

Lopez-Alvarez B, Martin-Laez R, Farinas MC, et al. Multidrug-resistant Acinetobacter baumannii ventriculitis: successful treatment with intraventricular colistin. Acta Neurochir (Wien) 2009;151:1465-72.
Lutsar I, McCracken GH, Jr., Friedland IR. Antibiotic pharmacodynamics in cerebrospinal fluid. Clin Infect Dis 1998;27:1117-27, quiz 28-9.

MacNeil JR, Cohn AC, Farley M, et al. Current epidemiology and trends in invasive Haemophilus influenzae disease--United States, 1989-2008. Clin Infect Dis 2011;53:1230-6.

Margetis K, Dimaraki E, Charkoftaki G, et al. Penetration of intact blood-brain barrier by doripenem. Antimicrob Agents Chemother 2011;55:3637-8.

Mendes RE, Biek D, Critchley IA, Farrell DJ, Sader HS, Jones RN. Decreased ceftriaxone susceptibility in emerging (35B and 6C) and persisting (19A) Streptococcus pneumoniae serotypes in the United States, 2011-2012: ceftraoline remains active in vitro among β-lactam agents. Antimicrob Agents Chemother 2014;58:4923-7.

Miller AD, Ball AM, Bookstaver PB, Dornblaser EK, Bennett Cl. Epileptogenic Potential of Carbapenem Agents: Mechanism of Action, Seizure Rates and Clinical Considerations. Pharmacotherapy 2011;31:408-23.

Miranda J, Tunkel AR. Strategies and new developments in the management of bacterial meningitis. Infect Dis Clin N Am 2009;23:925-43.

Nath A, Tyler KL. Novel approaches and challenges to treatment of CNS viral infections. Ann Neurol 2013;74:412-22.

Nau R, Prange HW, Muth P, et al. Passage of cefotaxime and ceftriaxone into cerebrospinal fluid of patients with uninflamed meninges. Antimicrob Agents Chemother 1993;37:1518-24.

Nau R, Sorgel F, Eiffert H. Penetration of drugs through the blood-cerebrospinal fluid/blood-brain barrier for treatment of central nervous system infections. Clin Microbiol Rev 2010;23:858-83.

Nevrekar S, Cunningham KC, Greathouse KM, et al. Dual intraventricular plus systemic antibiotic therapy for the treatment of Klebsiella pneumoniae carbapenemase-producing Klebsiella pneumoniae ventriculitis. Ann Pharmacother 2014;48:274-8.

Nuorti JP, Whitney CG, Centers for Disease Control and Prevention. Prevention of pneumococcal disease among infants and children - use of 13-valent pneumococcal conjugate vaccine and 23-valent pneumococcal polysaccharide vaccine - recommendations of the Advisory Committee on

Immunization Practices (ACIP). MMWR Recomm Rep 2010;59:1-18.

Patel AR, Alton TB, Bransford RJ, Lee MJ, Bellabarba CB, Chapman JR. Spinal epidural abscesses: risk factors, medical versus surgical management, a retrospective review of 128 cases. Spine J 2014;14:326-30.

Pouplin T, Pouplin JN, Van Toi P, et al. Valacyclovir for herpes simplex encephalitis. Antimicrob Agents Chemother 2011;55:3624-6.

Pradilla G, Ardila GP, Hsu W, Rigamonti D. Epidural abscesses of the CNS. Lancet Neurol 2009;8:292-300.

Rand K, Houck H, Lawrence R. Real-time polymerase chain reaction detection of herpes simplex virus in cerebrospinal fluid and cost savings from earlier hospital discharge. J Mol Diagn 2005;7:511-6.

Ricard JD, Wolff M, Lacherade JC, et al. Levels of vancomycin in cerebrospinal fluid of adult patients receiving adjunctive corticosteroids to treat pneumococcal meningitis: a prospective multicenter observational study. Clin Infect Dis 2007;44:250-5.

Seehusen DA, Reeves MM, Fomin DA. Cerebrospinal fluid analysis. Am Fam Physician 2003;68:1103-9.

Shin SH, Kim KS. Treatment of bacterial meningitis: an update. Expert Opin Pharmacother 2012;13:2189-206.

Sierra-Hoffman M, Iznaola O, Goodwin M, Mohr J. Combination therapy with ampicillin and daptomycin for treatment of Enterococcus faecalis endocarditis. Antimicrob Agents Chemother 2012;56:6064.

Smith JP, Weller S, Johnson B, et al. Pharmacokinetics of acyclovir and its metabolites in cerebrospinal fluid and systemic circulation after administration of high-dose valacyclovir in subjects with normal and impaired renal function. Antimicrob Agents Chemother 2010;54:1146-51.

Steadman E, Raisch DW, Bennett CL, et al. Evaluation of a potential clinical interaction between ceftriaxone and calcium. Antimicrob Agents Chemother 2010;54:1534-40.

Stenehjem E, Armstrong WS. Central nervous system device infections. Infect Dis Clin North Am 2012;26:89-110.

Stucki A, Cottagnoud M, Acosta F, et al. Efficacy of doripenem against Escherichia coli and Klebsiella pneumoniae in experimental meningitis. J Antimicrob Chemother 2012;67:661-5.

Studahl M, Lindquist L, Eriksson BM, et al. Acute viral infections of the central nervous system in immunocompetent adults: diagnosis and management. Drugs 2013;73:131-58.

Takhar SS, Ting SA, Camargo CA, Jr., et al. U.S. emergency department visits for meningitis, 1993-2008. Acad Emerg Med 2012;19:632-9.

Thigpen MC, Whitney CG, Messonnier NE, et al. Bacterial meningitis in the United States, 1998-2007. N Engl J Med 2011;364:2016-25.

Tompkins M, Panuncialman I, Lucas P, et al. Spinal epidural abscess. J Emerg Med 2010;39:384-90.

Tunkel AR, Glaser CA, Bloch KC, et al. The management of encephalitis: clinical practice guidelines by the Infectious Diseases Society of America. Clin Infect Dis 2008;47:303-27.

Tunkel AR, Hartman BJ, Kaplan SL, et al. Practice guidelines for the management of bacterial meningitis. Clin Infect Dis 2004;39:1267-84.

U.S. Food and Drug Administration (FDA). Anti-Infective Drugs Advisory Committee. Dalbavancin for Injection (Briefing Document, March 31 2014).

Wong SS, Daka S, Pastewski A, et al. Spinal epidural abscess in hemodialysis patients: a case series and review. Clin J Am Soc Nephrol 2011;6:1495-500.

World Health Organization. Global Health Observatory (GHO), 2014 [home page on the internet].)

Yaita K, Komatsu M, Oshiro Y, et al. Postoperative meningitis and epidural abscess due to extended-spectrum β-lactamase-producing *Klebsiella pneumoniae*: a case report and a review of the literature. Intern Med 2012;51:2645-8.

SELF-ASSESSMENT QUESTIONS

1. A 65-year-old man presents to the emergency department with a 3-day history of headache, malaise, nausea, and subjective fevers. He also reports a 1-week history of nasal congestion and rhinorrhea. Physical examination reveals some confusion, repetitive questioning, temperature 102.1°F, heart rate 105 beats/minute, blood pressure 98/64 mm Hg, and respiratory rate 18 breaths/minute. Cerebrospinal fluid (CSF) results from a lumbar puncure (LP) are as follows: opening pressure 470 mm Hg, WBC 3300 cells/mm^3, 75% polymorphonuclear cells, protein 160 mg/dL, glucose 48 mg/dL (serum glucose 160 mg/dL). Which one of the following types of meningitis does this patient most likely to have?

   A. Bacterial.
   B. Viral.
   C. Fungal.
   D. Aseptic.

Questions 2 and 3 pertain to the following case.

J.G. is a 9-month old girl who presents to the pediatrician with a 2-day history of high fever (103°F), lethargy, irritability, poor appetite, and vomiting. Her mother reports that yesterday, a red rash appeared on the infant's stomach and back. Physical examination reveals an ill-appearing infant, temperature 102.5°F, with a diffuse petechial rash. J.G. was born at 38 weeks gestation to a mother positive for group B *Streptococci*, and had a 3-day neonatal intensive care unit (ICU) stay for meconium aspiration. She has received vaccinations according to the recommended schedule. Based on her presentation, she is sent to the emergency department for LP and further work-up for meningitis.

2. Which one of the following bacteria is the most likely cause of meningitis in J.G.?

   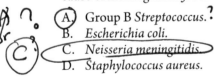
   A. Group B *Streptococcus*. ?
   B. *Escherichia coli.*
   C. *Neisseria meningitidis.*
   D. *Staphylococcus aureus.*

3. Which one of the following would be the best empiric therapy to initiate in J.G.?

   A. Cefotaxime and vancomycin.
   B. Cefepime and vancomycin.
   C. Cefotaxime, vancomycin, and ampicillin.
   D. Ceftriaxone, vancomycin, and ampicillin.

4. Which of the following immunizations has the most impact on reduction of the incidence of meningitis?

   A. Pneumococcal vaccination.
   B. Streptococcal vaccination.
   C. Influenza vaccination.
   D. Herpes zoster vaccination.

Questions 5 and 6 pertain to the following case.

M.L. is a 45-year-old man who presents to the emergency department with a 3-day history of nausea, vomiting, headache, and fever. Upon questioning, he also endorses photophobia and has nuchal rigidity on examination. M.L. reports that 1 week ago he received a prescription for penicillin VK for a dental abscess and began taking naproxen and acetaminophen to treat his pain. His other home drugs include lisinopril 20 mg orally daily and omeprazole 20 mg orally daily. Based on signs and symptoms, a LP is performed and results are pending. The resident inquires you regarding the possibility of aseptic meningitis.

5. Should M.L. have aseptic meningitis, which of the following medications is the most likely cause?

   A. Acetaminophen.
   B. Lisinopril.
   C. Naproxen.
   D. Penicillin VK.

6. After further review of M.L.'s chart with the finalized LP results, the resident suspects bacterial meningitis. Which one of the following would be the most likely cause of M.L.'s infection?

   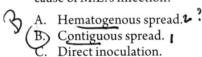
   A. Hematogenous spread. ?
   B. Contiguous spread. 1
   C. Direct inoculation.
   D. Trauma.

7. A 5-year-old boy is brought to the emergency department by paramedics after a 24-hour history of fever (104°F at home), vomiting, and headache. Upon arrival he is intubated for airway protection because of depressed mental status/obtundation. An LP is performed and is consistent with bacterial meningitis with a Gram stain demonstrated gram-positive cocci. Based on the severity of his condition, his mother is concerned about the spread of the disease to his 3-year-old sister. Which one of the following is best to recommend for this patient's 3-year-old sister?

   A. Ciprofloxacin.
   B. Ceftriaxone.
   C. Ampicillin.
   D. No prophylaxis.

Questions 8–10 pertain to the following case.

Seventeen days ago, J.R., a 19-year-old man, was admitted to the neurosurgery ICU after a motor vehicle collision. J.R. sustained multiple injuries including an epidural hematoma. A craniotomy was emergently performed and an external ventricular drain (EVD) was placed to remove excess CSF. After some initial improvement, his mental status has declined and he is febrile (Tmax 101.9°F). J.R. is pan-cultured including blood, urine, respiratory, and CSF from the EVD.

8. Which one of the following regimens is best recommendation for the treatment of possible meningitis in J.R.?

    A. Ceftriaxone and vancomycin.
    B. Cefotaxime, tobramycin, and vancomycin.
    C. Cefepime and vancomycin.
    D. Cefepime, tobramycin, and vancomycin.

9. Given J.R.'s decline in mental status, the resident asks if steroid therapy would help mitigate the inflammation in the CNS. Which one of the following is the best recommendation for J.R.?

    A. Adjunctive dexamethasone.
    B. Adjunctive methylprednisolone.
    C. Adjunctive prednisone.
    D. No adjunctive steroid therapy.

10. After two days, J.R.'s culture results are positive for ESBL-positive *Acinetobacter baumannii*. The team request intraventricular therapy in addition to systemic therapy. Which one of the following is best to recommend for intraventricular administration for J.R.?

    A. Daptomycin.
    B. Vancomycin.
    C. Meropenem.
    D. Amikacin.

Questions 11–13 pertain to the following case.

S.C. is a 24-year-old man (weight 73 kg, height 67 inches) who presents to the emergency department with headache, altered mental status, and lethargy. His medical history shows no comorbid conditions or medications. S.C. has a documented vancomycin allergy (red man's syndrome). Computed tomography (CT) and magnetic resonance imaging (MRI) scans suggest possible encephalitis. Vital signs are normal except for a temperature of 102.3°F. An LP is performed after CT scan and routine diagnostic lab tests are ordered on CSF. Blood cultures, complete blood count, and basic metabolic panel are obtained. LP results are still pending.

11. Which one of the following is best to recommend as empiric therapy for S.C.?

    A. Ceftriaxone, vancomycin, and acyclovir.
    B. Ceftriaxone, linezolid, and acyclovir.
    C. Ceftriaxone, linezolid, and valacyclovir.
    D. Ceftriaxone, acyclovir, and dexamethasone.

12. The analysis of S.C.'s CSF return 2 hours later as opening pressure 390 mm Hg, WBC 3500 cells/mm^3 (24% neutrophils), protein 160 mg/dL, glucose 64 mg/dL (serum glucose 120 mg/dL), RBC 1100 cells/mm^3. A basic metabolic panel is normal, with SCr 1.0 mg/dL. A CBC is normal except for a WBC 13.2 x 10^3 cells/mm^3. Bacterial antigen and CSF Gram stain were negative. A CSF herpes simplex virus (HSV) polymerase chain reaction (PCR) test is positive, and blood cultures are pending. Which one of the following is best to recommend for S.C.?

    A. Continue all antimicrobials until blood cultures have finalized.
    B. Acyclovir 700 mg intravenously every 8 hours for 14 days.
    C. Acyclovir 700 mg intravenously every 8 hours for 14 days and dexamethasone 10 mg intravenously every 6 hours for 3 days.
    D. Ceftriaxone 2 g intravenously every 12 hours and acyclovir 1000 mg intravenously every 8 hours for 14 days.

13. On day 4 of therapy, S.C. has returned to baseline and is eager to go home. The primary team inquires about the possibility of oral therapy for the remaining duration of therapy. Which one of the following is best to recommend for S.C.?

    A. Oral treatment options for HSV encephalitis are not available.
    B. Oral valacyclovir offers good bioavailability and adequate CSF penetration; however, clinical data are very sparse, limiting its routine use for HSV encephalitis.
    C. Oral valacyclovir would be an appropriate option in this patient to avoid the risk associated with a peripherally inserted central catheter line.
    D. Oral valacyclovir should be initiated at the end of a 14-day intravenous acyclovir course to prevent recurrence.

Questions 14–17 pertain to the following case.

H.T. is a 57-year-old man (weight 80 kg), height 70 inches) status post neurosurgery (10 days ago) secondary to head trauma sustained from a motor vehicle crash. An EVD remains in place after the surgery. H.T. is intubated and sedated but has spiked multiple fevers (Tmax 103.1°F) over the past 24 hours. There is no change in oxygen requirements or secretions and laboratory test values are stable with normal renal function. Blood and urine cultures are obtained. Initial blood Gram stain shows gram-positive cocci in clusters.

14. Given the concern for a possible CNS source, which one of the following is best to recommend as empiric treatment for H.T.?

    A. Meropenem 2 g intravenously every 8 hours plus vancomycin 1500 mg intravenously every 12 hours.
    B. Piperacillin/tazobactam 4.5 g intravenously every 6 hours plus gentamicin 7 mg/kg intravenously daily plus vancomycin 1500 mg intravenously every 12 hours.
    C. Cefepime 2 g intravenously every 8 hours plus metronidazole 500 mg intravenously every 6 hours plus vancomycin 1500 mg intravenously every 12 hours.
    D. Linezolid 600 mg intravenously every 12 hours.

15. On day 2, H.T.'s blood culture results show vancomycin-resistant *Enterococcus faecium* (susceptibilities pending). An LP is performed and a CSF Gram stain shows gram-positive cocci. Given the high likelihood of vancomycin-resistant Enterococcus meningitis, which of the following therapies is most appropriate for H.T.?

    A. Discontinue the current antibiotic regimen and initiate quinupristin/dalfopristin 600 mg intravenously every 8 hours.
    B. Discontinue the current antibiotic regimen and initiate ceftriaxone 2 g intravenously every 12 hours plus ampicillin 12 g intravenously every 24 hours by continuous infusion.
    C. Discontinue the current antibiotic regimen and initiate linezolid 600 mg intravenously every 12 hours.
    D. Discontinue the current antibiotic regimen and initiate tigecycline 100 mg intravenously every 12 hours plus gentamicin 500 mg intravenously daily.

16. Susceptibilities are available for H.T.'s culture and show the following: ampicillin, MIC >32 mcg/mL (R); gentamicin synergy (R); streptomycin synergy (R); daptomycin, MIC = 2 mcg/mL (S); linezolid, MIC=2 mcg/mL (S); rifampin, MIC = 4 mcg/mL (S); quinupristin/dalfopristin (S) no MIC available. S.C. is currently receiving daptomycin 800 mg intravenously every 24 hours. The primary team inquires about combination therapy. Which one of the following is best to recommend for H.T.?

    A. Ampicillin and aminoglycosides are viable options because of enhanced activity in combination.
    B. Rifampin demonstrated in vitro synergy with daptomycin but is contraindicated in patients with an EVD.
    C. Ampicillin has shown in vitro synergy with daptomycin and may be viable option in this patient.
    D. Linezolid and quinupristin-dalfopristin is the recommended combination therapy for H.T. because of the susceptibilities resistant patterns.

17. On Day 5, H.T.'s clinical status has not improved despite therapy. The EVD is still in place and the team is inquiring about direct therapy to ensure adequate CSF concentrations. Which one of the following would be the best choice for intraventricular administration in H.T.?

    A. Ampicillin.
    B. Daptomycin.
    C. Vancomycin.
    D. Linezolid.

18. Which of the following regimens would be the best empirical management for an acute brain abscess in a 73-year-old woman secondary to an oral abscess?

    A. Vancomycin plus ceftriaxone.
    B. Vancomycin plus ceftriaxone plus ampicillin.
    C. Penicillin plus clindamycin plus tobramycin.
    D. Ceftriaxone plus metronidazole.

19. A 45-year-old man had a gunshot wound to the head and has undergone numerous surgical procedures because of the trauma. He subsequently develops a brain abscess confirmed by CT. It is known that the patient has an allergy to vancomycin (facial swelling). The surgical team is prepared to drain the abscess, and empiric antibiotic therapy is initiated with ceftriaxone and metronidazole. While culture is pending, which one of the following is best to recommend for this patient?

    A. Discontinue metronidazole and initiate daptomycin and gentamicin.
    B. Discontinue ceftriaxone and initiate meropenem.
    C. Discontinue ceftriaxone and initiate linezolid and cefepime.
    D. Initiate daptomycin and ciprofloxacin.

20. A local university student health center and associated health clinics are updating protocols and antimicrobial inventory to manage meningitis postexposure prophylaxis. Given their patient population, which one of the following is best to recommend?

A. Maintain ceftriaxone and ciprofloxacin on protocol for prophylaxis of the most common bacterial pathogens.

B. Maintain ceftriaxone, rifampin, and acyclovir on protocol for prophylaxis of the most common bacterial and viral pathogens.

C. Maintain ceftriaxone, ciprofloxacin, and intravenous immunoglobulin on protocol for prophylaxis of the most common pathogens.

D. Postexposure prophylaxis should be filtered through state or local health departments, pre-empting the need for local antimicrobial therapy protocols.

Learner Chapter Evaluation: CNS Infections in Immunocompetent Hosts.

As you take the posttest for this chapter, also evaluate the material's quality and usefulness, as well as the achievement of learning objectives. Rate each item using this 5-point scale:

- Strongly agree
- Agree
- Neutral
- Disagree
- Strongly disagree

1. The content of the chapter met my educational needs.
2. The content of the chapter satisfied my expectations.
3. The author presented the chapter content effectively.
4. The content of the chapter was relevant to my practice and presented at the appropriate depth and scope.
5. The content of the chapter was objective and balanced.
6. The content of the chapter is free of bias, promotion, or advertisement of commercial products.
7. The content of the chapter was useful to me.
8. The teaching and learning methods used in the chapter were effective.
9. The active learning methods used in the chapter were effective.
10. The learning assessment activities used in the chapter were effective.
11. The chapter was effective overall.

Use the 5-point scale to indicate whether this chapter prepared you to accomplish the following learning objectives:

12. Use patient demographics, risk factors, and results of a lumbar puncture to distinguish the common pathogens associated with meningitis.
13. Assess a patient for medications associated with drug-induced aseptic meningitis.
14. Using the impact of immunization practices on national epidemiologic trends in meningitis and encephalitis, justify antimicrobial prophylaxis of meningitis.
15. Design a treatment regimen and monitoring plan for a patient with community- or hospital-acquired bacterial meningitis, bacterial brain abscess, or viral meningoencephalitis.
16. Using an understanding of medication penetration into central nervous system compartments, justify the use of intraventricular or intrathecal administration of antimicrobials.
17. Please provide any specific comments relating to any perceptions of bias, promotion, or advertisement of commercial products.
18. Please expand on any of your above responses, and/or provide any additional comments regarding this chapter:

Food- and Waterborne Illnesses

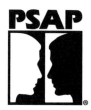

By Allana J. Sucher, Pharm.D., BCPS; and Elias B. Chahine, Pharm.D., BCPS (AQ-ID)

Reviewed by Katie J. Suda, Pharm.D., M.S.; Kari A. McCracken, Pharm.D., BCPS; and Jennifer Phillips, Pharm.D., BCPS

Learning Objectives

1. Analyze the epidemiology of food- and waterborne illnesses, including risk factors for acquisition, causative pathogens, and modes of transmission.
2. For a given patient, classify the most likely etiology of a food- or waterborne illness.
3. Assess a patient's risk of developing complications from a food- or waterborne illness.
4. Given a specific scenario, demonstrate the best means by which to diagnose a food- or waterborne illness.
5. Design appropriate pharmacotherapy for a suspected food- or waterborne illness.
6. Compose a prevention strategy and plan of self-treatment for a given patient at risk of a food- or waterborne illness.

Introduction

Food- and waterborne illnesses cause significant morbidity and mortality, with diarrhea accounting for about 800,000 deaths annually in children younger than 5 years of age worldwide (Liu 2012). Food- and waterborne illnesses result from ingestion of foods and water contaminated with bacterial, viral, or parasitic pathogens acquired domestically or through travel. Traveler's diarrhea (TD), the most common travel-associated disease, occurs in 30% to 70% of travelers after arrival at their destinations (Connor 2014).

Etiology

Bacterial Pathogens

Campylobacter jejuni is a microaerophilic, motile, non-spore-forming, oxidase-positive, gram-negative rod that causes infection after ingestion of 10,000 organisms. Foods associated with this pathogen include raw or undercooked poultry, unpasteurized milk, contaminated water, and produce that has come in contact with contaminated water.

Baseline Knowledge Statements

Readers of this chapter are presumed to be familiar with the following:
- Basic food-handling practices to prevent food and waterborne illnesses
- Basic hygiene practices to prevent food and waterborne illnesses
- Guidelines for the administration of rehydration therapy
- Pharmacology, including mechanisms of action, adverse effects, and drug interactions of antimicrobials used in the treatment of food- and waterborne illnesses
- Interpretation and appropriate use of the immunization schedules of the Advisory Committee on Immunization Practice

Additional Readings

The following free resources are available for readers wishing additional background information on this topic.
- Centers for Disease Control and Prevention. Food Safety.
- Centers for Disease Control and Prevention. Healthy Water.
- U.S .Food and Drug Administration. Bad Bug Book: Foodborne Pathogenic Microorganisms and Natural Toxins Handbook, 2nd ed., 2012.
- Brunette GW, Kozarsky PE, Cohen NJ, et al, eds. CDC Health Information for International Travel 2014: The Yellow Book. New York: Oxford University Press, 2014.

Escherichia coli, a member of the Enterobacteriaceae family, is a facultative anaerobic, glucose-fermenting, oxidase-negative, gram-negative rod that colonizes the gastrointestinal tract. *E. coli* is further categorized based on virulence properties and mechanism of causing disease. Enterotoxigenic *E. coli* (ETEC) is the most common cause of traveler's diarrhea and the most common type of *E. coli* infection. In adults, ingestion of more than 10 million organisms causes infection; children can be infected after ingestion of fewer particles. Shiga toxin–producing *E. coli* (STEC), also known as enterohemorrhagic *E. coli* (EHEC), is named for its cytotoxic toxins, which are referred to as Shiga-like toxin 1 and Shiga-like toxin 2. Serotypes are further classified by their lipopolysaccharide (O) and flagellar (H) antigens, with *E. coli* 0157:H7 the most common type in the United States. Ingestion of 10 to 100 organisms causes infection in humans. In developing countries and in patients with HIV, enteroaggregative *E. coli* produces a Shiga-like toxin and a hemolysin and is responsible for causing acute and chronic diarrhea lasting more than 14 days. Enteropathogenic *E. coli* adheres to small-bowel mucosal cells and is responsible for causing diarrhea in infants in developing countries. Enteroinvasive *E. coli* strains are nonlactose or late-lactose fermenting and invade the epithelial cells of the intestinal mucosa, producing diarrhea most commonly in children or travelers in developing countries after ingestion of 200 to 5000 organisms. Because *E. coli* is part of the normal intestinal flora, it is found in water or food that has been contaminated with animal or human feces. In addition, STEC may also be contracted from ingestion of undercooked beef or unpasteurized milk.

Listeria monocytogenes is a motile, catalase-positive, oxidase-negative, facultative anaerobic, non-spore-forming gram-positive rod that enters the human body through the gastrointestinal tract after the ingestion of contaminated foods. The infective dose is undetermined because it varies with the strain of the pathogen, the host's susceptibility, and the type of food ingested. Foods associated with this pathogen include unpasteurized milk, deli meats, soft cheeses, produce, refrigerated pâtés, and smoked seafood.

Salmonella spp. are motile, non-spore-forming, facultative anaerobic, enteric gram-negative rods of the Enterobacteriaceae family that ferment glucose and mannose. There are more than 2500 serotypes of *salmonellae*; these include more than 1400 group I serotypes, which are responsible for most cases of human illness. Although the infective dose varies with the strain of the pathogen and the host's age and immune status, ingestion of one organism may cause infection. Foods associated with this pathogen include beef, poultry, eggs, dairy, unpasteurized milk, contaminated water, and produce that came in contact with contaminated water.

Shigella spp. are nonmotile, aerobic, glucose-fermenting, gram-negative rods of the Enterobacteriaceae family that colonize the gastrointestinal tract. *Shigella* spp. infections are easily spread from person to person because only 1000 organisms are required for infection. Infection from this pathogen can be caused by water or food contaminated with human feces or by ingestion of ready-to-eat foods such as produce, egg or potato salad, or sandwiches that have been touched by an infected food handler.

Vibrio cholerae is an aerobic, motile, non-spore-forming, oxidase-positive, gram-negative rod that appears in the shape of a comma on Gram stain. *V. cholerae* is classified by O lipopolysaccharide antigen groups; serogroups O1 and O139 are responsible for the typical presentation of cholera, the cause of several worldwide pandemics. Ingestion of 10 billion organisms from water or 100 to 10,000 organisms from food causes infection. Foods associated with this pathogen include contaminated water, fish, and shellfish.

Vibrio vulnificus and *Vibrio parahaemolyticus* are aerobic, motile, non–spore-forming, halophilic, oxidase-positive, gram-negative rods found in undercooked or raw seafood such as fish or shellfish or in contaminated water. *V. vulnificus* is also found in oysters, particularly in warm months. The estimated median infective dose of *V. parahaemolyticus* is 100 million organisms, but ingestion of 1000 organisms of *V. vulnificus* can cause infection.

Bacteria That Cause Enterotoxigenic Food Poisoning

Bacillus cereus is a saprophytic, nonmotile, aerobic, spore-forming, gram-positive rod that produces two different toxins that cause either an emetic or diarrheal form of disease. Ingestion of 100,000 to 100 million organisms causes infection. Foods associated with this pathogen include fried rice, meats, and vegetables.

Clostridium botulinum is an anaerobic, spore-forming, gram-positive rod that is found in soil. It produces seven different types of toxin (A through G); types A, B, and E are responsible for most human infections. Spores of *C. botulinum* germinate in home-canned, smoked, or vacuum-packed foods with low acid content and transform into vegetative forms that produce preformed toxin that is subsequently ingested. The production of only a few nanograms of toxin can cause illness. Because the toxins are destroyed by heating at 212°F (100°C) for about 20 minutes, infection is caused by uncooked or undercooked food. Most cases of infection in infants are caused by ingestion of foods such a honey that contains spores of *C. botulinum*.

Clostridium perfringens is an anaerobic, spore-forming, gram-positive rod. Strains that produce enterotoxin cause intense diarrhea after ingestion of 100 million vegetative cells. Foods associated with this pathogen include beef, poultry, and gravy.

Staphylococcus aureus is a catalase-positive, coagulase-positive, aerobic, gram-positive coccus that appears in irregular grapelike clusters on Gram stain. Infection can occur from a toxin level less than 1 mcg. About one-half of *S. aureus* strains produce at least one enterotoxin. Enterotoxins are heat-stable superantigens that are formed in carbohydrate and protein-rich foods such as unrefrigerated or improperly refrigerated meats, egg or potato salads, or cream-filled pastries.

Viral Pathogens

Hepatitis A is an RNA virus of the Picornavirus family; it can be destroyed by boiling in water for 5 minutes or by heating food to above 185°F (85°C) for at least 1 minute. Ingestion of 10 to 100 viral particles causes infection. The virus is spread by the fecal-oral route through close personal contact or by a single source of fecal contamination, such as contaminated water or foods that are not reheated after contact with an infected food handler. In addition, ingestion of shellfish harvested from water polluted with sewage has caused disease outbreaks.

Norovirus is an RNA virus of the Calciviridae family that causes infection after ingestion of as few as 10 viral particles. It is spread by way of the fecal-oral route through close personal contact in settings such as restaurants, nursing homes, hospitals, schools, day care centers, and cruise ships or by fecal contamination of a single source, such as contaminated water or ready-to-eat foods that are touched by an infected food handler. In addition, ingestion of shellfish harvested from water polluted with sewage has caused disease outbreaks.

Rotavirus is an RNA virus of the Reoviridae family that is a major cause of diarrhea in infants and children worldwide. Ingestion of 10 to 100 viral particles causes infection that gets spread by the fecal-oral route through close personal contact such as in day care centers or by fecal contamination of a single source, such as contaminated water or ready-to-eat foods that are touched by an infected food handler.

Parasitic Pathogens

Cryptosporidium spp. is an intracellular intestinal parasite that is ubiquitous in the environment and causes infection after ingestion of 30 organisms. It is further classified as sporozoa, which are parasites that undergo a complex life cycle that includes both sexual and asexual reproductive phases. Infection is spread by way of the fecal-oral route from contaminated water or food or from

fecal contamination of a single source, such as food that has been touched by an infected food handler.

Giardia lamblia is an omnipresent flagellate intestinal protozoa that exists in both trophozoite and cyst forms. Ingestion of one or more cysts causes infection that gets spread by way of the fecal-oral route from ingestion of water or food that contains cysts or by direct fecal contamination in settings such as day care centers or from a single source, such as contaminated water or foods that are touched by an infected food handler. Animal feces may also spread infection to humans, as evidenced by outbreaks among campers and hikers in the wilderness.

Entamoeba histolytica is an amebic intestinal protozoa that is found wherever there is fecal contamination in the environment. *E. histolytica* exists in ameboid trophozoite form in tissues and in cyst form in the lumen of the colon and in feces. Ingestion of fewer than 10 cysts causes infection that is spread by way of the fecal-oral route from ingestion of water or food that contains cysts or by direct fecal contamination in settings such as day care centers or from a single source, such as an infected food handler.

EPIDEMIOLOGY

Burden

According to estimates from the Centers for Disease Control and Prevention (CDC), about 1 person in 6 in the United States (equivalent to 48 million people) annually becomes ill from a foodborne pathogen, resulting in 128,000 hospitalizations and 3000 deaths. The pathogens responsible for the majority of cases of domestically acquired illness include norovirus (58% of cases), nontyphoidal *Salmonella* spp. (11%), *Clostridium perfringens* (10%), *Campylobacter* spp. (9%), and *Staphylococcus aureus* (3%).

The CDC also estimates that 4 million to 32 million cases of acute gastrointestinal illness occur annually in the United States from public drinking water systems; *Campylobacter* spp. causes 78% of those illnesses (MMWR 2013). *Cryptosporidium* spp. is the most common cause of recreational water–associated disease outbreaks in the United States (MMWR 2014).

Around 70% of travelers experience at least one episode of diarrhea; symptoms typically appear within the first week of travel. Bacterial pathogens (particularly ETEC ,*Campylobacter* spp., *Shigella* spp., and nontyphoidal *Salmonella* spp.) cause 80%–90% of TD; parasites account for 10% of cases; and viral pathogens account for 5% –8% (Connor 2014).

Surveillance Systems and Trends in Disease

Box 2-1 describes CDC surveillance systems used to assess the incidence of food- and waterborne illnesses. It includes a list of foodborne illnesses that are required to be reported. One system, the Foodborne Diseases Active

Surveillance Network (FoodNet), has conducted active, population-based surveillance since 1996 for laboratory-confirmed infections caused by nine foodborne pathogens: *Campylobacter, Cryptosporidium, Cyclospora, Listeria, Salmonella*, STEC, *Shigella, Vibrio*, and *Yersinia*. The FoodNet surveillance area comprises 46 million individuals in the United States, which is equivalent to 15% of the population. According to 2013 FoodNet data, the percentage of infections caused by *Salmonella* spp. significantly (9%) whereas those caused by *Vibrio* increased by 32% from 2010 to 2012. These data show continued need for improved prevention of foodborne infections (Figure 2-1).

TRANSMISSION

Food- and waterborne illnesses are contracted through the fecal-oral route or after ingestion of contaminated food or water, including recreational water. Most cases of food- and waterborne illnesses are caused by improper food handling. Contaminated produce is the most common food source of diarrhea, with leafy green vegetables accounting for 22% of all cases (DuPont 2014). *Campylobacter* spp. and nontyphoidal *Salmonella* can be contracted after contact with infected animals. Cholera is rare in countries that have advanced water and sanitation systems but can be seen in areas of the world with inadequate treatment of sewage and drinking water.

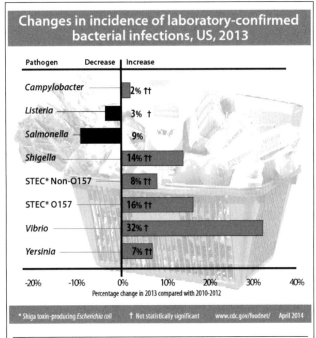

Figure 2-1. Changes in incidence of laboratory-confirmed bacterial infections in the United States, as captured by FoodNet, 2013.

Reprinted from the Centers for Disease Control and Prevention. FoodNet [homepage on the Internet].

RISK FACTORS

In general, immunosuppression, lack of gastric acidity (from surgery or use of proton pump inhibitors or histamine 2-receptor antagonists), or altered gut flora (from antibiotic use) are risk factors for acquiring a food- or

Box 2-1. U.S. Food- and Waterborne Illness Surveillance Systems

Foodborne Disease Active Surveillance Network (FoodNet)
- Active, population-based surveillance for 9 infections commonly transmitted through food; provides insights into incidence and trends of disease

National Antimicrobial Resistance Monitoring System – enteric bacteria (NARMS)
- Surveillance for antimicrobial resistance among foodborne bacteria in humans, retail meat, and animals; increases capability to detect, respond, and prevent antimicrobial resistance of foodborne bacteria

National ELectronic Norovirus Outbreak Network (CaliciNet)
- Electronic norovirus outbreak surveillance network with state and local public health laboratories; can quickly link norovirus outbreaks with a common food source and identify emerging strains

National Molecular Subtyping Network for Foodborne Disease Surveillance (PulseNet)
- Uses standardized methods to perform pulsed-field gel electrophoresis on foodborne bacterial pathogens; has revolutionized the detection and investigation of foodborne disease outbreaks; monitored by CDC and FDA's Coordinated Outbreak Response and Evaluation (CORE) network

National Notifiable Diseases Surveillance System (NNDSS)
- Health care providers and laboratory personnel are required by law to report the following foodborne infections: botulism, hemolytic uremic syndrome, listeriosis, salmonellosis, shiga toxin-producing *E. coli*, and vibriosis; local public health agencies report this information to the state or territorial agency, which voluntarily submits to NNDSS

National Outbreak Reporting System (NORS)
- Conducts analyses of data reported by health agencies; improves understanding of the foods, settings, and contributing factors of outbreaks

Environmental Health Specialists Network (EHS-Net), contributing factor surveillance
- Investigators from local and state public health agencies report contributing environmental factors of foodborne outbreaks to the CDC

Waterborne Disease and Outbreak Surveillance System (WBDOSS)
- Collects data in order to capture outbreaks associated with recreational water, drinking water, and other water exposures and is working to develop a comprehensive estimate of waterborne diseases in the United States in order to ensure effective disease prevention strategies are in place

waterborne illness. Patients with suppressed immune function include those who are younger than 5 years of age, 65 years or older, pregnant, or receiving immunosuppressive therapy; or who have chronic medical conditions such as HIV infection, AIDS, end-stage kidney disease, cirrhosis, or inflammatory bowel disease. Patients with suppressed immune function are at risk of developing more severe symptoms of infection such as bacteremia. In addition, travel destination, age 15 to 30 years, lack of avoidance of potentially contaminated food and water, and coming from a country with high sanitation standards are risk factors for TD.

Travel destination affects the risk of TD, with countries grouped into three risk categories (Box 2-2). The risk of TD varies with the water, sanitation, hygiene, food preparation, and food-handling practices in the travel destination, as well as the traveler's level of awareness of potentially contaminated food and water.

DIAGNOSTIC CONSIDERATIONS

A thorough medical history, travel history, and physical examination should be conducted, including an assessment of when the illness started, the specific foods consumed before symptom onset, relative time between consumption of food and onset of symptoms, and whether others have fallen ill. If two or more individuals experience a similar illness after ingestion of a common food, the clinician should consider a foodborne disease outbreak that may need to be reported to the health department (see Box 2-1). Additional information about reporting a foodborne illness is available on the CDC Web site. Frequency, consistency, and quantity of stool and intensity of vomiting should be assessed. The patient should be evaluated for dehydration and other signs of severe infection, including fever, presence of blood in stool, significant weight loss, lethargy, voluminous diarrhea, neurologic changes, and abdominal pain.

Because most cases of acute diarrhea or food poisoning are self-limited, a complete laboratory evaluation is not recommended for all patients. Laboratory testing should be considered for those who are older, are immunocompromised, recently used antibiotics (especially within the past month), have had diarrhea of any severity for more than 1 week or diarrhea for more than 1 day accompanied by fever of 101.3°F (38.5°C) or higher, bloody stools, or signs of sepsis or dehydration. Testing for the causative pathogen should also be considered when identification is important from a public health perspective, such as in the investigation of a suspected outbreak or when diarrhea is present in a food preparer or handler, a day care attendee or employee, a health care worker, or a resident of an institutional facility.

Stool cultures are used to identify and assess susceptibility of the infecting bacterial pathogen. Immunoassays or polymerase chain reaction (PCR) are used in testing for Shiga toxins or the genes that encode them. Newer, culture-independent testing methods use immunoassays or PCR to detect the presence of an antigen or toxin. A qualitative multiplex PCR assay that simultaneously detects 15 different pathogens from a stool sample was recently approved. In most laboratories, routine stool cultures include screening for *Salmonella* spp., *Shigella* spp., *Campylobacter* spp., and *E. coli* 0157:H7, which is the most common type of STEC in North America. Additional testing for viruses or other bacterial pathogens should be performed on the basis of the patient's prominent symptoms and history of food ingestion.

Testing for *Clostridium difficile* toxins should be performed if diarrhea develops after 3 days of hospitalization or recent antimicrobial exposure. Ova and parasites examination of stool (or antigen detection with immunofluorescence, immunoassays, or PCR testing for parasites) should be considered if the patient is immunocompromised, has a history of travel, or has diarrhea for more than 7 to 14 days. Testing for white blood cells or lactoferrin in stool may provide additional evidence of an inflammatory process in the colon. However, neither of those tests is specific for infection. Fecal white blood cells are not present with infections caused by viruses, parasites, or bacterial pathogens that cause watery diarrhea, because those organisms target the small intestine.

PATHOPHYSIOLOGY, PRESENTATION, AND COURSE OF ILLNESS

Table 2-1 describes the incubation period, duration of illness, and typical clinical presentation of food- and waterborne pathogens.

Bacterial Pathogens That Cause Watery Diarrhea

Enterotoxigenic *E. coli*, *L. monocytogenes*, *V. cholerae*, and *V. vulnificus* cause secretory diarrhea. The predominant symptoms of watery diarrhea are caused by excessive mucosal secretion of fluids and electrolytes and inhibition of absorption of sodium chloride in the small intestine.

Table 2-1. Characteristics of Food and Waterborne Illnesses

Etiology	Incubation Period	Duration of Illness	Clinical Syndrome
Bacteria			
Campylobacter jejuni	2–4 days	5–7 days	Diarrhea (may be bloody), fever, cramps[a]
EHEC	2–4 days	5–7 days	Diarrhea (often bloody), vomiting, severe cramps; HUS in 5%–10%
ETEC	6–48 hours	3–4 days	Profuse watery diarrhea, cramps
Listeria monocytogenes	1–2 days[a]	1–3 days[a]	Fever, nausea, vomiting, watery diarrhea; invasive disease (bacteremia, meningitis)b, fetal loss during pregnancy
Salmonella, nontyphoidal	6–48 hours	1–5 days	Diarrhea (may be bloody), fever, cramps[b]
Shigella spp.	2–4 days	1–7 days	Diarrhea (watery or bloody), fever, severe abdominal pain
Vibrio cholerae	2–4 days	1–3 days	Profuse watery diarrhea, vomiting
Vibrio parahaemolyticus	6–24 hours	2–5 days	Diarrhea (may be bloody), vomiting, fever, cramps[b]
Vibrio vulnificus	1–7 days	2–8 days	Watery diarrhea, vomiting, fever, cramps[b]
Bacteria that Cause Enterotoxigenic Poisonings			
Bacillus cereus	1–6 hours	1 day	Nausea, vomiting
	6–24 hours	1–2 days	Diarrhea
Clostridium botulinum	6–48 hours	Variable[c]	Visual changes, dropping eyelids, slurred speech, difficulty swallowing, muscle weakness
Clostridium perfringens	6–24 hours	1–2 days	Diarrhea, cramps
Staphylococcus aureus	1–6 hours	1 day	Nausea, vomiting, diarrhea, cramps
Viruses			
Hepatitis A	28 days	7 days[e]	Fatigue, anorexia, nausea, vomiting, diarrhea, jaundice, dark urine
Norovirus	6–48 hours	1–3 days	Watery diarrhea, fever, vomiting, cramps
Rotavirus	48 hours	3–7 days	Watery diarrhea, fever, vomiting, cramps
Parasites			
Cryptosporidium spp.	7 days[d]	2–14 days[e]	Watery diarrhea, fever, nausea, vomiting, cramps
Entamoeba histolytica	2–4 weeks[f]	Several weeks	Asymptomatic; mild diarrhea to severe bloody diarrhea; fever, pain, nausea, weight loss with liver abscess
Giardia lamblia	7 days[d]	2–6 weeks	Watery diarrhea, nausea, cramps, gas

[a]For gastroenteritis; incubation period of 2–6 weeks and duration of illness up to 3 months for invasive disease.
[b]Can cause systemic infection in immunocompromised host.
[c]Symptoms may last for up to 6 months.
[d]Range is 2 to 28 days.
[e]May lead to prolonged, chronic disease in immunocompromised.
[f]May reside in intestine for years without causing symptoms.
EHEC = enterohemorrhagic *Escherichia coli*; ETEC = enterotoxigenic *Escherichia coli*; HUS = hemolytic uremic syndrome.

Severe dehydration and electrolyte imbalances are possible complications.

Enterotoxigenic *E. coli* adheres to intestinal epithelial cells of the small bowel and produces toxins that ultimately cause prolonged hypersecretion of water and chloride as well as inhibition of sodium reabsorption, resulting in diarrhea for several days' duration.

L. monocytogenes has adhesion proteins that facilitate entry into host cells, a cell wall surface protein that enhances phagocytosis into epithelial cells, and filopods, all of which ultimately allow the organism to move from cell to cell while evading the host's immune system. Because *L. monocytogenes* causes an intracellular infection, patients with impaired cell-mediated immunity (e.g., those who are pregnant, recipients of organ transplants, patients with AIDS or lymphoma) are at risk of systemic infection.

V. cholerae attaches to microvilli of the brush border of epithelial cells; it produces a heat-labile enterotoxin, which ultimately results in hypersecretion of water and electrolytes as well as impaired absorption of sodium and chloride. Infection results in profound dehydration and a mortality rate of 25%–50% without treatment. The incubation period varies with the number of organisms ingested. Symptoms of infection include sudden onset of nausea and vomiting, abdominal cramps, and profuse, so-called rice water diarrhea, which typically contains mucus and epithelial cells.

V. vulnificus is the most virulent of the noncholera vibrios because of its polysaccharide capsule, extracellular proteins, and cell wall lipopolysaccharide. *V. vulnificus* causes gastroenteritis or wound infections in those who come into contact with contaminated water. Bacteremia, which is associated with a 50% mortality rate, may occur in those who are immunocompromised, have liver disease, or are in a state of iron overload. Infection with *V. vulnificus* progresses quickly, with bullous skin lesions or systemic infection developing in a few hours. It is often necessary to initiate treatment with antibiotics based on patient history and before confirmation of the etiology of infection.

Bacterial Pathogens That Cause Bloody Diarrhea

Pathogens associated with dysentery (bloody stools) include *C. jejuni*, STEC, nontyphoidal *Salmonella* spp., *Shigella* spp., and *V. parahaemolyticus*. These pathogens invade and destroy the colonic mucosa, triggering an intense inflammatory response. Patients with dysentery usually have fever and pass more than 10 stools per day. Severe complications associated with dysentery include tenesmus, rectal prolapse, and seizures.

Once ingested, *C. jejuni* multiplies in the small intestine and invades the epithelium, causing inflammation. Symptoms of gastroenteritis include profuse diarrhea (which may be bloody), cramping, abdominal pain, and fever. Symptoms are usually self-limited, with a 5- to 7-day duration. In patients with immunocompromise, *C. jejuni* can cause invasive disease that may last for up to 3 months.

Shiga toxin–producing *E. coli*, or enterohemorrhagic *E. coli*, produces Shiga-like toxin 1 and Shiga-like toxin 2, which are also referred to as verocytotoxins. These toxins cleave ribosomal RNA, interfering with protein synthesis. Shiga-like toxins cause apoptosis of intestinal epithelial cells and locally damage the colon, resulting in bloody diarrhea or hemorrhagic colitis. Shiga-like toxins may be carried to the kidneys through the bloodstream, where they damage renal endothelial cells and cause inflammation.

Nontyphoidal *Salmonella* multiplies in the small intestine and invades the epithelium, causing inflammation. Symptoms of gastroenteritis include diarrhea (which may be bloody), cramping, abdominal pain, and fever. Symptoms are usually self-limited, with a duration of 1 to 5 days. Nontyphoidal *Salmonella* can cause systemic infection in patients with immunocompromise.

Shigella spp. invades mucosal epithelial cells, forming microabscesses and a pseudomembrane on the affected areas of the intestinal tract. All species of *Shigella* release lipopolysaccharide endotoxin, which contributes to bowel wall irritation; *S. dysenteriae* type 1 produces a heat-labile exotoxin that acts as a neurotoxin in the central nervous system and affects the gastrointestinal tract. In the gut, it initially acts as an enterotoxin on the small intestine, producing watery diarrhea. Subsequently, infection progresses to the ileum and colon, producing recurring diarrhea that contains mucus or blood. Symptoms are usually self-limited, with a duration of illness of 1 to 7 days.

V. parahaemolyticus produces an enterotoxin that invades small bowel mucosal epithelial cells, causing inflammation and ultimately resulting in hypersecretion of water and electrolytes. Symptoms of gastroenteritis include diarrhea (which may be bloody), vomiting, cramping, abdominal pain, and fever. Symptoms are usually self-limited, with a duration of 2 to 5 days.

Pathogens That Cause Food Poisoning

Foodborne illness results from ingestion of enteric pathogens that cause gastrointestinal infections (commonly *Campylobacter* spp., *E. coli*, nontyphoidal *Salmonella*, *Shigella* spp., or norovirus) or from food poisoning, which is the ingestion of food contaminated by a preformed toxin produced by bacteria (e.g., *B. cereus*, *C. botulinum*, *C. perfringens*, *S. aureus*). Food poisoning caused by toxin-producing organisms typically has a swift onset of gastrointestinal symptoms (including vomiting) and a short duration of illness.

A preformed enterotoxin, produced when *B. cereus* spores germinate, causes nausea and vomiting within 1 to 6 hours of ingestion of improperly refrigerated cooked or fried rice. The diarrheal enterotoxin, which is either preformed or produced in the intestine, causes profuse diarrhea and abdominal cramping within 6 to 24 hours of ingestion of contaminated meats or gravies. Both types of infection are self-limited, usually lasting for about 1 day.

After absorption from the gut, *C. botulinum* toxin binds to presynaptic membranes of motor neurons; this inhibits the release of acetylcholine and hampers muscle contraction, causing paralysis. Symptoms of infection include vomiting, diarrhea, blurred or double vision, difficulty swallowing, and descending muscle weakness that occurs 6–48 hours after ingestion. Duration of illness may be up to several months in cases that are complicated by respiratory failure. In infants, ingested spores germinate in the intestinal tract after a 3- to 30-day incubation period and produce toxin that is absorbed into the bloodstream. The toxin inhibits the release of acetylcholine and causes flaccid paralysis with associated symptoms of poor feeding and weakness.

Some strains of *C. perfringens* produce an enterotoxin that causes hypersecretion of fluids and electrolytes in the jejunum and ileum, causing intense diarrhea 6–24 hours after ingestion of contaminated food. The illness is self-limited, lasting about 1–2 days.

The enterotoxin of *S. aureus* acts on neural receptors in the gut to stimulate the vomiting center, causing the sudden onset of severe nausea and vomiting 1–6 hours after ingestion of contaminated food. The infection is self-limited, with a duration of illness of about 1 day.

Viral Pathogens

Hepatitis A replicates in the liver after it is acquired through the fecal-oral route. It is excreted fecally through the biliary system 2 weeks before and 1 week after the onset of symptoms. Symptoms of infection include fever, anorexia, fatigue, vomiting, diarrhea, jaundice, or dark urine that occurs after an incubation period of 15–50 days. Hepatitis A virus is a self-limited infection that does not cause chronic liver disease. The duration of illness is variable and may last for up to 6 months.

Norovirus causes histologic changes in epithelial cells of the intestinal mucosa, apoptosis of enterocytes, and transient malabsorption of D-xylose, fat, and lactose that correlates with shortened microvilli and decreased activity of enterocyte brush border enzymes. Symptoms of infection include nausea, vomiting (more prevalent in children), watery diarrhea (more prevalent in adults), abdominal cramping, fever, and myalgia after an incubation period of 6–48 hours. The duration of illness is 1–3 days.

Rotavirus infects small intestinal villi, damaging the transport mechanisms of enterocytes. Enterocytes are then replaced by immature crypt cells that are unable to absorb sodium and glucose. Rotavirus also contains a protein called NSP4, which acts as an enterotoxin and induces secretion. After an incubation period of 1–3 days, symptoms of infection with rotavirus include watery diarrhea, fever, vomiting, and cramps that last for 3–7 days. Patients may also have temporary lactose intolerance.

Parasitic Pathogens

Cryptosporidium spp. is spread through oocysts that are passed in large amounts in human or animal feces. Once ingested, oocysts transform into sporozoites that invade intestinal cells, where they multiply asexually and infect other intestinal cells. The parasites also reproduce sexually, ultimately resulting in the formation of oocysts. Symptoms of infection in those who are immunocompetent include watery diarrhea that lasts for 1–2 weeks and occurs 2–28 days (average of 7 days) after exposure to the organism. Older people and those who are immunocompromised may have severe and prolonged diarrhea that can remit and relapse during a period of weeks to months. Because immune status affects severity and duration of symptoms from *Cryptosporidium* spp., potentially fatal infections can occur in immunocompromised patients.

G. lamblia exists in two forms; the trophozoite form has flagella and a sucking disk to help it adhere to the intestine; the cyst is formed in the colon and passed into stool. *G. lamblia* is not considered to be highly pathogenic in humans because large numbers of cysts have been found in stools of those who are asymptomatic. If the organism attaches to the mucosa of the duodenum or jejunum, it causes inflammation and subsequent epithelial cell damage, as well as watery diarrhea that lasts 2–28 days (average 7 days) after exposure. In addition to diarrhea, patients have symptoms of nausea, abdominal cramps, and flatulence for 2–6 weeks. Although infection caused by *G. lamblia* is typically self-limited, those without secretory IgA in the intestinal lumen may have chronic infection characterized by dehydration, malabsorption syndrome, and weight loss.

Invasive disease from *E. histolytica* occurs when trophozoite forms invade intestinal epithelial cells to form discrete ulcers, allowing mucus, necrotic cells, and amebae to pass. Extraintestinal infection occurs directly from the bowel or from microembolism of trophozoites to the liver through the portal circulation. The majority of patients exposed to *E. histolytica* are asymptomatically colonized; about 10% of patients have symptoms, predominantly with diarrhea. Invasive or disseminated disease is less common. Symptoms of infection vary with the site and extent of intestinal lesions, the number of microorganisms ingested, pathogenicity of ingested strain, and immune status of the host. Patients may develop symptoms ranging from mild diarrhea to severe bloody diarrhea, abdominal cramping, and loss of appetite within days to weeks after exposure. Patients with amebic liver abscess have fever, right upper quadrant pain that is persistent and dull, liver tenderness, nausea, and weight loss. The duration of illness from *E. histolytica* is variable and may last for several weeks to months.

Traveler's Diarrhea

Most patients with untreated TD caused by a bacteria or virus have symptoms of diarrhea of 4 or 5 loose or watery stools per day for 3–4 days, accompanied by abdominal cramping. Those infected with a parasite may have diarrheal symptoms that persist for weeks to months.

Although most patients fully recover from food- or waterborne illnesses, there are potential short- and long-term complications of infection. An acute episode of infectious gastroenteritis increases the risk of developing functional bowel disorders (e.g., irritable bowel syndrome) and for precipitating reactive arthritis. Nontyphoid *Salmonella* spp., *Campylobacter* spp., and *V. parahaemolyticus* may cause bacteremia in those with suppressed immune function, whereas *L. monocytogenes* can cause meningitis or bacteremia in neonates; older patients; or those with altered cellular immune function, including women who are pregnant. In addition, *L. monocytogenes* can cause miscarriage or stillbirth if acquired during pregnancy. About 8% of patients infected with *E. coli* O157:H7 or other STEC develop hemolytic uremic syndrome (HUS) (MMWR 2009). Hemolytic uremic syndrome is characterized by a triad of acute renal failure, thrombocytopenia, and hemolytic anemia, as well as the long-term sequelae of hypertension, chronic kidney disease, or end-stage renal disease. About 30% of cases of Guillain-Barré syndrome are estimated to occur after infection with *Campylobacter* spp. (Poropatich 2010), with patients noting ascending weakness starting 10 days to 3 weeks after the onset of diarrhea.

TREATMENT

The general approach to the management of a patient with diarrhea caused by a food- or waterborne illness is described in Figure 2-2. Patients who only exhibit symptoms of vomiting within 1–6 hours of ingestion likely have food poisoning caused by preformed enterotoxins of *S. aureus* or *B. cereus*. These patients typically do not require further diagnostic testing. Patients should be counseled to seek medical attention if they have diarrhea for 3 or more days or diarrhea accompanied by bloody stools, oral temperature higher than 101.3°F (38.5°C), or signs of dehydration. In addition, testing should be considered in children younger than 5 years, older patients, patients with immunocompromise, and pregnant women.

Therapeutic Goals

The main goals of therapy are to prevent and treat dehydration and to reduce the severity and duration of illness.

Supportive Care

To prevent and treat dehydration, fluid replacement is used routinely in all patients with diarrhea or vomiting caused by a food- or waterborne illness. For patients with mild to moderate dehydration, oral rehydration therapy (ORT) is recommended to replace ongoing fluid losses. Patients with severe dehydration are initially treated with intravenous fluids until they are hemodynamically stable, followed by ORT as soon as it is tolerated.

Aggressive rehydration is required to manage fluid and electrolyte losses in patients with cholera. Table 2-2 contains available oral rehydration solutions and their components. Glucose, a necessary component of oral rehydration

solutions, promotes the absorption of sodium and water in the small intestine. The potassium component prevents hypokalemia that could be caused by loss of potassium in diarrhea, and the base component prevents or corrects acidosis. If a premade solution is not available, patients can make their own by mixing 2 tablespoons of sugar, one-half teaspoon of salt, and one-half cup of orange juice or mashed banana per liter of water (Steiner 2013). Patients should not rehydrate with overly sweet beverages (e.g., carbonated soft drinks with sugar, apple juice, sports drinks) because these contain high carbohydrate-sodium ratios that can lead to osmotic diarrhea and increase intestinal fluid losses.

Antiemetics and antimotility agents provide symptomatic relief. Antimotility agents are not effective in the high-volume secretory diarrhea seen with cholera, and in general, they are not recommended in patients with signs of dysentery (fever higher than 101.3°F [38.5°C] or bloody diarrhea). These agents slow transit time in the gut, allowing for greater exposure to invasive pathogens and potentially increasing the risk of complications.

Zinc supplementation is recommended by the World Health Organization for children younger than 5 years who have diarrhea. The evidence for using zinc supplementation is stronger in children in developing countries, where zinc deficiency is more common. Typically, a 10-day course of 10 mg/day of elemental zinc for children younger than 6 months and 20 mg/day of elemental zinc for children aged 6 months to 5 years is used.

The role of probiotics for the treatment of infectious diarrhea is not clearly defined. A Cochrane review found that probiotics shortened the duration of diarrhea by about 16 to 34 hours in otherwise healthy individuals with no reported adverse events (Allen 2010). However, there are not enough data to recommend a specific probiotic regimen (agent, dose, duration of therapy) that would benefit a defined patient group. Future trials are needed that adhere to and apply standardized definitions for diarrhea and resolution of illness, ensure dosage of the probiotic being tested, and separately assess data for patient subgroups. Because most episodes of acute diarrhea are self-limited, cost-effectiveness studies would also help identify patient groups in which probiotics would be most beneficial. A theoretical concern is the potential for probiotic organisms to move outside the gastrointestinal tract and cause systemic infections. Overall, although probiotics are well tolerated in healthy individuals, they should be used with caution in patients who are immunosuppressed because bacteremia and fungemia have been reported with their use in immunosuppressed patient populations.

Pathogen-Specific Therapy

Because antibiotics are not useful for the treatment of toxin-mediated food- or waterborne illnesses or for viruses, their treatment is primarily supportive. *C. botulinum* can be treated with antitoxin to block circulating toxin and stop the progression of symptoms. Common

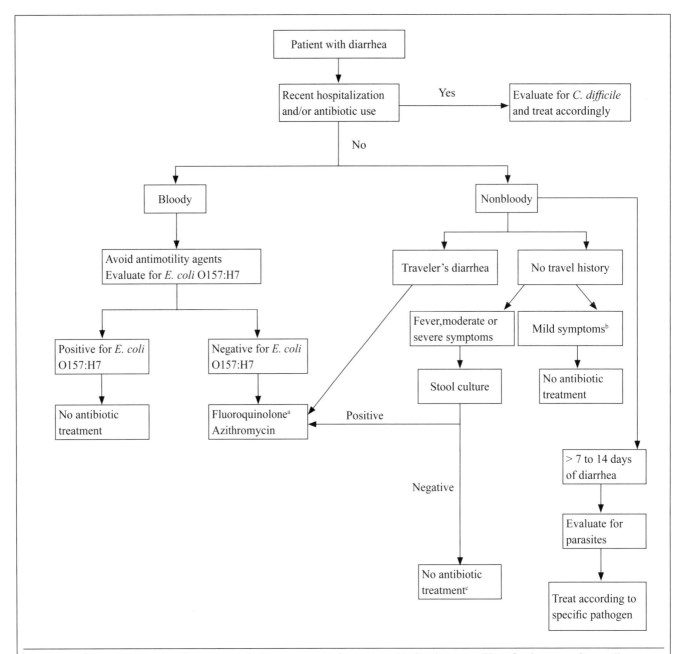

Figure 2-2. General approach to the antimicrobial management of a patient with diarrhea caused by a food- or waterborne illness.

[a]Not recommended for travel to southeast Asia or India.
[b]Likely food poisoning if accompanied by vomiting and started within 2 to 7 hours of food ingestion.
[c]Likely a viral etiology.

antibiotic and antiparasitic agents used for treating food- and waterborne illnesses caused by select bacteria and protozoa are listed in Table 2-3 and Table 2-4. Issues related to the antimicrobial treatment of those types of infections are detailed in the following.

Campylobacter

Antibiotics are recommended for patients with severe disease (including bloody diarrhea, fever, or extraintestinal manifestations) and for those at high risk of complications (including older patients, pregnant women, and those with immunocompromise). Antibiotic therapy in uncomplicated cases shortens the duration of intestinal symptoms by 1.32 days if used within the first 3 days of symptom onset (Ternhag 2007); because that time frame is likely missed by the time culture results return, most clinicians do not advocate treatment in this patient population. When indicated, macrolides are recommended as first-line therapy because of increasing rates of resistance to fluoroquinolones in *Campylobacter* spp..

A 55-year-old man reports to the primary care clinic with a 2-day history of fever of 101.5°F and bloody diarrhea. He reports no history of travel, no recent antibiotic use, and no contact with other sick individuals. He is allergic to sulfa

A stool culture is performed with the following results:
Negative for *Campylobacter* spp.
Negative for *E. coli* O157:H7
Negative for *Salmonella* spp.
Positive for *Shigella* spp.

medications. His past medical history is significant for uncontrolled type 2 diabetes mellitus, and his current medications include a daily multivitamin, glyburide 20 mg orally daily, and metformin 1000 mg orally twice daily.

His clinician must decide on the most appropriate course of treatment for this patient.

Answer

Because most cases of acute diarrhea are self-limiting, routine stool cultures are not recommended for all patients, but should be considered in certain situations, including the presence of fever ≥ 101.3°F or bloody stools. Routine stool cultures include testing for *Salmonella* spp., *Shigella* spp., *Campylobacter* spp., and *E. coli* O157:H7. It is important to rule out Shiga toxin producing *E. coli* in patients with bloody diarrhea because this pathogen should only be treated with supportive therapy and not with an antibiotic agent. There is no need to order testing for *C. difficile* or parasites because the patient does not have a history of recent antibiotic use, travel, or hospitalization and has not had symptoms of diarrhea for greater than 7 days. Based on stool results, this patient is infected with *Shigella* spp. and should be treated

with an antibiotic in order to prevent the spread of infection. Treatment options include a fluoroquinolone, azithromycin, or trimethoprim/sulfamethoxazole.

Trimethoprim/sulfamethoxazole should be avoided in this patient because he is allergic to sulfa medications. Ciprofloxacin or levofloxacin are effective for this type of infection; however, fluoroquinolones may cause alterations in blood glucose levels and this patient has diabetes mellitus. This leaves azithromycin 500 mg orally once daily for 3 days as the best treatment option for this patient. This case illustrates the role of diagnostic testing in evaluating a patient with suspected infectious diarrhea and the importance of taking into account patient-specific factors when selecting an antibiotic regimen.

1. Centers for Disease Control and Prevention. Shigellosis.
2. DuPont HL. Acute infectious diarrhea in immunocompetent adults. N Engl J Med 2014;370:1532-40.
3. Hatchette TF, Farina D. Infectious diarrhea: when to test and when to treat. CMAJ. 2011;183:339-44.

Escherichia coli

The treatment of EHEC infection consists primarily of supportive care because antibiotics do not alter the duration of acute diarrhea and may cause harm by increasing the release of Shiga toxin and the risk of HUS. The treatment of ETEC infection consists of supportive care, with antibiotics for moderate to severe cases. Because ETEC is the most common cause of TD, their treatment regimens are similar.

Listeria monocytogenes

Antibiotics are not routinely recommended for gastroenteritis caused by *L. monocytogenes* because the disease is usually self-limited. However, antibiotics can be considered for those at risk of invasive disease (e.g., pregnant women, those with immunocompromise) or those who have ingested a food implicated in an outbreak. Because this microorganism has an affinity for the central nervous system, patients with invasive disease may develop meningitis and should be treated according to those guidelines.

Salmonella

Antibiotics are not routinely recommended in otherwise healthy patients with diarrhea caused by nontyphoidal *Salmonella* because they do not provide any clinical benefit

and have been shown to increase the likelihood of shedding the microorganism for up to 1 month after completion of treatment. The risk of bacteremia from nontyphoidal *Salmonella* is about 8% in healthy people but is higher in patients younger than 3 months, age 65 years or older, corticosteroid users, with inflammatory bowel disease, hemodialysis recipients, with hemoglobinopathy (including sickle cell disease), and with immunocompromise (DuPont 2009). In addition, those with an abdominal aneurysm or a prosthetic heart valve are at risk of a focal infection. Antibiotic treatment of nontyphoidal *Salmonella* is recommended for patients with positive blood cultures, risk factors for bacteremia, or severe infection.

Shigella

Although mild *Shigella* infections are typically self-limited, antibiotic therapy for all patients with positive stool cultures is recommended from a public health perspective to decrease person-to-person transmission.

Vibrio cholerae

Antibiotics are considered to be adjunctive therapy to rehydration in patients with moderate to severe dehydration. Antibiotic therapy decreases both the volume and the duration of diarrhea by up to 50% and reduces the

Table 2-2. Common Oral Rehydration Solutions

Product	Na (mEq/L)	K (mEq/L)	Base (mEq/L)	Carbohydrate (mmol/L)	Osmolarity (mOsm/L)
Infalyte	50	25	30	70	200
Naturalyte	45	20	48	140	265
Pedialyte	45	20	30	140	250
Rehydralyte	75	20	30	140	250
WHO/UNICEF recommended solution	75	20	30	75	245

K = potassium; Na = sodium; UNICEF = United Nations Children's Fund; WHO = World Health Organization.

duration of shedding of organisms in stool (Harris 2012). The selection of antibiotics should be based on local resistance patterns and host characteristics.

Vibrio parahaemolyticus

Antibiotics are not typically recommended because they do not affect duration or severity of illness. However, an antibiotic may be considered for patients with diarrhea for more than 5 days.

Parasitic Infections

Although metronidazole has historically been the recommended treatment for *G. lamblia*, the newer agents tinidazole and nitazoxanide may be better tolerated because of their shorter duration of therapy. Chronic infections are usually refractory to drug therapy with any agent.

Nitazoxanide has FDA-approved labeling for the treatment of immunocompetent patients with diarrhea caused by *Cryptosporidium* spp.; however, most cases in this population are self-limited even without treatment. Nitazoxanide and paromomycin are considered to be partially active agents that have limited effectiveness for the treatment of cryptosporidiosis in patients with HIV/AIDS. Patients with HIV/AIDS should also be managed with combination antiretroviral therapy, which usually causes remission as long as therapy is continued. However, it is unclear whether treatment with nonprotease inhibitor–containing regimens are beneficial and whether the addition of an antiparasitic agent improves clinical response.

The type of infection caused by *E. histolytica* affects the selection of treatment. To prevent the progression to intestinal or disseminated amebiasis, patients who are asymptomatic carriers should be treated with either paromomycin or iodoquinol, which are luminal agents that achieve high concentrations of drug in the bowel. Patients with symptomatic intestinal infection or extraintestinal disease should be treated with either metronidazole or tinidazole—which are systemically absorbed and achieve high tissue concentrations—followed by a luminal agent.

Traveler's Diarrhea

Patients with TD should start fluid and electrolyte replacement by increasing their intakes of fluids and salt-containing foods. Oral rehydration therapy is recommended for infants, young children, older people, and those with chronic medical conditions. Most cases of TD do not require medical evaluation. Patients can self-treat with an antimotility agent and a prescribed antibiotic after communicating with their health care providers. Patients should purchase those agents before leaving the United States because the purity and integrity of medications purchased abroad cannot be ensured. Patients with bloody diarrhea should seek medical attention to monitor for complications and to determine the etiology, because EHEC should be treated only with supportive care.

Antimotility agents that reduce symptoms of TD include bismuth subsalicylate 524 mg every 30 minutes for up to 8 doses; or loperamide 4 mg once, then 2 mg after each loose stool up to a maximal daily dosage of 16 mg. Loperamide should be used for a maximal duration of therapy of 48 hours. In adults, loperamide is preferred because of its faster onset of action, greater efficacy and tolerability, and more convenient dosing schedule. Bismuth subsalicylate should not be used either in patients allergic to salicylates or in children because of the risk of Reye syndrome. There are also concerns about the safety of loperamide in young children. A meta-analysis of randomized trials of children younger than 12 years with acute diarrhea found an increased incidence of serious adverse events (e.g., ileus, lethargy, death) with the use of loperamide in children younger than 3 years (Li 2007).

Of the antibiotic classes used for the treatment of TD, a fluoroquinolone is usually recommended for those traveling to most parts of the world. Patients should receive a 3-day course of a fluoroquinolone but can stop therapy after the initial 24 hours if their symptoms have resolved. Azithromycin is preferred in patients allergic to or unable to tolerate fluoroquinolones, children, pregnant women, and those in areas of the world with fluoroquinolone-resistant *Campylobacter* spp. (e.g., Southeast Asia, India). Rifaximin is an alternative agent that can be used in patients with TD caused by ETEC. Because ETEC is found predominantly in Mexico, rifaximin

Table 2-3. Common Antibiotics Used in the Treatment of Selected Bacterial Food- and Waterborne Illnesses

Bacteria	Adult Regimen	Pediatric Regimen
Campylobacter spp.	[a]Azithromycin 500 mg PO daily for 3 days [b]Erythromycin 500 mg PO four times daily for 3–5 days [b]Ciprofloxacin 500 mg PO two times daily for 5–7 days	[a]Azithromycin 10 mg/kg/day PO daily for 3–5 days [a]Erythromycin 30 mg/kg/day PO divided into 2–4 doses for 3–5 days

Enterotoxigenic *Escherichia coli*	[a]Ciprofloxacin 750 mg PO daily or 500 mg
	   PO two times daily for 1–3 days
	[b]Rifaximin 200 mg PO three times daily for 3 days
	[b]Azithromycin 1000 mg PO single dose
	   or 500 mg PO daily for 3 days
	[b]Norfloxacin 400 mg PO two times daily for 3–5 days
		[a]Azithromycin 10 mg/kg/day PO daily for 3 days
		[b]Ceftriaxone 50 mg/kg/day IV daily for 3 days

Listeria monocytogenes gastroenteritis[c]	[a]Amoxicillin 500 mg PO three times daily or
	   875 mg PO two times daily for 7 days
	[a]Trimethoprim/sulfamethoxazole: trimethoprim
	   160 mg and sulfamethoxazole 800 mg
	   PO two times daily for 7 days
		[a]Amoxicillin
		Children >3 months and <40 kg: 20–100 mg/
		   kg/day in 2 or 3 divided doses for 7 days
		Children >3 months and ≥40 kg: see adult dosing
		[a]Trimethoprim/sulfamethoxazole: trimethoprim 8
		   mg/kg/day PO in 2 divided doses for 7 days

Nontyphoidal *Salmonella*	[a,d]Ciprofloxacin 750 mg PO daily for 7–10 days [a,d]Levofloxacin 500 mg PO daily for 7–10 days [b,d]Azithromycin 500 mg PO daily for 7 days [b,d]Ceftriaxone 1–2 g IV daily for 7–10 days	[a]Azithromycin 20 mg/kg/day PO daily for 7 days [b]Ceftriaxone 100 mg/kg/day IV divided into 2 doses for 7–10 days

Shigella spp.	[a]Ciprofloxacin 750 mg PO daily for 3 days
	[a]Levofloxacin 500 mg PO daily for 3 days
	[a]Azithromycin 500 mg PO daily for 3 days
	[b]Trimethoprim/sulfamethoxazole: trimethoprim
	   160 mg and sulfamethoxazole 800 mg
	   PO two times daily for 3 days
		[a]Azithromycin 10 mg/kg/day PO daily for 3 days
		[b]Ceftriaxone 50 mg/kg/day IV daily for 3 days
		[b]Trimethoprim/sulfamethoxazole: trimethoprim 8
		   mg mg/kg/day PO in 2 divided doses for 3 days

Traveler's diarrhea	[a]Ciprofloxacin 750 mg PO single dose or 500
	   mg PO two times daily for 1–3 days
	[a]Levofloxacin 1000 mg PO single dose
	   or 500 mg PO daily for 3 days
	[a]Norfloxacin 400 mg PO two times daily for 3 days
	[a]Ofloxacin 200 mg PO two times daily for 3 days
	[b]Rifaximin 200 mg PO three times daily for 3 days
	[b]Azithromycin 1000 mg PO single dose
	   or 500 mg PO daily for 3 days
		[a]Rifaximin (children ≥12 years) 200 mg
		   PO three times daily for 3 days
		[a]Azithromycin 10 mg/kg PO single
		   dose (maximum 1000 mg)
		[b]Ciprofloxacin 20–30 mg/kg/day PO in 2 divided
		   doses for 3 days (maximum 500 mg per dose)
		[b]Levofloxacin 10 mg/kg PO daily for 3
		   days (maximum 500 mg per dose)
		[b]Ofloxacin 7.5 mg/kg PO two times daily for
		   3 days (maximum 200 mg per dose)

Vibrio cholerae	[a]Doxycyline 300 mg PO single dose
	[b]Tetracycline 500 mg PO four times daily for 3 days
	[b]Erythromycin[b] 250 mg PO three times daily for 3 days
	[b]Azithromycin 500 mg PO daily for 3 days
	[b]Ciprofloxacin 500 mg PO two times daily for 3 days
	[b]Trimethoprim/sulfamethoxazole: trimethoprim
	   160 mg and sulfamethoxazole 800 mg
	   PO two times daily for 3 days
		[a]Erythromycin 30 mg/kg/day PO
		   divided into 3 doses for 3 days
		[a]Azithromycin 10 mg/kg/day PO daily for 3 days
		[b]Trimethoprim/sulfamethoxazole: trimethoprim 8
		   mg mg/kg/day PO in 2 divided doses for 3 days

Vibrio parahaemolyticus	[a]Ciprofloxacin 750 mg PO daily for 3 days [a]Azithromycin 500 mg PO daily for 3 days	[a]Azithromycin 10 mg/kg/day PO daily for 3 days

[a]Drug of choice.
[b]Alternative.
[c]Patients with meningitis should be treated with parenteral therapy according to guidelines for bacterial meningitis.
[d]Duration of therapy for immunocompromised patients is 14 days.
IV = intravenously; PO = by mouth.

should not be used routinely in patients traveling to other parts of the world. In addition, it should not be used in those with fever, bloody stools, or any systemic symptoms, because it is less effective in those types of infections.

Monitoring

Patients should be monitored for resolution of diarrhea, adverse effects from medications, and complications associated with their specific type of infection. Adverse effects and drug interactions of commonly used antimicrobials are listed in Table 2-5. Repeat stool analysis is not typically performed but may be used for public health purposes in certain individuals (e.g., food handlers, day care workers).

PREVENTION

Patient Education

Avoiding foods and beverages likely to be contaminated is the best strategy to prevent TD. Travelers should avoid tap water (including when brushing teeth), ice cubes, unpeeled fruits, fruit juices, salads, raw vegetables, unpasteurized dairy products, condiments in open bottles, open buffets, undercooked or incompletely reheated foods, and beverages in unsealed containers. The expression "Peel it, boil it, cook it, or forget it" can help travelers remember which foods and beverages should be avoided. However, that strategy is not entirely effective, because basic health precautions also need to be followed by food handlers.

Pharmacologic Measures

Although bismuth subsalicylate has been shown to be about 65% effective in preventing TD, some travelers may find its dosing schedule of 2 tablets or 30 mL (524 mg) orally four times a day to be inconvenient. Bismuth subsalicylate should be used for a maximal duration of 3 weeks because of the potential for adverse effects. In addition, bismuth subsalicylate may cause temporary blackening of the stools, which may make stools appear bloody.

Table 2-4. Common Antiparasitic Agents Used in the Treatment of Selected Protozoan Food- and Waterborne Illnesses

Protozoa	Adult Regimen[a]	Pediatric Regimen
Cryptosporidium spp.	[b,c]Nitazoxanide 500 mg PO two times daily for 3 days [b]Paromomycin 500 mg PO four times daily for 14–21 days	Nitazoxanide: • [b,c]Age 1–3 years: 100 mg PO two times daily for 3 days • [b,c]Age 4–11 years: 200 mg PO two times daily for 3 days • Age ≥12 years: see adult regimen
Entamoeba histolytica	[d]Paromomycin 25–35 mg/kg/day PO divided in 3 doses for 7 days [d]Iodoquinol 650 mg PO three times daily for 20 days [e]Metronidazole 750 mg PO/IV three times daily for 10 days [e]Tinidazole 2 g PO daily for 5 days	[d]Paromomycin 25–35 mg/kg/day PO divided in 3 doses for 7 days [d]Iodoquinol 30–40 mg/kg/day PO divided in 3 doses (maximum 650 mg/dose) for 20 days [e]Metronidazole 35–50 mg/kg/day PO/IV divided in 3 doses (maximum 750 mg/dose) for 10 days [e]Tinidazole (age > 3 years) 50 mg/kg/day (maximum 2 g) for 3–5 days
Giardia lamblia	Metronidazole 250 mg PO three times daily for 5–10 days Tinidazole 2 g PO single dose Nitazoxanide 500 mg PO two times daily for 3 days	Metronidazole 15 mg/kg/day PO divided in 3 doses (maximum 250 mg/dose) for 5–10 days Tinidazole (age > 3 years) 50 mg/kg PO single dose (maximum 2 g) Nitazoxanide • Age 1–3 years: 100 mg PO two times daily for 3 days • Age 4–11 years: 200 mg PO two times daily for 3 days • Age ≥12 years: see adult regimen

[a]Doses listed are based on normal kidney and liver function.
[b]In addition to optimized antiretroviral therapy in patients with HIV/AIDS.
[c]May consider increasing duration of therapy up to 14 days in patients with HIV/AIDS.
[d]Luminal agent.
[e]Followed by a course of one of the luminal agents for the treatment of intestinal amebiasis or liver abscess.
IV = intravenously; PO = by mouth.

The routine use of antibiotics as prophylaxis for TD is no longer recommended for most travelers but can be considered for those at high risk of complications from TD or for those taking critical trips such as athletes or politicians. Typically, a course of a fluoroquinolone such as norfloxacin 400 mg daily or ciprofloxacin/levofloxacin 500 mg daily for a maximal duration of 2–3 weeks is used. Rifaximin dosed at 200 mg once or twice daily for 2 weeks has been shown to be effective in preventing TD, but it has been studied only in regions of the world where ETEC is the most common pathogen.

Table 2-5. Selected Antimicrobials Used in the Treatment and Prevention of Food- and Waterborne Illnesses

Drug	Adverse Effects	Drug Interactions
Amoxicillin	Hypersensitivity reactions, nausea, vomiting, diarrhea	None significant
Azithromycin	Nausea, vomiting, diarrhea, QT prolongation	Inhibitor of CYP-mediated metabolism, QT prolonging agents
Bismuth subsalicylate	Darkening of the tongue, grayish black stools, hearing loss, tinnitus, muscle spasms, anxiety, confusion, headache, not recommended for pregnant women	Aspirin, warfarin, tetracyclines
Ceftriaxone	Hypersensitivity reactions, nausea, vomiting, diarrhea	None significant
Ciprofloxacin	Dysglycemia, QT prolongation, tendon rupture, peripheral neuropathy, not recommended for pregnant women, not routinely recommended for children	Oral cations, QT prolonging agents
Doxycycline	Nausea, vomiting, photosensitivity, permanent tooth discoloration in children < 8 years, not recommended for pregnant women and children < 8 years	Oral cations
Erythromycin	Nausea, vomiting, diarrhea, QT prolongation	Potent inhibitor of CYP-mediated metabolism, QT prolonging agents
Iodoquinol	Nausea, vomiting, diarrhea, abdominal cramps, rash, pruritus, peripheral neuropathy, optic neuritis, thyroid gland enlargement, limited data on use in pregnancy	None significant
Levofloxacin	Dysglycemia, QT prolongation, tendon rupture, peripheral neuropathy, not recommended for pregnant women, not routinely recommended for children	Oral cations, QT prolonging agents
Metronidazole	Headache, metallic taste, dizziness, nausea, diarrhea, not recommended during first trimester of pregnancy	Alcohol, warfarin
Nitazoxanide	Headache, abdominal pain, diarrhea, nausea, vomiting	None significant
Norfloxacin	Dysglycemia, QT prolongation, tendon rupture, peripheral neuropathy, not recommended for pregnant women, not routinely recommended for children	Oral cations, QT prolonging agents
Ofloxacin	Dysglycemia, QT prolongation, tendon rupture, peripheral neuropathy, not recommended for pregnant women, not routinely recommended for children	Oral cations, QT prolonging agents
Paromomycin	Abdominal cramps, diarrhea, heartburn, nausea, vomiting	None significant
Rifaximin	Nausea, vomiting, constipation, headache, flatulence	None significant
Tinidazole	Metallic taste, nausea, anorexia, flatulence, not recommended during first trimester of pregnancy	Alcohol
Trimethoprim/sulfamethoxazole	Hypersensitivity reactions, nausea, vomiting, myelosuppression, hyperkalemia, hepatotoxicity, not recommended for women in the third trimester of pregnancy	Warfarin, renin-angiotensin-aldosterone system inhibitors

CYP = cytochrome P450.

Immunizations

Table 2-6 lists immunizations available in the United States to prevent the food- and waterborne illnesses discussed in this chapter. Cholera vaccines are available in other parts of the world but are not commercially available in the United States because they do not fully protect against infection.

Hepatitis A

Immunization against hepatitis A virus is part of the routine immunization schedule for children in the United States and is recommended for susceptible people seeking protection against hepatitis A or who are at increased risk of infection, including those working in or traveling to areas with intermediate or high hepatitis A endemicity. The first dose of vaccine should be administered as soon as travel is considered. One dose of single-antigen vaccine given any time before departure provides adequate protection for most healthy people 40 years of age and younger; older adults should receive the first dose of vaccine at least 2 weeks before departure. Adults older than 40 years, those with immunocompromise, and those with chronic liver disease planning to depart the United States in 2 weeks or less should simultaneously receive the initial dose of vaccine and immune globulins against hepatitis A (0.02 mL/kg).

All patients should complete a vaccine series in order to achieve long-term protection against the virus. Children younger than 12 months and those who are allergic to the vaccine should receive a single dose of immune globulins. Because the duration of protection from immune globulins is limited to 3 months, a higher dose of 0.06 mL/kg should be used for travel longer than 2 months' duration, with repeat administration for travel longer than 5 months.

Situations in which postexposure prophylaxis is recommended include close personal contact (household member, sexual contact, illicit-drug sharer) with those with serologically confirmed hepatitis A and selected situations in which hepatitis A has been confirmed in a child care center or in a food handler. Postexposure prophylaxis should be given as soon as possible because there are no data on its efficacy when given longer than 2 weeks after exposure. For postexposure prophylaxis in those who are not vaccinated, administration of a single-antigen vaccine in those aged 12 months to 40 years is recommended. Immune globulins against hepatitis A are recommended in those younger than 12 months or older than 40 years, those with contraindications to the vaccine, those with immunocompromise, and those with chronic liver disease.

Rotavirus

Immunization against rotavirus is part of the routine immunization schedule for children in the United States. Almost all infants who receive the full vaccine series are protected against severe diarrhea, and most will not get infected. Because it is a live vaccine, it is contraindicated in infants with immunocompromise and contraindicated in infants with histories of intussusception.

CONCLUSION

Pharmacists have key roles in the treatment and prevention of food- and waterborne illnesses. Pharmacists can educate patients on preventive measures, including raising

Table 2-6. Available Vaccines for the Prevention of Selected Food- and Waterborne Illnesses

Vaccine Type	Brand	Dosing	Route of Administration
Hepatitis A			
Inactivated virus	Havrix	Adults: two-dose series at 0 and 6–12 months	IM
	Vaqta	Adults: two-dose series at 0 and 6–18 months	
	Twinrix[a]	Adults: three-dose series at 0, 1, and 6 months; four-dose series at day 0, 7, 21 to 30, and at month 12	
	Havrix or Vaqta	Children: two-dose series at 12 through 23 months separated by 6–18 months	
Rotavirus			
Live attenuated virus RV1	Rotarix[b]	Children: two-dose series at ages 2 and 4 months	PO
Live attenuated virus RV5	RotaTeq	Children: three-dose series at ages 2, 4, and 6 months	

[a]Combined hepatitis A and hepatitis B vaccine.
[b]May cause allergic reactions in latex-sensitive individuals.
IM = intramuscularly; PO = by mouth.

awareness of potentially contaminated foods and beverages. Pharmacists can advocate for and provide immunizations against hepatitis A virus and rotavirus. They also can ensure that patients carry antimicrobial and antimotility agents for the treatment of food- and waterborne illnesses when traveling outside the United States. For those with a confirmed food- or waterborne illness, pharmacists should actively work with providers to select the most proper antimicrobial agent or regimen based on patient-specific characteristics. Finally, pharmacists can counsel patients on the proper administration of antimicrobial agents, agents' most common adverse effects, and ways of managing adverse effects.

REFERENCES

Allen SJ, Martinez EG, Gregorio GV, et al. Probiotics for treating acute infectious diarrhoea. Cochrane Database Syst Rev 2010:CD003048.

Centers for Disease Control and Prevention. Food safety.

Centers for Disease Control and Prevention. Recommendations for diagnosis of Shiga toxin-producing Escherichia coli infections by clinical laboratories. Morbid Mortal Wkly Rep 2009;58:1-14.

Centers for Disease Control and Prevention. Recreational water-associated disease outbreaks– United States, 2009-2010. Morbid Mortal Wkly Rep 2014;63:6-10.

Centers for Disease Control and Prevention. Surveillance for waterborne disease outbreaks associated with drinking water and other nonrecreational water – United States, 2009-2010. Morbid Mortal Wkly Rep 2013;62:714-20.

Centers for Disease Control and Prevention. Trends in foodborne illness in the United States, 2006-2013.

Connor BA. Traveler's diarrhea. In: Brunette GW, Kozarsky PE, Cohen NJ, et al., eds. CDC Health Information for International Travel 2014: The Yellow Book. New York, NY: Oxford University Press; 2014.

DuPont HL. Acute infectious diarrhea in immunocompetent adults. N Engl J Med 2014;370:1532-40.

DuPont HL. Clinical practice. Bacterial diarrhea. N Engl J Med 2009;361:1560-9.

Harris JB, LaRocque RC, Qadri F, et al. Cholera. Lancet 2012;379:2466-76.

Li ST, Grossman DC, Cummings P. Loperamide therapy for acute diarrhea in children: systematic review and meta-analysis. PLoS Med 2007;4:e98.

Liu L, Johnson HL, Cousens S, et al. Global, regional, and national causes of child mortality: an updated systematic analysis for 2010 with time trends since 2000. Lancet 2012;379:2151-61.

Poropatich KO, Fischer Walker CL, Black RE. Quantifying the association between Campylobacter infection and Guillain-Barré syndrome: a systematic review. J Health Popul Nutr 2010;28:545-52.

Steiner T. Treating foodborne illness. Infect Dis Clin N Am 2013;27:555-76.

Ternhag A, Asikainen T, Giesecke J, et al. A meta-analysis on the effects of antibiotic treatment on duration of symptoms caused by infection with Campylobacter species. Clin Infect Dis 2007;44:696-700.

Practice Points

In determining the optimal treatment for a patient with a food- or waterborne illness, the clinician should consider the following important points:

- Most cases are self-limited.
- Fluid replacement should be recommended to all patients to prevent and treat dehydration.
- It is important to rule out EHEC in patients with bloody diarrhea because this bacterial pathogen should only be treated with supportive care.
- The treatment of toxin-mediated pathogens, viral pathogens, or mild infections is primarily supportive.
- Stool cultures should be performed in patients with fever or moderate to severe illness.
- Antimotility agents are generally not recommended for patients with bloody diarrhea or fever > 101.3°F (38.5°C).
- To prevent traveler's diarrhea, travelers should be counseled to avoid foods and beverages that are most likely to be contaminated.
- Patients should be counseled to travel with an antimotility agent and an antibiotic, especially if going to a geographic location that has an intermediate-risk or high-risk for traveler's diarrhea. Travelers should seek medical attention if they have bloody diarrhea. Without bloody diarrhea, most travelers can be treated with 1 dose of a fluoroquinolone, with the duration extended to 3 days if symptoms have not improved within 24 hours. Azithromycin is an alternative agent.
- Keep in mind safety and drug interaction concerns when selecting an antimicrobial agent or pharmacologic agent for supportive care.
- In the absence of contraindications, encourage parents to have their child receive hepatitis A and rotavirus vaccines as part of routine childhood immunizations.
- Encourage patients to receive the hepatitis A vaccine to decrease the risk for infection from this pathogen.

SELF-ASSESSMENT QUESTIONS

Questions 21-24 pertain to the following case.

J.P., a 44-year-old man, presents with a 24-hour history of diarrhea, vomiting, and cramps. His symptoms started about 8 hours after eating a meal of raw oysters, baked clams, fresh green beans, and potato salad. His vital signs are blood pressure 130/72 mm Hg, heart rate 70 beats/minute, respiratory rate 22 breaths/minute, and temperature 100.4°F (38°C). His medical history is significant for alcoholic liver disease. His current drugs include nadolol 40 mg orally daily. He is employed as a short order cook in a neighborhood restaurant. He has no history of recent antibiotic use and no history of travel.

21. Which one of the following pathogens is the most likely cause of J.P.'s symptoms?

    A. *Listeria monocytogenes.*
    B. *Shigella* spp.
    C. *Staphylococcus aureus.*
    D. *Vibrio parahaemolyticus.*

22. Which one of the following is the best next step in the diagnostic assessment of J.P.?

    A. Test for ova and parasites in stool.
    B. Stool cultures.
    C. Test for hepatitis A.
    D. Test for white blood cells in stool.

23. Which one of the following is the best treatment option for J.P.?

    A. Amoxicillin 875 mg orally every 12 hours for 7 days in addition to fluid replacement.
    B. Ciprofloxacin 750 mg orally daily for 3 days in addition to fluid replacement.
    C. Fluid replacement.
    D. Rifaximin 200 mg orally every 8 hours for 3 days in addition to fluid replacement.

24. In addition to resolution of J.P.'s symptoms, which one of the following laboratory parameters is best to monitor?

    A. Complete blood cell count.
    B. Liver function tests.
    C. Stool cultures.
    D. Renal function tests.

25. A 24-year-old man presents with a 2-day history of watery diarrhea, fever, and cramps. His symptoms started 1 day after eating at a local fast food restaurant. He is allergic to tetracycline and has no significant medical history. Which one of the following is the most likely cause of this patient's symptoms?

    A. *Campylobacter jejuni.*
    B. Enterohemorrhagic *Escherichia coli.*
    C. Hepatitis A.
    D. Norovirus.

26. A family consisting of a 34-year-old woman, a 52-year-old man, and a 7-month-old girl present to the travel medicine clinic. They are leaving in 4 weeks for a vacation to Ecuador, where they will stay for 14 days. All family members have previously completed the hepatitis B vaccine series and they do not have any significant medical history. Which one of the following measures is best for the prevention of hepatitis A virus infection in this family?

    A. All family members should each receive a dose of hepatitis A immune globulins now.
    B. The mother and father should each receive the first dose of hepatitis A vaccine now and return in 6 months for the second dose of hepatitis A vaccine. The 7-month-old girl should receive hepatitis A immune globulins now.
    C. The man and woman should each receive the first dose of hepatitis A vaccine now and return in 6 months for a second dose; the girl should receive hepatitis A immune globulins now and return in 5 months for a second dose.
    D. The woman should receive the first dose of hepatitis A vaccine now and return in 6 months for a second dose; the man should receive the first dose of hepatitis A vaccine now and hepatitis A immune globulins now, then return in 6 months for a second dose of hepatitis A vaccine; the girl should receive hepatitis A immune globulins now.

27. A 35-year-old woman presents with a 36-hour history of bloody diarrhea that started 48 hours after eating a meal of lobster, mashed potatoes, and salad. All of her vital signs are within normal limits. She has no known drug allergies and no history of travel. She has a medical history significant for bronchitis for which she received a 5-day treatment course of azithromycin 10 months ago. Which one of the following is the best next step for this patient?

    A. Assess for weight loss.
    B. Perform blood cultures.
    C. Perform stool cultures.
    D. Test for *Clostridium difficile* toxins.

28. A 68-year-old woman presents with a 1-day history of bloody diarrhea that began 2 days after eating seafood, pasta, and egg salad at a buffet restaurant. A stool culture is performed and is positive for *Shigella* spp. She

is allergic to sulfa (rash). Her medical history is significant for dyslipidemia and hypertension. Her home drugs are atorvastatin 40 mg at bedtime and furosemide 20 mg/day. Which one of the following is the best treatment option for this patient?

A. Azithromycin 500 mg orally daily for 3 days.
B. Levofloxacin 750 mg orally daily for 3 days.
C. Supportive care only.
D. Trimethoprim/sulfamethoxazole 160 mg/800 mg orally twice daily for 3 days.

29. A 28-year-old woman presents with a 9-day history of watery diarrhea and nausea. Her symptoms started a few days after returning from a domestic camping trip, during which she swam in a lake. She is allergic to penicillins and has no significant medical history. Which one of the following is the most likely cause of this patient's symptoms?

A. Bacteria that cause enterotoxigenic poisoning.
B. Bacteria that produce Shiga toxins.
C. Parasite.
D. Virus.

30. A 60-year-old man presents with a 2-day history of bloody diarrhea that began after eating eggs. A stool culture is performed and is positive for nontyphoidal *Salmonella*. He is allergic to fluoroquinolones (rash). His medical history is significant for hypertension, dyslipidemia, type 2 diabetes mellitus, and end-stage kidney disease. His current drugs include lisinopril 40 mg/day, furosemide 40 mg twice daily, metoprolol 100 mg twice daily, insulin glargine 80 units at bedtime, atorvastatin 80 mg at bedtime, sevelamer 800 mg twice daily, and erythropoietin 7500 units intravenously three times/week after each hemodialysis session. Which one of the following is the best treatment option for this patient?

A. Azithromycin 500 mg orally daily for 7 days.
B. Cefazolin 1 g intravenously every 8 hours for 7 days.
C. Levofloxacin 750 mg orally daily for 7 days.
D. Supportive care only.

31. A 34-year-old woman receives a diagnosis of infectious diarrhea caused by *Giardia lamblia* after returning from Mexico. She is allergic to sulfa drugs, and her medical history includes alcoholism. Her laboratory values are within normal limits, including a negative pregnancy test. Which one of the following is the best treatment option for this patient?

A. Iodoquinol 650 mg orally three times daily for 20 days.
B. Metronidazole 250 mg orally three times daily for 10 days.
C. Nitazoxanide 500 mg orally twice daily for 3 days.
D. Tinidazole 2 g orally as a single dose.

Questions 32–34 pertain to the following case.

P.W. is a 32-year-old man who is leaving the United States for a vacation to Peru in 2 weeks. He experienced traveler's diarrhea on a trip to Thailand last year and does not want to have it happen again. His medical history is significant for asthma and gastroesophageal reflux disease. His home drugs are fluticasone propionate and salmeterol 100 mcg/50 mcg per inhalation 1 inhalation twice daily, levalbuterol 2 puffs every 4 hours as needed for shortness of breath, and famotidine 20 mg orally twice daily. P.W. has a history of hives caused by salicylates.

32. How many risk factors does P.W. have for contracting traveler's diarrhea?

A. 0
B. 1
C. 3
D. 5

33. Which one of the following is best for P.W. to have on his trip to Peru?

A. Ciprofloxacin and bismuth subsalicylate.
B. Ciprofloxacin and loperamide.
C. Rifaximin and bismuth subsalicylate.
D. Rifaximin and loperamide.

34. P.W. is on day 5 of his vacation in Peru and calls you to report that he has had nausea, abdominal cramps, and watery diarrhea for the past 36 hours. He denies having any vomiting or dizziness when standing. Which one of the following is best to recommend to P.W.?

A. Seek immediate medical attention.
B. Start taking the antibiotic agent that you are travelling with.
C. Start taking the antimotility agent that you are travelling with.
D. Start taking the antibiotic and antimotility agents that you are travelling with.

35. A 58-year-old woman is leaving for a 10-day mission trip to Ethiopia. She is allergic to sulfa drugs (rash) and has a medical history significant for atrial fibrillation and dyslipidemia. Her current drugs are warfarin 2.5 mg/day, atorvastatin 40 mg at bedtime, a multivitamin daily, and calcium citrate 1200 mg/vitamin D 400 international units daily. Which one of the following is best for this patient to have on her trip?

A. Amoxicillin and bismuth subsalicylate.
B. Azithromycin and loperamide.
C. Levofloxacin and bismuth subsalicylate.
D. Rifaximin and loperamide.

36. A food handler who works in a popular restaurant was recently found to be infected with hepatitis A virus. A 35-year-old man with no significant medical history ate at this restaurant's buffet 5 days ago. He has never received a hepatitis vaccine, and he is concerned about contracting the virus. Which one of the following is best to recommend for this patient?

    A. One dose of immune globulins against hepatitis A as soon as possible.
    B. One dose of single-antigen hepatitis A vaccine as soon as possible.
    C. One dose of single-antigen hepatitis A vaccine and one dose of immune globulins against hepatitis A as soon as possible.
    D. One dose of bivalent hepatitis A and hepatitis B vaccine and one dose of immune globulins against hepatitis A as soon as possible.

37. A 40-year-old woman complains of vomiting, diarrhea, double vision, and difficulty swallowing. She lives in a rural community and has a garden from which she eats home-canned fruits and vegetables. Which one of the following is best to recommend for this patient?

    A. Test for *C. botulinum*; report a positive result to the health department.
    B. Test for *C. botulinum*; no need to report a positive result to the health department.
    C. Test for *L. monocytogenes*; report a positive result to the health department.
    D. Test for *L. monocytogenes*; no need to report a positive result to the health department.

38. You are counseling a woman in her first trimester of pregnancy at her first prenatal visit. Which one of the following counseling points regarding foodborne illness caused by *L. monocytogenes* would be best for this patient?

    A. Avoid eating canned tuna fish.
    B. Do not change a cat's litter box.
    C. Do not put feta cheese on salads.
    D. Wash your hands thoroughly after gardening.

39. A 37-year-old woman (height 65 inches, weight 50 kg) received a diagnosis of amebic liver abscess after traveling to Africa. She has no known drug allergies. Her medical history is significant for HIV infection currently controlled on a regimen of raltegravir 400 mg twice daily and tenofovir 300 mg/emtricitabine 200 mg once daily. Which one of the following is best to recommend for this patient?

    A. Metronidazole 250 mg orally three times daily for 5 days.
    B. Metronidazole 750 mg orally three times daily for 10 days, followed by paromomycin 500 mg orally three times daily for 7 days.
    C. Tinidazole 2 g orally daily for 5 days.
    D. Tinidazole 2 g orally daily for 5 days, followed by paromomycin 250 mg orally three times daily for 7 days.

40. Which one of the following patients is most at risk of bacteremia from a foodborne illness?

    A. A 1-year-old girl with no significant medical history who is infected with nontyphoidal *Salmonella*.
    B. A 15-year-old adolescent taking albuterol as needed for asthma who is infected with *Campylobacter jejuni*.
    C. A 28-year-old woman in the third trimester of pregnancy who is infected with *Listeria monocytogenes*.
    D. A 60-year-old woman taking mesalamine for Crohn's disease who is infected with *Shigella* spp.

Learner Chapter Evaluation: Food- and Waterborne Illnesses.

As you take the posttest for this chapter, also evaluate the material's quality and usefulness, as well as the achievement of learning objectives. Rate each item using this 5-point scale:

- Strongly agree
- Agree
- Neutral
- Disagree
- Strongly disagree

19. The content of the chapter met my educational needs.
20. The content of the chapter satisfied my expectations.
21. The author presented the chapter content effectively.
22. The content of the chapter was relevant to my practice and presented at the appropriate depth and scope.
23. The content of the chapter was objective and balanced.
24. The content of the chapter is free of bias, promotion, or advertisement of commercial products.
25. The content of the chapter was useful to me.
26. The teaching and learning methods used in the chapter were effective.
27. The active learning methods used in the chapter were effective.
28. The learning assessment activities used in the chapter were effective.
29. The chapter was effective overall.

Use the 5-point scale to indicate whether this chapter prepared you to accomplish the following learning objectives:
30. Analyze the epidemiology of food- and waterborne illnesses, including risk factors for acquisition, causative pathogens, and modes of transmission.

31. For a given patient, classify the most likely etiology of a food- or waterborne illness.
32. Assess a patient's risk of developing complications from a food- or waterborne illness.
33. Given a specific scenario, demonstrate the best means by which to diagnose a food- or waterborne illness.
34. Design appropriate pharmacotherapy for a suspected food- or waterborne illness.
35. Compose a prevention strategy and plan of self-treatment for a given patient at risk of a food- or waterborne illness.
36.   Please provide any specific comments relating to any perceptions of bias, promotion, or advertisement of commercial products.
37. Please expand on any of your above responses, and/ or provide any additional comments regarding this chapter:

Quality and Safety in Antimicrobial Practice

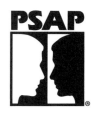

By Monica V. Mahoney, Pharm.D., BCPS (AQ-ID);
and Christopher McCoy, Pharm.D., BCPS

Reviewed by Kimberly Luk, Pharm.D.; Carol Heunisch, Pharm.D., BCPS; and Michael C. Ott, Pharm.D., BCPS

Learning Objectives

1. Evaluate recent antimicrobial U.S. Food and Drug Administration (FDA) drug interaction warnings and implement strategies to mitigate adverse drug reactions.
2. Assess for antimicrobial adverse drug events and recommend therapy adjustments.
3. Assess legislation and the several national support programs for the establishment of antimicrobial stewardship endeavors across health care systems.
4. Compose strategies to meet Centers for Medicare & Medicaid Services (CMS) and QualityNet goals for pneumonia treatment, the Surgical Care Improvement Project, and immunization rates.
5. Develop strategies that comply with CMS and its National Healthcare Safety Network's reporting requirements involving catheter-related infections, surgical-site infections, resistant organisms, and health care personnel influenza vaccination.
6. Design strategies that limit antimicrobial exposure in feed animals.

Introduction

An estimated 25%–40% of inpatients receive an anti-infective while hospitalized. Most use is empiric, and upwards of 50% is prescribed inappropriately (John 1997). With such widespread use, safety is a major concern, and the U.S. Food and Drug Administration (FDA) releases warnings regarding drug interactions and adverse reactions related to antimicrobials. In addition, antimicrobials are costly, constituting up to 30% of an inpatient pharmacy's annual budget. Antimicrobial stewardship programs (ASPs) are designed to optimize clinical outcomes, minimize unintended adverse effects, decrease selection of pathogenic organisms, and prevent emergence of resistance.

As more and more national and governmental organizations come to require public reporting of antimicrobial use and health care–associated infections (HAIs), ASPs become vital to the success and reimbursement of institutions. Quality of care has become increasingly important as well, with infection-related measures high on the list of standards; quality measures now allow for tracking of and compliance with national standards for individual hospitals.

Baseline Knowledge Statements

Readers of this chapter are presumed to be familiar with the following:
- Common doses and adverse reactions associated with azithromycin, cefepime, daptomycin, linezolid, and tigecycline

Additional Readings

The following free resources are available for readers wishing additional background information on this topic.
- Dellit, TH, Owens, RC, McGowan JE, et al. Infectious Diseases Society of America and the Society for Healthcare Epidemiology of America guidelines for developing an institutional program to enhance antimicrobial stewardship. Clin Infect Dis (2007) 44(2):159-77.
- American Society of Health-System Pharmacists. ASHP statement on the pharmacist's role in antimicrobial stewardship and infection prevention and control. Am J Health Syst Pharm (2010) 67:575-7.

ABBREVIATIONS IN THIS CHAPTER

ASP	Antimicrobial stewardship program
CAUTI	Catheter-associated urinary tract infections
CLABSI	Central line–associated bloodstream infection
EP	Eosinophilic pneumonia
HAI	Health care–associated infection
HAP	Hospital-acquired pneumonia
HICPAC	Healthcare Infection Control Practices Advisory Committee
MDRO	Multidrug-resistant organism
MRSA	Methicillin-resistant *Staphylococcus aureus*
NHSN	National Healthcare Safety Network
SCIP	Surgical Care Improvement Project
SS	Serotonin syndrome
VAP	Ventilator-associated pneumonia
VRE	Vancomycin-resistant *Enterococcus*

Financial incentives are offered to institutions that score high on Centers for Medicare & Medicaid Services (CMS) measures, and these data are shared with consumers so they can make informed decisions about where to seek care.

FDA Warnings

After gathering information from postmarketing reports, large-population publications, and registration trials, the FDA provides notifications on new warnings and safety information. The drug manufacturer then complies with any necessary labeling changes. Pharmacists should review the data carefully and implement changes as necessary. Some recent antimicrobial communications follow.

Drug Interactions
Azithromycin and Cardiovascular Death

In May 2012, the FDA released a statement regarding the risk of cardiovascular death with 5 days of azithromycin use compared with other antibiotics (FDA 2012a). A study team retrospectively reviewed 3.5 million patient records, including patients aged 30–74 years without histories of life-threatening cardiovascular disease who were prescribed azithromycin, amoxicillin, levofloxacin, ciprofloxacin, or no antibiotics from 1992 to 2006. End points encompassed cardiovascular death and death from any cause. Compared with no antibiotic use, azithromycin had increased risks of cardiovascular death (hazard ratio [HR] 2.88; 95% confidence interval [CI], 1.79–4.63; p<0.001) and death from any cause (HR 1.85, 95% CI, 1.25–2.75, p=0.002). Those mortality risks were also elevated compared with amoxicillin use (cardiovascular death HR 2.49, 95% CI 1.38–4.50, p=0.002; death from any cause

HR 2.02, 95% CI, 1.24–3.30, p=0.005). The risk was increased for cardiovascular death only, when compared to ciprofloxacin use (HR 3.49, 95% CI 1.32–9.26, p=0.01). There was no difference in risk of death compared with levofloxacin use. The difference in cardiovascular deaths was most prominent in patients with higher baseline risks for cardiovascular diseases (Ray 2012).

After reviewing additional manufacturer data, the FDA cautioned in March 2013 that azithromycin use may lead to potentially fatal heart rhythm abnormalities (FDA 2013a). Patients with pre-existing QTc interval prolongation, uncorrected hypomagnesemia or hypokalemia, bradycardia, or taking concomitant Class IA or Class III antiarrhythmic agents were at increased risk. The azithromycin prescribing information was updated related to QTc prolongation and torsades de pointes.

Two additional studies compared azithromycin use and the risk of death. One team retrospectively compared more than 1 million exposures to azithromycin, penicillin, or no antibiotics from 1997 to 2010 in younger Danish patients (average age 40 years), most of whom were women. Compared with no antibiotics, azithromycin use had a higher risk of death from cardiovascular causes (rate ratio 2.84, 95% CI, 1.13–7.24), but there was no difference compared with penicillin (rate ratio 0.93, 95% CI, 0.56–1.55). The authors concluded that the increased risk of death associated with antibiotics was likely an indicator of acute infection rather than because of the antibiotic (Svanström 2013). Another team retrospectively reviewed electronic health records at Veterans Health Administration (VHA) medical centers from 1999 to 2012, focusing on azithromycin (n=594,792), amoxicillin (n=979,380) and levofloxacin (n=201,798) use in older white men (average age 56.8 years). Compared with amoxicillin, both azithromycin use and levofloxacin use were associated with statistically higher hazard ratios for all-cause mortality (HR 1.48, 95% CI, 1.05–2.09, and HR 2.49, 95% CI, 1.70–3.64, respectively) (Rao 2014).

Clarithromycin and erythromycin are associated with QTc prolongation, but this was the first strong evidence regarding azithromycin. Discrepancies in study findings and varied patient populations highlight the important role pharmacists have in evaluating risks. Azithromycin, other macrolides, and other antibiotics (e.g., fluoroquinolones) all have the potential for QTc prolongation. Inpatient pharmacists can evaluate baseline risk factors for cardiovascular disease, request baseline QTc readings, and correct underlying electrolyte abnormalities. Outpatient pharmacists may discuss alternatives with providers. Azithromycin is sometimes prescribed inappropriately for viral upper respiratory infections, which presents an ideal opportunity for intervention. If azithromycin is necessary, pharmacists can evaluate drug interaction potential and monitor the QTc interval. In patients developing QTc prolongation or torsades de pointes, the offending drugs should be discontinued immediately and intravenous magnesium administered. Alternative medications (e.g., doxycycline) can then be recommended.

Linezolid and Serotonin Syndrome

Linezolid, an oxazolidinone antibiotic, is active against gram-positive organisms, including methicillin-resistant *Staphylococcus aureus* (MRSA) and vancomycin-resistant *Enterococcus* (VRE). According to the package insert, linezolid also weakly but reversibly binds to monoamine oxidase (MAO). Dopamine, epinephrine, norepinephrine, and serotonin are metabolized by MAO enzymes; therefore, inhibition of MAOs can lead to accumulation, potentially resulting in serotonin syndrome (SS). This is characterized by autonomic dysfunction (fever, shivering, tachycardia), neuromuscular hyperactivity (clonus, tremor), and mental status changes (confusion, agitation), which may present hours to days after medication ingestion/interaction (Tisdale 2010).

In July and October 2011, the FDA released statements regarding reports of SS in patients concomitantly taking linezolid and serotonergic psychiatric medications. The majority of case reports involved selective serotonin reuptake inhibitors (SSRIs) or serotonin norepinephrine reuptake inhibitors (SNRIs). It is unclear whether psychiatric drugs with lesser degrees of serotonergic activity pose a comparable risk to patients (FDA 2011a, 2011b). Table 3-1 lists drugs with serotonergic properties.

A recent publication reviewed 20 phase 3 and phase 4 studies, comparing SS risk with serotonergic drugs and concomitant use of linezolid or comparators (Butterfield 2012). In addition to the agents in Table 3-1, the authors included analgesics (e.g., codeine, fentanyl, meperidine, propoxyphene, tramadol), anti-Parkinson drugs (amantadine, bromocriptine, levodopa, selegiline), migraine drugs (dihydroergotamine, rizatriptan, sumatriptan, zolmitriptan), atypical antipsychotics (clozapine, risperidone, ziprasidone), and antiemetics (dolasetron, granisetron, ondansetron, droperidol, metoclopramide). Clinical signs of SS were identified by word search algorithms and evaluated using two common SS diagnostic criteria: the Sternbach criteria and the Hunter criteria.

The Sternbach criteria require all of the following for a diagnosis of SS: recent addition of a serotonergic medication; at least three serotonergic symptoms (mental status changes, agitation, myoclonus, hyperreflexia, diaphoresis, shivering, tremor, diarrhea, incoordination, and/or fever); no new neuroleptic drugs started or doses increased; and other causes ruled out (Sternbach 1991). The Hunter criteria, purportedly more sensitive and more specific, require recent addition of a serotonergic medication and at least one of the following: spontaneous clonus, inducible clonus plus agitation or diaphoresis, ocular clonus plus agitation/diaphoresis, tremor plus hyperreflexia, and/or hypertonia plus temperature higher than 38°C (100.4°F) plus ocular clonus or inducible clonus (Dunkley 2003).

In a review of more than 10,000 patients who had received at least one serotonergic medication and who satisfied the

---

Patient Care Scenario

A 73-year-old woman with chronic kidney disease is diagnosed with a vancomycin-resistant *Enterococcus* (VRE) liver abscess. She is febrile, tachycardic, with a WBC of 16.5 x10³ cells/mm³. The abscess is successfully drained but the patient still requires some "mop up" antibiotic therapy. To avoid a peripherally inserted central catheter line, the prescriber would like to start the patient on oral linezolid. The patient is also taking codeine as needed for cough, metoclopramide 10 mg every 6 hours for peristalsis, and citalopram 20 mg daily for major depression. Which one of the following is best to recommend for this patient?

A. Discontinue codeine and metoclopramide, start linezolid immediately, and closely monitor the patient.

B. Discontinue codeine, metoclopramide, and citalopram, start linezolid in 1 week, and closely monitor the patient.

C. Discontinue codeine, metoclopramide, and citalopram, start linezolid in 5 weeks, and closely monitor the patient.

D. Switch linezolid to daptomycin 4 mg/kg intravenous every 24 hours

Answer

The patient is acutely ill (febrile, tachycardiac, elevated WBC) and the abscess has been surgically managed, but the patient still requires antibiotic therapy. Linezolid has the potential to interact with the patient's SSRI (citalopram), and to a lesser degree, the codeine and metoclopramide. Because the codeine is only as-needed, after discussion with the patient, it would be best to discontinue this. Additionally, the need for metoclopramide should also be discussed, and if possible, discontinued or changed to an alternative agent such as erythromycin. The patient is on citalopram for major depression, and this may not be discontinued as easily, plus it optimally would require a week for washout (half-life of 24-48 hours). However, the more pressing issue is the timing of linezolid initiation. The patient is acutely ill, therefore immediate initiation of linezolid is recommended (Answer A is correct). Daptomycin has activity against VRE and may potentially be an option, however, intravenous access is an issue with this patient, and the dose of 4 mg/kg is arguably too low for this indication.

1. Ramsey TD, Lau TTY, Ensom MHH. Serotonergic and adrenergic drug interactions associated with linezolid: A critical review and practical management approach. Annals Pharmacother 2013;47:543-60
2. Casapao AM, Kullar R, Davis SL, et al. Multicenter study of high-dose daptomycin for treatment of enterococcal infections. Antimicrob Agents Chemother 2013;57:4190-6

---

requirements of at least one diagnostic method of SS, no difference was found between linezolid and comparator groups (12 patients [0.54%] vs. 4 patients [0.19%], respectively; relative risk [RR] 2.79, 95% CI, 0.90–8.65). Compared with patients receiving one or two serotonergic medications, patients receiving three or more drugs had a slightly higher proportion of satisfying criteria for SS (p=NS). Use of SSRIs was implicated in only 2 patients with SS. Patients meeting SS criteria had comorbidities such as hepatic failure, cerebrovascular events, or renal failure (Butterfield 2012).

Most of the SS literature is retrospective in nature, and causality cannot be determined. However, the prescribing information for linezolid and serotonergic medications has been updated for SS and possible management strategies, such as discontinuing serotonergic medications during linezolid treatment.

Table 3-1. Drugs with Serotonergic Properties

Agent	Half-life (hours)
Selective Serotonin Reuptake Inhibitors (SSRIs)	
Citalopram	24–48
Escitalopram	27–32
Fluoxetine	96–144 (parent drug), 220 (metabolite)
Fluvoxamine	15–16
Paroxetine	21
Sertraline	26
Vilazodone	25
Serotonin Norepinephrine Reuptake Inhibitors (SNRIs)	
Desvenlafaxine	10–11
Duloxetine	12
Venlafaxine	5 (parent drug), 11 (metabolite)
Tricyclic Antidepressants (TCAs)	
Amitriptyline	9–27
Clomipramine	19–37 (parent), 54–77 (metabolite)
Desipramine	15–24
Doxepin	15 (parent), 31 (metabolite)
Imipramine	8–21
Nortriptyline	28–31
Protriptyline	54–92
Trimipramine	16–40
Monoamine Oxidase Inhibitors (MAOIs)[a]	
Isocarboxazid	Not available
Phenelzine	12
Selegiline	10 (oral), 18–25 (transdermal)
Tranylcypromine	1.5–3
Other Psychiatric Medications	
Amoxapine	8 (parent), 4–6 and 30 (metabolites)
Bupropion	14 (parent), 20–37 (metabolites)
Buspirone	2–3
Maprotiline	27–58
Mirtazapine	20–40
Nefazodone	2–4 (parent), metabolites longer
Trazodone	7–10

[a]Although the half-life of the MAOIs is only several hours, many irreversibly bind to MAO with effects persisting for several weeks.

Information from: U.S. Food and Drug Administration (FDA). FDA Drug Safety Report. 2011.

Pharmacists can determine the risk and significance of potential interactions by evaluating the qualities of serotonergic agents, linezolid indications, and planned durations. Although most clinicians recognize SSRIs and SNRIs, pharmacists can help identify lesser-known serotonergic drugs. In a nonemergent situation, the pharmacist may recommend holding the serotonergic agent while the patient is receiving linezolid. Serotonergic drugs have varying half-lives, which may be associated with serotonin withdrawal or require longer tapering periods. For example, a patient would ideally stop taking fluoxetine at least 5 weeks before starting linezolid. Serotonergic drugs may be resumed 24 hours after the last dose of linezolid. If pre-emptive discontinuation is not possible and no alternatives to linezolid exist, the recommendation is to immediately stop the serotonergic drug, administer linezolid, and monitor the patient for 2 weeks (5 weeks if on fluoxetine) (FDA 2011b). If serotonergic drugs cannot be stopped and concomitant administration occurs, the patient should be monitored for signs and symptoms of SS and the offending agent(s) stopped immediately if SS is suspected. Treatment strategies for SS include supportive measures and, potentially, administering benzodiazepines and/or cyproheptadine.

Adverse Drug Events

Tigecycline and Increased Rates of Death

Tigecycline is a glycylcycline antibiotic similar to the tetracyclines but with a broader spectrum of activity encompassing gram-positive (including MRSA and VRE), gram-negative, and anaerobic organisms. Tigecycline has FDA label approval for the treatment of complicated skin and skin structure infections (cSSSIs), complicated intra-abdominal infections (cIAIs), and community-acquired bacterial pneumonia (CABP). It lacks activity against *Pseudomonas aeruginosa*. Because of its large volume of distribution, tigecycline has a limited role in treating primary bloodstream infections, because it rapidly and extensively distributes into tissue.

In September 2010, the FDA released a safety announcement about increased risk of mortality with tigecycline compared with other antibiotics (FDA 2010a). The FDA reviewed 13 studies of approved and nonapproved indications, including cSSSI, cIAI, CABP, hospital-acquired pneumonia (HAP), ventilator-associated pneumonia (VAP), nonVAP, resistant pathogens, and diabetic foot infections (DFI). Although mortality was not higher for tigecycline in any individual infection, pooled results indicated death in 4.0% of patients on tigecycline (150/3788 patients) versus 3.0% of comparator-treated patients (110/3646 patients) (adjusted risk difference 0.6%, 95% CI, 0.1%–1.2%). Two characteristics drove the increased mortality: VAP infection and baseline bacteremia, with mortality of 50.0% in the tigecycline subgroup compared with 7.7% in the comparator subgroup (McGovern 2013).

Outcome discrepancies were first seen in patients with HAP who were receiving standard-dose tigecycline (100-mg load, then 50-mg intravenous every 12 hours) with or without ceftazidime (for *Pseudomonas* coverage) versus imipenem with or without vancomycin (for MRSA coverage). Overall cure rates were lower for tigecycline (67.9% vs. 78.2%), with an increased discrepancy among VAP subgroups (47.9% tigecycline vs. 70.1% imipenem). A nonsignificant trend toward increased mortality was also seen in this tigecycline subgroup (Freire 2010).

A potential confounder is the 15% lower tigecycline area under the curve observed in the VAP population. A phase 2 trial compared higher tigecycline doses versus imipenem in patients with HAP (70% being VAP). Based on early termination with enrollment difficulties, 108 patients were randomized to tigecycline (150-mg load, then 75-mg intravenously every 12 hours), tigecycline (200-mg load, then 100-mg intravenously every 12 hours), or imipenem. Additional antibiotics targeting *Pseudomonas* or MRSA were allowed. Clinical cure was numerically higher in the tigecycline 100-mg group (85.0%) compared with tigecycline 75 mg (69.6%) and imipenem (75.0%). As expected, patients in the tigecycline groups often reported adverse gastrointestinal events (Ramirez 2013). Although the results are promising, providers must remember that tigecycline lacks activity against *Pseudomonas*, a key pathogen in this patient population.

In September 2013, the FDA released a stronger warning regarding the increased risk of death associated with tigecycline (FDA 2013b). A review of 10 clinical trials for FDA-approved indications only (cSSSI, cIAI, CABP) also showed a higher risk of death in the tigecycline group (66/2640 patients [2.5%]) versus comparators (48/2628 patients [1.8%]) (adjusted risk difference 0.6% (95% CI, 0.0–1.2%). Deaths were caused by worsening infections, complications of infection, or other underlying medical conditions.

As a result, tigecycline's prescribing information has been updated. A boxed warning cautions that higher all-cause mortality was seen in patients treated with tigecycline, although the cause is unknown. Tigecycline should be reserved for situations in which alternative treatments are unavailable.

Pharmacists can be instrumental in determining when tigecycline may be clinically appropriate. Tigecycline retains activity against many resistant organisms, so it may be a last resort for *Acinetobacter*, third-generation cephalosporin-resistant Enterobacteriaceae or carbapenem-resistant Enterobacteriaceae (CRE) infections, or in patients with extensive drug allergies. The cause of the higher mortality rate has not been fully elucidated. That higher rate may be secondary to tigecycline's use as salvage therapy in refractory infections and critically ill patients. On-label use in less critically ill patients may result in a lower mortality risk. Pending further study, pharmacists may adjust doses to achieve higher area under the curve concentrations for multidrug-resistant organisms

(MDROs). Alternative agents should always be considered for the treatment of bacteremia.

Cefepime and Seizure Risk

Cefepime, a fourth-generation cephalosporin antibiotic, is active against gram-positive and gram-negative organisms, including *P. aeruginosa*. Similar to other β-lactams, cefepime is excreted renally and requires dosage adjustment in patients with renal dysfunction. The manufacturer recommends a dose reduction if CrCl is less than 60 mL/minute. Table 3-2 lists doses and adjustments for various infections.

Since its introduction in 1996, cefepime has been used extensively in critically ill patients, offering broad empiric antibacterial coverage. In 2012, the FDA warned of cefepime-induced nonconvulsive status epilepticus (NCSE)—seen in patients with renal impairment who were not receiving appropriate dosage adjustments (FDA 2012b). A thorough review of the FDA's Adverse Event Reporting System (AERS) identified 59 cases of NCSE during cefepime administration, occurring mostly in people 65 years or older (56%) and in women (69%). Renal dysfunction was present in 58 patients (information missing for one patient), with the dose not appropriately adjusted in 56/58 patients. In most cases, NCSE resolved after cefepime discontinuation. After searching for additional cases of cefepime-associated seizure activity, the FDA identified three cofactors significantly increasing cefepime-associated neurotoxicity: (1) patients older than 50 years with (2) the presence of renal dysfunction and (3) dosing inappropriate for their individual levels of renal function.

Investigators at the Mayo Clinic reviewed 100 adult ICU patients receiving at least 3 days of cefepime: 15 met criteria for neurotoxicity, ranging from impaired consciousness (n=13) to NCSE (n=1). The authors found that inappropriate renal dosing had contributed to neurotoxicity, although some neurotoxicity was also seen in patients receiving appropriate doses. The authors commented that even though cefepime-associated seizures are rare, other manifestations such as unexplainable "altered mental status" may be more common, and a change in antimicrobial therapy may be warranted to alleviate those symptoms (Fugate 2013).

Many β-lactam antibiotics cross the blood-brain barrier. Most are excreted renally, necessitating dosage adjustment in cases of renal impairment. It is not unexpected that inappropriately high doses of cefepime can lead to neurotoxic events. Drug manufacturers are required to perform dose-finding studies of various degrees of renal dysfunction, with most using the Cockcroft-Gault equation to estimate renal function. Alternative equations have been developed to more accurately stage renal dysfunction, including the Modification of Diet in Renal Disease (MDRD) equation. Clinicians may use the readily calculated estimated glomerular filtration rate to determine medication

Table 3-2. Cefepime Dosing Recommendations

Indication	Dose and Frequency
Febrile neutropenia	2 g IV q8h
Intra-abdominal infections, complicated	2 g IV q8h–12h
Pneumonia, moderate to severe (including *Pseudomonas*)	1–2g IV q8h–12h
Skin and soft tissue infection, moderate to severe, uncomplicated	2 g IV q12h
Urinary tract infection, mild to moderate, uncomplicated or complicated	500 mg–1 g IV q12h
Urinary tract infection, severe, uncomplicated or complicated	2 g IV q12h

Dose Reduction for Impaired Renal Function

CrCl (mL/minute)				
Greater than 60	500 mg IV q12h	1 g IV q12h	2 g IV q12h	2 g IV 8h
30–60	500 mg IV q24h	1 g IV q24h	2 g IV q24h	2 g IV q12h
11–29	500 mg IV q24h	500 mg IV q24h	1 g IV q24h	2 g IV q24h
Less than 11	250 mg IV q24h	250 mg IV q24h	500 mg IV q24h	1 g IV q24h
CAPD	500 mg IV q48h	1 g IV q48h	2 g IV q48h	2 g IV q48h
HD	1 g IV once, then 500 mg IV q24h	1 g IV once, then 500 mg IV q24h	1 g IV once, then 500 mg IV q24h	1 g IV q24h

Information from cefepime package information. 2012.

CAPD = continuous ambulatory peritoneal dialysis; h = hours; HD = hemodialysis; IV = intravenous; q = every.

doses. Studies comparing dosing recommendations between equations recognize higher recommendations using the MDRD equation in 20%–35% of cases. Some manufacturers provide dosing recommendations by using both equations for newer medications. However, the use of either equation has inherent limitations: controversies exist regarding extremes of weight or age and rapidly changing or unstable renal function.

Pharmacists can be instrumental in assessing renal function and dosing by calculation and evaluation of urine output, severity of illness, and site of infection. Patients with underlying seizure disorders or patients at high risk of seizure (e.g., status post-neurosurgery) may require monitoring more often, including daily renal function assessment. Microbiologic culture results should be followed for de-escalation because most use is empiric in nature. If patients show signs or symptoms of neurotoxicity, pharmacists can evaluate the likelihood that it is associated with cefepime versus other medications or disease states. Because NCSE is difficult to diagnose symptomatically, electroencephalography is recommended for diagnosis and follow-up. If cefepime is deemed responsible, it should be stopped immediately, switching to alternative antibiotics as needed. Most cases of cefepime-induced NCSE resolve after discontinuation.

Daptomycin and Eosinophilic Pneumonia

Daptomycin, a rapidly acting bactericidal lipopeptide antibiotic, is active against gram-positive organisms, including MRSA and VRE; it has FDA label approval for the treatment of cSSSI and bacteremia, including right-sided endocarditis. As noted in the package insert, daptomycin should not be used to treat pneumonia because it is inactivated by pulmonary surfactant. In July 2010, the FDA warned of potential daptomycin-associated eosinophilic pneumonia (EP) (FDA 2010b).

Eosinophilic pneumonia is a rare but serious condition in which white blood cells migrate to lung tissue. Clinical symptoms include fever, cough, shortness of breath, and difficulty breathing. Peripheral eosinophilia (>6%) is common, but pulmonary eosinophilia (>25%) obtained by bronchoalveolar lavage is necessary for diagnosis. The FDA reviewed its AERS database and conducted a literature search for daptomycin-associated EP, including in its case definition concurrent daptomycin exposure, fever, dyspnea with increased oxygen requirement or requiring mechanical ventilation, new infiltrates on chest radiography or computed tomography scan, bronchoalveolar lavage with greater than 25% eosinophils, and clinical improvement after daptomycin discontinuation. Forty-three cases were identified: 7 were deemed definite and 36 were considered probable. Of the definite cases, all patients received daptomycin off-label. Patients were older (60–87 years), mostly male (6/7), received doses of 4.4–8.0 mg/kg daily, and developed EP 2–4 weeks after daptomycin exposure (Kim 2012, FDA 2010b). All cases improved or

resolved following daptomycin discontinuation. Systemic steroids were often administered. Two patients rechallenged with daptomycin developed recurrence of EP.

The daptomycin prescribing information was updated with this information. Language was also added to the patient information section asking patients to report to their health care provider (HCP) any signs of cough, breathlessness, or fever.

Pharmacists have an important educational role regarding this adverse event. If patients are suspected of developing EP, other causes of eosinophilia such as parasitic infections or allergic bronchopulmonary aspergillosis should be ruled out. Other drugs associated with EP include nitrofurantoin, minocycline, meropenem, clarithromycin, dapsone, and azithromycin (Kim 2012). Pharmacists can evaluate the event, make sure that daptomycin is stopped immediately, and recommend systemic steroids and alternative antibiotic therapy. Common courses of steroids included methylprednisolone 60–125 mg intravenously every 6 hours for 1–3 days until resolution of respiratory failure, followed by several weeks of oral prednisone 40–60 mg with tapering. Because this reaction reappeared upon rechallenge, daptomycin should be documented as an allergy in the medical record.

ANTIMICROBIAL STEWARDSHIP LEGISLATION AND SUPPORT

Since the 1950s, infectious disease (ID) providers have recognized the consequences of antibiotic overprescribing. Worldwide, antibiotic overprescribing, poor antibiotic selection, and inadequate dosing remain problematic. Antimicrobial resistance has spread across multiple drug classes (Boucher 2009, Valencia 2009), and superinfections with *Clostridium difficile* and fungi continue to rise (Redelings 2007, McDonald 2006). Antimicrobial misuse contributes to high rates of adverse drug events (Weiss 2013), worsening clinical outcomes, and higher costs (Roberts 2009, DiazGranados 2005, Cosgrove 2003, Engemann 2003).

The antimicrobial pipeline has slowed in the past decade, leaving providers with very few new therapeutic options. Therefore, more-toxic medications (e.g., polymyxins) are used, doses are pushed higher than approved, and combinations of three and four drugs are used. Limiting antibiotic exposure is critical across all populations in academic and nonacademic centers, as well as inpatient and outpatient settings. However, changing patient and provider behavior is not an easy task.

Recognition of the benefit and need for antimicrobial stewardship activities across the health care spectrum (Paterson 2006) prompted professional societies, government policy makers, and third-party payers to endorse, and, in some cases, mandate, these activities. Antimicrobial stewardship programs are considered among the most-effective ways to improve antimicrobial utilization and to slow an impending maelstrom.

Box 3-1. CDC List of Successful Elements for Stewardship

Leadership: Dedicating necessary human, financial, and information technology resources.

Accountability: Appointing a single leader responsible for program outcomes. Experience with successful programs has shown that a physician leader is effective.

Drug Expertise: Appointing a single pharmacist leader responsible for working to improve antibiotic use.

Action: Implementing at least one recommended action, such as systemic evaluation of ongoing treatment need after a set period of initial treatment (e.g., antibiotic "time out" after 48 hours)

Tracking: Monitoring antibiotic prescribing and resistance patterns.

Reporting: Regular reporting information on antibiotic use and resistance to doctors, nurses and relevant staff members.

Education: Educating clinicians about resistance and optimal prescribing.

CDC Get Smart Program

In 1992, the Institute of Medicine (IOM) reported concerns over increasing resistance among several common pathogens. More than 95% of patients with *S. aureus* infections failed to respond to then first-line antibiotics penicillin and ampicillin. Over 15% of *S. aureus* isolates were resistant to methicillin. Erythromycin resistance was rising in *Streptococcus,* and penicillin resistance had surpassed 10% (IOM 1992). In 1995, the Centers for Disease Control and Prevention (CDC) launched an antibiotic-abuse community awareness program, renamed in 2003 as Get Smart: Know When Antibiotics Work. That media campaign aimed to reduce antibiotic-resistance rates by promoting "intelligent" antimicrobial prescribing by health care providers and thoughtful demand by patients.

The initial target was to decrease outpatient prescribing and consumer demand for antibiotics for upper respiratory infections. The CDC estimates that more than 75% of outpatient antibiotic prescriptions are for otitis media, the common cold, sinusitis, and bronchitis caused by viral pathogens. As a campaign, primary delivery methods are in the forms of examination room posters and prescription pads touting symptom relief medications, not antibiotics. Additionally, the CDC encourages, supports, and promotes evidence-based guidelines for coughs and acute bacterial sinusitis. Using those materials, the outpatient pharmacist is key in educating both the public and prescribers about unnecessary antibiotics.

Through the Get Smart program, the CDC endorses institutional ASPs as means of promoting efficient controls. For optimal program success and institutional (physician) buy-in, a physician leader is considered best practice, although clinical pharmacist expertise is also emphasized. A dashboard is encouraged for the tracking

of pneumonia days of therapy or of de-escalation rates of broad empiric prescribing. The CDC recommends goals be geared toward local problems, such as ICU antifungal overuse or increased rates of *C. difficile* infection (CDI).

In 2014, the CDC updated its core list of successful ASP elements (Box 3-1). Dedicated staff support, technology funding, expanded pharmacist leadership, action plans (including retrospective reviews at 48–72 hours) and specific reporting are listed as important.

Stewardship continues to be called "the single most-important action needed to slow down the development and spread of antibiotic-resistant infections" (CDC 2013). The 2013 CDC report found that at least half of patients receive one antibiotic during hospitalization and that antibiotics are used for too long or for treating colonizing or contaminating microorganisms. Data from the CDC's Emerging Infections Program further pointed out general antibiotic misuse and overuse in hospitals. Secondary analyses demonstrated regular, inappropriate prescribing for urinary tract infections (UTIs), particularly for asymptomatic bacteriuria, as well as long vancomycin courses despite negative cultures or lack of cultures. A 30% reduction in antibiotic use (fluoroquinolones, β-lactam/β-lactamase inhibitors, and extended-spectrum cephalosporins) can lead to a 26% decrease in CDI rates, accomplished by (1) avoiding treatment of asymptomatic bacteriuria, (2) ruling out noninfectious pulmonary processes before or during treatment of presumptive pneumonia, and (3) ruling out MRSA and de-escalating vancomycin for colonization or when identified as methicillin-susceptible *S. aureus* (MSSA). The inpatient pharmacist is uniquely poised to implement those interventions.

Pharmacists may also look to the 2012 Institute for Healthcare Improvement (IHI) Drivers and Change Package, which outlines best practices from pilot projects (IHI 2012). The package sets forth suggested processes, divided into "primary" and "secondary" drivers that can lead to optimal antibiotic use. The package lists specific interventions, which should be thoroughly evaluated before embarking on a multifaceted intervention protocol. The package also encourages facilities to prioritize the interventions by their individual needs, resources, and perceived barriers.

IDSA/SHEA Stewardship Guidelines

In 2007, the Infectious Diseases Society of America (IDSA), with the Society for Healthcare Epidemiology of America (SHEA), detailed evidence-based, best-practice strategies for established and burgeoning ASPs (Dellit 2007). Activities include prospective audit with intervention and feedback, formulary restriction, and pre-authorization (Table 3-3).

However, the presence of an ASP does not ensure a controlled environment of antimicrobial prescribing because behavioral change can be challenging. When attempts at modifications to antimicrobial-prescribing behavior are not fully vetted through division chiefs and house staff, the perception of forced control can result in pushback and failure (Charani 2011). Even guidelines with institutional buy-in and agreement may be underused by providers (Cortoos 2008).

In 2012, the IDSA, the SHEA, and the Pediatric Infectious Diseases Society (PIDS) recommended that legislation such as the Strategies to Address Antimicrobial Resistance (STAAR) Act (U.S. Congress 2009) establish within the U.S. Department of Health and Human Services (DHHS) an Antimicrobial Resistance Office and a Public Health Antimicrobial Advisory Board (SHEA/IDSA/PIDS 2012). They recommended enlisting nongovernment experts to support the existing task forces and to strengthen the coordination, prioritization, and accountability of federal efforts. Furthermore, they recommended specific fund allocations: $30 million in fiscal year 2012, $44 million in fiscal year 2013, and $80 million in fiscal year 2014. They cited a fiduciary responsibility whereby all health care institutions would establish and maintain policies to control antibiotic overuse.

The IDSA policy statement for saving lives urges congressional leaders to support the establishment and long-term support of ASPs in all health care settings (IDSA 2011). The statement says ASPs "should be required as a condition of participation in the federal CMS programs or through another regulatory mechanism." Funding recommendations for each agency and program are detailed,

Table 3-3. Core Strategies from the IDSA/SHEA Guidelines

Strategy	Rationale	Recommendation
Prospective audits with intervention and feedback to the prescriber	Performed by ID physician or clinical pharmacist with ID training	AI
	Can assist in reducing inappropriate use of antimicrobials	
Formulary restrictions	Can lead to immediate and significant reductions in use and cost of antimicrobials	AII
	Role of pre-authorization requirements has not been established and may shift use to other antimicrobial agents leading to increased resistance	BII
	Where pre-authorization is used, monitoring is necessary	BIII
Strategies for Consideration Based on Local Practice Patterns		
Education	Provides foundation to influence prescribing behaviors and accept antimicrobial stewardship	AIII
	Education alone has marginal effect in changing behavior	BII
Guidelines and Clinical Pathways	Develop using multidisciplinary approach and local microbiological information (e.g., resistance patterns to improve utilization)	AI
	Implement through education and provider feedback	AII
Antimicrobial Order Forms	Can be an effective component of a stewardship program and assist with practice guidelines	BII
Streamlining or De-escalating Therapy	Used on the basis of microbiology culture reports and pharmacokinetic and pharmacodynamic drug characteristics	AIII
	Can result in decreased antimicrobial exposure and cost savings	AII
Optimizing Antibiotic Dose	Based on the individual patient characteristics, causative organism, site of infection, and characteristics of the drug	AII
Converting from Parenteral to Oral	Determined by patient condition; can decrease length of stay and costs	AIII
Strategies with Insufficient Data for Strong Recommendations		
Antimicrobial Cycling	Insufficient data to recommend as routine procedure over long periods of time	CII
Combination Therapy	Insufficient data to recommend for routine use to prevent emergence of resistance	CII

including research to define inappropriate antimicrobial prescribing and enable behavioral change. Benchmarking is also covered regarding how and why antibiotic use per patient hospital day should be monitored and publicly reported. There is also a pay-for-implementation proposal of federal incentives to institutions that successfully implement and maintain ASPs. This should form the basis for new CMS quality measures for hospital incentives.

The policy also describes how industry should be supported in antibiotic research and development. One proposal has to do with implementation of an antibiotic innovation and conservation fee. The fee would be a flat fee (e.g., $3 per daily dose) charged against the wholesale purchase of antibiotics for human, animal, and plant agriculture use and would be paid by the dispensing entity (e.g., pharmacy, animal feed mill) at the time of purchase from the supplier. Of the flat fee, 75% would fund the research and development of antibiotics and 25% would fund ASPs.

Problems surrounding wide-scale empiricism can be resolved only by more-sensitive and more-affordable point-of-care testing, including rapid molecular diagnostics. Gains in the development of matrix-assisted laser desorption/ionization time-of-flight (MALDI-TOF), procalcitonin, and other diagnostic platforms are supported for that purpose. Additional regulatory strategies include postapproval audits by the industry to ensure that newly marketed antibiotics are being used appropriately.

CMS Stewardship Requirements/ Recommendations

Drafted work sheets for CMS surveyors list a number of ASP-related measures, including that (1) facilities demonstrate multidisciplinary processes to review antimicrobial use, local susceptibility patterns, and formulary management; (2) clinical decision support focuses on using appropriate antimicrobial agents; (3) interpretive comments are present in microbiology susceptibility reports, with notifications for clinical pharmacists; (4) formulary restrictions exist; (5) active endorsement of evidence-based guidelines are present; (6) antimicrobial orders include an indication and are reassessed at 72 hours; and (7) automated intravenous to oral substitution programs are in place.

Those drafted measures have yet to be implemented. However, the CMS fiscal year 2015 performance budget includes the following statement (DHHS 2015): *The Committee encourages CMS to collaborate with participating healthcare institutions to develop and implement ASPs in all healthcare facilities, including hospitals, long-term care facilities, long-term acute-care facilities, ambulatory surgery centers, and dialysis centers.*

The report details that CMS is engaged with infection prevention/epidemiologic organizations (1) to gather supporting evidence and information on effective actions and interventions and (2) to focus on regulatory changes to the CMS requirements that promote ASPs in hospitals and long-term acute care facilities. The potential for pharmacist involvement in any of the above interventions is far-reaching.

California and Veterans Health Administration ASP Initiatives

In February 2010, the California Department of Public Health (DPH) HAI Program developed its statewide ASP initiative for facilities. The purpose was to promote appropriate antimicrobial use across the entire state to curb CDI and the emergence of MDROs. Resource-limited settings have struggled with ASP implementation, so the advisory committee recently drafted three tiers of ASP activities: basic, intermediate, and advanced (CA DPH 2014) (Box 3-2).

In January 2014, VHA Directive 1031 required ASPs at all VHA medical facilities by July 2014. The document stated that administrative and clinical leadership support, as well as access to local data and clinical informatics, are vital to a successful program. The directive stipulates (1) how the National ASP Central Office Core Team—consisting of ID providers and clinical pharmacists—will oversee generation of standardized initiatives and guidance documents and (2) how it will collect and analyze data at the local and national levels. Leadership is defined as a medical director and a pharmacist, both of whom can perform or facilitate day-to-day operations. With centralized informatics, the group seeks to perform advanced

---

Box 3-2. California Antimicrobial Stewardship Program (ASP) Guidance

Basic Program
- Hospital antimicrobial stewardship policy/procedure
- Physician-supervised multidisciplinary antimicrobial stewardship committee, subcommittee, or workgroup
- Program support from a physician or pharmacist who has attended specific training on antimicrobial stewardship (e.g., continuing education program offered by the CDC and SHEA or other recognized professional organization, or post-graduate training with concentration in antimicrobial stewardship)
- Reporting of ASP activities to hospital committee involved in quality improvement activities

Intermediate Program
- Annual antibiogram developed using Clinical Laboratory Standards Institute guidelines with distribution to and education of the medical staff
- Institutional guidelines for the management of common infection syndromes (e.g., order sets, clinical pathways, empiric antimicrobial therapy guide, etc)
- Monitoring of usage patterns of antibiotics determined to be of importance to the resistance ecology of the facility, using defined daily dosing (DDD) or days of therapy (DOT)
- Regular education to hospital staff/committees about antimicrobial stewardship

Advanced Program
- Antimicrobial formulary that is reviewed annually with changes made based on local antibiogram
- Prospective audits with intervention/feedback
- Formulary restriction with pre-authorization

utilization reviews, make inferences about resistance patterning, and offer subsequent decision support. As this directive is fulfilled, the demand for pharmacists adequately trained in ID and ASPs will increase.

Other Legislation and Support

Much support is born out of defining the evolving resistance problem. The establishment of the Antimicrobial Resistance Task Force in 1999 was an initial step. Unfortunately, the task force was unable to effect legislation or bring public action. The STAAR legislation was introduced to enhance the program and to further recommend combating resistance, including a plan for the VHA Directive (U.S. Congress 2009).

In 2010, the American Society of Health-System Pharmacists (ASHP) published a position statement on pharmacists' roles in stewardship and infection prevention. The statement recognizes the unique qualifications of trained pharmacists to influence and direct proper antimicrobial use—largely through multidisciplinary work groups and committees (ASHP 2010). Such committees should oversee activities described in the IDSA/SHEA/PIDS guidelines, such as the development of restricted antimicrobial use procedures, therapeutic interchange, treatment guidelines, and clinical care plans. The statement stresses active participation in antimicrobial-related patient care, focusing on pharmacists' strengths (e.g., empiric selection, pharmacokinetic and dynamic dosing, cost-effective monitoring, prospective de-escalation). The statement also details collaboration with microbiology department leadership around susceptibility test results tailored for formulary concordance and cascaded based on resistance. Infection prevention recommendations are not limited to patient care units, and collaboration (e.g., with the IV room pharmacy) is important to limit drug product contamination and to encourage single-dose sterile products over multiple-dose containers. Finally, the statement describes a variety of educational formats and platforms whereby clinical pharmacists can develop guidance for providers and patients. The formats and platforms include newsletters, patient counseling sessions, and didactic sessions for house staff trainees and students.

In the past several years, ASP endorsement has strengthened; some states or institutions mandate ASP existence. Program funding has not been completely fulfilled, but there have been pushes for tax breaks, reimbursement incentives, and grants.

ANTIMICROBIAL RESTRICTIONS IN AGRICULTURE

Similar to the CDC's undertaking to tackle inappropriate antibiotic use, IDSA and other organizations aim to curb antibiotic overuse in food animals. Many factors contribute to the development of antimicrobial resistance, including inappropriate use—and abuse—in human and animal medicine and in food animal production. Although ASPs are well-accepted practices in human medicine, they are still novel concepts in the agricultural setting.

Antibiotics have been used in agriculture for decades and for many reasons. They have growth-promoting and disease-fighting capabilities, and they promote greater feed efficiency. Farmers claim that without routine use of antibiotics, pathogen loads in animals would increase, leading to more human foodborne illnesses. Plus, animals would contract more infections, leading to more antibiotic use for disease treatment rather than disease prevention. Increased animal infection rates and the inability to quickly isolate the sick would lead to losses in productivity and national food shortages (Aarestrup 2010, IDSA 2010). Animals typically implicated include swine, poultry, cattle, and fish.

In 1977, the FDA concluded that low antibiotic doses given to feed animals could lead to resistance; however, the agency failed to act. Additional studies followed, linking antibiotic-resistant *Salmonella, Campylobacter,* and *Escherichia coli* foodborne infections in humans to antibiotic use in feed animals. Pathogens such as VRE were also linked to animal antibiotic consumption. Tetracyclines, macrolides, bacitracin, penicillins, and sulfonamides are routinely used in farm water and feed. In 2010, an estimated 3.3 million kilograms of antibiotics was used for human health and 13.5 million kilograms of antibiotics in feed animals. In other words, 80% of antibiotic consumption in the United States was for feed animals (PAMTA 2013).

In the 1960s, several European countries banned antibiotic use in food animals if the antibiotics were also used to treat human infections. Veterinary antibiotics were not included in the same therapeutic class, and in 1995, glycopeptide-resistant *enterococci* were discovered in pigs and poultry, tracing back to the use of avoparcin, a vancomycin-like antibiotic. Since 2006, the European Union phased out all antibiotic growth promoters. Denmark voluntarily banned antibiotic use in swine in 2000 and summarized its findings in 2010. Contrary to farmers' beliefs, the elimination of antibiotics as growth promoters did not have a negative impact on herds. The opposite was found: following a short-term increase in mortality the year after the ban, mortality rates are lower than before. And swine productivity has increased by 40%. Most notably, antibiotic resistance has decreased in animal agriculture, in meat, and in healthy and infected humans (Aarestrup 2010).

The Danes implemented several key interventions: First, all antibiotic use in feed animals must be pursuant to a veterinarian-client-patient relationship (i.e., the veterinarian must prescribe antibiotics for specific individual animals only, not for whole herds). Secondly, the veterinarian may prescribe only up to 5 days of therapy unless a specific herd health contract allows prescribing up to 35 days. Lastly, farmers, veterinarians, and pharmacies must report the use and sale of animal antibiotics; these reports are audited and inspected regularly.

Encouraged by the European interventions, the IDSA and other organizations are lobbying for tighter regulation of feed-animal antibiotic use in the United States. In 2010, the IDSA testified before a House committee, urging support of the FDA's Preservation of Antibiotics for Medical Treatment Act (PAMTA 2013). The act would phase out seven medically significant classes of antibiotics currently approved for nontherapeutic uses in animals (i.e., for growth promotion). It would also require manufacturers to apply for approval of new animal medications that are medically important antibiotics and demonstrate no harm to human health and no development of resistance if they are used nontherapeutically. If antibiotics are necessary in feed animals, they should be prescribed pursuant to veterinary consultation or oversight (PAMTA 2013, IDSA 2010).

The IDSA also recommends a revision of FDA Guidance #152, which outlines the approval process for new animal antibiotics (FDA 2003). The IDSA urged avoidance of approval of antibiotics deemed "critically important" to human health, expansion of the list of antibiotics classified as such, and a ban on their use as growth promoters. The IDSA also encouraged the development of vaccines to decrease reliance on antibiotics.

Overall, even improvement in the judicious use of antibiotics in humans will only partially tackle the larger issue of antibiotic resistance. Because the majority of antibiotic use is in feed animals, any efforts to curb antibiotic use in humans must be collaborated with efforts to eliminate unnecessary use of antibiotics in animals. The European Union has proved this can be done successfully without compromising the productivity and vitality of feed animals.

MEASURING QUALITY

National Healthcare Safety Network and Healthcare Infection Control Practices Advisory Committee

Previously, mandatory reporting and public disclosure of HAI rates were limited to individual-state legislation, which few states had enacted. Legislators, infection prevention practitioners, and public watchdogs encouraged a national mandate for reporting and disclosure to oblige institutions to invest in more significant improvements in resources and reduce HAIs. The secondary aim was to improve overall health care quality and enable consumers to make better informed choices. Patient advocates say the right to know is critically important. Health care–associated infections have now been classified as preventable-harm events by CMS and others.

Concerns about possibly unreliable public reporting systems was recognized early because there was variability in not just HAI definitions but also how data were collected and reported. A 2005 Healthcare Infection Control Practices Advisory Committee (HICPAC) guidance document based on established principles for public health and HAI-reporting systems recommended:

- Using established public health surveillance methods to design and implement mandatory reporting systems
- Creating multidisciplinary, expert panels to monitor the planning and oversight of reporting systems
- Choosing appropriate process and outcome measures based on facility type
- Developing regular and confidential performance feedback data for HCPs

Identified preventable events were surgical-site infections (SSIs), central line–associated bloodstream infections (CLABSIs), and catheter-associated urinary tract infections (CAUTIs). Best-practice suggestions include preventive central line insertion protocols, surgical antimicrobial prophylaxis guidelines, and broader influenza vaccination among patients and HCPs. The CDC's National Healthcare Safety Network (NHSN) includes non-ICU areas and limits reports to device- and procedure-associated HAIs. The benefits of the NHSN are real-time reporting and analysis, as well as benchmarking with health departments or quality improvement organizations. The data analysis is compliant with CMS's infection reporting requirements.

Antimicrobial Use Option: CDC

Through the Antimicrobial Use Option (AUO), the NHSN began receiving antibiotic-use data in 2012. The national public health infrastructure had previously lacked a means for real-time assessments of antimicrobial consumption in hospitals to quantify usage patterns, make inferences about resistance patterns, or facilitate benchmarking. Prior reports used order or dispensing data across networks of hospitals, but because of variations in reporting systems, usage patterns between facilities could not be easily compared.

Development of a revised AUO led to the monitoring of national and facility-specific antimicrobial use. Roughly 6000 acute-care hospitals are enrolled in the electronic, real-time, prospective surveillance system. The antimicrobial-resistance tracking feature enables facilities to specifically analyze data regarding HAI pathogens, including individual and cumulative susceptibility data. The feature also qualifies the criteria necessary to participate in national quality improvement programs for health care settings other than acute-care hospitals, including outpatient dialysis and long-term acute care facilities.

Currently, participation in either HICPAC or the AUO requires data configuration to import into NHSN (CMS 2014). The primary metric reported is antimicrobial days per 1000 days present. As such, an electronic medication administration record (eMAR) and/or bar-coding medication administration record is required. Days present are defined as the aggregate number of patients housed at a patient-care location anytime throughout a day during a calendar month. Facilities must report data specific for adult and pediatric medical and surgical ICUs, adult and pediatric medical and surgical units, and at least one specialty care area, if present.

Table 3-4. Hospital Inpatient Quality Reporting and Potential Role of the Pharmacist

Measurement	Collected for:	Reported on Hospital Compare	Included in HVBP Beginning	Potential Role of Pharmacist
PN-3a Blood cultures performed within 24h of hospital arrival	CMS/TJC	No	No	Emergency room pharmacist can encourage blood cultures be performed Design automated pathways or protocols
PN-6 Initial antibiotic selection for CAP in Immunocompetent patient	CMS	Yes	FY 2013	Tailor institutional antibiotic formulary to reflect CMS choices Design automated pathways or protocols
PN-6a Initial antibiotic selection for CAP in Immunocompetent patient – ICU	TJC	No	No	Tailor institutional antibiotic formulary to reflect CMS choices Design automated pathways or protocols Ensure first dose is intravenous
PN-6b Initial antibiotic selection for CAP in Immunocompetent patient – nonICU	TJC	No	No	Tailor institutional antibiotic formulary to reflect CMS choices Design automated pathways or protocols IV to PO conversion as appropriate
SCIP-Inf-1 Prophylactic antibiotic received within 1h before surgical incision	CMS/TJC	Yes	FY 2013	Ensure appropriate antibiotics are available in the OR pharmacy or automated dispensing cabinets
SCIP-Inf-2 Prophylactic antibiotic selection for surgical patients	CMS/TJC	Yes	FY 2014	Tailor institutional antibiotic formulary to reflect CMS choices Design peri-operative prophylaxis guidelines
SCIP-Inf-3 Prophylactic antibiotics d/c within 24h after surgery end time	CMS/TJC	Yes	FY 2013	Implement automatic stop dates or decision support
SCIP-Inf-4 Cardiac surgery patients with controlled post-operative glucose	CMS/TJC	Yes	FY 2013	Review and/or develop finger stick protocols with sliding scales and recommend appropriate insulin and other regimens Consider insulin order sets for basal insulin infusions
SCIP-Inf-6 Surgery patients with appropriate hair removal	CMS/TJC	No	No	Ensure peri-operative guidelines include appropriate hair removal procedures
SCIP-Inf-9 Urinary catheter removal on POD1 or POD2 with day of surgery being day 0	CMS/TJC	Yes	FY 2014	Review patient catheter status Recommend catheter removal in eligible patients. Develop online decision support
IMM-1a Pneumococcal immunization – Overall rate	CMS/TJC	Yes	No	Screen patients eligible for pneumococcal vaccination Design automated pathways or protocols Administer pneumococcal vaccines in appropriate patients

Table 3-4. Hospital Inpatient Quality Reporting and Potential Role of the Pharmacist *(continued)*

Measurement	Collected for:	Reported on Hospital Compare	Included in HVBP Beginning	Potential Role of Pharmacist
IMM-1b Pneumococcal immunization – High risk populations (age 5-64 years)	CMS/TJC	No	No	Screen patients eligible for pneumococcal vaccination Design automated pathways or protocols Administer pneumococcal vaccines in appropriate patients
IMM-1c Pneumococcal immunization – age 65 and older	CMS/TJC	No	No	Screen patients eligible for pneumococcal vaccination Design automated pathways or protocols Administer pneumococcal vaccines in appropriate patients
IMM-2 Influenza immunization	CMS/TJC	Yes	FY 2016	Screen patients eligible for influenza vaccination Design automated pathways or protocols Administer influenza vaccines in appropriate patients
Healthcare Associated Infection (HAI) data submitted to the CDC's National Healthcare Safety Network (NHSN)				
MRSA bacteremia	CMS	Yes	No	Participate in CLABSI prevention bundle development, education and monitoring
SSI-colon, SSI-abdominal hysterectomy	CMS	Yes	FY 2016	Participate in SCIP protocol development Design peri-operative prophylaxis guidelines
CLABSI	CMS	Yes	FY 2015	Participate in CLABSI prevention bundle development, education and monitoring
CAUTI	CMS	Yes	FY 2016	Review patient catheter status Recommend catheter removal in eligible patients. Develop online decision support
Clostridium difficile	CMS	Yes	No	Review CDI rates and potential relationships to formulary antibiotics, prolonged duration by service and relapse rates Participate in the development of Infection Control protocols for curbing spread through improved hand hygiene and isolation Investigate prolonged duration antibiotic courses through daily reports and review
Health care personnel influenza vaccination	CMS	Dec 2014	No	Participate in vaccine brand selection, ordering, development of educational materials, algorithms for product selection by HCP medical status and workforce category

CAP = community-acquired pneumonia; CAUTI = catheter-associated urinary tract infection; CDI = *Clostridium difficile* infection; CLABSI = central line-associated bloodstream infection; CMS = Centers for Medicare and Medicaid Services; d/c = discontinue; FY = fiscal year; HCP = health care personnel; ICU = intensive care unit; MRSA = methicillin-resistant *Staphylococcus aureus*; POD = post-operative day; SSI = surgical site infection; TJC = the Joint Commission.

Quality Net and Hospital Quality Alliance

The Joint Commission (TJC) and CMS aligned measurement specifications for TJC-accredited hospitals in 2002, detailing measures in the _Specifications Manual for National Hospital Inpatient Quality Measures_. The manual is updated often for institutions to use as guidance for common national hospital performance measures. The CMS and TJC reviewers can standardize compliance with those measures during chart review. The manual contains in-depth algorithms for processes of care and the documentation to be used by coders. Preventive quality of care is defined for each measure, such as timing of antibiotic doses before surgical incision for prevention of surgical site infections (SSIs) (Jarret 2013). The Surgical Care Improvement Project (SCIP) defines the necessary components of surgical prophylaxis, including antibiotic choices, need for redosing, and duration of prophylaxis (Stulberg 2010).

The Hospital Quality Initiative aims to standardize measures for national public-reporting activities. For CLABSI, CAUTI, SSI, and VAP, CMS requires that institutions enrolled in the Hospital Inpatient Quality Reporting (IQR) payment program publicly report their data. In turn, the public can access the Hospital Care Web site, search for hospitals, and select up to three quality measures to compare on a graded scale. Detailed information is available for comparison, such as patient satisfaction surveys, spending per Medicare patient, and rates of preventable events. In addition to comparing hospitals selected, state and national averages are also presented.

The Optional Public Reporting network (formally Hospital Quality Alliance), is a quality measure program that can be publicly reported and is not required for the Hospital IQR payment program. Even hospitals that are not part of the Hospital IQR payment program may submit quality measures for public reporting. Table 3-4 summarizes measures available through the Hospital IQR payment program.

Central Line–Associated Bloodstream Infection

A CLABSI is a bloodstream infection in which a central line or umbilical catheter was in place for more than 2 days. Organisms cultured from the blood are attributed to the central line when no other site of infection is evident (e.g., a secondary bloodstream infection [BSI]). Catheter tip cultures do not determine whether a patient has a primary CLABSI alone, but clinical signs or symptoms of localized infection at a vascular access site when no other infection can be found is considered a primary BSI. The CLABSIs are differentiated by the type of central line: permanent versus temporary. Peripheral line–associated BSIs are not counted toward CLABSIs. The rates of CLABSIs are adjusted for 1000 catheter-days.

Agencies such as the IHI have introduced bundle programs to prevent infections. The programs include promotion of aseptic technique for insertion; detailed instructions for hub care, including chlorhexidine; and daily line site assessments. One center that initiated the bundle documented a reduction in CLABSI rates per catheter-days from 19/3784 to 3/1870 after implementation (1.60 vs. 5.02 CLABSIs per 1000 days; rate ratio 0.32 [.08 to .99, p<0.05]). In a control ICU where no bundles were implemented, there was no change in CLABSI rates (Sacks 2014).

Pharmacists may become involved in tracking CLABSI rates and can ensure that central line bundles are practiced and unnecessary lines removed. Combining another ASP activity, pharmacists may evaluate patients for intravenous to-oral switch, potentially eliminating the need for IV access.

Catheter-Associated Urinary Tract Infections

A CAUTI is a UTI in which an indwelling urinary catheter was in place for more than 2 days. A urinary catheter is inserted into the urinary bladder through the urethra (i.e., Foley catheter). This definition includes indwelling urethral catheters used for intermittent or continuous irrigation. The CAUTI rates should be adjusted and reported for 1000 patient-days.

Urinary catheters can easily get overlooked, with studies quoting up to 50% of providers unaware their patients retain urinary catheters. By identifying patients who may no longer require catheterization or by suggesting a switch to straight catheterization, pharmacists can help decrease CAUTI rates. Pharmacists also can discourage the use of more-expensive, silver-coated or impregnated catheters, which have not been shown to decrease CAUTI rates.

Surgical-Site Infections

An SSI is a major complication of surgical procedures; it occurs in 30,000 to 75,000 cases in the United States annually and leads to increased hospital stays and associated costs. More than one-half of all HAIs are SSIs, the majority of which are preventable (Anderson 2008). The NHSN/CDC defines SSIs according to their depth. Deep incisional SSIs must have occurred within 30 or 90 days after the procedure (where day 1 = the procedure date) and must involve deep soft tissues of the incision (e.g., fascial and muscle layers). The patient must have at least one of the following:

- Purulent drainage from the deep incision
- Spontaneous dehiscence or deliberate opening by an HCP with culture positivity
- At least one constitutional symptom (including fever higher than 38°C (100.4°F), localized pain, or tenderness)
- An abscess or other evidence of infection involving the deep incision and detected on direct examination, during invasive procedure, or by histopathologic examination or imaging test

Complex SSIs, including deep-skin or organ/space infections, require hospitalization. Organ/space infections are those that either match the area opened or are manipulated during the operative procedure and have at least one of the following:

- Purulent drainage from a drain placed into the organ/space
- Organisms isolated from aseptically obtained fluid culture or tissue in the organ/space
- An abscess or other evidence of infection involving the organ/space detected either on direct examination, during invasive procedure, or by histopathologic examination or imaging test. Superficial infections are not captured as SSIs.

The SCIP was an IHI initiative intended to prevent SSIs, venous thromboembolism, and other complications. Nine items are reported to TJC/CMS and available for public viewing. Seven core infection prevention items included in SCIP are listed in Table 3-4. The SCIP specifically focuses on coronary artery bypass grafts, other cardiac surgery, hip and knee arthroplasty, colon surgery, hysterectomy, and vascular surgery.

Antibiotics must be initiated 1 hour before surgical incision to deliver the highest concentration of drug at the time of surgery (Silver 1996). Because fluoroquinolones and vancomycin require 1 hour for infusion, and because tissue levels remain optimized for a longer duration, these antibiotics may be initiated within 2 hours of surgical incision.

The short antibiotic duration is intended to avoid untoward effects. Forty-eight hours (for cardiac surgery) is the longest recommended perioperative duration, although the data are not compelling (Edwards 2006). This includes patients with tubes in place (e.g., intra-abdominal, chest, genitourinary). Methods to improve compliance include automated stop dates in POE programming, eMAR signals for antibiotics exceeding 24–48 hours' duration, and distributing-division report cards that highlight outliers.

Surgical infections have been temporally related to elevated blood glucose levels (higher than 180 mg/dL). Hyperglycemia increases infection risk in both diabetic and nondiabetic patients, with the rate proportional to hyperglycemia level. Intensive insulin therapy can reduce related in-hospital mortality by decreasing the risk of BSIs, acute renal failure, red cell transfusions, ventilator support, and intensive care. Guidelines highlight the need for perioperative glucose control in cardiac surgery patients. The Society of Thoracic Surgeons Workforce guidelines recommend all cardiac surgery patients maintain serum glucose levels of less than 180 mg/dL (Lazar 2009).

For hair removal, a depilatory or the use of electric clippers immediately before surgery is preferred to reduce microabrasions associated with razor shaving. No hair removal is also an option (Kjonniksen 2002).

Indwelling urinary catheterization is often initiated before surgical procedures, particularly for prolonged procedures. The longer the catheter remains, the higher the risk of CAUTI, up to 24% higher after just 2 days (Wald 2008). Patients developing CAUTIs postoperatively are significantly less likely to be discharged to home, and they have significantly increased mortality at 30 days. In 2006, an interventional protocol limiting the use and duration of postoperative catheterization decreased from 10.4 to 3.9 episodes per 100 patients (incidence-density ratio, 0.41; 95% CI, 0.20–0.79) (Stephan 2006).

Hypothermia can impair wound healing and increase culture-positive SSIs rates. Active warming to at least 36°C (96.8°F) intraoperatively and immediately postoperatively is recommended (Hooper 2009). Studies on SCIP participation support its implementation. In one study, adherence to SCIP measures decreased SSI risk from 14.2 to 6.8 per 1000 discharges (adjusted odds ratio, 0.65; 95% CI, 0.76–0.95). When all infection prevention measures were followed, postoperative infection rates fell from 11.5 to 5.3 per 1000 discharges (p=NS) (Stulberg 2010).

Pharmacists can initiate many interventions to meet SCIP goals by selecting appropriate perioperative antibiotics and creating guidelines or protocols. It is important that drugs be available at the point of care in the preoperative area, and that clinicians work with anesthesia and nursing to give reminders about when to start the infusion and how to confirm documentation. Antibiotic selection is based on common pathogens relative to surgical procedures, including skin colonizers (e.g., *Staphylococcus*, *Streptococcus*) and colonizers of the surgical area (e.g., anaerobes for colon surgery, gram-negatives for hysterectomies). Vancomycin is not recommended unless the patient has a serious β-lactam allergy or is colonized with MRSA. The need for vancomycin must be clearly documented in the medical record, and the guidelines specify that pharmacists may perform the documentation. Pharmacists are also uniquely positioned to make recommendations on antibiotic dosing and redosing to maintain adequate tissue concentrations during surgery. A number of published guidelines review the data behind the antibiotic and intervention recommendations (Bratzler 2013). Protocols may be adjusted to deal with local resistance patterns (e.g., use of ceftriaxone over cefazolin) with adequate rationale documentation.

The IHI recommends that ASPs assist in writing institution-specific guidelines; in bringing in infection prevention practitioners to analyze types of procedures, pathogens, and resistance profiles; and in handling other aspects of the preventive bundle. Surgical leadership buy-in is important to drive compliance, as are education and report cards.

The American College of Surgeons and the CDC have worked with CMS and Hospital Compare to develop specific SSI outcome measures for colon surgery and abdominal hysterectomy. This prototype measure is the first step toward a more comprehensive SSI measure that includes additional surgical-procedure categories and expanded SSI risk adjustment by procedure type. The information is available underlined but lists only SSI rates for these surgical types. Hospitals must report deep incisional primary and organ/space SSIs during the 30-day postoperative period among patients older than 18 years who undergo inpatient colon surgeries or abdominal hysterectomies. No details are included about specific SCIP performance measures (e.g., appropriate ordering, administration, and discontinuation of preoperative prophylactic antibiotics), proper surgical site preparation, optimal glucose control in certain surgical patients, or maintenance of patient normothermia during surgery.

Laboratory-Identified Events

For NHSN surveillance in the acute-care setting, an HAI is a localized or systemic condition resulting from an adverse reaction to the presence of an infectious agent or its toxins that was not present on admission to the facility. For an HAI, that means either the onset happened on at least day 3 of admission or symptoms of the infection were present during the first 2 hospital days as long as they are also present on or after day 3.

1. MDRO including MRSA

Facilities may choose to monitor the following MDROs: MRSA, MRSA and MSSA, VRE, cephalosporin-resistant (ceph-R)-*Klebsiella* spp., CRE-*Klebsiella* spp., CRE-*E. coli*, and/or multidrug-resistant *Acinetobacter* spp. For *S. aureus*, both MRSA and MSSA phenotypes can be tracked to provide concurrent measures of the susceptible pathogens as a comparison with those of the resistant pathogens in a setting of active MRSA prevention efforts. Reported pathogens should not include active surveillance culture/testing results such as nasal swabs. Ceph-R-*Klebsiella* includes those intermediate or resistant to ceftazidime, cefotaxime, ceftriaxone, or cefepime. CRE-*Klebsiella* spp. are those testing nonsusceptible (i.e., resistant or intermediate) to imipenem, meropenem, or doripenem by standard susceptibility testing methods or by a positive result for any FDA-approved method for carbapenemase detection. Multidrug-resistant *Acinetobacter* includes any isolates testing nonsusceptible (i.e., resistant or intermediate) to at least one agent in at least three antimicrobial classes (β-lactam/β-lactamase inhibitor, cephalosporins, sulbactam, aminoglycosides, carbapenems, or fluoroquinolones). With the exception of unique blood isolates, if an MDRO from the same patient is isolated within the same calendar month, the isolate should not be counted. New blood isolates identified at least 14 days after the first isolate should be counted

.

2. Clostridium difficile

Hospital-associated cases of CDI are defined by positive *C. difficile* toxin results, including toxin-producing gene (i.e., polymerase chain reaction) or other laboratory means from a stool sample. All *C. difficile*–positive events must be reported separately and independently. The CDI events are classified according to community onset, community onset health care–facility associated, and health care–facility onset. Prevention and process measures that should be implemented and tracked include hand hygiene and gown and glove use. Hospitals can use the NHSN Laboratory identified system to calculate rates per 10,000 patient-days and benchmark. If an institution uses standard surveillance methods and converts to the NHSN method, there may be rate discordance. Recognizing the change in some definitions and adjusting for the conversion year should balance that phenomenon. Pharmacists can gain from access to such data for stewardship activities. Tracking antibiotic utilization trends and consequent changes in CDI rates is an important part of this evaluation.

Health Care Provider/Health Care Personnel Influenza Vaccination

Protecting patients against communicable diseases is one of the most basic preventive concepts. Protecting the health care workforce is necessary in anticipation of outbreaks such as recent influenza and SARS pandemics. The CDC and HICPAC worked with the Advisory Council on Immunization Practices (ACIP) to develop guidance for immunizing otherwise healthy workforces (MMWR 2011). The guidance recommends immunization and/or confirmation of immunity for hepatitis B, measles/mumps/rubella, varicella, tetanus/diphtheria/pertussis, *Neisseria meningitides,* and influenza.

Annual influenza vaccine—typically, the inactivated trivalent injectable containing two influenza A strains (H1N1 and H3N2) and an influenza B strain—should be administered to HCPs. Intranasal live attenuated influenza vaccine is acceptable for low-risk, nonpregnant employees younger than 50 years. However, because of potential live-virus shedding, these workers should not—for 7 days after administration—provide direct care for patients who are most at risk. Previously, at-risk groups included many kinds of patients but now are limited to immunocompromised patients in isolation (e.g., stem cell transplant recipients before engraftment). A high dose (60 mcg of hemagglutinin antigen per influenza vaccine virus) may be used for workers 65 years or older. All institution personnel regardless of patient-care duties should be immunized against influenza. Exceptions may include egg hypersensitivity, prior severe hypersensitivity reaction to influenza vaccine, and history of Guillain-Barré syndrome, although recombinant egg-free vaccine is available, as are non–thimerosal-containing products.

There are few well-controlled randomized trials of the protective effect of the vaccine in HCPs. One study identified a small decrease in absenteeism; another found a decrease in serologically confirmed disease (Saxen 1999, Wilde 1999). Much of the supportive data are linked to reports of low vaccination rates in health care facilities and observational studies.

Under 2007 TJC regulations, accredited health care facilities are required to track and report HCP influenza vaccination rates. The CMS requires that HCP vaccination rates be reported alongside inpatient rates. Despite the requirements, institutions have struggled with tracking, administration, and employee compliance. Many employees have declined vaccination based on (1) their beliefs that there is a very low risk of getting ill from influenza, (2) their previous experiences with vaccine adverse effects (e.g., muscle soreness, general malaise), or (3) their fears of unusual reactions (e.g., Guillain-Barré syndrome). Successful campaigns promoting better compliance include "Protect Your Patients" messages and senior management "Lead by Example" slogans. Other helpful strategies include removing barriers such as (1) cost (by providing free vaccine) and (2) logistics (by operating on-site clinics during multiple days and shifts). Some states have enacted laws that specify that employees must document vaccination. As of now, no state legally enforces that employees are not permitted to report to the workplace without documentation, but a state may mandate masks for unvaccinated HCPs. Alternately, "ensure" clauses for health care facilities also exist, meaning that each institution must have documentation that vaccine was offered. National CDC reports from institutions with mandatory vaccination requirements report vaccination rates of 89%; institutions with no recommendations or requirements report rates of only 44%. Average rates increased from 63.5% in 2010–2011 to 66.9% in 2011–2012, to 72% in 2012–2013. However, the DHHS goal for Healthy People 2020 is 90%. The current Internet Panel Survey of the CDC (n=1985 HCP) identifies the lowest compliance rates among assistants, aides, nonclinical support staff, and HCP working in long-term care. The highest compliance rates are among pharmacists, physicians, and nurses.

Acquisition of adequate vaccine supply can be challenging. Large health care systems may have the advantage of increased buying power, leaving smaller facilities struggling. Supply chain and production delays have historically hampered early vaccine delivery. Vaccine strain inclusion is based on epidemiologic modeling and the prevalence of prior strains by hemispheric spread. Pharmacists have played a role in the selection of product supply mix to ensure steady supply streams in case of delays at a particular manufacturer and to meet the special needs of those receiving the vaccine (e.g., products without thimerosal, latex, and/or egg content).

Many pharmacists are called on to participate in test-and-treat algorithms during peak weeks, as well as vaccine administration clinics within the institution. Pharmacists can access the latest information from the CDC online at FluVaxView. New this season was the availability of quadrivalent vaccine containing four strains of influenza (two influenza A and two influenza B strains) to improve the likelihood of antigen match. The ACIP has yet to issue an opinion on the additional benefit of this vaccine—because of the lack of large databases to confirm—but the future of vaccine development may swing toward only quadrivalent product.

CONCLUSION

Health care quality—including a focus on safety, improving health outcomes, decreasing preventable events, and curbing costs—has evolved from a secondary process to a mandatory endeavor. Institutions are now responsible for maintaining high performance scores to secure and maintain accreditation, to obtain reimbursement from CMS, and to remain appealing to consumers/patients in an increasingly competitive marketplace. Pharmacists can participate in the process of ensuring safety, enhanced quality, and antimicrobial stewardship to help achieve the basic requirements and to look for ways of ensuring high scores—from the most-basic bedside endeavors such as renal dose adjustment of cefepime to the highest level of clinical acumen in directing an institution's ASPs or guiding its SCIP procedures.

REFERENCES

Aarestrup FM, Jensen VF, Emborg HD, et al. Changes in the use of antimicrobials and the effects of productivity of swine farms in Denmark. Am J Vet Res 2010;71:726-33.

Advisory Committee on Immunization Practices (ACIP). Immunization of Health-Care Personnel: Recommendations of the Advisory Committee on Immunization Practices (ACIP). MMWR 2011; 60(RR-7).

Anderson DJ, Kaye KS, Classen D, et al. Strategies to prevent surgical site infections in acute care hospitals. Infect Control Hosp Epidemiol 2008;29(Suppl 1):S51-61.

American Society of Health-System Pharmacists (ASHP). ASHP Statement on the pharmacist's role in antimicrobial stewardship and infection prevention and control. Am J Health Syst Pharm 2010;67:575-7.

Boucher H, Talbot GH, Bradley JS, et al. Bad bugs, no drugs: no ESKAPE! An update from the Infectious Diseases Society of America. Clin Infect Dis 2009;48:1-12.

Bratzler DW, Dellinger EP, Olsen KM, et al. Clinical practice guidelines for antimicrobial prophylaxis in surgery. Am J Health Syst Pharm 2013;70:195-283.

Butterfield JM, Lawrence KR, Reisman A, et al. Comparison of serotonergic toxicity with concomitant use of either linezolid or comparators and serotonergic agents: An analysis of phase III and IV randomized clinical trial data. J Antimicrob Chemother 2012;67:494-502.

California Department of Public Health (CA DPH). The California Antimicrobial Stewardship Program Initiative. 2014.

Practice Points

U.S. Food and Drug Administration warnings:

Drug Interactions
- Through drug interactions and QTc prolongation, azithromycin has been linked with fatal rhythm abnormalities. Patients most at risk include those with bradycardia or pre-existing QTc prolongation, electrolyte abnormalities, and on Class IA or III antiarrhythmic agents.

Adverse Drug Reactions
- Tigecycline, when used for labeled and unlabeled indications, has been shown to have a higher mortality rate compared to comparable therapies. Patients must be carefully selected for receipt of tigecycline, if no suitable alternatives exist.
- Cefepime, when not properly adjusted for renal function, has led to cases of nonconvulsive status epilepticus. Elderly

- Concomitant linezolid and strong serotonergic medication (SSRIs, SNRIs) use has been linked to cases of serotonin syndrome. If discontinuation of these medications is not possible, patients must be monitored for signs and symptoms of this interaction.

patients, women, and patients predisposed to seizures may be at higher risk.
- Daptomycin use has been linked to cases of eosinophilic pneumonia. Patients should be counseled to report signs of cough, breathlessness, or fever to their health care provider immediately.

Stewardship and Legislature concerns:

The need for expanded and standardized antimicrobial stewardship programs and activities are quickly being recognized by a larger group of professional societies, local and national legislators and regulatory bodies.
- The CDC continuously updates the successful practice elements for programs and has expanded educational endeavors through the Get Smart program.
- The IDSA, SHEA, PIDS, ASHP, SIDP continue to update best practice strategies as well as endorsement of legislation such as the STAAR act.
- The CMS has drafted stewardship requirements for inclusion in surveys for reimbursement for all participating health care facilities.
- State programs (e.g., California) and the Veterans Affairs system have drafted mandatory stewardship program activi-

ties.
- The highest level activities include: (1) review of the antimicrobial formulary at least annually with changes made based on local antibiogram (2) prospective audits with intervention/feedback and (3) formulary restriction with pre-authorization.
- Stewardship in the human realm must be coupled with tougher antibiotic legislature and more judicious consumption in the agricultural world, in order to make a lasting impact.

Quality measurements, documentation and benchmarking have become increasingly important as they relate to infectious diseases, particularly preventable hospital-acquired infections.
- Identified preventable events include surgical site infections (SSI), central line-associated bloodstream infections (CLABSI), and catheter-associated urinary tract infections (CAUTI).
- The NHSN continues to track antibiotic consumption through the antimicrobial use option (AUO) also allowing institutions to track antimicrobial days per 1000 days pres-

ent locally and against a national benchmark.
- The Hospital Inpatient Quality Reporting (IQR) system allows patients to view quality measures in infectious diseases across institutions to make consumer decisions.
- Surgical site infection rates, health care worker influenza vaccination rates, rates of C. difficile and multidrug resistant pathogens are all reportable events.

Centers for Disease Control and Prevention (CDC). Antibiotic resistance threat reports. 2013

Centers for Disease Control and Prevention (CDC). 2014. Core elements of hospital antibiotic stewardship programs. Atlanta, GA: U.S. Department of Health and Human Services.

Centers for Medicare & Medicaid Services (CMS). Survey & Certification Focus on Patient Safety and Quality - Draft Surveyor Worksheets. 2012.

Centers for Medicare & Medicaid Services (CMS). Antimicrobial Use and Resistance (AUR) Module. 2014.

Charani E, Edwards R, Sevdalis N, et al. Behavior change strategies to influence antimicrobial prescribing in acute care: a systematic review. Clin Infect Dis 2011;53:651–62.

Cortoos PJ, Witte KD, Peetermans WE, et al. Opposing expectations and suboptimal use of a local antibiotic hospital guideline: a qualitative study. J Antimicrob Chemother 2008;62:189–95.

Cosgrove SE, Sakoulas G, Perencevich EN, et al. Comparison of mortality associated with methicillin-resistant and methicillin-susceptible Staphylococcus aureus bacteremia: A meta-analysis. Clin Infect Dis 2003;36:53–9.

Dellit TH, Owens RC, McGowan JE Jr, et al. Infectious Diseases Society of America and the Society for Healthcare Epidemiology of America guidelines for developing an institutional program to enhance antimicrobial stewardship. Clin Infect Dis 2007;44:159-77.

Department of Health and Human Services (DHHS) 2015. Fiscal year 2015 justification of estimates for appropriations committees. Centers for Medicare & Medicaid Services.

DiazGranados CA, Zimmer SM, Klein M, et al. Comparison of mortality associated with vancomycin-resistant and vancomycin susceptible enterococcal bloodstream infections: A meta-analysis. Clin Infect Dis 2005;41:327-33.

Dunkley EJ, Isbister GK, Sibbritt D, et al. The Hunter serotonin toxicity criteria: Simple and accurate diagnostic decision rules for serotonin toxicity. Q JM 2003;96:635-42.

Edwards FH, Engelman RM, Houck P, et al. The Society of Thoracic Surgeons practice guideline series: Antibiotic prophylaxis in cardiac surgery, Part I: Duration. Ann Thoracic Surg 2006;81:397-404.

Engemann JJ, Carmeli Y, Cosgrove SE, et al. Adverse clinical and economic outcomes attributable to methicillin resistance among patients with Staphylococcus aureus surgical site infection. Clin Infect Dis 2003;36:592-8.

Freire AT, Melnyk V, Kim MJ, et al. Comparison of tigecycline with imipenem/cilastatin for the treatment of hospital-acquired pneumonia. Diagn Microbiol Infect Dis 2010;68:140-51.

Fugate JE, Kalimullah EA, Hocker SE, et al. Cefepime neurotoxicity in the intensive care unit: A cause of severe, underappreciated encephalopathy. Critical Care 2013;17:R264-9.

Hooper VD, Chard R, Clifford T, et al. ASPAN's evidence-based clinical practice guideline for the promotion of perioperative normothermia: second edition. J Perianesth Nurs 2010;25:346-65.

Infectious Diseases Society of America (IDSA) 2010. Statement on antibiotic resistance: Promoting judicious use of medically important antibiotics in animal agriculture.

Infectious Diseases Society of America (IDSA). Combating antimicrobial resistance: Policy recommendations to save lives. Clin Infect Dis 2011;52(Suppl5):S397-428.

Institute for Healthcare Improvement (IHI). Antibiotic Stewardship Driver Diagram and Change Package. 2012. Institute of Medicine (IOM). Emerging Infections: Microbial Threats to Health in the United States. National Academy Press, Washington, D.C.: 1992

Jarret N. Evidence-based Guidelines for Selected and Previously Considered Hospital-Acquired Conditions. 2013.

John JF, Fishman NO. Programmatic role of the infectious diseases physician in controlling antimicrobial costs in the hospital. Clin Infect Dis 1997;24:471–85.

Kim PW, Sorbello AF, Wassel RT, et al. Eosinophilic pneumonia in patients treated with daptomycin. Drug Saf 2012;35:447-57.

Kjonniksen I, Andersen BM, Sondenaa VG, et al. Preoperative hair removal- a systematic literature review. AORN J 2002;75:928-38, 940.

Lazar H, McDonnell M, Chipkin S, et al. The Society of Thoracic Surgeons practice guideline series: Blood glucose management during adult cardiac surgery. Ann Thorac Surg 2009;87;663-9.

McDonald LC, Owings M, Jernigan DB. Clostridium difficile infection in patients discharged from US short-stay hospitals, 1996–2003. Emerg Infect Dis 2006;12:409-15.

McGovern PC, Wible M, El-Tahtawy A, et al. All-cause mortality imbalance in the tigecycline phase 3 and 4 clinical trials. Int J Antimicrob Agents 2013;41:463-7.

PAMTA 2013. Preservation of Antibiotics for Medical Treatment Act of 2013

Paterson DL. The role of antimicrobial management programs in optimizing antibiotic prescribing within hospitals. Clin Infect Dis 2006;42 Suppl 2: S90-5.

Ramirez J, Dartois N, Gandjini H, et al. Randomized phase 2 trial to evaluate the clinical efficacy of two high-dosage tigecycline regimens versus imipenem-cilastatin for treatment of hospital-acquired pneumonia. Antimicrob Agents Chemother 2013;57:1756-62.

Rao GA, Mann JR, Shoaibi A, et al. Azithromycin and levofloxacin use and increased risk of cardiac arrhythmia and death. Ann Fam Med 2014;12:121-7.

Ray WA, Murray KT, Hall K, et al. Azithromycin and the risk of cardiovascular death. N Engl J Med 2012;366;1881-90.

Redelings M, Sorvillo F, Mascola L. Increase in Clostridium difficile-related mortality rates, United States, 1999-2004. Emerg Infect Dis 2007;13:1417-9.

Roberts RR, Hota B, Ahmad I, et al. Hospital and societal costs of antimicrobial-resistant infections in a Chicago teaching hospital: implications for antibiotic stewardship. Clin Infect Dis 2009;49:1175-84.

Sacks GD, Diggs BS, Hadjizacharia P, et al. Reducing the rate of catheter-associated bloodstream infections in a surgical intensive care unit using the Institute for Healthcare Improvement central line bundle. Am J Surg 2014; doi: 10.1016/j.amjsurg.2013.08.041

Saxen H, Virtanen M. Randomized, placebo-controlled double blind study on the efficacy of influenza immunization on absenteeism of health care workers. Pediatr Infect Dis J 1999;18:779.

SHEA/IDSA/PIDS 2012. Policy statement on antimicrobial stewardship by the Society for Healthcare Epidemiology of America (SHEA), the Infectious Diseases Society of America (IDSA), and the Pediatric Infectious Diseases Society (PIDS). Infect Control Hosp Epidemiol 2012;33:322-7.

Silver A, Eichorn A, Kral J, et al. Timeliness and use of antibiotic prophylaxis in selected inpatient surgical procedures. Am J Surg 1996;171:548-52.

Stéphan F, Sax H, Wachsmuth M. Reduction of urinary tract infection and antibiotic use after surgery: a controlled, prospective, before-after intervention study. Clin Inf Dis 2006; 42:1544-51.

Sternbach H. The serotonin syndrome. Am J Psychiatry 1991;148:705-13.

Stulberg JJ, Delaney CP, Neuhaser DV, et al. Adherence to surgical care improvement project measures and the association with postoperative infections. JAMA 2010;303:2479-85.

Svanström H, Pasternak B, Hviid A. Use of azithromycin and death from cardiovascular causes. N Engl J Med 2013;368:1704-12.

Tisdale JE, Miller DA. Drug-Induced Diseases. American Society of Health-System Pharmacists. Bethesda, MD. 2010. Pages 659-65.

U.S. Congress. Strategies to Address Antimicrobial Resistance (STAAR) Act (H.R. 2400 in the 111th Congress). 2009.

U.S. Food and Drug Administration (FDA). Guidance #152. Evaluating the safety of antimicrobial new animal drugs with regard to their microbiological effects on bacteria of human health concern. 2003.

U.S. Food and Drug Administration (FDA) 2010a. Drug Safety Communication: Increased risk of death with Tygacil (tigecycline) compared with other antibiotics used to treat similar infections.

U.S. Food and Drug Administration (FDA) 2010b. Drug Safety Communication: Eosinophilic pneumonia associated with the use of Cubicin (daptomycin).

U.S. Food and Drug Administration (FDA) 2011a. Drug Safety Communication: Serious CNS reactions possible when linezolid (Zyvox) is given to patients taking certain psychiatric medications.

U.S. Food and Drug Administration (FDA) 2011b. Drug Safety Communication: Updated information about the drug interaction between linezolid (Zyvox) and serotonergic psychiatric medications.

U.S. Food and Drug Administration (FDA) 2012a. Statement regarding azithromycin (Zithromax) and the risk of cardiovascular death.

U.S. Food and Drug Administration (FDA) 2012b. Drug Safety Communication: Cefepime and risk of seizure in patients not receiving dosage adjustments for kidney impairment.

U.S. Food and Drug Administration (FDA) 2013a. Drug Safety Communication: Azithromycin (Zithromax or Zmax) and the risk of potentially fatal heart rhythms.

U.S. Food and Drug Administration (FDA) 2013b. Drug Safety Communication: FDA warns of increased risk of death with IV antibacterial Tygacil (tigecycline) and approves new Boxed Warning.

Valencia R, Arroyo LA, Conde M, et al. Nosocomial outbreak of infection with pan-drug-resistant Acinetobacter baumannii in a tertiary care university hospital. Infect Control Hosp Epidemiol 2009;30:257–63.

Wald HL, Ma A, Bratzler DW, et al. Indwelling urinary catheter use in the postoperative period: Analysis of the national surgical infection prevention project data. Arch Surg 2008;143:551-7.

Weiss AJ, Elixhauser A. Characteristics of adverse drug events originating during the hospital stay, 2011. Healthcare Cost and Utilization Project Statistical Brief #164. Rockville, MD: Agency for Healthcare Research and Quality; 2013.

Wilde JA, McMillan JA, Serwint J, et al. Effectiveness of influenza vaccine in health care professionals: a randomized trial. JAMA 1999; 281:908–13.

SELF-ASSESSMENT QUESTIONS

41. A patient presents with a prescription for 5 days of azithromycin to treat a confirmed bacterial sinus infection. He heard on the news that azithromycin can increase the risk of death in patients taking the drug for 5 days or longer and asks you to speak with his prescriber. Which one of the following is best to recommend for this patient?

    A. The risk of death from any cause is increased in patients taking azithromycin for 5 days or longer and the prescription should be changed to 3 days.
    B. The risk of death from any cause is increased in patients taking azithromycin and the prescription should be changed to levofloxacin.
    C. The risk of death from any cause is increased in patients taking azithromycin and the prescription should be changed to amoxicillin.
    D. The risk of death from any cause is increased in patients taking azithromycin and the prescription should be changed to ciprofloxacin.

42. Which one of the following patients, if prescribed 5 days of azithromycin, would be at greatest risk of developing a fatal heart arrhythmia? Use the table for QTc intervals and their interpretation.

	Women	Men
Normal	<450 msec	<430 msec
Borderline	450–470 msec	430–450 msec
Prolonged	>470 msec	>450 msec

    A. A 72-year-old woman with a QTc interval of 450 msec, history of diabetes (hemoglobin A1C 8.4%) and hypokalemia (3.1 mEq/L), currently prescribed amiodarone.
    B. A 48-year-old man with a history of QTc prolongation (last measurement 450 msec), currently prescribed mexiletine for a ventricular tachyarrhythmia.
    C. A 62-year-old woman, with a QTc interval of 430 msec, osteoporosis, and longstanding uncorrected hypokalemia (3.3 mEq/L).
    D. A 78-year-old woman, with a QTc interval of 430 msec, currently prescribed flecainide.

Questions 43 and 44 pertain to the following case.

U.W. is a 68-year-old man who has been maintained on amiodarone for a history of atrial fibrillation. He presents with a prescription for azithromycin for 5 days for community-acquired pneumonia. Upon review of U.W.'s medication profile, he is also on metronidazole for a recently diagnosed *Clostridium difficile* infection. Pertinent

laboratory parameters include a WBC of 14.5 x 10³ cells/mm³, SCr 0.8 mg/dL, sodium 140 mEq/L, potassium 3.2 mEq/L, chloride 108 mEq/L, and magnesium 1.3 mEq/L. U.W.'s last QTc reading was 432 msec

43. According to the FDA review, which one of the following best describes the number of risk factors for fatal arrhythmia (other than azithromycin usage) present in U.W.?

    A. 2
    B. 3
    C. 4
    D. 5

44. Which one of the following is best to recommend for U.W.?

    A. Replete potassium and magnesium before administering azithromycin.
    B. Hold metronidazole and amiodarone until after completion of azithromycin.
    C. Switch to doxycycline.
    D. Replete magnesium and administer azithromycin for only 3 days.

45. Which of the following patients, if prescribed linezolid, would be at greatest risk of developing serotonin syndrome?

    A. A 24-year-old woman on oral contraceptives who is also maintained on fluoxetine 20 mg perimenstrually (14 days per cycle).
    B. An 84-year-old man with Parkinson's disease maintained on carbidopa/levodopa and amantadine.
    C. A 46-year-old man taking sumatriptan 50 mg as needed and metoclopramide 10 mg as needed for migraines.
    D. A 66-year-old man maintained on escitalopram 10 mg daily and quetiapine 25 mg at bedtime for depression and sleep disorder.

46. Four days ago, a 57-year-old man was prescribed linezolid 600 mg orally every 12 hours for treatment of a methicillin-resistant *Staphylococcus aureus* (MRSA) skin infection. Today, he complains of fever, diarrhea, agitation, and sweating. A *C. difficile* test is positive. Which one of the following statements best applies to the evaluation for serotonin syndrome (SS) in this patient?

    A. The patient meets the criteria for SS based on the Sternbach Criteria.

B. The patient meets the criteria for SS based on the Hunter Criteria.

C. The patient meets the criteria for SS based on both the Sternbach and Hunter Criteria.

D. The patient does not meet the criteria for SS based on either the Sternbach or Hunter Criteria.

47. In which one of the following patients would tigecycline therapy be most appropriate, according to the agent's FDA-approved labeling?

A. A 54-year-old patient with a doxycycline allergy being treated for an *E. coli* intra-abdominal abscess.

B. A 36-year-old patient with a history of bronchiectasis and pseudomonal colonization being evaluated for community-acquired pneumonia.

C. A 47-year-old patient with a β-lactam allergy for whom a course of vancomycin failed, now being treated for a complicated skin and skin structure infection.

D. A 60-year-old patient on a ventilator being treated for a pan-susceptible *H. influenza* ventilator-associated pneumonia.

48. A prescriber approaches you with concern over the FDA statements regarding the increased risk of death associated with tigecycline therapy for FDA-approved and non–FDA-approved indications. The prescriber has a 77-year-old patient who resides at an assisted living center, currently hospitalized for an *Acinetobacter* pneumonia; susceptibility results are listed in the table below. The patient has a history of anaphylaxis to penicillins and is currently receiving tigecycline (100 mg intravenous load, followed by 50 mg intravenous every 12 hours).

Antibiotic	Susceptibility Interpretation
Ampicillin/Sulbactam	S
Cefepime	S
Ceftazidime	S
Ciprofloxacin	I
Gentamicin	I
Levofloxacin	R
Meropenem	I
Tigecycline	S
Trimethoprim/Sulfamethoxazole	R

Which one of the following responses would be best to recommend for this patient?

A. Tigecycline use is appropriate in this patient because no other suitable alternatives exist.

B. Tigecycline should not be used for this indication because of the increased risk of death. The patient should be changed to ciprofloxacin 400 mg intravenous every 8 hours.

C. Tigecycline should not be used for this indication because of the increased risk of death. The patient should be changed to cefepime 2 g intravenous every 12 hours (dose adjusted for renal function).

D. Tigecycline can be used to treat this patient, but the dose should be increased to a load of 200 mg intravenous followed by a maintenance dose of 100 mg intravenous every 12 hours.

49. Which one of the following patients, if prescribed cefepime, would be at the highest risk of developing nonconvulsive status epilepticus according to the agent's FDA-approved labeling?

A. A 24-year-old, 65-kg woman with SCr of 1.8 mg/dL receiving cefepime 2 g intravenous every 8 hours for pseudomonal pneumonia.

B. A 54-year-old, 70-kg man with chronic kidney disease (SCr 3.4 mg/dL) receiving cefepime 500 mg intravenous every 24 hours for a moderate, uncomplicated urinary tract infection (UTI).

C. A 70-year-old, 50-kg man with cancer (SCr 1.2 mg/dL) receiving cefepime 2 g intravenous every 12 hours for the treatment of febrile neutropenia.

D. A 67-year-old, 60-kg woman with newly diagnosed renal insufficiency (SCr 2.0 mg/dL) receiving cefepime 1 g intravenous every 12 hours for a mild, complicated UTI.

50. A prescriber orders cefepime 2 g intravenous every 8 hours for a septic patient with ventilator-associated pneumonia. She states the computer calculated the patient's renal function as 69 mL/minute/1.73m³ using the MDRD equation. You calculate the patient's renal function as 44 mL/minute using the Cockcroft-Gault equation. Which one of the following is best to recommend for this patient?

A. Both equations are appropriate for dosing medications, therefore 2 g intravenous every 8 hours is appropriate.

B. The manufacturer recommends doses based on the MDRD equation; therefore 2 g intravenous every 8 hours is appropriate.

C. The manufacturer recommends doses based on the Cockcroft-Gault equation; therefore 2 g intravenous every 8 hours is appropriate.

D. The manufacturer recommends doses based on the Cockcroft-Gault equation; therefore the dose should be decreased to 2 g intravenous every 12 hours.

Questions 51 and 52 pertain to the following case.

L.G. is a man who has been receiving daptomycin 6 mg/kg intravenous every 24 hours for 16 days for the treatment of MRSA bacteremia. At a routine infectious diseases clinic follow-up, L.G. mentions that he's developed a fever and shortness of breath over the past 2 days. Chest radiography does not show infiltrates.

51. L.G.'s ID clinician is concerned about the possibility of eosinophilic pneumonia and asks you whether this patient meets the FDA definition. Which factor most rules out eosinophilic pneumonia in L.G.?

    A. The temporal relationship.
    B. The lack of chest infiltrates.
    C. The use of daptomycin for an FDA-approved indication.
    D. The lack of ventilator requirement.

52. Which one of the following laboratory parameters would best help evaluate eosinophilic pneumonia in L.G.?

    A. Peripheral WBC count.
    B. Peripheral eosinophil count.
    C. Bronchoalveolar lavage (BAL) eosinophil count.
    D. O$_2$ saturation.

53. You have been charged with developing the new antimicrobial stewardship program at your institution. On the basis of recent CDC recommendations, which one of the following would be the best first priority during the development phase?

    A. Implementing mandatory rapid respiratory viral panel studies for patients with suspected influenza-related pneumonia.
    B. Investigating antimicrobial resistance in your region of the country.
    C. Researching and documenting the most problematic prescribing patterns at your institution.
    D. Mandating pre-prescriptive restriction of vancomycin.

54. Which one of the following scenarios would be most aligned with the need for intervention according to the CDC Get Smart Campaign?

    A. A 28-year-old woman asks the community pharmacist to call her primary care physician for a refill of levofloxacin for her bronchitis.
    B. A 73-year-old man presents from home to the emergency department with pneumonia, including positive chest radiography, and the intern writes for ceftriaxone and doxycycline upon admission.

    C. An 83-year-old woman presents from a nursing home with symptomatic UTI and is being treated with trimethoprim/sulfamethoxazole for 3 days.
    D. A 26-year-old man is admitted to the intensive care unit with gram-negative sepsis and is initiated on cefepime and tobramycin.

55. The Centers for Medicare & Medicaid Services is performing an audit of your institution and is focusing on the new drafted antimicrobial stewardship requirements. Which one of the following scenarios is most likely to result in a citation?

    A. In a chart review, they find that a pharmacist transitioned a patient from intravenous to oral linezolid without a physician order, pursuant to hospital policy.
    B. An order was processed for a patient written for ceftriaxone 2 g intravenous every 12 hours but without an indication.
    C. In a documented note in a patient chart, a pharmacist recommended a change in antibiotics from piperacillin/tazobactam to ciprofloxacin for a patient with a UTI growing *E. coli* susceptible to ciprofloxacin.
    D. The pharmacy and therapeutics committee minutes note that provider order entry was enhanced with a warning about use of daptomycin for pneumonia.

56. In preparing drug use data for benchmarking across institutions, you realize that with your newly installed electronic medication administration record, you can prepare the data for National Healthcare Safety Network reporting. Which one of the following formats would best suit both needs?

    A. Patient days of linezolid therapy adjusted for 1000 patient days.
    B. Total number of grams of linezolid used per 1000 patient days.
    C. Total number of patients on linezolid per 1000 patient days.
    D. Patient days of linezolid therapy adjusted for grams of linezolid.

57. When looking to resources for establishing an antimicrobial stewardship program, which one of the following supportive documents would be most helpful to review for a checklist of activities?

    A. California Department of Public Health Guidance Document for Antimicrobial Stewardship.

B. *Specifications Manual for National Hospital Inpatient Quality Measures by the Joint Commission.*

C. The STAAR Act. Strategies to Address Antimicrobial Resistance.

D. Special Report CDC 2013. The threat of antibiotic resistance.

58. Which one of the following outpatient scenarios best aligns with the CDC's Get Smart program?

A. Calling prescribers to change to more cost-effective generic products.

B. Educating patients that antibiotics do not work against common illnesses caused by viral pathogens.

C. Providing coupons or incentives for patients to not fill antibiotic prescriptions.

D. Providing no-cost antibiotics for ailments such as otitis media, so patients may adequately and completely treat their infections and prevent the emergence of resistance.

59. Which one of the following is most likely to be a key component of the drafted worksheets for CMS surveyors, focusing on antimicrobial stewardship programs?

A. The infectious disease pharmacist is solely responsible for reviewing antimicrobial utilization and reporting results to the antimicrobial subcommittee.

B. Pharmacists contact prescribers to indicate a patient meets criteria for intravenous-to-oral interchange and recommend an interchange.

C. Prescribers must include an infectious indication for each antimicrobial agent ordered.

D. A pharmacist trained in antimicrobial stewardship should be the director of the stewardship program.

60. The chair of the orthopedic surgery department approaches you, the antimicrobial stewardship pharmacist, with some questions regarding the Surgical Care Improvement Project (SCIP). His practice leads the state in hip and knee replacement surgery. Recently, they have also been expanding their shoulder replacement program. Because there is a considerable rate of MRSA in the community, patients receive a weight-based dose of vancomycin before surgery, which is discontinued within 24 hours of the end of surgery time. The vancomycin infusion starts 2 hours before incision time. The department has not had any "fall outs" (e.g., deviations from SCIP guidelines) in the past 6 months. The chair is wondering how expanding their shoulder replacement program will impact their scores. Which one of the following is the best response to the chair's concerns?

A. If the same preventative measures are taken for shoulder replacement as for hip and knee, the department should not have any SCIP "fall outs" for shoulder replacement.

B. Because the shoulder replacement program is relatively new, it would not be subject to SCIP review until it has been in effect for 1 year.

C. Shoulder replacements are not subject to SCIP review.

D. Vancomycin should be re-evaluated as peri-operative prophylaxis.

61. Which of the following scenarios, if documented in the medical record of a patient undergoing a coronary artery bypass graft procedure, would best meet the criteria for vancomycin as peri-operative prophylaxis?

A. Colonization with MSSA.

B. Colonization with vancomycin-resistant *Enterococcus* (VRE).

C. Serious β-lactam allergy.

D. Patient preference.

62. According to the California Antimicrobial Stewardship Program Guidance document, which one of the following programs would best meet the criteria for an advanced program?

A. An infectious diseases or stewardship trained pharmacist is available to review restricted antimicrobial orders before patient administration, and recommend alternative therapies, if warranted.

B. An annual report is generated, outlined the top 10 utilized antibiotics, completed with days of therapy and defined daily doses.

C. Multidisciplinary institutional treatment guidelines are available for the five most common infectious etiologies, which are updated semi-annually.

D. Monthly antimicrobial subcommittee meetings where formulary decisions are made based on costs.

63. Based on the Danish experience, which of the following measures would be most likely to decrease antibiotic use in feed animals?

A. Veterinarians have a treating relationship with the animals.

B. Prescriptions may be prescribed for up to 1 month duration.

C. Pharmacies voluntarily report annual antibiotic prescriptions for feed animals.

D. Antibiotics must be purchased from a central wholesaler.

64. Which of the following interventions would have the greatest effect on decreasing antimicrobial use in agriculture but not affect feed animal production?

   A. Banning the use of antimicrobials with activity against MRSA and VRE.
   B. Banning the use of antimicrobials not approved for human use but in the same therapeutic class as those for human use.
   C. Banning the use of antimicrobials for feed production in swine only.
   D. Banning the use of antimicrobials for the treatment of infection in feed animals.

As you take the posttest for this chapter, also evaluate the material's quality and usefulness, as well as the achievement of learning objectives. Rate each item using this 5-point scale:

- Strongly agree
- Agree
- Neutral
- Disagree
- Strongly disagree

38. The content of the chapter met my educational needs.
39. The content of the chapter satisfied my expectations.
40. The author presented the chapter content effectively.
41. The content of the chapter was relevant to my practice and presented at the appropriate depth and scope.
42. The content of the chapter was objective and balanced.
43. The content of the chapter is free of bias, promotion, or advertisement of commercial products.
44. The content of the chapter was useful to me.
45. The teaching and learning methods used in the chapter were effective.
46. The active learning methods used in the chapter were effective.
47. The learning assessment activities used in the chapter were effective.
48. The chapter was effective overall.

Use the 5-point scale to indicate whether this chapter prepared you to accomplish the following learning objectives:

49. Evaluate recent antimicrobial U.S. Food and Drug Administration (FDA) drug interaction warnings and implement strategies to mitigate adverse drug reactions.
50. Assess for antimicrobial adverse drug events and recommend therapy adjustments.
51. Assess legislation and the several national support programs for the establishment of antimicrobial stewardship endeavors across health care systems.
52. Compose strategies to meet Centers for Medicare & Medicaid Services (CMS) and QualityNet goals for pneumonia treatment, the Surgical Care Improvement Project, and immunization rates.
53. \Develop strategies that comply with CMS and its National Healthcare Safety Network's reporting requirements involving catheter-related infections, surgical-site infections, resistant organisms, and health care personnel influenza vaccination.
54. Design strategies that limit antimicrobial exposure in feed animals.
55. Please provide any specific comments relating to any perceptions of bias, promotion, or advertisement of commercial products.
56. Please expand on any of your above responses, and/or provide any additional comments regarding this chapter:

Questions 57–59 apply to the entire learning module.

57. How long did it take you to read the instructional materials in this module?
58. How long did it take you to read and answer the assessment questions in this module?
59. Please provide any additional comments you may have regarding this module:

REFERENCE RANGES FOR COMMON LABORATORY TESTS[a]

Serum Chemistries	Reference Range	SI Units
Albumin	3.5–5.0 g/dL (adults); 3.4–4.2 g/dL (children 1–3 years)	35–50 g/L (adults); 34–42 g/L (children 1–3 years)
Ammonia	30–70 mcg/dL	17–41 μmol/L
Amylase	60–180 U/L	1–3 μkat/L
Alanine aminotransferase (ALT)	0–35 IU/L	0–0.50 μkat/L
Alkaline phosphatase (ALP)	Varies with age: 30–120 IU/L (adults); 150–420 IU/L (children)	0.50–2.00 μkat/L (adults); 2.51–7.01 μkat/L (children)
Aspartate aminotransferase (AST)	8–42 IU/L	0.133–0.700 μkat/L
Bilirubin, direct	0.1–0.3 mg/dL	1.7–5.0 μmol/L
Bilirubin, total	0.3–1.0 mg/dL	5–17 μmol/L
Blood urea nitrogen (BUN)	8–20 mg/dL (adults); Lower in children	2.9–7.1 mmol/L
Calcium, ionized	4.4–5.1 mg/dL	1–1.3 mmol/L
Calcium, total serum	8.5–10.8 mg/dL	2.1–2.7 mmol/L
Carbon dioxide (venous)	24–30 mEq/L	24–30 mmol/L
Chloride	96–106 mEq/L	96–106 mmol
C-reactive protein	<0.8 mg/dL	<0.76 nmol/L
Creatine kinase	25–90 IU/L (men); 10–70 IU/L (women)	0.42–1.50 μkat/L (men); 0.17–1.17 μkat/L (women)
Creatinine, serum (SCr)	0.7–1.5 mg/dL (adults); 0.2–0.7 mg/dL (children)	62–133 μmol/L (adults); 18–62 μmol/L (children)
Creatinine (clearance) (CrCl)	90–140 mL/minute/1.73m²	1.50–2.34 mL/second/m²
Ferritin	22–322 ng/mL	49–724 pmol/L
γ-Glutamyl transpeptidase	0–30 IU	0–30 IU
Glucose, serum	70–110 mg/dL	3.9–6.2 mmol/L
Hemoglobin A1C (glycolated hemoglobin)	4%–6%	0.04–0.06
Lactate dehydrogenase (LDH)	100–210 IU/L	1.7–3.5 μkat/L
Lipase	<160 U/L	<2.67 μkat/L or <160 U/L
Magnesium	1.5–2.2 mEq/L	0.75–1.1 mmol/L
Osmolality, serum	280–295 mOsm/kg	280–295 mmol/kg
Phosphorus (inorganic)	2.6–4.5 mg/dL (adults); 3.8–6.5 mg/dL (children)	0.84–1.45 mmol/L (adults); 1.22–2.1 mmol/L (children)
Potassium	3.5–5.0 mEq/L	3.5–5.0 mmol/L
Prealbumin	20–36 mg/dL	200–360 mg/L
Sodium	135–145 mEq/L	135–145 mmol/L
Uric acid, serum	3.4–7 mg/dL (men); 2.4–6 mg/dL (women)	202–416 μmol/L (men); 143–357 μmol/L (women)

Hematology/Coagulation	Reference Range	SI Units
Hematocrit	42%–50% (men); 36%–45% (women)	0.42–0.5 (men); 0.36–0.45 (women)
Hemoglobin	14–18 g/dL (men); 12–16 g/dL (women)	8.7–11.2 mmol/L (men); 7.5–10 mmol/L (women)
International normalized ratio (INR)	0.9–1.1	0.9–1.1
Mean corpuscular hemoglobin (MCH)	27–33 pg/cell	1.66–2.09 fmol/cell
Mean corpuscular hemoglobin concentration (MCHC)	33–36 g/dL	20.3–22 mmol/L
Mean corpuscular volume (MCV)	80–960 fL/cell	80–960 fL
Partial thromboplastin time (PTT)	21–45 seconds	21–45 seconds
Platelet count	150,000–450,000/mm³	150–450 × 10⁹/L
Prothrombin time (PT)	10–13 seconds	10–13 seconds
Red blood cell (RBC) count	$4.5–5.9 \times 10^6$ cells/mm³ (men); $4.1–5.1 \times 10^6$ cells/mm³ (women)	$4.5–5.9 \times 10^{12}$/L (men); $4.1–5.1 \times 10^{12}$/L (women)
Reticulocyte count	0.5%–2.5%	0.005–0.025
White blood cell (WBC) count	$4.4–11.3 \times 10^3$ cells/mm³	$4.4–11.3 \times 10^9$/L

Serum Lipids	Reference Range	SI Units
Cholesterol, total (TC)	<200 mg/dL	<5.18 mmol/L
High-density lipoprotein (HDL), cholesterol	>40 mg/dL	>1.04 mmol/L
Low-density lipoprotein (LDL) cholesterol	<130 mg/dL	<3.36 mmol/L
Triglycerides (TG)	<150 mg/dL	<1.26 mmol/L

Blood Gases	Arterial	Venous	Arterial	Venous
Partial pressure of carbon dioxide (PCO₂)	35–45 mm Hg	42–55 mm Hg	4.7–5.9 kPa	
Partial pressure of oxygen (PO₂)	>70 (80–100 mm Hg)	30–50 mm Hg	>9.3 (11–13 kPa)	
Oxygen saturation (SaO₂)	>90%	60%–85%	0.90 to fraction of 1	
Serum bicarbonate	24–30 mEq/L	24–28 mEq/L	24–30 mmol/L	24–28 mmol/L

Urinalysis	Reference Range	SI Units
Leukocyte esterase, nitrite, protein, blood, ketones, bilirubin, glucose	Negative	
pH	4.5–8.0	4.5–8.0
Specific gravity	1.010–1.025	m³/kg

[a]Values given in this table are commonly accepted reference ranges compiled from many sources. Patient-specific goals may differ depending on age, sex, clinical condition, and the laboratory methodology used to perform the assay.

...permission from the American College of Clinical Pharmacy (ACCP). Copyright Pharmacotherapy Self-Assessment Program (PSAP).